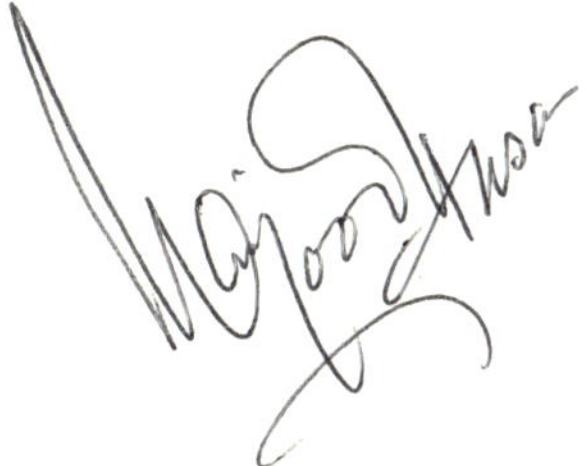

AF412816

RECENT ADVANCES
IN SURGERY

SELWYN TAYLOR

DM MCh FRCS
Senior Lecturer and Consultant Surgeon,
Royal Postgraduate Medical School,
Hammersmith Hospital, London

RECENT ADVANCES IN SURGERY

EDITED BY

SELWYN TAYLOR

NUMBER NINE

CHURCHILL LIVINGSTONE

Edinburgh, London and New York

1977

CHURCHILL LIVINGSTONE
Medical Division of Longman Group Limited

Distributed in the United States of America by
Longman Inc., 19 West 44th Street, New York,
N.Y. 10036, and by associated companies,
branches and representatives throughout
the world

ISBN 0 443 01506 6
Library of Congress Cataloging in Publication Data
Taylor, Selwyn Francis, ed. Recent advances in surgery, number nine.
Includes index.   1. Surgery—Addresses, essays, lectures.   I. Title.
RD39.T39   1977   617   76-21284

Printed in Great Britain

PREFACE

It is not possible to define what is 'recent' nor what is an 'advance', especially in a field like surgery and therefore in gathering together the contents of the present volume of Recent Advances I have used the same formula as before. I have chosen subjects in which there has been a complete change of approach, those in which the pattern of treatment has now emerged clearly, and finally I have included descriptions of new techniques which seem to me to have reasonably wide applications in surgery.

Take the subject of carcinoma of the rectum as an example. In the early days attempts were made to excise it through the perineum. Later a variety of operations were devised; first approaching it through an incision beside the sacrum, later via the perineum and finally through the abdomen. There used to be great arguments as to whether an abdominoperineal operation was better than a perineoabdominal one and for a period there was a vogue for anterior resection, no matter how low the lesion lay. Today it is possible to look back and hopefully forward, and review the best method available for tackling the disease at whatever level it lies and at whatever stage it is discovered. Who better could present such a review than John Goligher, whose opinion in these matters is respected all over the world. There are however, quite different advances in this field, and colonoscopy and the technique of removing polyps endoscopically is one of these as Christopher Williams explains.

In the field of malignant disease it is timely to review the treatment of tumours of the testis and John Blandy tackles this with his usual clarity. The gastrointestinal tract is well represented in this volume as John Dawson looks at portal hypertension, de Jode at pancreatitis and, in order to be thoroughly controversial, Michael Baddeley reviews his own experience in using an intestinal bypass for obesity. Finally in this section Ivan Johnston gives an excellent up-to-the-minute account of parenteral alimentation; I imagine in the United States this chapter would have been headed hyperalimentation but then they have a tradition of overstatement.

In each issue of Recent Advances I have tried to introduce a central theme and on this occasion it is the place of immunology in surgery. There is practically no part of the body now into which the immunologist has not introduced his expertise and for those of us who were not brought up in this field it is necessary to go back to school. It would be difficult to find a better guide than the Professor of Pathology at the Royal College of Surgeons, John Turk, and he has been ably abetted in his task by John Castro who has been as active in the tumour immunology field as he has in renal transplantation. The language being difficult, I persuaded the authors to include a jargon-box to which the reader can rapidly refer when he temporarily forgets the meaning of one of the basic new words in this subject.

For good measure I have included on this occasion another subject of universal importance to surgeons, mainly because it has been giving me concern in the management of patients. This is the investigation and management of disorders of bleeding and clotting. One of my erstwhile Hammersmith colleagues, R. Mibashan, in collaboration with Milica Brozovic of the Central Middlesex Hospital, has produced a guide which I believe will be a standard reference for a long time.

Professor Welbourn and Stephen Joffe have reviewed the apudomas, those fascinating endocrine tumours that have so much influence on the bowel and also on the rest of the endocrine system. In the field of locomotion there is a splendid account of low backache, which is such a problem in the outpatient clinic and consulting room, and it is very appropriately written by the collaboration of a physical medicine expert with an orthopaedic surgeon.

The cardiovascular system is represented by a masterly account of the treatment of stroke by Professor Taylor and John Lumley, a field in which surgery plays a special part. Coronary bypass, which takes up so much operating time today and offers such rewards in the right patients, is discussed by cardiac surgeon and cardiologist, William Cleland and Celia Oakley. The anterior tibial syndrome, so often misdiagnosed, is neatly portrayed by Georges Jantet.

Turning to the newer techniques, Professor Walder writes about the use of hyperbaric oxygen in surgery where it is now an essential part of the treatment for certain afflictions. It has been brought to the fore recently as a result of the diving hazards associated with drilling for oil in the North Sea. Another technique that has certainly come to stay and will certainly impinge on more and more surgical fields is microsurgery. In this country it was Terence Cawthorne who pioneered the use of magnification and later the microscope in middle ear surgery; however it is an ophthalmic surgeon, Walter Rich of Exeter, whom I have invited to contribute what is a particularly exciting chapter.

The contribution on SI units, the Système Internationale, was essential as we all have to make the transition to these new units of measurement, confusing though it will undoubtedly be. Finally, I make no apology for the clash with tradition in writing about surgical education. For all of my professional life I have been involved in teaching and latterly closely concerned with the evolution of the Higher Surgical Training Scheme and Accreditation. I hope that every reader will turn to this chapter as it is so important that the working of the scheme is understood throughout the surgical world.

This, the ninth in the series, like its predecessors is not a new edition but an entirely new book. It is for this reason that I have included a list of contents of Number Eight since in many ways it complements the present volume. So do earlier volumes in the series, but sadly they are all long out of print.

I could not have produced this, the ninth Recent Advances in Surgery, without the help, advice and wisdom of many colleagues and friends. In particular my assistant John Cooke has given yeoman assistance as well as contributing the chapter about SI units.

London, 1976   SELWYN TAYLOR

CONTRIBUTORS

R. M. BADDELEY ChM FRCS
Consultant Surgeon, Birmingham General Hospital, Birmingham

J. P. BLANDY DM MCh FRCS
Professor of Urology and Consultant Surgeon, The London and St Peter's Hospitals, London

MILICA BROZOVIC MD MRCPath
Consultant Haematologist, Central Middlesex Hospital, London

J. E. CASTRO PhD MS FRCS
Lecturer in Urology, Royal Postgraduate Medical School and Consultant Surgeon, Hammersmith Hospital, London

W. P. CLELAND FRCP FRCS
Director of Surgery, Institute of Diseases of the Chest, Brompton Hospital, and Consultant Surgeon, Royal Postgraduate Medical School, Hammersmith Hospital, London

T. J. C. COOKE MB BS FRCS
Senior Surgical Registrar and Surgical Tutor, Royal Postgraduate Medical School, Hammersmith Hospital, London

J. L. DAWSON MS FRCS
Consultant Surgeon, King's College Hospital, London

L. R. J. de JODE MS FRCS
Consultant Surgeon, Whipps Cross Hospital, Leytonstone, London

J. C. GOLIGHER ChM FRCS
Professor of Surgery, University of Leeds, and Consultant Surgeon, The General Infirmary, Leeds

G. JANTET MB FRCS
Lecturer in Surgery (Vascular), Royal Postgraduate Medical School, and Consultant Surgeon, Hammersmith and King Edward Memorial Hospitals, London

S. N. JOFFE BSc FRCS
Senior Lecturer in Surgery, St Mungo Department of Surgery, and Consultant Surgeon, Royal Infirmary, Glasgow

I. D. A. JOHNSTON MCh FRCS
Professor of Surgery and Consultant Surgeon, Royal Victoria Infirmary, Newcastle upon Tyne

J. S. P. LUMLEY MB BS FRCS
Assistant Director, Surgical Unit, and Consultant Surgeon, St Bartholomew's Hospital, London

J. A. MATHEWS MB BChir MRCP
Consultant Physician, Department of Rheumatology, St Thomas's Hospital, London

R. S. MIBASHAN BSc MD FRCP
Senior Lecturer in Haematology and Consultant Haematologist, King's College Medical School

CELIA M. OAKLEY MD FRCP
Senior Lecturer in Cardiology, Royal Postgraduate Medical School, Hammersmith Hospital, London

D. A. REYNOLDS MB BS FRCS
Consultant Orthopaedic Surgeon, St Thomas's Hospital, London, and Queen Victoria Hospital, East Grinstead

W. J. RICH FRCS DO
Consultant Ophthalmologist, West of England Eye Infirmary, Exeter

G. W. TAYLOR MS FRCS
Professor of Surgery and Director of Surgical Unit, St Bartholomew's Hospital, London

SELWYN TAYLOR DM MCh FRCS
Senior Lecturer and Consultant Surgeon, Royal Postgraduate Medical School, Hammersmith Hospital, London

J. L. TURK DSc MD FRCPath
Sir William Collins Professor of Pathology, Royal College of Surgeons, Lincoln's Inn Fields, London

D. N. WALDER MD ChM FRCS
Professor of Surgical Science and Consultant Surgeon, Royal Victoria Infirmary, Newcastle upon Tyne

R. B. WELBOURN MD FRCS
Professor and Director, Department of Surgery, Royal Postgraduate Medical School, and Consultant Surgeon, Hammersmith Hospital, London

J. E. A. WICKHAM BSc MS FRCS
Consultant Urologist, St Bartholomew's Hospital and St Peter's Hospital Group, London, and Senior Lecturer, Institute of Urology, London

CHRISTOPHER B. WILLIAMS BM BCh MRCP
Physician, St Mark's and St Bartholomew's Hospitals, London

CONTENTS

1

CURRENT TRENDS IN THE RADICAL MANAGEMENT OF CARCINOMA OF THE RECTUM

J. C. Goligher

THE OVERALL CONTEMPORARY ACHIEVEMENTS OF RADICAL SURGERY

There are few other forms of malignant disease about which we possess such detailed information regarding the outcome of surgical treatment as we do in relation to carcinoma of the rectum. Thanks mainly to the comprehensive and meticulous analyses of Gabriel (1932, 1957, 1963), Dukes (1940, 1957), Morgan (1965), Bussey (1963) and Bussey, Dukes and Lockhart-Mummery (1960) at St Mark's Hospital, London, of Grinnell (1953) at the Presbyterian Hospital, New York City, and of Waugh, Block and Gage (1955), Mayo, Lee and Davis (1951), Mayo, Laberge and Hardy (1958) and Vandertoll and Beahrs (1965) and their colleagues at the Mayo Clinic, a vast fund of accurate data has been amassed regarding the prospects of cure after rectal excision for cancer. The general impression derived from a study of this information is of steady improvement in the results over the past three or four decades culminating in a standard of accomplishment at the present time that is vastly superior to that of surgical treatment for several other common cancers, such as those of the bronchus, oesophagus or stomach.

Nowhere is this continued improvement better demonstrated than in Dukes' (1957) chronicle of the rising resectability, falling operative mortality and increasing five year survival rate at St Mark's Hospital between the years 1928 and 1952 (Table 1.1). Morgan (1965) has shown that there has been a further rise in resectability rate to 96.5 per cent and fall in operative mortality

Table 1.1 Resectability, operative mortality and five-year survival in patients with rectal carcinoma at St Mark's Hospital 1928 to 1952 (based on data from Dukes, 1957)

Period	Resectability rate (per cent)	Operative mortality (per cent)	Crude five-year survival rate of immediate survivors of operation (per cent)	Corrected five-year survival rate of immediate survivors of operation (per cent)
1928–32	46.5	12.8	49.3	56.5
1933–37	57.6	11.0	46.2	54.5
1938–42	69.4	11.1	46.8	54.9
1943–47	79.0	7.9	53.7	63.9
1948–52	92.7	6.8	46.2	56.1

rate to 2.6 per cent at St Mark's Hospital during the period 1958 to 1963. That these excellent results are not confined to a specialist centre like St Mark's is attested by many published reports from general hospitals, such as Butler's (1971) from the London Hospital and my own (Whitaker and Goligher, 1975) from the General Infirmary at Leeds. Though we have a resectability rate of 90 per cent it should be pointed out that, as at St Mark's Hospital in more recent years (Morgan, 1965), roughly 18 per cent of the 90 or so in every 100 patients who proceed to removal of their growths have purely palliative excisions in the presence of hepatic deposits or other unremovable extensions, for it has long been established that excision of the main primary growth under these circumstances has an important contribution to make towards relief of symptoms (Goligher, 1941).

Published results of surgical treatment tend to be better than the much more common unpublished results and it may be questioned how accurately the statistics referred to from leading centres reflect the average experience of the majority of surgeons throughout the country. A more accurate impression of mean achievements of surgery in the country at large is conveyed by the reports of various Cancer Registries which relate to all the cases of cancer in a particular region of the country. One of the largest of these in Britain is the Birmingham Regional Cancer Registry, which has followed up 5800 cases of rectal carcinoma treated in that area between 1950 and 1961 inclusive (Slaney, 1971): 3005 or 52 per cent underwent radical resection. The crude and corrected five-year survival rates for resected cases were 37.8 and 48.6 per cent respectively and for all cases registered 21.9 and 29.2 per cent. During the years 1962 to 1964 inclusive the South-Western Regional Cancer Bureau (Walker, 1971) registered 1346 patients with cancer of the rectum; 923 or 68.6 per cent had excision. The crude five-year survival rate in resected cases was 34.1 per cent and for all cases registered 23.5 per cent.

These reports show what a discrepancy there is between the results that are possible under specially favourable circumstances and those regularly obtained in various regions of the country, including all grades of hospital. Perhaps the main cause of the poorer results in regional surveys is the lower average operability rate, which is not compensated for by any improvement in the survival rate amongst those undergoing resection. In turn this may reflect partly differences in the type of patients presenting for treatment and partly a less determined approach towards eradication of adherent lesions by many of the surgeons concerned. Clearly at a national level there are no grounds for complacency in the management of rectal cancer.

THE VALUE OF PREOPERATIVE RADIOTHERAPY IN IMPROVING THE RESULTS OF RADICAL SURGERY

In 1959 Stearns, Deddish and Quan reported that a retrospective survey of the patients treated for carcinoma of the rectum and sigmoid at the Memorial

Hospital, New York City, during the years 1939 to 1951 showed that those who had had preoperative irradiation prior to radical surgery obtained a significantly better five-year survival rate than did those who were treated solely by operation. As a consequence of these observations it was decided at that hospital to set up a prospective, properly controlled trial of preoperative irradiation at a dose of approximately 2000 rad. Only patients who underwent an ostensibly curative operation, who had no obvious evidence of residual or metastatic cancer in distant sites, were included. Stearns et al (1974) have now reported that during the years 1957 to 1967 790 patients were entered in the trial. The crude five-year survival rate in the 376 control patients was 65 per cent and in 414 treated patients 67 per cent. The incidence of nodal metastasis in the control cases was 37 per cent and in the treated cases 35 per cent. The five-year survival rate for cases without nodal involvement in the treated group was 78 per cent and for similar cases in the untreated group 79 per cent. When nodes were involved the survival rate was 40 per cent in both groups. This trial would thus seem to demolish the hopes of improvement of the achievements of surgical treatment of rectal cancer by means of supplementary radiotherapy.

However, more encouraging results from preoperative irradiation have been reported by Dwight et al (1972) in a controlled trial in 700 cases treated in Veterans Administration Hospitals in USA. Approximately half the patients were randomly allocated to radiotherapy at a dose of between 2000 and 3000 rad (usually delivered by conventional 180–400 kV equipment) and half were exempted from this treatment. Roughly the same number of patients underwent removal of their growths in the two groups, most of them by abdominoperineal resection, some by anterior resection. At first the operative mortality was slightly higher in the irradiated cases but later this difference diminished. A striking feature was that the proportion of patients showing lymph node metastases was higher in the non-irradiated than the irradiated group, suggesting that radiotherapy had, as it were, sterilised some nodes of their metastases in the latter patients. Survival curves constructed by life table methods for the two groups showed a five-year survival rate of 44 per cent for cases having excision after irradiation and 35 per cent for those having excision without radiotherapy—a difference that is statistically significant. The better survival rate of preoperative irradiation applied only to patients whose lesions were removed by abdominoperineal excisions and not to those who were submitted to anterior resection.

In view of the contradictory results as to the value of preoperative radiotherapy recorded by these two trials, the Medical Research Council has recently instituted a study in several centres in Britain in which patients with growths up to 15 cm from the anal verge on sigmoidoscopy are being randomised to three groups—one of which is given no radiotherapy, one receives 2000 rad of preoperative irradiation, and one has only 500 rad. This trial has only been running for 12 months so that no reliable data are yet available.

At the present time therefore, the usefulness of preoperative radiotherapy remains sub judice and, in my opinion, till the controversy is resolved by further controlled studies, it would not be justifiable to employ this treatment as a routine measure in the radical surgical management of rectal cancer.

ADJUVANT CYTOTOXIC DRUG THERAPY

In the belief that malignant cells are particularly liable to be exfoliated into the portal circulation by handling of growths during operation, Warren Cole's group (Cruz, McDonald and Cole, 1956; Mrazek et al, 1959), introduced the practice of injecting a cytotoxic agent into a tributary of the portal vein during operation and into a peripheral vein in the early postoperative period in the hope of minimising the risks of distant metastases. They employed nitrogen mustard for this purpose but had to report no significant improvement of the results in the cases so treated. Dwight, Higgins and Keehn (1969) and Holden and Dixon (1962), preferred to use triethylenethiophosphosamide in their controlled trials of this form of adjuvant chemotherapy for rectal (and colonic) cancer, but were equally unsuccessful. More recently Nadler and Moore (1964) commenced similar trials with 5-fluorouracil—which is currently believed to be the most effective cytotoxic agent against alimentary neoplasms—and in one report (Higgins et al, 1971) there was evident a slight trend in favour of the treated group, but no significant difference had yet emerged.

The information so far available thus provides no inducement to engage in routine adjuvant chemotherapy in operable, ostensibly curable cases of rectal cancer.

SPECIAL ANTIBACTERIAL MEASURES

Because of the infective nature of the colonic contents patients undergoing operations for carcinoma of the colon and rectum, particularly those involving opening of the bowel and establishment of an anastomosis, are predisposed to develop septic complications (Goligher, 1975). In an effort to lessen the incidence and severity of such complications special antibacterial measures have been much used in recent years with encouraging results.

Bowel Preparation and Intestinal Antiseptics

Surgeons are fairly generally agreed—not so much on the basis of good objective data as on common-sense grounds—that thorough mechanical preparation of the bowel by aperients, enemas and wash-outs is desirable before major operations on the colon and rectum. But despite many careful studies there is no consensus of opinion on the value in such cases of pre-operative medication with oral antibiotics and other drugs in securing a reduction in the bacterial population of the stools and a lowering of the incidence of septic complications. Each report in the literature favourable to these agents seems to be followed by yet another casting doubt on their efficacy (Yale and Peet, 1971; Nichols and Condon, 1971; Goligher, 1975).

In the last few years the importance of faecal anaerobic bacteria in pathogenesis has been emphasised, and unquestionably the most fashionable organism in this connection at the moment is *Bacteroides fragilis* (Drasar, 1968; Gorbach et al, 1967; Moore, Cato and Holdeman, 1969). More recently, therefore, in the evaluation of preoperative oral antibiotic regimes of bowel preparations the special attention directed to the use of drugs effective against a wide range of organisms has been particularly interesting (Nichols et al, 1973; Washington et al, 1974).

In Nichols et al's (1973) study the antibiotics used were neomycin and erythromycin which were given in three doses of 1 g of each at 1 p.m., 2 p.m. and 11 p.m. of the day before operation. A comparison of cultures from stools obtained before commencement of the preoperative antibiotic regime and from faeces aspirated from the resected specimen at laparotomy in the treated group showed a considerable reduction in the numbers of aerobes and anaerobes, amounting to virtually complete suppression in many instances. A similar comparison in the control patients given mechanical preparations alone disclosed no significant change in the numbers of aerobic and anaerobic organisms. In terms of septic complications the difference between treated and untreated groups was of the same order, but its significance was lessened by the small size of the two series.

In Washington et al's (1974) trial the patients were randomly allocated to three groups, all of which were given mechanical preparation (saline purgatives and enemas) for 48 h before operation, one had in addition neomycin medication during the same period, and another neomycin and tetracycline. As is shown in Table 1.2 the incidence of wound infection was significantly less in the neomycin-tetracycline group than in the other two groups. There were no instances of staphylococcal or pseudomembranous enterocolitis in the entire study. Among the bacteria isolated from the infected wounds (mainly in Groups 1 and 2) *Bacteroides fragilis* was a frequent offender. This trial seems to show beyond question the advantage of neomycin-tetracycline preparation for elective colorectal surgery. It is, however, arguable that a neomycin-clindamycin combination might be even more valuable, because of clindamycin's particular effectiveness against Bacteroides.

Total Gut Irrigation for Mechanical Preparation

An interesting development in the last year or two in the mechanical preparation of the bowel for rectal or colonic resection has been the attempt by Hewitt et al (1973) to replace the conventional methods of aperients, enemas and wash-outs spread out over several days by an orthograde irrigation of the entire gastrointestinal tract from above downwards in a period of $2\frac{1}{2}$ to 3 h. The irrigation is delivered into the stomach via a nasogastric tube whilst the patient sits on a commode. The solution used consists of sodium chloride (6.14 g), potassium chloride (0.75 g) and sodium bicarbonate (2.94 g) in distilled water (1000 ml) warmed to 37°C in a water bath. It is delivered to the stomach tube by a peristaltic pump at the rate of 75 ml/min. The first bowel action usually occurs about 40 to 60 min after the start of the irrigation. Almost clear fluid is passed from about 90 min onwards and the irrigation is continued for a further hour after this stage has been reached. The total irrigation time is therefore 2 to 3 h and the amount of irrigant in the region of 11 litres.

The originators of this method advise against its use in elderly patients, in those with impaired heart or kidney function, or in those with stenosing carcinomas. The irrigation is surprisingly well tolerated by patients and can produce a most effective cleansing of the large bowel, affording excellent conditions for large bowel surgery. Our experience confirms these claims and shows also that the method is an excellent way of preparing patients for barium enema studies or for colonoscopy. But further experience with it is necessary to define its safety and convenience under a variety of circumstances.

Local Antiseptic Applications to the Parietal Wound or Abdominal Cavity

Parietal wound. As is well shown in Table 1.2, one of the commonest manifestations of sepsis after colorectal surgery is infection in the parietal abdominal wound. Realisation of this fact has induced many surgeons to adopt the practice of placing a deposit of an antiseptic agent in the parietal wound immediately before suturing it at the conclusion of the operation. There is good evidence from controlled trials with several different antiseptic drugs that the incidence of wound sepsis can thereby be reduced. This holds for ampicillin 1 g in powdered form (Nash and Hugh, 1967; Mountain and Seal, 1970; Anderson, Korner and Østergaard, 1972; Stoker and Ellis, 1972), ampicillin 0.5 g and cloxacillin 0.5 g in powdered form (Jensen et al, 1975) cephaloridine 1 g in solution (Evans, Pollock and Rosenberg, 1974) and povidone iodine as a spray (Gilmore and Sanderson, 1975).

Peritoneal cavity. When a major degree of contamination with faecal matter has occurred at operation—as may occasionally happen during the conduct of an anastomosis when the bowel is more heavily loaded than usual or if the colon or rectum is accidentally torn at the site of the growth or elsewhere, it is natural to consider the use of some form of antiseptic irrigation. In Britain at the present time the popular solution for this purpose is noxythiolin. Not an antibiotic, but a chemotherapeutic agent, it is said to be effective against practically all Gram-positive and Gram-negative bacteria. It is introduced

Table 1.2 Postoperative complications after three different regimes of bowel preparation (from Washington et al, 1974)

	Group 1 (mechanical preparation alone)	Group 2 (mechanical preparation and neomycin)	Group 3 (mechanical preparation and neomycin/ tetracycline)
Wound infection[a]	27	28	3
Peritonitis	5	1	0
Wound separation	0	4	0
Septicaemia	4	4	2
Faecal fistula	7	1	0
Staphylococceal enterocolitis	0	0	0
Pseudomembranous enterocolitis	0	0	0
Ileus	1	0	0
Urinary tract infections	12	8	6
Cardiac	3	2	2
Pneumonia	3	1	0
Pulmonary embolus	0	0	0
Renal failure	0	0	0
Hepatic failure	0	0	0

[a] Difference between incidence of wound infection between group 3 and groups 1 and 2 is significant ($P < 0.01$).

into the peritoneal cavity (5 g in 200 ml of fluid) immediately before the abdomen is closed and removed subsequently by a suction drain which is set in action as soon as the wound closure has been completed. The best documented report on the use of noxythiolin for faecal contamination of the peritoneal cavity is that of Browne and Stoller (1970). Apparently it is relatively ineffective in combating parietal wound sepsis (Bird et al, 1971; Stoker and Ellis, 1972).

Systemic Antibiotic Therapy

Surgical opinion has been sharply divided on the wisdom of administering prophylactically to patients undergoing surgical operations a full course of systemic antibiotics in order to lessen the risk of septic complications, particularly when there has been some degree of contamination of the operative field as is not infrequent at any rate in anastomotic procedures for carcinoma of the rectum and colon. Probably the majority of surgeons have hitherto been opposed to the practice of systemic antibiotic therapy in 'clean-contaminated' cases partly because of doubts as to its efficacy and partly because of the fear that antibiotics given in this way over a period of several days might lead to the development of strains of bacteria that would be resistant to the particular antibiotics used. More recently, however, several convincing experiences have been recorded with shorter prophylactic courses of antibiotics confined to the phase of operation itself and to the first few hours after it in order to avoid the emergence of resistant strains and retain the efficacy of the prophylactically used antibiotics for subsequent treatment if necessary. Using cephaloridine in two or three 1 g doses immediately before and up to 12 h after operation in a controlled clinical trial Polk and Lopez-Mayer (1969) and Evans and Pollock (1973) have reported a significant reduction in the frequency of wound sepsis. In the prophylaxis of post-operative infections Stokes et al (1974) have argued a persuasive case for combined therapy with two antibiotics together to secure a wide range of cover against commonly encountered organisms. They recommend tobramicin (or gentamicin) for its potency against aerobic and Gram-negative bacilli including *Pseudomonas aeruginosa* and against staphylococci including those resistant to penicillin, and lincomycin for its effect on nearly all the non-sporing anaerobes and clostridia which inhabit the intestine (including *Bacteroides fragilis*) and on many staphylococci and streptococci. Patients are given intramuscularly two doses of lincomycin 600 mg plus either tobramicin or gentamicin 80 mg, one dose being administered in the anaesthetic room before operation, the second dose in the ward or recovery room 8 h later. In a controlled trial Stokes et al (1974) had only one instance of sepsis in 85 treated cases, but 8 in 90 control cases—a difference that is significant at the 5 per cent level.

But whatever may be the attitude towards prophylactic systemic antibiotic therapy in mildly or dubiously contaminated cases, when there has been massive faecal contamination—which is rare in the surgery of rectal carcinoma compared with colitis surgery—there would be general agreement as to the desirability of vigorous systemic antibiotic therapy with agents possessing a broad spectrum of activity likely to be effective against the common intestinal organisms, such as ampicillin, cephaloridine, cephalothin, gentamicin and lincomycin. Depending on the amount of soiling, it may be thought wise to commence with a loading dose (e.g. 2–4 g of cephalothin) given intravenously during the operation, and to continue thereafter with normal dosage intra-venously or intramuscularly.

ABDOMINOPERINEAL EXCISION

The operation most commonly employed by the majority of surgeons at the present time for the radical treatment of rectal carcinoma is abdominoperineal excision, which is now largely a standardised procedure, regarding which two comments alone may suffice—one on the management of the perineal wound and the other on the care of the colostomy.

Management of the Perineal Wound

In recent years many surgeons have turned from open drainage or packing of the perineal wound after abdominoperineal excision to primary suture and suction drainage, the ischiorectal and perianal fat being sutured with two layers of chromic catgut and the skin with silk or other non-absorbable material. The advantage of this technique is that, if successful, primary healing of the perineum is obtained, which minimises the discomfort to the patient and might expedite the convalescence. Of course, the method may fail to attain its objective due to the accumulation of blood clot in the pelvis or the occurrence of pelvic infection—the latter often as a sequel to the former— but it is hoped that the provision of efficient suction drainage of the pelvic cavity by means of two or more tubes inserted either through the skin of each ischiorectal fossa or suprapubically and connected to one of the several closed systems of drainage now available (or operated on the open sump drainage plan) would lessen the risks of these complications. Various authors have reported rates of primary healing with primary suture of the perineum ranging from 60 to over 90 per cent (Ruckley, Smith and Balfour, 1970; Hultén et al, 1971; Dencker, Norryd and Tranberg, 1973; Broader et al, 1974; Walton and Mallik, 1974; Altemeier et al, 1974). My own controlled study of this technique (Irvin and Goligher, 1975) includes patients suffering from inflammatory bowel disease as well as cases of rectal carcinoma, which doubtless partly explains why complete primary healing was secured in only roughly half the patients treated. In another quarter of the cases one or two sutures had to be removed to allow escape of blood clot or infective material, but healing was adjudged eventually to have taken place more rapidly than if the wound had been managed by open drainage ab initio, whilst in the remaining quarter considerably more opening up of the wound was necessary and it was not clear that any advantage had resulted from using primary suture.

One of the variants in the practice of primary closure of the perineal wound is to leave the pelvic peritoneum unsutured so that coils of small intestine and the greater omentum may gravitate into the pelvis and help to obliterate the pelvic space. It had been claimed by Haxton (1970) that this modification further lessens the incidence of complications with primary suture and greatly enhances the prospects of obtaining primary union. In our trial (Irvin and Goligher, 1975) patients were randomly allocated to two groups, in one of which the pelvic peritoneum was sutured, in the other it was left open. No significant difference was noted in the frequency with which primary union was obtained in these two groups. From this point of view, therefore, it seems immaterial whether the pelvic peritoneum is sutured or not.

On the basis of these reported experiences it appears reasonable to employ primary suture of the perineal wound together with suction drainage of the pelvic cavity, unless it is specifically contraindicated because of inadequate control of bleeding at the conclusion of the dissection—when packing of the pelvic cavity with naked gauze should be adopted—or because of the occurrence of gross contamination of the perineal wound during the operation as from tearing of the rectum—when open drainage should preferably be established. If primary suture is performed it is probably wise always to administer systemic antibiotic cover.

Colostomy Care

Earlier attempts to make colostomies continent by various modifications of operative technique (as, for example, by taking the colon obliquely through the musculo-aponeurotic layers of the abdominal wall or by rotating the bowel during its passage through the parietes) proved quite ineffective (Goligher, 1975) and it has come to be accepted that a colostomy must inevitably be an incontinent opening. However in May 1975 Feustel and Hennig of Erlangen in West Germany revived the hope of rendering colostomies continent by their introduction of a new magnetic device. The principle of this method is that at the time of the operation a magnetic ring of Samarium-cobalt is buried in the abdominal wall around the emerging colon. After the wound has soundly healed a magnetic cap with an obturator is fitted to the colostomy, being held in position by magnetic attraction to the metal ring. The force of the magnet is sufficiently strong to ensure firm but not injurious contact of the cap and obturator with the skin and bowel, and an additional precaution to render the apposition even more secure is the wearing of a thin rubber washer between the cap and the skin, with a coating of karaya powder on the surface that is in contact with the skin.

Certainly this ingenious new device holds out the promise of conferring continence on at least some of the patients who have to have a colostomy, but clearly much further critical experience with it will be required to assess its reliability, complications and full potential. Meanwhile the management of most colostomy patients will follow the lines that have evolved over the years in the care of an incontinent stoma. Basically, there are two routines available for this purpose—namely the wash-out regime and the spontaneous action regime. The former is used by the majority of colostomy patients in USA, the large intestine being washed out daily by two or more pints of tap water or soapy fluid delivered from a douche-can or other container through tubing and a catheter into the stoma, the subsequent evacuation from the bowel being conveyed by a chute or other device into the lavatory basin. In the intervals between irrigations the colon remains relatively inactive as a rule and the colostomy is covered with a piece of gauze and adhesive strapping. The main disadvantages of this method are the length of time often required for the wash-out, which may take an hour or even longer in some cases, the risk—slight but definite—of perforating the colon during the irrigation, and the fact that really good lavatory and bathroom accommodation are necessary for convenient application of the method (Goligher, 1975).

It is perhaps partly because these latter facilities are not so generally available in Britain that this regime has never enjoyed the same degree of popularity in this country, a notable exception being the Gordon Hospital, London, which has always used the wash-out routine (Seargeant, 1966). Most British surgeons and their colostomy patients have preferred the spontaneous action regime, by which the colostomy is allowed to develop its own rhythm of action, which may result in it acting anything from one to four or more times a day. According to Dukes (1947) and Gabriel (1945, 1963), a regular pattern of colostomy actions is eventually achieved in the great majority of cases, so that the patients can usually predict with confidence when the motion is going to be passed and thus repair to the toilet in time to deal with this event in an orderly fashion. Thereafter the colostomy site is cleansed and covered with a dressing and belt or bag. A certain amount of dieting, with avoidance of excess fruit and vegetables and other foods and drinks with a somewhat aperient action is claimed to be helpful in establishing this routine, as also is the taking of hydrophilic drugs such as methyl-cellulose, Isogel, Celevac and Normacol, which may assist in making the faeces firmer in consistence.

However, in my experience (Goligher, 1975) and that of Grier et al (1964) who surveyed some of my cases, most patients are a good deal less successful in regulating the actions of their colostomy than is implied by these accounts of Dukes (1947) and Gabriel (1945, 1963). Whilst a very few individuals may achieve the ideal of one colostomy action every 24 h, occurring with the utmost regularity at exactly the same time each day, much commoner is a more frequent and irregular state of affairs. But, as patients following the regime of spontaneous colostomy actions now always wear a plastic bag over their stomas, it is really immaterial whether they are able to anticipate exactly when the colostomy action is going to take place or not. Instead the bowel is simply allowed to act incontinently into the bag and at a convenient moment soon afterwards the opportunity is taken to empty or change the bag.

As regards provision of colostomy appliances (Goligher and Pollard, 1972), a wealth of proprietary disposable plastic bags is now available (e.g. Chiron, Coloplast, Hollister, Meredith, Shaw, Simpla-Sassco, Translet). In some of them non-adherent bags are held in position solely with a belt, in others the bag is stuck to the skin with adhesive plaster, karaya gum washers, or a combination of the two, and often reinforced with a supporting belt. Some of the bags are blind pouches which when full are removed and discarded. Others have an opening at the lower end controlled by a clip, release of which allows the faeces to be milked out as required without having to disturb the adhesive and take off the appliance. The latter plan is an advantage in so far as frequent changes of ordinary adhesive plaster may lead to the development of soreness of the skin, which, besides being uncomfortable for the patient, may make it difficult to secure firm fixation of the appliance to the skin. On the other hand, if the faeces are rather stiff, it may be difficult to expel them from the chute type of bag in situ. An alternative solution, if a blind pouch bag is preferred and several changes of appliance are necessary each day, is to use one which incorporates a karaya gum washer as the means of sticking it to the skin, for karaya is a non-irritating, soothing, adhesive. But some of the more sophisticated bags containing karaya gum washers are quite expensive (at least 40p each), so that if the patient changes the bag three or four times in the 24 h, the cost will come to over £1 per day! Another very agreeable adhesive to use on an inflamed skin is Stomahesive, which is applied as a washer between the bag and the sore skin, but it also is expensive, each square costing approximately 60p.

A small matter worthy of comment in connection with adherent colostomy appliances is the escape of intestinal flatus. The Simpla-Sassco bag incorporates an air vent to allow of automatic deflation. With other appliances the upper part of the bag may be pricked with a pin just before it is applied to the stoma to provide egress for wind. Or if the appliance is fixed by a karaya gum washer and the bag becomes distended with flatus, it is often possible for the patient to grasp the more rigid upper part of the bag through his clothing and lift it slightly off the skin at one point for a moment or two so that the bag may deflate itself.

A closely related question that greatly exercises the minds of most patients with a colostomy is how to minimise the possibility of malodour arising from their stoma. The resistance to odour of the material used in the construction of different plastic bags varies considerably and some appliances are thus more effective in containing odour than others. But whatever appliance is used it is probably a good principle to empty or change the bag as soon as possible after a colostomy action. In addition deodorants can be prescribed, either to be taken by mouth or to be applied to the bag. Oral drugs that have been recommended are chlorophyll or powdered charcoal given in a dose of 20 mg and 1 to 2 g respectively four times daily. Locally applied deodorants that have been used are Dor (made by Simpla-Sassco) and Stomogel (made by C. G. Thackeray); a drop or two of either fluid is smeared with the finger on the inside of the bag immediately before use. Patients' opinions on the efficacy of all these deodorants are very mixed and mostly unflattering. More recently bismuth subgallate 400 mg in capsules orally before each meal has been found moderately effective in lessening odour from colostomies or ileostomies (Sparberg, 1974).

The disposal of plastic colostomy appliances is something of a problem. It is difficult to dispose of even purely flimsy plastic bags down the toilet, for they tend to float on the surface of the water and not to submerge, whilst appliances such as the Hollister, part of which is rigid, are quite unsuitable for this form of disposal. The alternative is to empty the bag into the lavatory and then to wrap it up in paper or place it in sanitary-style envelope, so that it may be taken and burnt in an AGA or similar sort of kitchen stove or in a garden incinerator. Plastic bags are not easily burnt in an ordinary domestic hearth. If necessary, they may be disposed of with household rubbish.

Enterostomal therapy

The detailed attentions to colostomy management just outlined are a most important part of the treatment of rectal carcinoma. In recent years in all centres with a special interest in colorectal surgery it has become the practice to have a so-called 'enterostomal therapist' to be responsible for such care to colostomy and ileostomy patients, as we have been doing in my department at the Leeds General Infirmary for over 20 years. I believe that there is a real need for such a person at every medium sized or larger hospital. The position is ideal for a suitably dedicated married nurse who is returning to hospital work after her children have grown up. After a course of training or a period of apprenticeship she can take up stoma therapy on a part-time basis—say four or five half days a week. She sees all patients with a stoma in the wards and again in conjunction with the surgeon when they report to the outpatient department.

Medical and social care of colostomy patients

The social conditions of patients who have had a colostomy operation, particularly those of advanced years and in impoverished circumstances, often leave much to be desired, as Devlin et al (1971) have stressed. Accordingly there may be a great deal for the medical social worker to do for them. To start with, she has usually to arrange convalescence in a suitable convalescent home, which may be quite difficult to organise, as not all such homes are willing to accept patients who have a colostomy. The conditions in the patient's own home require to be investigated, for not a few houses in Britain are sadly deficient in proper sanitary facilities in the form of a proper bathroom or inside toilet. Such circumstances are hard enough for fit individuals to bear, but for colostomy patients they are well nigh intolerable and constitute particularly strong grounds for rehousing. A major problem with older patients with a colostomy is their tendency to feel isolated and depressed and to lose all interest in feeding and looking after themselves. This needs to be combated as far as possible by relatives, friendly neighbours or the community services.

RADICAL TREATMENT WITHOUT PERMANENT COLOSTOMY

Though a properly managed colostomy is generally compatible with a full and active life, the fact remains that virtually all patients faced with the prospect of an operation for cancer of the rectum fervently hope and pray that it will not leave them with a permanent colostomy. Even after they have surmounted this ordeal and have found, as is usually the way, that the colostomy is much less of an inconvenience than they had feared, most of them would still give a great deal to have restored to them natural anorectal function.

Almost since the start of effective surgical treatment for rectal carcinoma in the latter part of the nineteenth century a number of surgeons tried to reconcile the requirements of radical removal of the growth with the preservation of the sphincter mechanism in suitable cases (Hochenegg, 1889; Mandl, 1929). These efforts received further impetus from the pathological researches of Westhues (1934) and Dukes (1930, 1940) in the 1930s, showing that spread of carcinoma of the rectum is often less extensive than had been depicted in the authoritative work of Ernest Miles (1908, 1926). In the last few years there has been a fresh quickening of interest in the possibilities of sphincter preservation in the radical management of rectal cancer. A host of methods is available for the attainment of this objective (Goligher, 1975), but they can be divided in the first instance into two main categories—*rectum-saving forms of local destruction or excision* of well localised, specially favourable growths, and *sphincter-saving forms of rectal resection* applicable to more ordinary growths.

Rectum-saving Forms of Local Destruction or Excision of Specially Favourable Lesions

The crucial consideration in regard to these methods of purely local treatment is the choice of patients appropriate for their use. Obviously these techniques are directed solely at the primary lesion itself in the bowel wall and cannot be expected to deal effectively with metastases in nodes, nor indeed with any deep local extramural spread. [This would certainly be the opinion of most surgeons, though Strauss et al (1965) and Madden and Kandalaft (1971) have postulated that, if the primary lesion is destroyed by diathermy, nodal metastases may subsequently regress.] Consequently these local treatments are only suitable for cases with growths in Dukes' categories A or early B. Unfortunately, there is no way of telling for certain the Dukes' status of a rectal carcinoma till after the rectum has been excised and submitted to pathological dissection. We do know that routine pathological examination according to the manner of Dukes (1940) of rectal excision specimens from 100 consecutive cases of rectal carcinoma will show that roughly 50 have nodal metastases (i.e. are in category C). By comparison, similar pathological examination of rectal excision specimens from 100 patients with polypoid or small sessile carcinomas—the sort of lesions that might be considered for local therapy—will show nodal metastases in only 11 according to Morson (1966), or even fewer by Jackman's (1961) estimate. If purely local treatment instead of rectal excision had been used on these 100 more favourable carcinomas there would almost certainly have been no operative mortality, but the 11 cases with lymph node metastases would have been failures (though they might in certain circumstances have been salvaged by a secondary rectal excision). However, if these 100 favourable cases had all been treated by primary rectal excision, according to average experience, at least three or four would have succumbed as operative deaths, and amongst the 11 who had lymph node metastases (six cases) no more than three or four would have been cured and seven would have developed recurrences. Furthermore most of the 100 patients treated by rectal excision would also have incurred a permanent colostomy as part of the price of cure. Clearly, therefore, local therapy can just compete with more extensive forms of surgical treatment in patients with specially favourable carcinomas, but, if in addition the patients being considered are in particularly poor general health so that the operative mortality of major rectal excision could well be 10 or 15 per cent, the relative advantages of local treatment might be greatly strengthened.

It may be helpful to summarise the clinical characteristics of rectal carcinomas that may be regarded as suitable for purely local methods of treatment. They should be situated in the lowermost 10 cm of the rectum, should be small in size (not more than 5 or 6 cm in diameter and preferably smaller), should project into the lumen rather than ulcerate deeply, and should be mobile on the underlying muscle coat of the rectum and unassociated with any indurated nodes palpable through the rectal wall. Biopsy should show a well-differentiated growth. Obviously the poorer the patient's general condition the more liberal the surgeon can be in interpreting the suitability of the lesion for any form of local treatment. Personally I have always been reluctant to employ such methods on any patient who is well fitted to stand a major cancer operation and have reserved them for very carefully selected poor risk individuals or for those who have refused rectal excision because of their abhorrence of a colostomy.

Electrocoagulation

This method of local treatment for rectal carcinoma was introduced by Strauss et al (1935) of Chicago and has been strongly advocated also by Jackman (1961), Madden and Kandalaft (1971) and Crile and Turnbull (1972). It is probably the most convenient technique of local therapy for the average surgeon.

Technique. Access to the lesion is obtained through a wide bore operating sigmoidoscope, such as Lloyd-Davies's, equipped with a suction tube to remove the smoke and maintain a clear field of vision. A general or caudal anaesthetic is necessary. The diathermy current is best applied by a needle electrode which is inserted into the growth at different points in turn. As the coagulation proceeds the superficial coagulum formed can be scraped away with a uterine curette till a bleeding surface is reached. In turn the latter is coagulated and the process is repeated as required till it is considered that all the tumour has been destroyed or that coagulation has been taken as far as it is safe to go at that session. The operation may last from 15 to 50 min or longer depending on the size of the tumour and other considerations.

The patient reports for digital palpation and resigmoidoscopy under anaesthesia in three weeks time and attempt is made to gauge whether any areas in the zone of ulceration resulting from the electrocoagulation represent persisting growth. If necessary further fulguration is carried out, preceded possibly by biopsy and frozen section histological examination. Thereafter the patient attends at monthly intervals up to six months for repeat rectal palpation and sigmoidoscopy, doubtful areas being subjected to further electrocoagulation. Usually the ulcer is healed in three or four months, and the follow-up is maintained at six-monthly intervals for five years or longer.

Results. Crile and Turnbull (1972) obtained a 68 per cent crude five year survival rate in 62 patients after electrocoagulation. They noted that the prognosis was better the smaller the tumour. In eight patients in whom the growth was not controlled by this treatment a subsequent rectal excision was performed with five year survival in seven.

Endocavitary contact irradiation

This form of treatment has been developed by Papillon (1973) of Lyons and involves administering a dose of 4000 rad directly to the primary growth in the bowel for 3 min at a time.

Technique. An old-fashioned low voltage (50 kV) short focal distance (4 cm), high output (19500–2000 rad/min in the air) Philips machine is used. It has a narrow light tube, easy to handle and capable of being introduced through a sigmoidoscope. The treatment is conducted on an outpatient basis and no anaesthetic is necessary as a rule. The sigmoidoscope is inserted and the growth brought into view. The x-ray tube is then passed up through the scope and the lesion irradiated. The patient re-attends at intervals of seven to ten days and further irradiation is given as required. Usually the tumour has undergone considerable shrinkage after the first two applications, but often a third or fourth is required to complete the regression. Thereafter the patient is kept under regular follow-up supervision as after electrocoagulation.

Results. Papillon (1973) reported on 123 patients treated by this method: 34 died in less than five years, 16 from intercurrent disease, 18 from rectal cancer. Eighty-nine patients (72 per cent) were alive and well after more than five years; five underwent subsequent rectal excision for failure, and 84 were disease-free after irradiation alone.

Local excisions

Both Parks (1972) and York-Mason (1972) have practised purely local excision of early favourable rectal carcinomas, using the techniques which they have respectively developed for excising villous papillomas. Parks (1972) performs the excision through the anus using a bivalve speculum, and York-Mason (1972) uses a posterior transsphincteric approach, dividing the anal sphincters and wall of the rectum in the midline posteriorly and after excising the growth resutures these structures. For the sort of small early carcinomas now being considered it is difficult to see the advantage of these methods for the average surgeon over electrocoagulation or endocavitary irradiation, for they are both technically more difficult than the latter two methods and York-Mason's is more destructive. Furthermore no sizeable series has yet been followed up for five years after local excision, so that their value is still sub judice.

Sphincter-saving Forms of Rectal Resection

These operations differ in their scope and application from the foregoing forms of purely local treatment in that they are intended not solely for use in connection with specially early and favourable lesions, but for the treatment of most ordinary rectal carcinomas, provided that they are so situated as to make preservation and use of the terminal portion of the anorectum patho-logically acceptable and technically feasible.

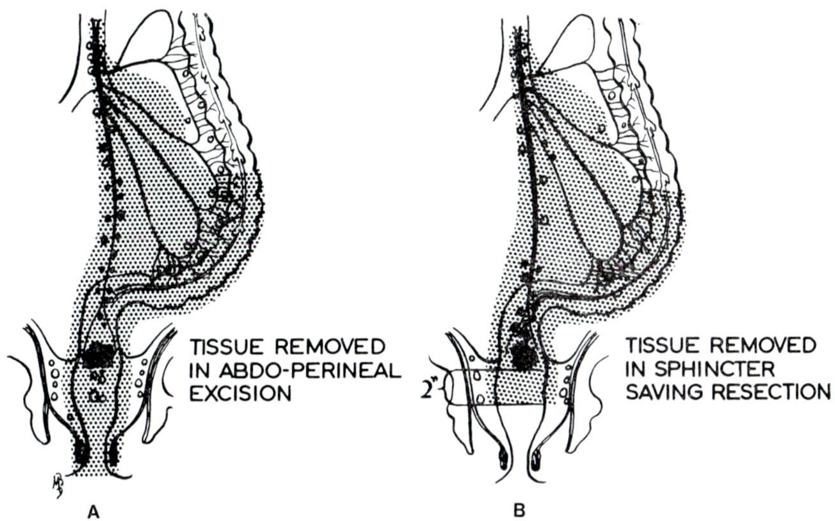

Figure 1.1 Diagram indicating the respective scopes of combined abdominoperineal excision *A*, and a modern radical sphincter saving resection, *B*. Stippled areas indicate the tissues to be removed. (Reproduced from Goligher, J. C. (1975) *Surgery of the Anus, Rectum and Colon*, 3rd edn. London: Baillière Tindall, by kind permission)

The amount of tissue that can be removed in a radical sphincter-saving resection of the rectum is in all directions except distally just as extensive as in a combined abdominoperineal excision (Fig. 1.1). As for the distal extent, Westhues (1934), Pannett (1935) and Wangensteen (1945) claimed that a 2.5 cm margin of macroscopically normal bowel wall distal to the lower edge of the growth would suffice for adequate clearance in this direction. But a reinvestigation of this point by Goligher, Dukes and Bussey (1951), Quer, Dahlin and Mayo (1953) and Grinnell (1954) suggested the advisability as a rule of a 2 in. (5 cm) margin of bowel and perirectal fat, vessels and lymphatics beyond the carcinoma.

These distances are as measured on the straightened out—but not tautly stretched—bowel, after the rectum has been freely mobilised by dissection. It is important to emphasise, too, that the process of mobilisation of the rectum, particularly the thorough division of the lateral ligaments, allows of considerable lengthening. Take the example of a growth which lies with its lower edge 7.5 cm from the anal verge on a preoperative sigmoidoscopy. It might seem at first sight that this lesion would be too low for a sphincter-saving

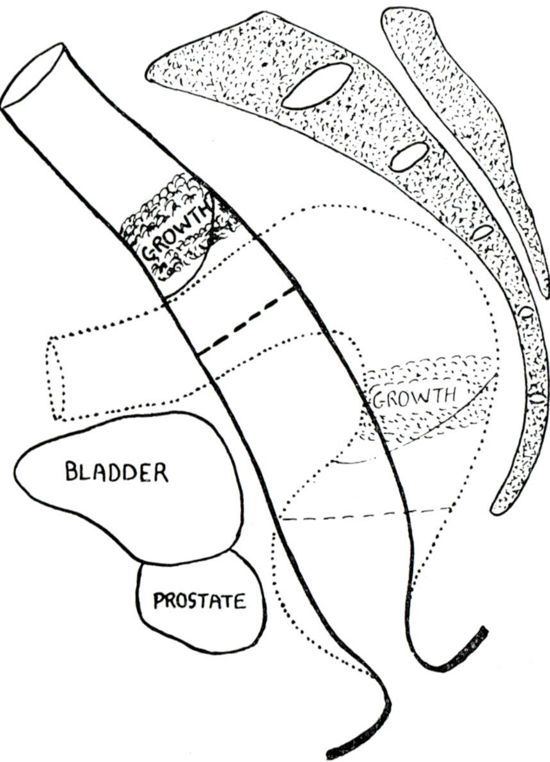

Figure 1.2   Diagram illustrating that, when the lateral ligaments are divided and the rectum is thoroughly mobilised from the sacral concavity, a growth lying at 7.5 cm from the anal verge may rise to 12.5 cm or higher.

resection, for a 5 cm margin of clearance distally would take the lower line of the resection through the top of the anal canal at 2.5 cm. Actually, after the rectum has been fully mobilised by the abdominal dissection carried down to the pelvic floor, this growth will usually be elevated to 11 or 12 cm (Fig. 1.2), which would permit of its resection with a distal margin of 5 cm of normal bowel and yet leave an anorectal stump of 6 or 7 cm beyond, which would be worthwhile conserving if technical considerations are conducive to anastomosing the colon stump to it.

Of course other factors besides the amount of elevation of the growth after dissection influence the decision in an individual case as to whether resection with restoration of continuity will be possible and which technique of operation should be used. The sex and physique of the patient are very important for the wider female pelvis facilitates any form of pelvic anastomosis and it is much easier to carry out all these operations on thin individuals. Another very important consideration is the activity of the growth, for the guidelines given above in regard to the distal margin of clearance necessary in resection operations apply only to carcinomas of average histological differentiation or well differentiated. It is known that with poorly differentiated or anaplastic carcinomas malignant cells may occasionally be found in the bowel wall three or more inches away from the macroscopic edge of the primary lesion (Goligher et al, 1951; Quer et al, 1953). If, therefore, the preoperative biopsy of the growth shows a very active tumour, a sphincter-saving resection is better avoided unless a very wide margin of clearance can be achieved. In this connection it should be added that in dealing with growths found at operation to be associated with extensive local spread, most surgeons would be deterred from performing a resection with restoration of continuity for fear of eventual recurrence in the pelvis implicating the anastomotic site, and in such cases would prefer to do an abdominoperineal excision with iliac colostomy. A further factor that bears strongly on the decision whether to adopt a sphincter-saving type of resection or not is the experience of the surgeon with this form of operation and his ability to perform it especially when circumstances for its application are less than optimal.

Low anterior resection

This is the form of sphincter-saving resection that has secured widest acceptance and it is now a well-established operation in the repertoire of virtually all surgeons treating colorectal carcinoma. If it is reserved for growths well within its scope and the resection is performed in a thoroughly radical manner, this operation is capable of yielding very satisfactory immediate and long-term results including normal continence, as the reports of Morgan (1965), Vandertoll and Beahrs (1965), Cullen and Mayo (1963), Goligher (1975) fully testify. On the technical side, whatever may be the relative merits of single and double-layer suture techniques of suture for colonic anastomoses in general, it would seem from recent experience, and particularly from Everett's (1974) controlled trial on the subject, that a one layer suture for low anterior resection is less likely to be followed by anastomotic dehiscence (Fig. 1.3A, B) than is a two-layer suture in this situation. A suitable technique of one layer suture is illustrated in Figures 1.4 to 1.7; the actual suture material may be silk, Ethiflex, stainless steel wire, or any other non-absorbable material that ties good knots. Perhaps even chromic catgut inserted in the same way might do equally well. Most surgeons now leave the pelvic peritoneum unsutured at the conclusion of the operation so that the coils of small intestine and the tail of the greater omentum can drop down into the pelvis and surround the anastomosis. In addition suction drainage of the site is usually instituted with two or three suction drains brought out through the abdominal wall in the suprapubic region.

Another debatable technical point that should be mentioned is that of proximal decompression of the large bowel. In the past some surgeons such as myself have quite often used a complementary transverse colostomy in connection with low anterior resection in order to lessen the incidence of

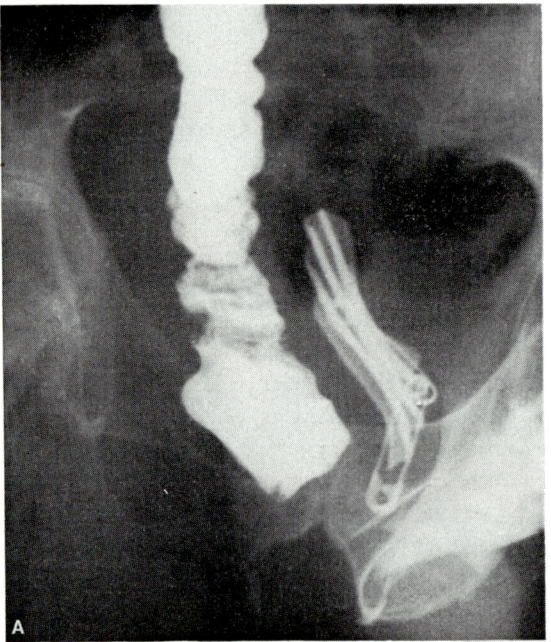
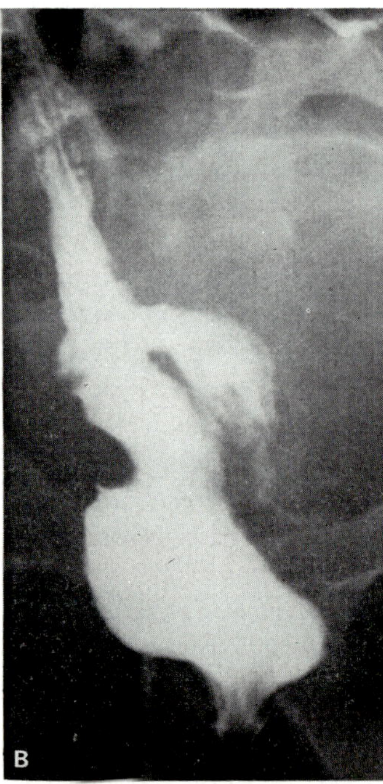

Figure 1.3   X-ray plates after gastrografin enemas two weeks following low anterior resection: *A*, showing intact anastomosis, and *B*, showing a posterior anastomotic dehiscence with extravasation of the opaque medium into the presacral space

anastomotic dehiscence—or more correctly to diminish the hazard of such leakage if it occurred. But other surgeons such as Turnbull (1974) and Beahrs (1975), who have had an extensive experience of anterior resection, have only occasionally made use of colostomy in this way. With the improved results following use of a single layer suture technique for the anastomosis, surgeons who have hitherto frequently favoured colostomy may now have greater confidence in dispensing with it.

Anterior resection is indeed a very valuable operation in the treatment of rectal carcinoma, and it is fair to say that where it can be conveniently applied it is preferable to any other method of resection with preservation of the sphincters. Unfortunately its application even in expert hands is limited to but a proportion of the growths that might on purely pathological grounds be deemed treatable by a sphincter-saving type of resection. Thus, whilst a surgeon specially experienced with this operation may be able with it to remove carcinomas with their lower edges as low as 7.5 or 8 cm from the anal verge on preoperative sigmoidoscopy in thin female patients, in the average

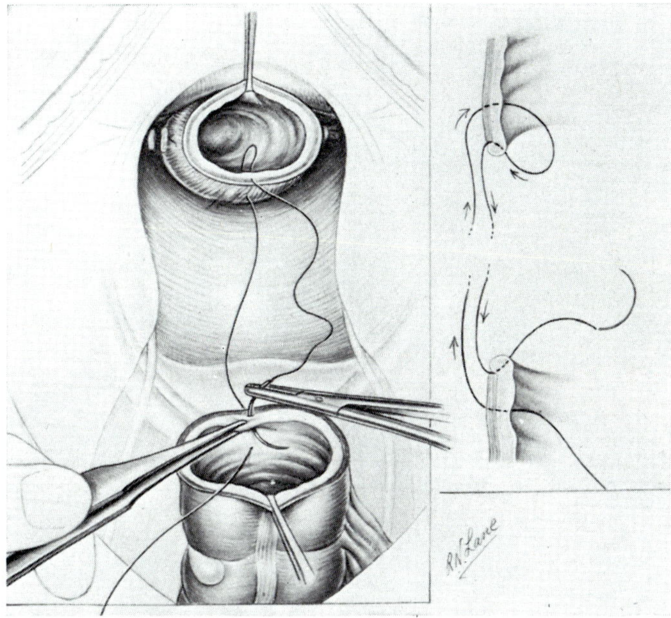

Figure 1.4   One layer suture technique for low anterior resection. View obtained by surgeon standing on left side of patient and looking down into pelvis. Whilst colonic and rectal stumps are about 6 in. apart the first silk stitch is placed loosely in the posterior midline of both stumps. It is inserted from the mucosal aspect of the colonic stump through all coats, transfixes the rectal wall from without inwards and on the return journey catches the cut edges of rectal and colonic mucosae (insert: diagrammatic representation of course of suture). (Figures 4 to 7 from Goligher, J. C. (1975) *Amer. J. Surg.*, by kind permission)

man or in obese women he would find it quite difficult to deal with growths at 10 cm with it, and in obese men he would be lucky to be able to remove lesions at 12 or 13 cm. Obviously a number of carcinomas in the middle third of the rectum in males or obese females, which are eligible for removal without sacrifice of the sphincters, for technical reasons cannot be treated by anterior resection—at least by ordinary suture technique. Whether it may be possible with the aid of a suture machine such as the Russian circular stapling apparatus (Fain, Patin and Morgenstern, 1975) remains to be established. Unless this device does prove helpful, it would seem that, if sphincter-saving resection

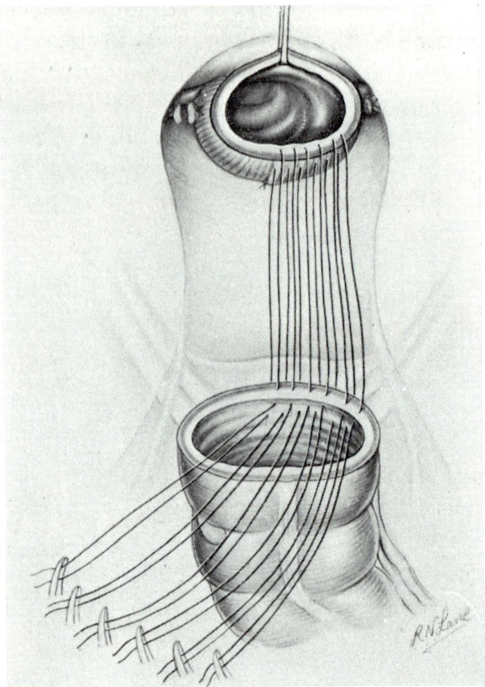

Figure 1.5 One layer suture technique for low anterior resection. Sutures corresponding to right posterior quarter (or preferably third) of the circumference of bowel loosely placed

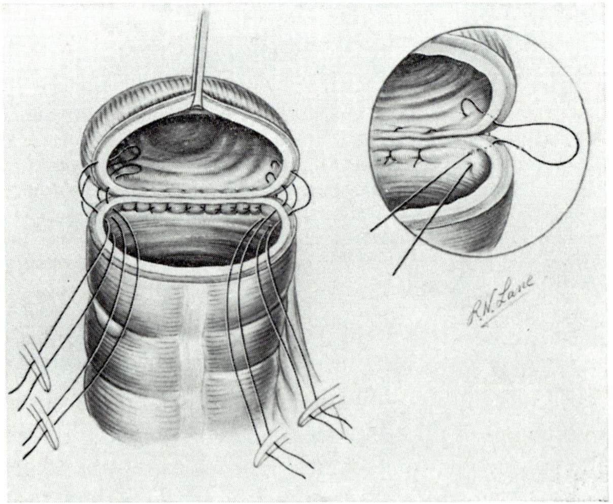

Figure 1.6 One layer suture technique for low anterior resection. After sutures corresponding to posterior two-thirds of circumference have been loosely placed, the colon stump is slid down on the silks to make contact with the rectal stump and the sutures are tied with the knots on the mucosa

is to be practised in these less favourable subjects, it must take the form of one of the several other more complex methods of achieving this type of excision, such as an abdominoanal pull-through resection or abdominosacral resection. During the past couple of decades the majority of surgeons, including some very experienced colorectal surgeons such as Beahrs (1975), have taken the view that these alternative techniques are not sufficiently reliable in their results to be worth adopting, and that the best practical policy in treating rectal carcinoma is to use anterior resection to the limit of technical feasibility and to relegate all the remaining cases to abdominoperineal excision. But in the last few years several surgeons have been turning again to these other methods of sphincter-saving resection.

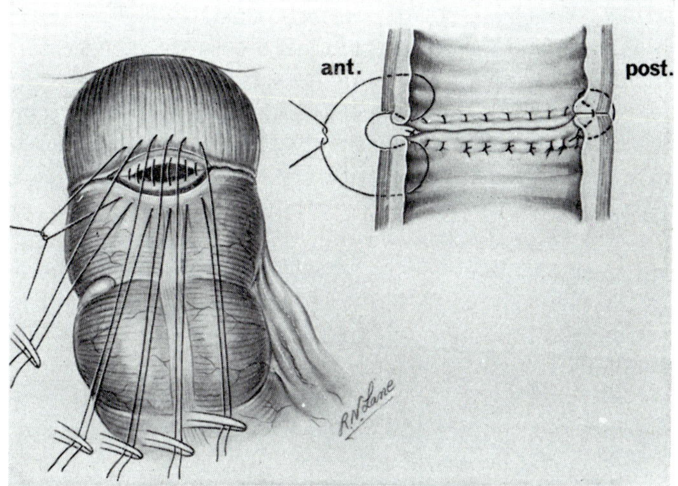

Figure 1.7 One layer suture technique for low anterior resection. The gap in the anterior third of the circumference of the anastomosis is being closed with vertical (or, if more convenient, horizontal) mattress sutures

Abdominoanal pull-through resection

In this type of operation the resection of the growth is conducted from the abdomen as in an anterior resection, leaving a long colonic and a very short anorectal stump, the latter consisting of little more than the anal canal and its sphincters. These stumps are brought into continuity not by a difficult sutured anastomosis deep in the pelvis but by pulling the colon through the anal canal from below. There are many variants of the operation (Goligher, 1975) depending on exactly how the colon and anorectum are co-apted—whether the colonic stump is simply made to project through the anal canal (possibly denuded of its lining), or whether the intact anorectal remnant is everted before the colon is drawn through and the cut edges of the latter and the colon are united by suture, as in the Swenson (1958) operation for Hirschsprung's disease, or by a two-stage modification of this technique.

Septic complications, necrosis of bowel or leakage are recognised mishaps in a proportion of the patients after this operation, but in the hands of surgeons with special familiarity with the procedure it is clear that it may have an acceptably low operative morbidity and mortality (Bacon, 1956; Black and Botham, 1958; Waugh and Turner, 1958; Hughes, Cuthberton and Carden, 1962; Goligher et al, 1965; Kratzer, 1967; Kennedy et al, 1970; Wenckert, 1970). It also seems reasonably well established that the long-term survival rate is quite competitive with that after other radical operations. Perhaps the main point of contention about the pull-through method is the quality of functional results afforded by it. Estimates have varied from 9 per cent of perfect continence (Waugh and Turner, 1958) to 90 per cent (Black and Botham, 1958; Wenckert, 1970), the differences being perhaps explained partly by variations in operative technique and partly by different standards of assessment. In my own series (Goligher et al, 1965) and in that surveyed by Kennedy et al (1970), in both of which the same operative method was used and the same general criteria of evaluation of the results were employed, about 30 per cent of the patients had roughly normal continence and 23 per cent were completely incontinent. It was noticeable however that many of the 47 per cent who suffered partial incontinence were reasonably happy with the outcome of their operation and reckoned that it was preferable to having a colostomy. As Kennedy et al (1970) and Bennett, Hughes and Cuthberton (1972) have stressed, too, there is often considerable improvement in control over a period of 12 months or so after the operation.

The fact remains that the abdominoanal pull-through operation has never been popular in this country and has had only limited support in the USA, but perhaps it should be looked at afresh.

Abdominotransanal resection. Recently Parks (1972) has devised a new operative method which is similar to the pull-through procedure, though he hopes that it will be an improvement on it. With the patient in the modified lithotomy-Trendelenburg position to allow of simultaneous access to the abdomen and the anal region, the affected segment of bowel is removed through the abdomen by a resection extending from the mid-descending colon down almost to the anorectal ring, the splenic flexure being mobilised in the process. Continuity is then restored by opening up the anal canal from below by means of a bivalve speculum to expose the top of the anorectal remnant and allow the cut edge of the colon stump to be drawn down to it. The two edges of bowel are then united by a single row of fine through-and-through sutures of non-absorbable material, the speculum being gradually rotated round to expose the various sectors of the bowel circumference in turn (Fig. 1.8). A special handled urethroplasty needle may be used to place the sutures in this rather inaccessible situation, but I have found that very small $\frac{5}{8}$ circle atraumatic needles on an ordinary needle holder do equally well. A complementary transverse colostomy or caecostomy is probably advisable in most cases after this very low anastomosis.

The advantages claimed for this method are that it does not involve damaging the anal canal mechanism by turning it inside out or by removing its lining. On the other hand, the sphincters are quite considerably stretched by the speculum. Parks (1972) reports favourably on the results obtained by him to date, but insufficient cases have as yet been done by this method and followed up for a substantial period of time to permit of a proper appraisal.

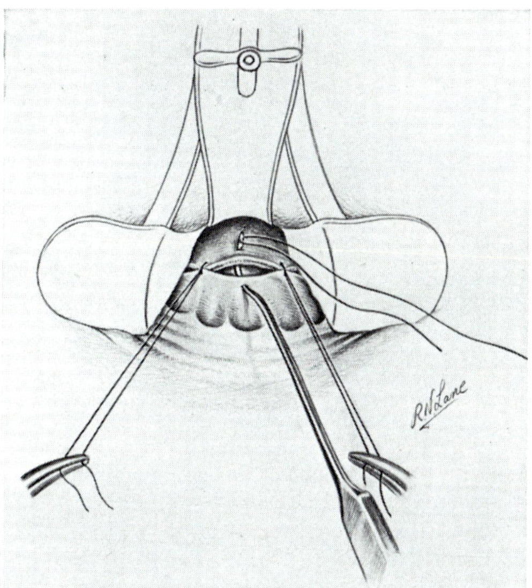

Figure 1.8   Parks (1972) method of coloanal anastomosis conducted from below through the anal canal by means of a bivalve anal speculum, which is rotated to expose all sectors of the bowel circumference in turn

Abdominosacral resection

In this operation the rectum and left colon are fully mobilised, but not divided, through an abdominal approach and pushed down into the pelvis. The abdomen is then closed and the patient is turned on his right or left side in a Sims position and the coccyx and exceptionally rarely the terminal piece of the sacrum are resected through a transverse or curved oblique incision (Fig. 1.9). The resulting gap provides access to the pelvis, from which the previously freed rectum and sigmoid colon are drawn out as a loop (Fig. 1.10). After some further dissection, if necessary to isolate the rectum right down to the anorectal ring, the loop is doubly clamped above and below and resected. The colonic and distal anorectal stumps are then anastomosed, preferably by a single layer suture as described in Figures 1.4 to 1.7 for anterior resection and shown in this context in Figure 1.11.

Abdominosacral resection was extensively practised some years ago by Finsterer (1941), Goetze (1944) and particularly by d'Allaines (1951). It was also the first method used by Pannett (1935) one of the pioneers of sphincter-saving resection in this country. But it has fallen out of vogue in more recent times. However, Donaldson, Rodkey and Behringer (1966) and Localio

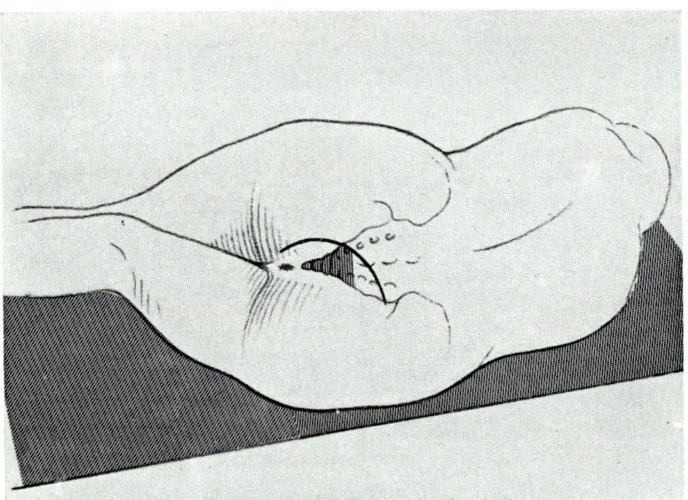

Figure 1.9 Abdominosacral resection. Patient in right lateral slightly prone position for the sacral phase of this operation. Note outline of incision

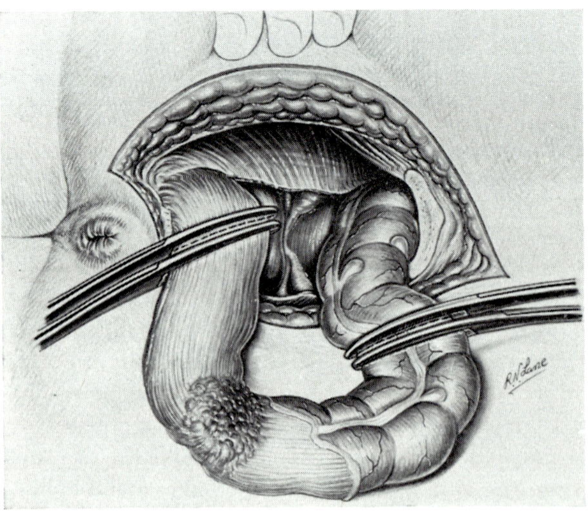

Figure 1.10 Abdominosacral resection. Coccyx has been excised and levators partly incised to give access to pelvic cavity and allow previously mobilised rectum and sigmoid colon to be withdrawn as a loop. Lines of proposed resection indicated

(Localio and Stahl, 1969; Localio and Baron, 1973; Localio, 1975) have stimulated some interest in it again in America. The latter has developed a technique for the operation in which the patient is placed on his left side throughout, so that the abdominal and sacral phases can be performed to some extent simultaneously, which is a convenience for bringing the colon down for accurate anastomosis to the anorectal remnant.

One of the complications previously encountered with abdominosacral resection was that of anastomotic dehiscence, with the development of a faecal fistula through the sacral wound. Localio (1975) has only had this trouble in technically difficult heavily built male patients; in this group he now always

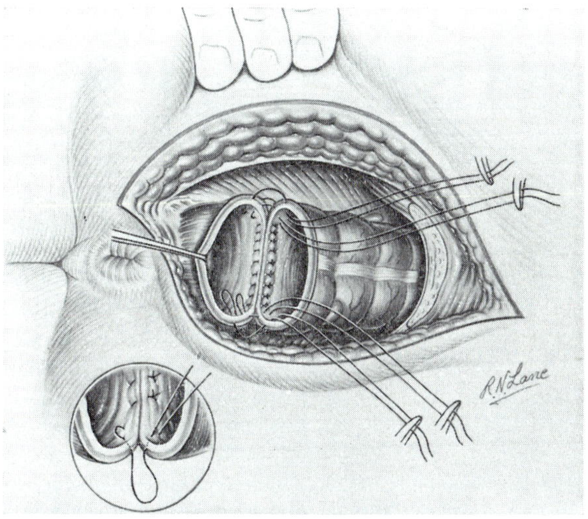

Figure 1.11   Abdominosacral resection. Colonic and rectal stumps being anastomosed by a single layer of inverting silk sutures

performs a complementary transverse colostomy to protect the anastomosis. But in all other patients having this operation he does not use a colostomy and has had virtually no leaks. His immediate results are excellent and the functional state of the patients even with an anastomosis as low as 4 cm from the anal verge is after four to six months most impressive. There is no doubt that with this method it is possible to treat by spincter-saving resection growths that would be too low, particularly in the male, for anterior resection. Unfortunately though the later results are so far encouraging, a longer follow-up period will be necessary before they can mean very much.

Abdominotranssphincteric resection. York-Mason (1972) has evolved an operation which possesses many features in common with the abdominosacral resection. However, instead of obtaining access from below by means of a para- or transcoccygeal incision with removal of the coccyx and possibly the terminal part of the sacrum, he incises the levators and the external sphincter, the patient being in the prone position, slightly flexed at the hips, for this phase (Fig. 1.12), York-Mason (1975) has reported good results as regards postoperative function and lack of serious morbidity, but the cases treated by him by this method are too few and too recent for its curative value to be fairly judged at the present time.

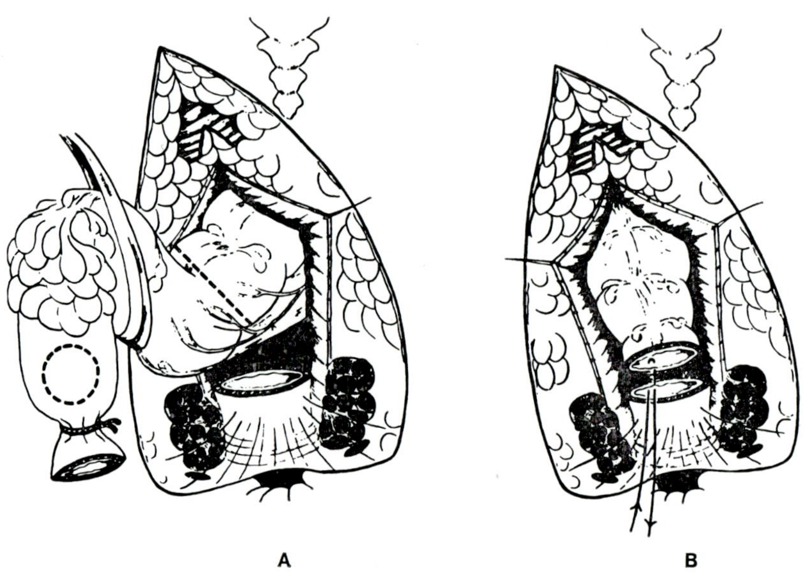

Figure 1.12   York-Mason's abdominotranssphincteric resection. The patient is in the prone position for the posterior incision through the levators and the external anal sphincter. *A*, The rectum has been resected down to the top of the intact anal sphincter, and *B*, the cut edge of the colon stump is being apposed to the top of the anal canal for suture. (Reproduced from York-Mason (1972) *Ann. roy. Coll. Surg. Engl.*, **51**, 320–331, by kind permission)

Conclusion

These efforts to expand the use of sphincter-saving methods in the radical management of rectal cancer are in the highest degree laudible—always provided that the surgeon does not allow his enthusiasm and that of his patient for this idea to deflect him from his main objective, which is permanent cure of the disease.

REFERENCES

Altemeier, W. A., Culbertson, W. R., Alexander, J. W., Sutorius, S. & Bossert, J. (1974) Primary closure and healing of the perineal wound in abdominoperineal resection of the rectum for carcinoma. *Amer. J. Surg.*, **127**, 215–219.
Anderson, B., Korner, B. & Østergaard, A. H. (1972) Topical ampicillin against wound infection after colorectal surgery. *Ann. Surg.*, **176**, 129–132.

Bacon, H. E. (1956) Abdominoperineal proctosigmoidectomy with sphincter preservation. Five-year and ten-year survival after pull-through operation for cancer of the rectum. *J. Amer. med. Ass.*, **160,** 628–634.

Beahrs, O. H. (1975) Personal communication.

Bennett, R. C., Hughes, E. S. R. & Cuthberton, A. M. (1972) Long-term review of function following pull-through operations of the rectum. *Brit. J. Surg.*, **59,** 723–725.

Bird, G. G., Bunch, G. A., Croft, C. B., Hoffmann, D. C., Humphrey, C. S., Rhind, J. R., Rosenberg, I. L., Whitaker, M., Wilkinson, A. R. & Hall, R. (1971) Topical noxythiolin antisepsis. Report of a controlled trial. *Brit. J. Surg.*, **58,** 447–448.

Black, B. M. & Botham, R. J. (1958) Combined abdominoendorectal resection for lesions of the mid and upper parts of the rectum. *Arch. Surg. (Chicago),* **76,** 688–696.

Broader, J. H., Masselink, B. A., Oates, G. D. & Alexander-Williams, J. (1974) Management of the pelvic space after proctectomy. *Brit. J. Surg.*, **61,** 94–97.

Browne, M. K. & Stoller, J. L. (1970) Intraperitoneal noxythionin in faecal peritonitis. *Brit. J. Surg.*, **57,** 525–529.

Bussey, H. J. R. (1963) The long-term results of surgical treatment of cancer of the rectum. *Proc. roy. Soc. Med.*, **56,** 494–496.

Bussey, H. J. R., Dukes, C. E. & Lockhart-Mummery, H. E. (1960) Results of the surgical treatment of rectal cancer. In *Cancer of the Rectum,* ed. Dukes, C. E., p. 267. London: Livingstone.

Butler, E. C. B. (1971) Treatment of carcinoma of the large intestine. *Brit. J. Surg.*, **58,** 29–32.

Crile, G. Jr & Turnbull, R. B. Jr (1972) The role of electrocoagulation in the treatment of carcinoma of the rectum. *Surg. Gynec. Obstet.*, **135,** 391–396.

Cruz, E. P., McDonald, G. O. & Cole, W. H. (1956) Prophylatic treatment of cancer: the use of chemotherapeutic agents to prevent tumor metastasis. *Surgery,* **40,** 291–296.

Cullen, P. K. Jr & Mayo, C. W. (1963) A further evaluation of the one-stage low anterior resection. *Dis. Colon Rect.*, **6,** 415–421.

d'Allaines, F. (1951) *Traitement Chirurgical du Cancer du Rectum,* 2nd edn. Paris: Editions Medicales Flammarion.

Dencker, H., Norryd, C. & Tranberg, K. G. (1973) Management of the perineal wound after rectal excision. *Acta chir. scand.*, **139,** 568–570.

Devlin, H. B., Plant, J. A. & Griffin, M. (1971) Aftermath of surgery for anorectal cancer. *Brit. med. J.*, **2,** 413–418.

Donaldson, G. A., Rodkey, G. V. & Behringer, G. E. (1966) Resection of the rectum with anal preservation. *Surg. Gynec. Obstet.*, **123,** 571–580.

Drasar, B. S. (1968) Cultivation of anaerobic intestinal bacteria. *J. Path. Bact.*, **94,** 417–427.

Dukes, C. E. (1930) The spread of cancer of the rectum. *Brit. J. Surg.*, **17,** 643–669.

Dukes, C. E. (1940) Cancer of the rectum: an analysis of 1000 cases. *J. Path. Bact.*, **50,** 527–539.

Dukes, C. E. (1947) Management of a permanent colostomy. *Lancet,* **2,** 12–14.

Dukes, C. E. (1957) Discussion on major surgery in carcinoma of the rectum with or without colostomy, excluding the anal canal and including the rectosigmoid. *Proc. roy. Soc. Med.*, **50,** 1031–1052.

Dwight, R. W., Higgins, G. A. & Keehn, R. J. (1969) Factors influencing survival after resection in cancer of the colon and rectum. *Amer. J. Surg.*, **117,** 512–522.

Dwight, R. W., Higgins, G. A., Roswit, B., Le Veen, H. H. & Keehn, R. J. (1972) Pre-operative radiation and surgery for cancer of the sigmoid colon and rectum. *Amer. J. Surg.*, **123,** 93–103.

Evans, C. & Pollock, A. V. (1973) The reduction of surgical wound infections by prophylactic parenteral cephaloridine. *Brit. J. Surg.*, **60,** 434–437.

Evans, C., Pollock, A. V. & Rosenberg, I. L. (1974) The reduction of surgical wound infections by topical cephaloridine: a controlled clinical trial. *Brit. J. Surg.*, **61,** 133–135.

Everett, W. G. (1974) A comparison of the one-layer and two-layer techniques for colorectal anastomosis. *Brit. J. Surg.*, **62,** 135–140.

Fain, S. N., Patin, C. S. & Morgenstern, L. (1975) Use of a mechanical suturing apparatus in low colorectal anastomosis. *Arch. Surg.*, **110,** 1079–1082.

Finsterer, H. (1941) Zur chirurgischen Behandlung des Rektumkarzinoms. *Arch. klin. Chir.*, **202,** 15–83.

Feustel, H. & Hennig, G. (1975) Kontinente kolostomie durch magnet verschluss. *Dtsch. med. Wschr.*, **100**, 1063–1064.

Gabriel, W. B. (1932) The end-results of perineal excision and of radium in the treatment of cancer of the rectum. *Brit. J. Surg.*, **20**, 234–248.

Gabriel, W. B. (1945) Discussion on the management of permanent colostomy. *Proc. roy. Soc. Med.*, **38**, 692–696.

Gabriel, W. B. (1957) Discussion on major surgery in carcinoma of the rectum with or without colostomy, excluding the anal canal and including the rectosigmoid. *Proc. roy. Soc. Med.*, **50**, 1041–1052.

Gabriel, W. B. (1963) *The Principles and Practice of Rectal Surgery*, 5th edn. London: Lewis.

Gilmore, O. J. A. & Sanderson, P. (1975) Prophylactic interparietal povidone-iodine in abdominal surgery. *Brit. J. Surg.* **62**, 792–799.

Goetze, O. (1944) Die abdominosakrale Resektion des Mastdarms mit Wiederherstellung der natürlichen Kontinenz. *Arch. klin. Chir.*, **206**, 293–337.

Goligher, J. C. (1941) Operability of carcinoma of the rectum. *Brit. med. J.*, **2**, 393–397.

Goligher, J. C. (1975) *Surgery of the Anus, Rectum and Colon*, 3rd edn. London: Ballière Tindall.

Goligher, J. C., Dukes, C. E. & Bussey, H. J. R. (1951) Local recurrences after sphincter-saving excision for carcinoma of the rectum and rectosigmoid. *Brit. J. Surg.*, **39**, 199–211.

Goligher, J. C., Duthie, H. L., de Dombal, F. T. & Watts, J. M. (1965) The pull-through abdomino-anal excision for carcinoma of the middle third of the rectum: a comparison with low anterior resection. *Brit. J. Surg.*, **52**, 323–334.

Goligher, J. C. & Pollard, M. (1972) *The Care of Your Colostomy*, 2nd edn. London: Baillière Tindall.

Gorbach, S. L., Nahas, L., Lerner, P. I. & Weinstein, L. (1967) Studies of intestinal microflora. I. Effect of diet, age, and periodic sampling on numbers of fecal microorganisms in man. *Gastroenterology*, **53**, 845–855.

Grier, W. R., Postel, A. H., Syarse, A. & Localio, S. A. (1964) An evaluation of colonic stoma management without irrigations. *Surg. Gynec. Obstet.*, **118**, 1234–1242.

Grinnell, R. S. (1953) Results in the treatment of carcinoma of the colon and rectum. *Surg. Gynec. Obstet.*, **96**, 31–42.

Grinnell, R. S. (1954) Distal intramural spread of carcinoma of the rectum and rectosigmoid. *Surg. Gynec. Obstet.*, **99**, 421–430.

Haxton, H. (1970) *Surgical Techniques*. Bristol: John Wright.

Hewitt, J., Rigby, Janet, Reeve, J. & Cox, A. G. (1973) Whole-gut irrigation in preparation for large-bowel surgery. *Lancet*, **2**, 337–340.

Higgins, G. A., Dwight, R. W., Smith, J. V. & Keehn, R. J. (1971) Fluorouracil as an adjuvant to surgery in carcinoma of the colon. *Arch. Surg.*, **102**, 339–343.

Hochenegg, J. (1889) Beiträge zur Chirurgie des Rektums und der Beckenorgane. *Wien. Klin. Wschr.*, **2**, 578–580.

Holden, W. D. & Dixon, W. J. (1962) A study of the use of triethylene-thiophosphoramide as an adjuvant to surgery in the treatment of colorectal cancer. *Cancer Chemother. Rep.*, **16**, 129–134.

Hughes, E. S. R., Cuthberton, A. M. & Carden, A. B. G. (1962) Pull-through operations for carcinoma of the rectum. *Med. J. Aust.*, **2**, 907–909.

Hultén, L., Kewenter, J., Knutsson, U. & Olbe, L. (1971) Primary closure of perineal wound after proctocolectomy or rectal excision. *Acta chir. scand.*, **137**, 467–469.

Irvin, T. T. & Goligher, J. C. (1975) A controlled clinical trial of three different methods of perineal wound management following excision of the rectum. *Brit. J. Surg.* **62**, 287–291.

Jackman, R. J. (1961) Conservative management of selected patients with carcinoma of the rectum. *Dis. Colon Rect.*, **4**, 429–434.

Jensen, M. T., McKenzie, R. J., Hugh, T. B. & Lake, B. (1975) Topical ampicillin-cloxacillin in the prevention of abdominal wound sepsis. *Brit. J. clin. Pract.*, **29**, 115–118.

Kennedy, J. T., McOmish, D., Bennett, R. C., Hughes, E. S. R. & Cuthberton, A. M. (1970) Abdomino-anal pull-through resection of the rectum. *Brit. J. Surg.*, **57**, 589–596.

Kratzer, G. L. (1967) The pull-through operation. *Dis. Colon Rect.*, **10**, 112–117.

Localio, S. A. (1975) Personal communication.

Localio, S. A. & Baron, B. (1973) Abdomino-sacral resection and anastomosis for mid-rectal cancer. *Ann. Surg.*, **178**, 540–546.

Localio, S. A. & Stahl, W. M. (1969) Simultaneous abdomino-transsacral resection and anastomosis for midrectal cancer. *Amer. J. Surg.*, **117**, 282–289.

Madden, J. L. & Kandalaft, S. (1971) Clinical evaluation of electrocoagulation in the treatment of cancer of the rectum. *Amer. J. Surg.*, **122**, 347–352.

Mandl, F. (1929) Uber 1000 sakrale Mastdarmkrebsexstirpationen. (Aus dem Hocheneggschen Material.) *Dtsch. Z. Chir.*, **219**, 3–40.

Mayo, C., Laberge, M. Y. & Hardy, W. M. (1958) Five-year survival after anterior resection for carcinoma of the rectum and rectosigmoid. *Surg. Gynec. Obstet.*, **106**, 695–698.

Mayo, C., Lee, M. J. & Davis, R. M. (1951) A comparative study of operations for carcinoma of the rectum and rectosigmoid. *Surg. Gynec. Obstet.*, **92**, 360–364.

Miles, W. E. (1908) A method of performing abdominoperineal excision for carcinoma of the rectum and of the terminal portion of the pelvic colon. *Lancet*, **2**, 1812–1813.

Miles, W. E. (1926) *Cancer of the Rectum.* London: Harrison.

Moore, W. E., Cato, E. P. & Holdeman, L. V. (1969) Anaerobic bacteria of the gastrointestinal flora and their occurrence in clinical infections. *J. infect. Dis.*, **119**, 641–649.

Morgan, C. N. (1965) Carcinoma of the rectum. *Ann. roy. Coll. Surg. Engl.*, **36**, 73–97.

Morson, B. C. (1966) Factors influencing the prognosis of early cancer of the rectum. *Proc. roy. Soc. Med.*, **59**, 607–608.

Mountain, J. C. & Seal, P. V. (1970) Topical ampicillin in gridiron appendicectomy wounds. *Brit. J. clin. Pract.*, **24**, 111–115.

Mrazek, R., Economou, S., McDonald, G. O., Slaughter, D. P. & Cole, W. H. (1959) Prophylactic and adjuvant use of nitrogen mustard in the surgical treatment of cancer. *Ann. Surg.*, **150**, 745–755.

Nadler, S. H. & Moore, G. E. (1964) Fluorouracil colon-rectum adjuvant chemotherapy. *Arch. Surg. (Chicago)*, **89**, 592–595.

Nash, A. G. & Hugh, T. B. (1967) Topical ampicillin and wound infection in colon surgery. *Brit. med. J.*, **1**, 471–472.

Nichols, R. L. & Condon, R. E. (1971) Preoperative preparation of the colon. *Surg. Gynec. Obstet.*, **132**, 323–337.

Nichols, R. L., Broido, P., Condon, R. E., Gorbach, S. L. & Nyhus, L. M. (1973) Effect of preoperative neomycin-erythromycin intestinal preparation on the incidence of infectious complications following colon surgery. *Ann. Surg.*, **178**, 453–462.

Pannett, C. A. (1935) Resection of the rectum with restoration of continuity. *Lancet*, **2**, 423–425.

Papillon, J. (1973) Endocavitary irradiation of early rectal cancers for cure: a series of 123 cases. *Proc. roy. Soc. Med.*, **66**, 1177–1190.

Parks, A. G. (1972) Transanal technique in low rectal anastomosis. *Proc. roy. Soc. Med.*, **65**, 975–976.

Polk, H. C. Jr & Lopez-Mayor, J. F. (1969) Postoperative wound infection: a prospective study of determinant factors and prevention. *Surgery*, **66**, 97–103.

Quer, E. A., Dahlin, D. C. & Mayo, C. W. (1953) Retrograde intramural spread of carcinoma of the rectum and rectosigmoid: a microscopic study. *Surg. Gynec. Obstet.*, **96**, 24–30.

Ruckley, C. V., Smith, A. N. & Balfour, T. W. (1970) Perineal closure by omental graft. *Surg. Gynec. Obstet.*, **131**, 300–302.

Seargeant, P. W. (1966) Colostomy management by the irrigation technique: review of 165 cases. *Brit. med. J.*, **2**, 25–26.

Slaney, G. (1971) Results of treatment of carcinoma of the colon and rectum. In *Modern Trends in Surgery*, 3rd edn, ed. Irvine, W. T. London: Butterworth.

Sparberg, M. (1974) Bismuth subgallate as an effective means for the control of ileostomy odor: a double blind study. *Gastroenterology*, **66**, 476–480.

Stearns, M. W. Jr, Deddish, M. R., Quan, S. H. Q. & Leaming, R. H. (1974) Preoperative roentgen therapy for cancer of the rectum and rectosigmoid. *Surg. Gynec. Obstet.*, **138**, 584–586.

Stearns, M. W. Jr, Deddish, M. R. & Quan, S. H. Q. (1959) Preoperative roentgen therapy for cancer of the rectum. *Surg. Gynec. Obstet.*, **109**, 225–229.

Stoker, T. A. M. & Ellis, H. (1972) Wound antibiotics in gastrointestinal surgery. Comparison of ampicillin with penicillin and sulphadiazine. *Brit. J. Surg.*, **59**, 184–186.

Stokes, E. J., Waterworth, P. M., Watson, B. & Clark, C. G. (1974) Short-term routine antibiotic prophylaxis in surgery. *Brit. J. Surg.*, **61**, 739–742.

Strauss, A. A., Strauss, S. F., Crawford, R. A. & Strauss, H. A. (1935) Surgical diathermy of carcinoma of rectum: its clinical end results. *J. Amer. med. Ass.*, **104**, 1480–1484.

Strauss, A. A., Appel, M., Saphir, O. & Rabinovitz, A. J. (1965) Immunologic resistance to carcinoma introduced by electrocoagulation. *Surg. Gynec. Obstet.*, **121**, 989–996.

Swenson, O. (1958) In *Paediatric Surgery*. New York: Appleton, Century, Crofts.

Turnbull, R. P. Jr (1974) Personal communication.

Vandertoll, D. J. & Beahrs, O. H. (1965) Carcinoma of rectum and low sigmoid. Evaulation of anterior resection of 1766 favourable lesions. *Arch. Surg.* **90**, 793–798.

Walker, R. M. (1971) Annual Report of South-Western Regional Cancer Bureau. UTF House, King Square, Bristol BS2 8HY.

Walton, P. & Mallik, M. K. (1974) Management of the perineal wound after excision of the rectum. *J. roy. Coll. Surg., Edinb.*, **19**, 251–254.

Wangensteen, O. (1945) Primary resection (closed anastomosis) of rectal ampulla for malignancy with preservation of sphincter function together with further account of primary resection of colon and rectosigmoid and note on excision. *Surg. Gynec. Obstet.*, **81**, 1–24.

Washington, J. A., Dearing, W. H., Judd, E. S. & Elveback, L. R. (1974) Effect of preoperative antibiotic regimen on development of infection after intestinal surgery: prospective, randomised, double-blind study. *Ann. Surg.*, **180**, 567–571.

Waugh, J. M., Block, M. A. & Gage, R. P. (1955) Three- and five-year survivals following combined abdominoperineal resection, abdominoperineal resection with sphincter preservation, and anterior resection for carcinoma of the rectum and lower part of the sigmoid colon. *Ann. Surg.*, **142**, 752–757.

Waugh, J. M. & Turner, J. C. Jr (1958) Abdominoperineal resection with preservation of the anal sphincter for carcinoma of the midrectum. *Surg. Gynec. Obstet.*, **107**, 777–783.

Wenckert, A. (1970) Endorectal (pull-through) resection for tumours of the rectum. *Acta chir. scand.*, **136**, 337–339.

Westhues, H. (1934) *Die pathologisch-anatomischen Grundlagen der Chirurgie des Rektumkarzinoms*. Leipzig: Thieme.

Whitaker, M. & Goligher, J. C. (1975) The early and late results of surgical treatment for carcinoma of the rectum (awaiting publication).

Yale, C. E. & Peet, W. J. (1971) Antibiotics in colon surgery. *Amer. J. Surg.*, **122**, 787–791.

York-Mason, A. (1975) Personal communication.

York-Mason, A. (1972) Transsphincteric exposure of the rectum. *Ann. roy. Coll. Surg. Engl.*, **51**, 320–331.

2
COLONOSCOPY AND COLONOSCOPIC POLYPECTOMY

Christopher B. Williams

At the present time, 10 years after the 'fibreoptic revolution' of the mid 1960s, colonoscopy is beginning to emerge from its position as the Cinderella of fibrendoscopic techniques. At first sight this is surprising because of the expense and relatively short life-span of the equipment, the difficulty of the examination, and the equal difficulty in most centres of persuading any established physician or surgeon to commit himself to regular colonoscopy. However, an increasing stream of review articles, clinical reports and presentations on the topic of colonoscopy (Wolff et al, 1972; Williams and Teague, 1973; Sivak, Sullivan and Rankin, 1974; Overholt, 1975) stress its rewards and in the earlier diagnosis and more correct management of colonic disease. Hospitals and clinics of any size are being forced, however unwillingly, to face the problems of introducing a colonoscopy service. The purpose of this chapter is to cover some of the practical problems of colonoscopy and to summarise broadly the conclusions reached by pioneer colonoscopists around the world, with particular emphasis on those aspects which must concern practising surgeons. Even for those who do not intend to be directly involved with colonoscopy or rarely look after patients with colonic disease it is important to be aware of the strengths and weaknesses of the technique. For the past 60 years since the barium enema was introduced there has been no practical diagnostic method in the colon after x-ray and before the surgeon's knife. All this has changed, as the following pages should show.

Equipment

The fibreoptic colonoscope is essentially the same instrument as the fibregastroscope, but slightly strengthened to stand up to the twisting stresses involved in manoeuvring the instrument round the colon. As techniques of colonoscopy evolve, the trend has been towards slightly stiffer instruments than the early models, which tended to curl up in the loops of bowel. All the major manufacturers of fibreoptic endoscopes (ACMI, Machida, Olympus) produce several models of colonoscope and since further variants are constantly being developed, it would be unrewarding to catalogue present models. All colonoscopes have air insufflation, lens washing, suction and biopsy facilities and four-way tip-angling controls. The main difference between them is the length of the instrument, either 110 cm or 165 to 185 cm, and known colloquially as 'medium' and 'long' colonoscopes respectively. The short colonoscopes (or fibresigmoidoscopes) which were originally introduced are little used at the time of writing, but it seems that as experience in handling fibrescopes becomes more widespread there may be a place for a short robust colonoscope to be used in the clinic for routine examinations. The medium colonoscope will reach at least to the splenic flexure or transverse colon and with skill it can often be made to reach to the caecum or terminal ileum (Gaisford, 1975). The long colonoscope is designed to reach the right colon but, because of its length, is more liable to both optical and mechanical damage. The commonest source of instrument failure and repair bills in colonoscopy is due to stretching or breaking of the angling wires but later models of colonoscope are significantly stronger. Like an automobile a colonoscope can be stripped down for repair and its components replaced for an indefinite period so that its 'life-span' will depend on how much money is spent on it. Similarly the way in which it is handled and the extent of examinations will greatly affect its durability; a medium colonoscope which is carefully handled by an experienced endoscopist for mainly limited examinations might perform over 500 colonoscopies without major repairs, whilst an instrument (medium or long) less skilfully handled or expected routinely to reach the caecum may require major expenditure after about 100 to 150 examinations.

In choosing an instrument of one make or another attention must be paid to the endoscopist's previous experience and to other instruments and light sources already in use. A very important factor is the relative attentiveness of the different companies' local agents with regard to repairs or loan-instruments. To set up a regular colonoscopy service it is almost mandatory to have more than one colonoscope. This is partly so that a back-up instrument is on the spot, which allows one that is damaged to be returned for early repair rather than to be used to destruction, and partly so that wherever possible a medium instrument is used rather than the more fragile long colonoscope. All but the fortunate few must choose one instrument first and it is difficult to give good advice about this. It is probably best to start with a medium colonoscope, provided that a long one can be purchased soon after. If a limited service has to be provided with one colonoscope a surgically orientated endoscopist will get better value from the medium instrument but the physician, due to his interest in the right colon and terminal ileum, should have the long instrument.

A further choice is required with the recently introduced two-channel 'operating' colonoscopes, which are designed for polypectomy and have a second channel which allows a polyp-grasping forceps and snare to be used simultaneously. The large additional channel is very convenient for suction and in most patients the increased diameter of the shaft of the instrument presents no problem and makes the instruments stronger. For children, or for frail or ill patients where a limited and gentle examination is required the single-channel instrument is still preferable and my own bias would be to have a medium length single-channel colonoscope and a 'long' two-channel colonoscope.

A range of invaluable accessories is produced by each company from biopsy forceps and cytology brushes to snares and grasping forceps. These accessories are usable with different makes of colonoscope and it is wise to take advice on the best individual accessories to use rather than to be bound

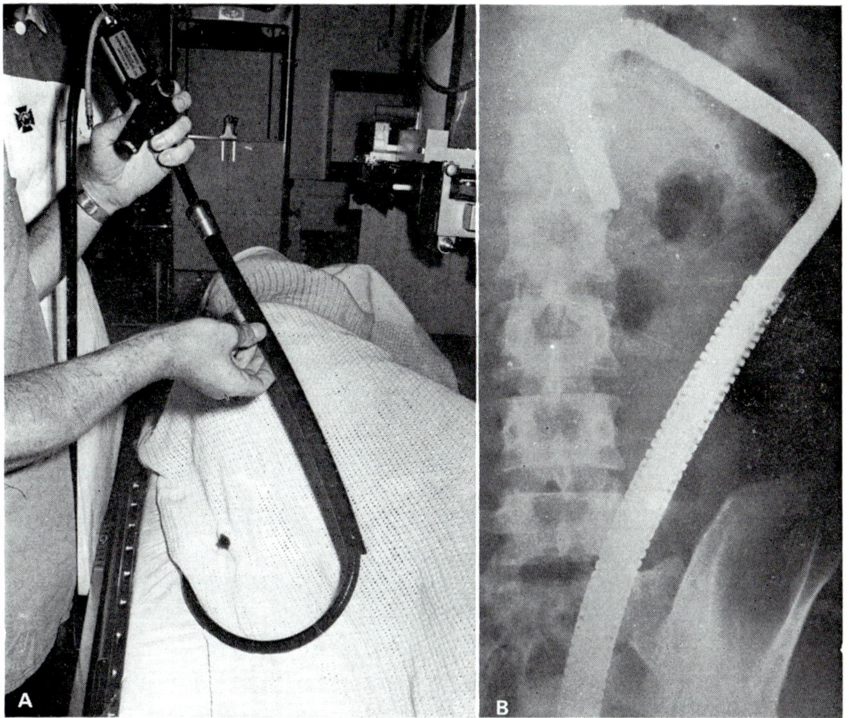

Figure 2.1   The stiffening tube, *A*, in position on the shaft of the colonoscope, *B*, inserted to the descending colon

by mistaken 'brand loyalty'. It is also economical to buy long rather than medium length accessories so that they can be used with either type of instrument. One frequently misunderstood but essential accessory for the colonoscopist is the stiffening or 'over'-tube (Fig. 2.1). This is a flexible sigmoidoscope which is passed over the colonoscope *before* starting and kept out of the way on the upper part of the shaft. It is only passed in over the colonoscope once the tip has already reached the upper descending colon and when, after straightening the colonoscope, a sigmoid loop tends to reform. The tube is thus used to stiffen an already straight colonoscope and is *not* used to straighten it. In colonoscopes with a large suction channel a stiffenable internal wire can be used. This is less effective in the sigmoid colon than the over-tube but is occasionally useful in the transverse colon.

Since colonoscopy is time consuming and frequently requires the help of an assistant in manipulating the instrument or its accessories a side-viewing attachment or 'teaching aid' is an advantage and should almost be counted as an 'essential'. With the long colonoscope the extra light required to view with the teaching aid may require the use of a high powered and more expensive light source. The introduction of polaroid photography will also necessitate extra light but will provide an invaluable objective record for the case notes. Good colonoscopy cannot be cheaply bought.

Organisation

The majority of colonoscopies can be performed on an outpatient or 'day-case' basis, with the patient taking the bowel preparation at home beforehand. Only old or ill patients need to be in hospital for preparation but if heavy sedation is used or if polypectomy has been performed the patient is kept in hospital overnight afterwards. Colonoscopy can therefore be very satisfactorily arranged in conjunction with a day-ward, a 'minor-ops' theatre or an existing gastroscopy list. It is cumbersome to include colonoscopies on a routine operating list and usually unnecessary to involve an anaesthetist in the procedure. Although not absolutely essential for colonoscopy, fluoroscopy with television image intensification greatly helps the procedure and speeds up the learning process. A mobile intensifier is suitable or a routine x-ray room can be used if one is available.

Colonoscopy as well as being a slow and difficult procedure involves a considerable entanglement of expensive tubes, wires and accessories, particularly during polypectomy with its additional equipment and added risks (Fig. 2.2). A would-be endoscopist needs mechanical aptitude as well as manual dexterity to cope with all this successfully. He also needs assistance by nursing and technical staff who are familiar with the equipment and know how to maintain and clean it. By training one or two assistants who are regularly available for the endoscopic sessions, repair bills are kept down and the whole procedure made easier and safer. Normally one nurse should supervise the patient and another look after the instrument and the endoscopist.

Bowel Preparation

The key to pleasant and successful colonoscopic examination lies in achieving a clean bowel beforehand. Since the normal bowel habit varies so much from patient to patient it is best to discuss the preparation with the individual patient beforehand. If the previous barium enema shows faecal residue or if the patient is constipated extra preparation will be necessary. As this is to be self-inflicted the patient needs to realise that without good preparation the examination will be impossible or inaccurate. The few minutes needed to explain the rationale of bowel preparation to the patient personally is time well spent.

The most widely used preparation regime starts with a day or two of diet excluding meat, vegetables and fruit and then 24 to 48 h of clear fluids before the examination. It is a solace to some patients to have it pointed out that nearly all alcoholic drinks are 'clear fluids'. A single 30 to 50 ml dose of castor

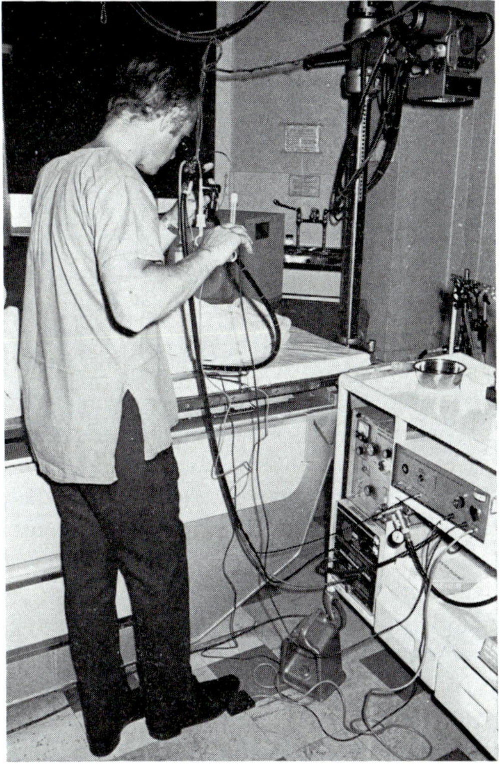

Figure 2.2   Colonoscopic polypectomy in progress

oil, mixed with fresh orange juice or beaten up quickly in an effervescent drink, is taken 12 to 18 h before the procedure followed by two large tap-water enemas 1 to 2 h beforehand. Adding a purgative agent such as oxyphen-isatin (Veripaque) or bisacodyl (Dulcolax) to the enema makes it more effective. Constipated patients need pretreatment, and patients with fluid diarrhoea or colitis may need no purgation at all.

Medication and Sedation

Most people favour the use of sedation during colonoscopy because, although some patients tolerate the procedure easily, others will find it unpleasant and painful. Only children or very nervous patients require premedication. For a limited colonoscopy it may be best to start with no sedation but for extensive examination a combination of intravenous diazepam (Valium) 5 to 20 mg and pethidine (Demerol, Dolantin) 25 to 75 mg produces satisfactory analgesia and amnesia for the 30 to 40 min needed to complete the examination. It is extremely important for the endoscopist to pay attention to any pain being experienced because this is his only warning of excessive stress on the bowel wall or the attachments of the colon. Antispasmodic agents are thought to be counter-productive during the insertion of the colonoscope because of the increased redundancy of the bowel, but they are useful if circular muscle spasm is interfering with examination during withdrawal.

Selection of Patients for Colonoscopy

If fibreoptic colonoscopy was easy it would be the obvious first-line screening procedure for colonic disease, as rigid proctosigmoidoscopy is in the anorectal region. Unfortunately, colonoscopy has its own problems, limitations and complications and at present it is regarded as a second-line procedure comparable to arteriography—though with broader applications. Colonoscopy is particularly indicated in any situation where radiography has given insufficient information or doubtful results, where there are unexplained colonic symptoms or signs or where tissue diagnosis is required. Some details of the clinical yield from diagnostic colonoscopy and polypectomy are given later in the chapter and provide an idea of some of the possible indications for the technique.

Absolute contraindications to colonoscopy are few and dictated by common sense. Colonoscopy is considerably less traumatic than surgery and there is no contraindication to examining any patient, however ill, who is otherwise likely to undergo operation but might avoid it through colonoscopy. Obviously the risks of the procedure are increased in a severely ill patient, if there has been recent myocardial infarction or if the patient is pregnant. In acute severe colitis from any cause, such as inflammatory or ischaemic disease, the risk of bowel perforation will be high and colonoscopy rarely justified. The instruments can only be sterilised with ethylene oxide, although glutaraldehyde (Cidex) is reasonably effective (Axon et al, 1974) and therefore patients with bacterial or parasitic diseases of the colon should not be examined if this can be avoided.

Examination Technique and Principles

The first essential is to be familiar with the handling of fibrendoscopes and to be sympathetic rather than aggressive to them. It is for this reason a definite advantage to have performed routine gastroscopies before starting colonoscopy. Colonoscopy technique can be considered at two levels: firstly the art of inserting the instrument through any length of convoluted bowel and secondly the anatomical manipulations of the colon required to reach the caecum, e.g. the 'alpha-manoeuvre' in the sigmoid colon.

The colon is an elastic tube which can be stretched and contorted by attempts at forceful endoscopy, but can also be shortened over the instrument like a collapsed balloon. Insertion along a length of bowel depends on small

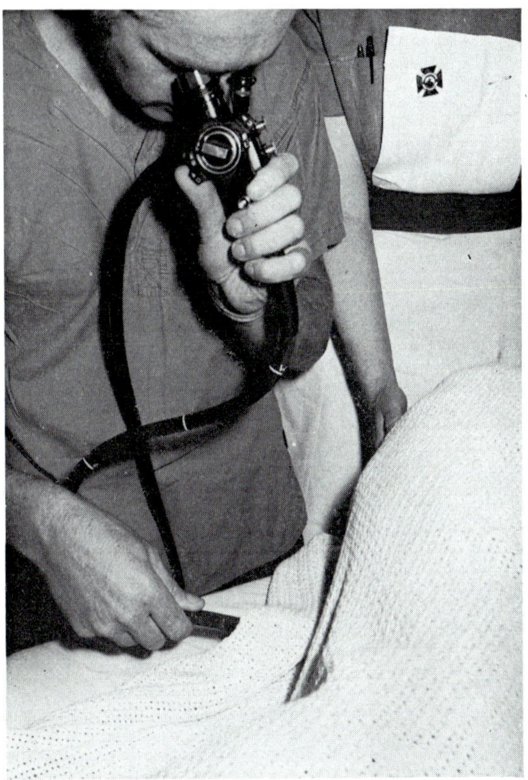

Figure 2.3   'Single-handed' manipulation of the colonoscope without an assistant

gentle movements around each successive bend, avoiding excessive air insufflation and keeping as good a view of the lumen as is possible without excessive angulation of the instrument tip. Each colonoscopy consists of passing a succession of bends in one direction or the other, and it is often difficult to see which direction is the right one. The natural tendency is to use force and to push blindly; occasionally this works, but usually it is the wrong thing to do and rarely can lead to bowel perforation. The most important manoeuvre in colonoscopy is to *pull back* the instrument each time the view is lost, for by this simple act the view is regained, the bowel is shortened and straightened and the way ahead is pulled into view. With a little practice manipulation of the colonoscope becomes easier if a single-handed 'corkscrew' technique is used, the endoscopist using his left hand to hold and move the up-down angling control and the right hand to twist or torque the shaft of the instrument (Fig. 2.3). This single-handed technique allows subtle and rapid movements, in, out, twisting and angling in a way that is impossible

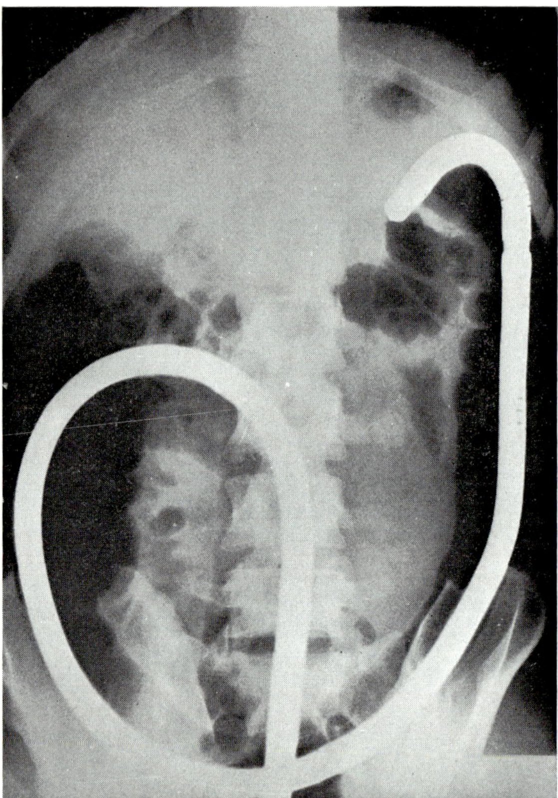

Figure 2.4   The sigmoid 'alpha loop' during colonoscopy

when trying to coordinate with an assistant. It is also particularly useful during withdrawal of the instrument to make a complete and rapid examination of every recess and bend.

Once one or more loops form in the colonoscope the resulting friction in the control wires and difficulty in torqueing the shaft mean that the endoscopist needs both hands on the controls and the assistant must advance and withdraw the instrument. Under these circumstances subtlety is lost and the instrument and patient are put under strain, so the instrument must always be withdrawn and straightened out as soon as possible. Straightening is obviously only feasible when the tip of the instrument is high enough up the colon or around a flexure so that it can be prevented from simply slipping out again. The tip may be hooked before pulling out or the shaft twisted in whichever direction is seen to keep the tip in position during straightening—manoeuvres which are easy and logical if x-ray screening is used. Providing fluoroscopy is television intensified and used for only a second or two at a time the x-ray dosage during colonoscopy is insignificant and the gain to the patient much greater than any theoretical hazard. Glass fibres discolour as their physical structure is altered by ionising radiations but when x-ray is used as described there is no danger of this.

A formal description of the 'alpha-manoeuvre' (Fig. 2.4) and the other anatomical tricks of colonoscopy is given elsewhere (Williams and Teague, 1973) and out of place in this account. In general terms the technique of insertion of the colonoscope remains unpredictable even after experience of some hundreds of examinations, some patients being easy to examine and some very difficult or impossible, for no very obvious reason. This unpredictability is reflected in the wide range of times taken to insert the colonoscope to the caecum even after considerable practice, the times varying from 2 to 40 min or more with a mean of almost 20 min (Williams, 1975a). In most cases the whole examination should be completed within an hour. Clearly 'total colonoscopy' to the caecum is not always needed but in a normal colon it is possible in over 95 per cent of cases and, if not diseased, the ileocaecal valve can be passed in the majority of these. To the less experienced endoscopist who performs only an occasional examination colonoscopy will remain too often frustratingly difficult and the clinical results equally unimpressive. If a hospital is to get good service for its patients it must find an enthusiast who will develop and then practice the technique regularly and over a long period.

Intraoperative Colonoscopy

The colonoscope can be rapidly inserted to the caecum during laparotomy with the help of the surgeon guiding the colon over it (Espiner, Salmon and Read, 1973), but it is a counsel of despair to suggest this as more than an occasional technique. Intraoperative colonoscopy is justified if normal colonoscopy has failed, if the patient has to come to laparotomy and there is some reason to avoid prior colonoscopy, or if during laparotomy it is unexpectedly necessary to examine the proximal colon. The colonoscope can also be inserted perorally through the small intestine in patients with unexplained bleeding (Dehyle et al, 1972). In any patient where peroperative colonoscopy is being considered full bowel preparation and large volume enemas must be given, since normal surgical bowel preparation is almost always inadequate and solid faeces become impacted in the instrument tip and halt the procedure. The ileum should be clamped in order to stop overinflation of the small intestine by the endoscopist. If the small intestine is to be examined (per-orally or per-rectum) air insufflation should be used only during withdrawal of the instrument and kept to a minimum, otherwise the intestine becomes unmanageably distended.

Polypectomy

Colonoscopic polypectomy is now a most important activity for the colonoscopist, since by this means almost all colon polyps can be removed without the need for surgery (Wolff and Shinya, 1975; Williams et al, 1974; Williams, 1975b). The technique presents few problems for anyone with experience of the colonoscope but it takes confidence to snare and electro-coagulate a large polyp endoscopically, often with an inadequate view. Although the snaring technique is essentially the same as used with the rigid proctosigmoidoscope it is easier for the colonoscopist to learn snare technique than for every colorectal surgeon to master colonoscopy.

The equipment used is simple, comprising an electrosurgical source, polypectomy snares and retrieval forceps and a source of carbon dioxide. The hazards of bleeding and bowel perforation during polypectomy are reduced by having a purpose-built electrosurgical source for fibrendoscopic use which will have a lower power range than those designed for urological or surgical purposes. Suitable sources are available from ACMI, Cameron-Miller, Machida, Martin (Elmed), Olympus and Valley-Lab, some producing a preblended current and others having separate cutting and coagulating circuits which can be blended by the operator. It is possible to snare polyps with a simple wire loop passed down the Teflon tube (Shinya snare) but the commercially available snares are more convenient and probably safer, since the position of the handle shows exactly how far the snare loop is closed. The different snares have different shaped loops and wire characteristics which suit them for different polyps, small and large, stalked or sessile, and it is useful to have a choice. Ideally for polypectomy one should use a two-channel 'operating' colonoscope so that an insulated retrieval forceps or grasper can hold the polyp head before it is severed, which saves the tedium of hunting for it afterwards.

There is dispute as to whether insufflation of carbon dioxide or other inert gas is necessary during colonic polypectomy. The methane produced by colonic bacteria should be removed during bowel preparation and the clean bowel has been shown to be safe (Ragins, Shinya and Wolff, 1974; Bond and Levitt, 1975); there have however been fatal explosions during rigid procotosigmoidoscopy and clandestine reports of catastrophe during colonoscopic polypectomy in the under-prepared bowel. Most endoscopists therefore favour the use of carbon dioxide, using either laparoscopy apparatus (Wisap) or an electrosurgical source (ACMI) with suitable gas flow and pressure characteristics.

Polypectomy technique in the colon is indicated by the need to ensure complete coagulation of the stalk vessels, since bleeding is difficult or impossible to control with the colonoscope due to its limited irrigation and suction facilities. Having closed the snare loop gently midway between the head of the polyp and the bowel wall there is a choice of two possible snare techniques. One is to apply a medium–high setting of the source (approximately that which would light a 40 W bulb) and pull the snare loop through the stalk in one movement. The other technique is slower but probably safer and involves closing the snare loop tightly and then giving 2 to 4 short bursts

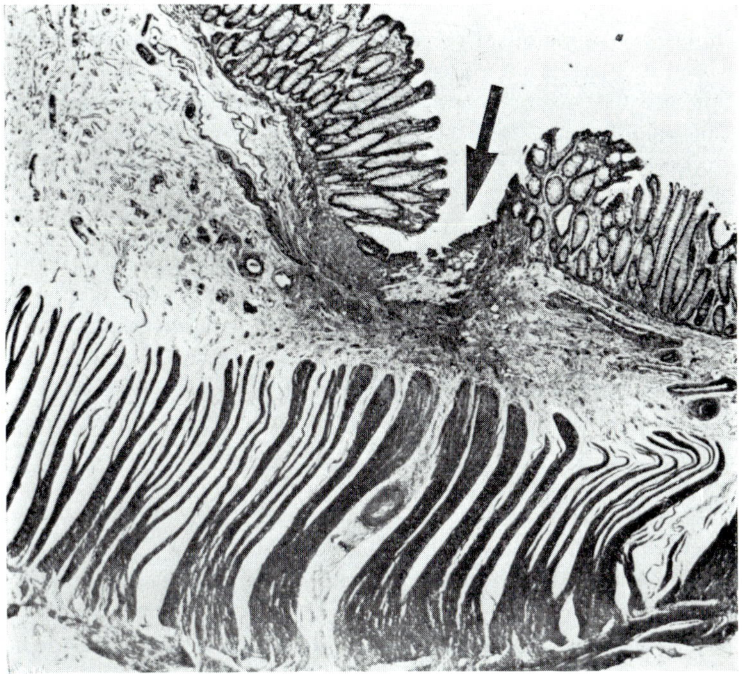

Figure 2.5   Photomicrograph showing the limited zone of ulceration and heat necrosis in the submucosa following colonoscopic polypectomy

of current, starting at a low power setting and working up so that there is visible coagulation of the stalk *before* the loop is pulled through or a higher current is applied to achieve cutting. The latter technique gives more time to check progress and also to stop if coagulation does not occur—which indicates that there is a problem, such as faulty snaring or circuitry. None the less polypectomy should not take more than 15 to 20 seconds of current application so as to avoid the risk of widespread tissue heating and bowel perforation (Fig. 2.5). A more detailed account of the principles and practice of polypectomy technique is given elsewhere (Williams et al, 1974) but four polyp problems which face the endoscopist deserve discussion—large polyps, small polyps, multiple polyps and malignant polyps.

Large polyps usually present little problem, for above the rectum most large polyps are pedunculated and it is unusual for the stalk to be more than 1.5 cm diameter. The size of the polyp head itself is relatively unimportant in snaring, although a larger head tends to require larger feeding vessels in the stalk. If the head diameter exceeds about 4 cm it may be difficult to pass an ordinary snare over it and the Shinya loop is useful for this purpose; if this is not available the polyp can be removed in several bits. If the polyp is large and the stalk is greater than 1 to 1.5 cm diameter there is a high probability of haemorrhage during even careful coagulation and transection and blood should be available before polypectomy. If a two-channel colonoscope is being used it is possible to have two snare loops in position, the upper one transecting and the lower available as a tourniquet if necessary. In our series of over 700 polypectomies only about one in a hundred polyps seen above the rectum has been broad based or sessile, if obviously malignant polyps and polypoid cancers are excluded. These broad based polyps over 2.5 cm or so in diameter should not usually be snared in one session; one or more large bits should be removed on the first occasion for histological examination and if the histology is benign the base area resnared several days later to reduce the danger of full thickness heat damage. On the second occasion it should be clear whether it is going to be possible to remove all tissue, and if this seems unlikely the patient is probably best referred for surgery since on top of the risks of snaring must be added the risk of subsequent malignancy in any residual tissue.

Solitary very small polyps are not infrequently seen in the colon and biopsies show that above the rectosigmoid region at least 70 per cent of these are adenomatous and merit destruction. This is not to say that every patient with a 5 to 6 mm 'ring-shadow' on barium enema needs colonoscopy and polypectomy for not infrequently the appearance is artefactual due to an air bubble or faecal blob; the x-ray should be repeated before considering colonoscopy. It is much more difficult to be sure on colonoscopy that the colon is normal and that such a small polyp has not been missed behind a fold or bend. Due to divergence of the x-ray beam the radiological measurement of a polyp overestimates its real size by at least 10 to 15 per cent, and more in some oblique and lateral views (Fig. 2.6). Colonoscopy is therefore probably not justified for a polyp less than about 7 to 8 mm in diameter on x-ray, which cannot cause symptoms and has almost no risk of malignancy; the barium enema should be repeated after a year or so and if the polyp is confirmed the decision for or against colonoscopy will depend on the age and clinical assessment of the patient, the site of the polyp, and on the availability of colonoscopy. A middle-aged patient with a family history of cancer and a 7 mm sigmoid polyp justifies polypectomy whereas an 80 year old with a similar shadow in the transverse colon probably does not.

If a polyp of this size, or even of 2 to 3 mm diameter, is seen *during* colonoscopy perhaps in a patient with another larger polyp, it does of course merit attention. Snaring is inconvenient and usually loses the tiny specimen and local diathermy destroys the evidence. A practical solution is to 'hot-biopsy' polyps up to 6 to 7 mm diameter, passing the electrosurgical current down insulated biopsy forceps. This destroys the base of the polyp but obtains a perfect biopsy (Williams, 1973, 1975c). Suitable insulated forceps are now coming on to the market.

Multiple polyps are another problem in polypectomy. Multiple small polyps can be dealt with by 'hot-biopsies' but if 20 or more small polyps are seen

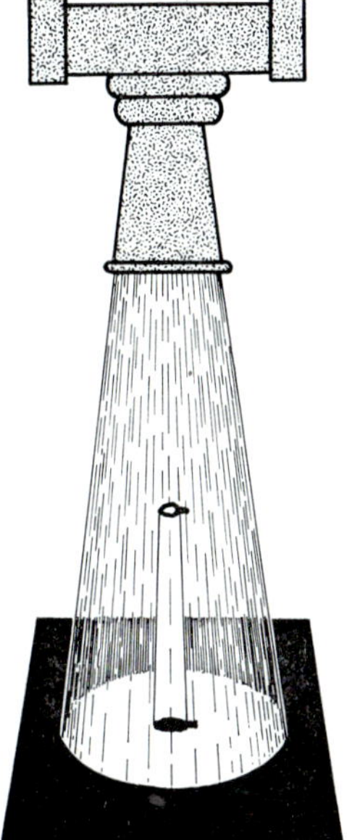

Figure 2.6   X-ray magnification of a polyp

the possibility that the patient has adenomatous polyposis coli should be considered. The tendency is inevitably to underestimate the number of small polyps present, particularly the smallest ones, which may be transparent and seen only in reflected highlights. To exclude polyposis in these patients one should therefore scrutinise the apparently *normal* areas of mucosa between the obviously visible polyps. If 40 to 50 polyps are seen, and biopsies of a representative number show them to be adenomatous, the patient has polyposis coli because at least an equal number will be found to have been missed on the formalin-fixed operation specimen. Biopsies are essential because there are rare patients with multiple metaplastic polyposis who have no cancer risk and do not require surgery. The multiple small, shiny, inflammatory or 'pseudo' polyps seen in patients with previous severe ulcerative or Crohn's colitis have no significance and can normally be distinguished visually from adenomatous polyps, representative biopsies showing normal mucosa. In ulcerative colitis there may be larger, soft, slough-covered inflammatory polyps composed of granulation tissue and because of their falsely frightening appearance radiologically and endoscopically (Fig. 2.7) these are best snared off.

Fortunately very few patients have more than one or two large adenomatous polyps so that the problem of retrieval of multiple snared polyps is uncommon. There is no easy solution. With a double channel instrument at least

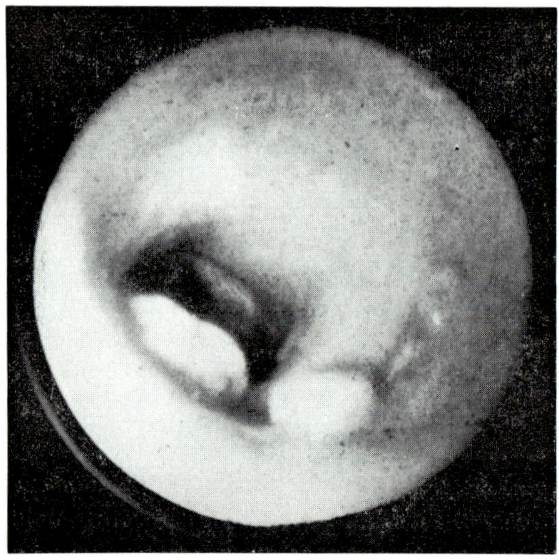

Figure 2.7   Large inflammatory polyps in ulcerative colitis

two polyps can be snared and retrieved at a time and several journeys must be made. If the colonoscopy has been excessively difficult or if polyps are lost after snaring then the largest polyps should be retrieved and the others washed out as soon as possible with a saline enema. It is so important to identify and localise any malignant polyp that normally the wash-out technique should be avoided.

A malignant polyp is one that has adenocarcinoma invading through the muscularis mucosae of the head of the polyp. 'Focal carcinoma' or 'carcinoma in situ' on the surface of a polyp cannot reach the lymphatics of the polyp stalk which extend only to the muscularis mucosae, and therefore these conditions cannot metastasise and clinically are not malignant (Fenoglio, Raye and Lane, 1973; Morson and Bussey, 1970). To diagnose or exclude invasive malignancy the pathologist must make multiple sections which must be in the correct plane so that any spread down the stalk is identified. It has been shown in the rectum (Carden and Morson, 1964) that unless the invasive carcinoma is of high grade malignancy (anaplastic) even spread into the upper part of the stalk is unlikely to be associated with local spread or metastasis providing that there is no cancer close to the point of section (Fig. 2.8).

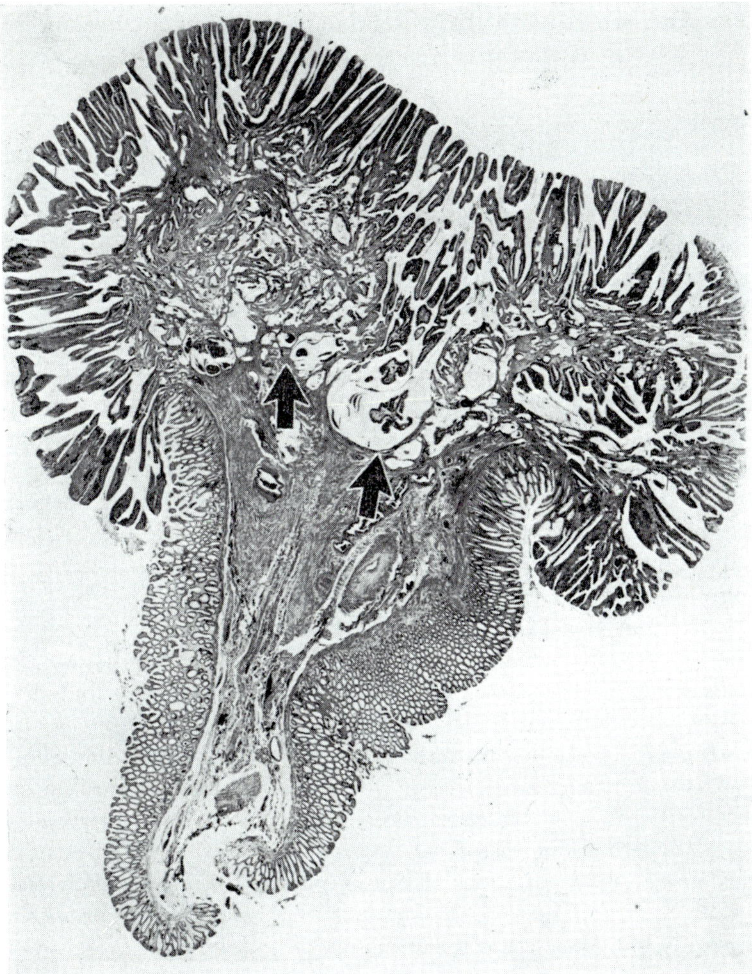

Figure 2.8   Photomicrograph showing carcinomatous tissue (arrowed) invading the upper stalk of an endoscopically removed polyp

Surgical intervention and resection of the local colon carries at least a 5 per cent mortality rate even in specialised centres so that the risks of advising surgery must be assessed in a patient with limited invasion of a polyp by carcinoma of low or average grade. In such a patient the risk of metastasis is small and the chance of resectable local spread even smaller. In the average elderly patient with moderately well-differentiated carcinoma invading only to the upper part of the stalk we do not recommend surgery.

The Clinical Yield from Diagnostic Colonoscopy

Colonoscopy proves particularly useful in a number of circumstances which will be considered separately.

Possible cancer on x-ray—strictures, diverticular disease, etc.
When x-ray shows stricturing, perhaps as a sequel to ulcerative colitis, or when there is severe diverticular disease with irregular narrowing, the radiologist cannot exclude malignancy and the patient is likely to be submitted to surgery. The colonoscope will not always pass through a stricture and unless it does so the endoscopist cannot give a useful opinion (Hunt et al, 1975). Diverticular disease causes particular difficulty because of pericolic adhesions, fixation of the bowel and the narrow tortuous lumen in which it is not easy to pick the right path. In these circumstances the endoscopist may overstress the angling mechanisms of the instrument and break it, but with patience it is possible to get through the abnormal area in two-thirds of patients with severe diverticular disease and to achieve an adequate examination. In the presence of diverticular disease even a good radiologist can miss polyps of any size. Severe diverticular disease is therefore difficult to examine colono-scopically, but highly rewarding when it is possible, both because of the pathology found and because the alternative procedure would be resection. Bleeding from an area of diverticular disease stems most commonly from a polyp or cancer, occasionally from localised mucosal inflammatory changes apparently related to the region of circular muscle hypertrophy, and only very rarely from a diverticulum itself.

The strictures of chronic ulcerative colitis are most commonly shown by x-rays as a smooth narrowing due to muscular hypertrophy, and on colono-scopy few of them show evidence of malignancy. They tend to occur in just those patients with a long history of extensive colitis where the fear of cancer is greatest and there has previously been a tendency to consider such strictures as an indication for surgery. Sometimes the radiological abnormality is exaggerated by the presence of inflammatory polyps, small or large, which are almost invariably benign but constitute a further 'red herring' which falsely persuades the surgeon that colectomy is indicated. Colonoscopy with poly-pectomy or multiple biopsies is an effective substitute for surgery in most of these cases and should pick out the few patients that are at risk for cancer (see inflammatory bowel disease).

Deformity of the caecum may either be due to spasm, poor bowel prepara-tion, cancer or inflammatory bowel disease. Unfortunately the caecum is difficult to prepare and may be difficult to demonstrate properly by x-rays although using antispasmodics intravenously (Buscopan) should allow diagnostic pictures to be obtained on a second examination. If there is still doubt the colonoscope can usually reach the caecum and get an adequate view. For the endoscopist also the caecum can be a difficult area to see fully; the appendix orifice and ileocaecal valve should be identified to prove the location of the instrument and a voluminous caecum must be painstakingly examined to see all parts of it. At least the endoscopist's colour vision can easily and accurately discriminate between faecal residue and cancer tissue! Not all patients with radiologically demonstrated colon cancer need colonoscopy, but if there is any doubt the area can be checked on the day before operation during the normal period of bowel preparation or possibly during the operation. In most patients an adequate view of colon proximal to a cancer can be obtained on barium enema, but if the x-ray is unsuccessful or any polyps are seen it may be wise to perform colonoscopy to be sure that there is no synchronous carcinoma.

Postoperative colonoscopy and 'ostomies'

During radiography following resection for carcinoma it can be impossible to be sure of the significance of irregularity or narrowing of the anastomosis. Endoscopically it is usually easy to discriminate between recurrent cancer, spasm and stitch-granulation tissue. Brushing or washing cytology specimens can be taken as well as biopsies to provide objective proof, which is important since in some cases the profusion of friable granulation tissue may simulate malignancy even to the endoscopist. Usually suture material can be seen and the extremely soft tissue suggests the true diagnosis.

The colon of patients with a colostomy is often difficult to prepare and to x-ray adequately and the faecal residue in the proximal bowel makes interpretation of the films impossible. Providing the stoma will admit the little finger it will take a colonoscope. Inserting the instrument for the first few centimetres through a stoma can be tedious and this part may be poorly seen but, since there is no sigmoid colon to negotiate, colonoscopy is usually easy and well tolerated. Ileostomies may be more difficult to examine for more than a few centimetres but useful information and biopsies can be obtained within either a conventional or 'continent' ileostomy that is malfunctioning or bleeding. Possibly because of the 'colonisation' that occurs in the ileum above an ileorectal anastomosis the instrument can often be passed 100 cm or more above the anastomosis, and since it is difficult to get satisfactory x-ray pictures of minor mucosal changes in this area, colonoscopy may be useful in picking up the ulcers of recurrent Crohn's disease or in excluding recurrence.

Normal barium enema but persistent bleeding or symptoms

Before colonoscopy every patient should have had full clinical assessment including conventional proctosigmoidoscopy and barium enema. There has been up till the present no way of checking on barium enema findings—

except by repeating the barium enema. Colonoscopy shows that the radiologist can miss cancer, polyps, Crohn's disease and colitis—and it is important too know which patients with a normal barium enema merit colonoscopy and which do not.

If a patient has no demonstrable haemorrhoids and passes altered blood per rectum, or if no cause can be found in the upper tract for persistent gastrointestinal blood loss, colonoscopy is indicated. About 10 per cent of these patients are found to have a missed carcinoma, usually in the sigmoid colon but occasionally in the caecum, and another 20 per cent have polyps, inflammatory bowel disease or a rarity such as haemangioma. This is an impressive pick-up rate, but 70 per cent of the group will undergo extensive colonoscopy with negative findings. True black melaena with no history of passage of blood is probably not an indication for colonoscopy. Fresh red blood, primarily on the toilet paper, is an indication for repeat proctoscopy in the first instance.

In a patient with a normal air contrast barium enema, abdominal pain alone or associated with a minor alteration of bowel habit or with mucus production indicates only a functional bowel disorder or 'irritable colon' and colonoscopy invariably also reveals morphologically normal colon. In many patients with an irritable colon the endoscopist will either see unusually frequent contractions or marked circular muscle spasms and these should be reported as possible evidence of functional disorder. Other patients are hypersensitive, especially to air insufflation, and may say that the pain they experience is identical to their normal symptoms. However, some patients with clinically undoubted functional disorder appear in all respects normal endoscopically.

Profuse diarrhoea or diarrhoea with abdominal pain may, even with a normal barium enema, be due to ulcerative or Crohn's colitis, but it is very unusual not to have some hint of this diagnosis on other investigations such as rectal biopsy or a raised sedimentation rate. No one would suggest routine colonoscopy in all patients with symptoms of functional bowel disorder, but colonoscopy has an occasional place as the final arbiter or to give a particularly anxious patient a chance to see the overactivity and normality of his own colon down the 'teaching' side-arm of the endoscope.

Selected patients with inflammatory bowel disease
Usually the well-tried combination of clinical history and examination, rectal biopsy and radiography, gives an accurate enough assessment of inflammatory bowel disease for clinical management, but in some circumstances colonoscopy can be highly useful. For the initial diagnosis of inflammatory bowel disease colonoscopy is useful, mainly in Crohn's disease where there may be rectal sparing or involvement of the proximal bowel or terminal ileum alone. In many of these patients even a normal looking rectum will show suggestive or diagnostic histological appearances on biopsy, but if the

x-ray pictures and the histology are equivocal it is preferable to proceed to colonoscopy rather than to make a wrong diagnosis of Crohn's disease in a patient with functional bowel disorder. The converse situation of the rare patient presenting with normal x-ray pictures and diarrhoea due to extensive very mild ulcerative or Crohn's colitis has been mentioned above.

The *differential diagnosis* between Crohn's and ulcerative colitis has long been a problem, and though colonoscopy has a great contribution to make it does not always succeed in making the distinction—there are cases where even the whole excised colon specimen does not enable the pathologist to be sure. The endoscopic appearance is the best discriminant, Crohn's disease showing a characteristic patchy distribution in the colon with apthoid or linear ulcers separated by areas of normal mucosa, whereas ulcerative colitis presents a uniform change. The small forceps biopsies obtained are sometimes inadequate and it is best to give the pathologist six to eight biopsies from the same area including apparently ulcerated and normal parts, and the 'patchiness' of the histological changes will suggest Crohn's colitis. The large 'hot-biopsy' forceps recently introduced for small polyps can also be used for mucosal biopsy to provide a view of the submucosa without increasing the risk of haemorrhage and should be useful in improving histological results.

It is important not to forget other specific causes of inflammatory change, including irradiation (pale mucosa, marked bleeding from petechial areas), antibiotics (pscudomembranous patches of slough), tuberculosis (appearances similar to Crohn's, very localised with bacilli on biopsy or brushing) or amoebiasis (very friable and haemorrhagic, parasites on biopsy).

Colonoscopy can also be very useful in assessing the exact extent of Crohn's disease or ulcerative colitis. Crohn's disease is frequently more extensive than x-ray suggests and it may be useful to know the exact extent in deciding whether surgical excision or intensified medical treatment is indicated for an apparently localised segment of disease. In at least a quarter of cases of ulcerative colitis, radiography underestimates the extent (Dilawari et al, 1973), and in a few the whole colon may be affected by mild disease although the barium enema looks normal, so if a patient with radiologically distal disease is not improving on adequate local treatment with steroid retention enemas it may be worthwhile checking the proximal colon with colonoscopy.

Colonoscopy is also useful in the management of patients with longstanding extensive total ulcerative colitis where the cancer risk is said to be high. Some of these patients have strictures (see above) which can be biopsied, and usually prove to be benign. Others have ugly looking inflammatory polyps, also benign, and others are at risk for 'prophylactic colectomy' because of the cancer fear. Colonoscopy with multiple (12–20) biopsies throughout the colon will show whether there is any overt malignancy or, more importantly, whether there are any precancerous changes at any point (Morson and Pang, 1967; Cook and Goligher, 1975). Carcinoma in colitis often starts invisibly in the submucosa but seems always to be associated with local epithelial precancer and colonoscopy now gives the hope that the occasional patient harbouring dysplastic change can be identified at an early stage and the others with a long history of extensive colitis can be spared unnecessary mutilation.

Conclusions

Most colonic disease starts in the mucosa and the fibreoptic colonoscope gives the most accurate view of this, takes biopsies which are usually adequate for histological diagnosis and can remove most polypoid lesions (including some cancers) without the need for laparotomy. Colonoscopy represents a considerable revolution in the diagnosis and management of colon disease but the technique is unfortunately sufficiently difficult that it will remain for the present a second-line investigation for patients where barium enema and proctosigmoidoscopy do not give sufficient information, or where surgery is the alternative. Colonic surgery is a major undertaking and the effectiveness of colonoscopy as a substitute means that it is highly cost-effective in spite of its apparent expense in time and repair bills. The equipment costs may gradually fall and the techniques will doubtless be refined, but the clinical rewards are so great that colonoscopy must be made generally available now.

REFERENCES

Axon, A. T. R., Phillips, I., Cotton, P. B. & Avery, S. A. (1974) Disinfection of gastro-intestinal fibre-endoscopes. *Lancet*, **1**, 656–658.

Bond, J. H. & Levitt, M. D. (1975) Factors influencing the concentration of combustible gases in the colon during colonoscopy. *Gastroenterology*, **68**, 1445–1448.

Carden, A. B. G. & Morson, B. C. (1964) Recurrence after local excision of malignant polyps of the rectum. *Proceedings of the Royal Society of Medicine*, **57**, 559–561.

Cook, M. G. & Goligher, J. C. (1975) Carcinoma and epithelial dysplasia complicating ulcerative colitis. *Gastroenterology*, **68**, 1127–1136.

Dehyle, P., Jenny, S., Ammann, R. & Siegenthaler, W. (1972) Ileoskopie. *Deutsche medizinische Wochenschrift*, **97**, 1679–1680.

Dilawari, J. B., Parkinson, C., Riddell, R. H., Loose, H. & Williams, C. B. (1973) (Abstr.) Colonoscopy in the investigation of ulcerative colitis. Proceedings of Spring Meeting of the British Society of Gastroenterology. *Gut*, **14**, 426.

Espiner, H. J., Salmon, P. R. & Read, A. E. (1973) Operative colonoscopy. *British Medical Journal*, **1**, 453–454.

Fenoglio, C. M., Raye, G. I. & Lane, N. (1973) Distribution of human colonic lymphatics in normal, hyperplastic and adenomatous tissue. *Gastroenterology*, **64**, 51–66.

Gaisford, W. D. (1975) Fibrendoscopy of the caecum and terminal ileum. *Gastrointestinal Endoscopy*, **21**, 13–18.

Hunt, R. H., Teague, R. H., Swarbrick, E. T. & Williams, C. B. (1975) Colonoscopy in the management of colonic strictures. *British Medical Journal*, **2**, 360–361.

Morson, B. C. & Pang, L. S. C. (1967) Rectal biopsy as an aid to cancer control in ulcerative colitis. *Gut*, **8**, 423.

Morson, B. C. & Bussey, H. J. R. (1970) Predisposing causes of intestinal cancer. In *Current Problems in Surgery* (February). Chicago: Year Book Medical Publishers.

Overholt, B. F. (1975) (Progress in gastroenterology). Colonoscopy: a review. *Gastroenterology*, **69**, 1308–1320.

Ragins, H., Shinya, H. & Wolff, W. I. (1974) The explosive potential of colonic gas during colonoscopic electrosurgical polypectomy. *Surgery, Gynecology and Obstetrics*, **138,** 554–556.

Sivak, M. V., Sullivan, B. H. & Rankin, G. B. (1974) Colonoscopy: a report of 644 cases and review of the literature. *American Journal of Surgery*, **128,** 351–357.

Williams, C. B. (1973) Diathermy-biopsy. A technique for the endoscopic management of small polyps. *Endoscopy*, **5,** 215–218.

Williams, C. B. & Teague, R. H. (1973) Progress report: colonoscopy. *Gut*, **14,** 990–1503.

Williams, C. B., Hunt, R. H., Loose, H., Riddell, R. H., Sakai, Y. & Swarbrick, E. T. (1974) Colonoscopy in the management of colon polyps. *British Journal of Surgery*, **61,** 673–682.

Williams, C. B. (1975a) Extent of ulcerative colitis. *Diseases of the Colon and Rectum*, **18,** 365–368.

Williams, C. B. (1975b) Colonoscopic polypectomy. In *Topics in Gastrointestinal Endoscopy*, ed. Salmon, P. R. and Schiller, K. E. R. London: Heinemann Medical.

Williams, C. B. (1975c) In *Surgical Endoscopy*, ed. Seifert E. Baden-Baden: G. Witzstrock.

Wolff, W. I., Shinya, H., Geffen, A. & Ozaktay, S. Z. (1972) Colonofiberoscopy. A new and valuable diagnostic modality. *American Journal of Surgery*, **123,** 180–184.

Wolff, W. I. & Shinya, H. (1975) Definitive treatment of 'malignant' polyps of the colon. *Annals of Surgery*, **182,** 516–525.

3

3
PORTAL HYPERTENSION

J. L. Dawson

The pressure in the portal venous system rises when there is an impedance to its flow through the liver. This impedance may be:

(a) extrahepatic

(b) intrahepatic

Portal hypertension is important clinically because it causes death as a result of haemorrhage from oesophageal varices.

Surgical treatment of patients with portal hypertension is fraught with difficulties and disadvantages. Operations are of two types, those that remove, occlude or thrombose the varices locally and those that attempt to lower the portal pressure. Direct operations on the varices are associated with a high incidence of further bleeding, and shunt operations hasten the onset of liver failure. Recent evidence suggests that even therapeutic shunts in cirrhotic patients do not affect the overall survival rate (Resnick et al, 1974).

Pathophysiology

The rise in portal pressure causes venous dilatation in the portal bed and the blood seeks alternative pathways back to the systemic venous system. The most important collateral channels to open up are those between the left gastric veins and the azygos system at the oesophageal diaphragmatic hiatus. The pressure gradient between the positive abdominal pressure and the negative intrathoracic pressure encourages collateral formation at this site. Dilated veins develop around and within the oesophagus. The veins in the submucosa may become hugely dilated and are seen on a barium swallow (see Fig. 3.1).

The rise in portal pressure causes splenic enlargement. In a few patients it is possible that idiopathic splenomegaly may so increase the portal blood flow that the portal radicals within the liver constitute a relative obstruction to flow and portal hypertension results (Banti's syndrome). Secondary fibrotic changes then occur in the liver around the portal branches contributing further to the obstruction of the flow.

EXTRAHEPATIC OBSTRUCTION

This condition occurs in the young and usually presents in childhood or adolescence. There is occlusion of the portal vein perhaps by a continuation of the physiological occlusion that occurs in the left umbilical vein at birth. Sometimes there is a clear history of umbilical sepsis, causing an infective thrombophlebitis which spreads into the portal vein and occludes it. A leash of collateral veins develop in the lesser omentum, endeavouring to return the portal blood to the hepatic parenchyma. This is known as portal cavernoma (Fig. 3.2). In some patients portal vein thrombosis undoubtedly follows a splenectomy for another condition, e.g. for thalassaemia.

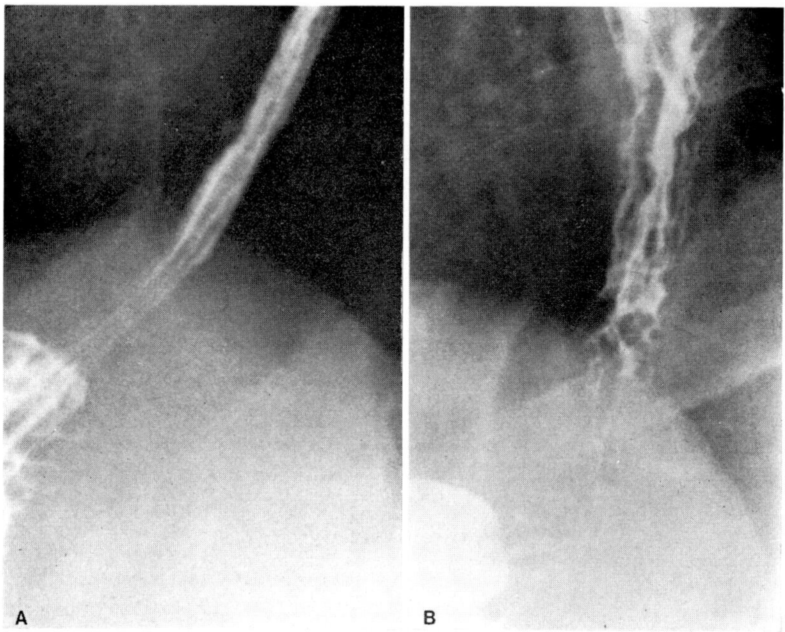

Figure 3.1   Radiograph of a standard barium swallow (A) before and (B) after the administration of Buscopan. Buscopan makes the oesophageal varices more obvious

Occasionally a secondary thrombosis develops in the portal vein in cirrhotic patients with a well-established intrahepatic obstruction. Rarely, carcinoma of the pancreas may cause thrombosis of the left gastric and splenic veins to produce varices.

INTRAHEPATIC OBSTRUCTION

The most common cause is cirrhosis of the liver, with the distorted architecture of the liver causing obstruction to the venous portal flow in the liver sinusoids. Cirrhosis itself causes a progressive decline in liver cell function, although the speed of this deterioration may vary considerably from patient to patient.

The overall picture is grim. In a series of 155 unselected patients with cirrhosis only 14.3 per cent survived five years after diagnosis (Stone, Islam

and Paton, 1968). Logistically oesophageal varices are a minor problem in
the cirrhotic population. In the above series, varices were found at autopsy
in 49 per cent and in 32.7 per cent on barium examination, but only 17 per
cent of the patients bled. Hepatoma was more common than bleeding varices
and developed in 18.4 per cent. Twenty-seven patients bled from their varices
but in 16 this was a terminal event associated with gross liver failure, and all
16 died within one month. Of the remaining 11, 5 had only mild haemorrhages and were only given supportive treatment, and of these 2 survived five

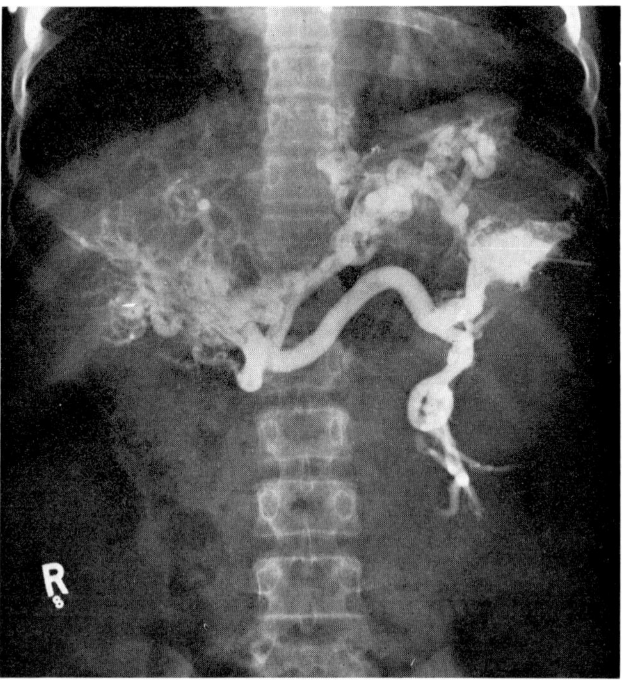

Figure 3.2   Radiograph of a splenic portogram which shows the portal vein to be obstructed
at the hilum of the liver where it is replaced by leash of collateral vessels many of which are
lying on the surface of the liver capsule

years. The remaining 6 had severe haemorrhage necessitating operation and
only 1 of these survived five years (Fig. 3.3).

Most other British series are selected, as they come from centres with a
special interest in portal hypertension, to which patients are referred from
afar. In one such report of these patients who survived a haemorrhage and
who were considered fit enough for a shunt operation, only 40 per cent
survived five years (Zeegen et al, 1973).

In schistosomiasis, portal hypertension may develop before the cirrhosis
becomes established. Occasionally obstruction of portal flow is mainly post-

sinusoidal, i.e. hepatic vein obstruction or thrombosis. This variety is usually associated with intractable ascites (Budd–Chiari syndrome). A congenital web in the suprahepatic vena cava is a rare but potentially curable cause of hepatic vein obstruction (Yamamoto et al, 1968).

Recently a group of patients has been identified in whom there is portal hypertension but no true cirrhosis (Zeegen et al, 1970). These patients did well after shunt surgery, with over three-quarters surviving for 10 years. Although there is fibrosis in the liver there is no true destruction of liver architecture and the parenchymal liver function is good. Whether the primary lesion is always hepatic, or whether in some cases it is the result of increased portal

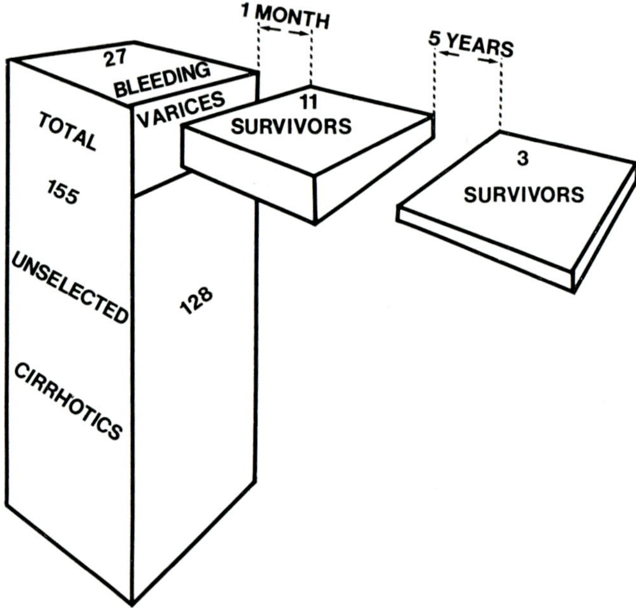

Figure 3.3   The natural history of cirrhosis in 155 unselected patients. Bleeding from oesophageal varices affected only a minority of patients (27 out of 155). In some of these it was associated with severe liver failure. Survival for five years after harmorrhage was rare despite treatment (3 out of 27 patients) (after Stone et al, 1968)

flow secondary to splenomegaly is not clear. Cirrhosis, however, is responsible for the majority of cases of intrahepatic portal hypertension and although 10 years ago the incidence of alcoholic cirrhosis was low in Britain, it is increasing and accounts for nearly 50 per cent of those admitted to hospital.

Haemodynamic changes

Three stages of haemodynamic change have been described in patients with portal hypertension.

Stage I. The portal blood flow to the liver (hepatopetal) is maintained at normal or near normal levels. There is little escape of blood through the collateral circulation.

Stage II. Portal flow to the liver is significantly reduced and the flow through the collaterals is high.

Stage III. Portal flow is zero or possibly reversed. The portal vein may therefore act as an outflow from the liver (hepatofugal flow). All of the portal circulation escapes through the collaterals in Stage III. Recently the existence of a spontaneous reversal of portal flow has been questioned (Moreno et al, 1975).

Indications for Elective Operation

Haemorrhage

Once patients bleed from oesophageal varices they usually bleed again. The risk of death during an episode of haemorrhage is considerable in cirrhotic patients, so that surgical treatment should be considered in any patient who is known to have bled from oesophageal varices. However, it is impossible to give an accurate prediction of the chance of rebleeding in any particular patient and even patients with intrahepatic obstruction may go a year or more between haemorrhages.

Hypersplenism

Although most patients with splenomegaly secondary to portal hypertension show mild to moderate pancytopenia, these haematological abnormalities are rarely symptomatic and operation is usually only considered if the patient has bled from associated varices.

Ascites

Intractable ascites is seen in the veno-occlusive disease (Budd–Chiari syndrome) and constrictive pericarditis. With modern drug therapy and a strict diet, ascites secondary to cirrhosis of the liver is rarely an indication for operation.

Portosystemic Encephalopathy (Hepatic Coma)

Neurological sequelae of experimental portosystemic operations were described by Eck in 1871. After creating portocaval shunts in the dog it was observed that meat precipitated severe neurological symptoms. These symptoms became progressively worse over several weeks and the dogs usually died within a month (Whipple, 1945; McDermott, 1972).

Similar neuropsychiatric disturbances are seen in man with severe liver disease and frequently develop after portosystemic shunt operations and are called portosystemic encephalopathy. Although the mental changes usually predominate, almost any neurological lesion, even with focal signs, may be mimicked. The changes range from minor EEG abnormalities, subtle changes of personality through to precoma and coma. The incidence of encephalopathy reported in any particular series depends very much upon the method of assessment and the criteria used in so doing.

Encephalopathy seems to be caused by at least one of three factors:

1. Diversion of portal blood from the liver.
2. Deteriorating liver cell function.
3. Haemodynamic changes precipitated by shunt operations.

Diversion of portal blood

The bacterial flora of the large intestine degrade the protein of the diet and produce substances (as yet unidentified) which pass through the liver where they are normally removed or detoxified. Although ammonia production also occurs in the large bowel as a result of the activity of urea splitting organisms it is clear that ammonia is not the only toxic substance of importance in producing encephalopathy. In portal hypertension the portal blood may circumvent the liver through the collateral veins to reach the systemic venous system and thus directly affect the brain.

As the toxic substances are produced mainly by the bacterial flora of the large intestine, clinical improvement in encephalopathic patients is achieved therefore by:

1. Decreasing the dietary protein,
2. Changing the bowel flora, and
3. Preventing absorption from the colon.

In patients with chronic encephalopathy reduction of dietary protein is the mainstay of treatment and considerably improves the patient's condition. Acute gastrointestinal haemorrhage frequently precipitates coma probably as a result of the protein load provided by the blood.

Efforts to change the bowel flora are effective clinically. Neomycin is the drug which is commonly used and even in small doses it may have a very satisfactory effect on changing the bowel flora. The disadvantage of this drug is that it allows opportunist infection by yeast and other organisms in the gut. Large doses of lactobacillus orally have also been reported as having been helpful. Lactulose is effective clinically, its action is complex and includes provision of a substrate which favours the lactobacillus, a lowering of gut pH and a purgative effect (Elkington, 1970).

Absorption of toxic substances from the colon may be reduced by purgation with magnesium sulphate and this is used routinely in patients with acute haemorrhage. In patients with chronic encephalopathy and stable liver disease, colonic exclusion with ileostomy or ileorectal anastomosis has been successfully reported, although the combination of an ileostomy stoma and encephalopathy is a formidable one to deal with if the operation does not succeed. The mortality of these procedures has been very high in some series (Resnick et al, 1968).

Liver cell function

Encephalopathy occurs more frequently in patients with severe parenchymal liver disease. However, portocaval shunting done in patients with normal livers during the course of other operations may produce severe and intractable encephalopathy (McDermott and Adams, 1954). Furthermore, long-term survivors after portosystemic shunt operations done for extrahepatic portal obstruction in childhood show evidence of increased neuropsychiatric disturbance as they become older (Vorhees and Price, 1974). Thus it appears that although hepatic cell function is an important factor in the production of coma, good liver function in itself will not protect the patient from this post-shunt complication (Mikkelsen et al, 1965).

Haemodynamic factors

The creation of a surgical portosystemic shunt clearly diverts portal blood away from the liver especially in those patients with significant prograde flow in the portal veins (Stages I and II). After a shunt operation the hepatic artery is usually able to augment its flow and perhaps the distorted architecture produced by the cirrhosis may facilitate this. It has been generally assumed in the literature on this subject that the patients who fare worst after operation are those who have the greatest reduction in liver blood flow after operation. Numerous measurements have been made to try and identify a poor risk group before operation. The following measurements have commonly been made in such investigations.

Preoperative Measurements

Estimated hepatic blood flow

Injected radioactive colloidal gold is removed from the blood stream by the liver. This estimated liver blood flow is measured by observing the isotope decay curve after the isotope is injected. After portocaval shunting there is a decrease in the estimated hepatic blood flow, but this bears no relationship to preoperative levels. Those with the greatest falls are, however, those who are most severely affected by encephalopathy (Bradley et al, 1951).

Portal flow

Estimation of the velocity of the portal flow has been made by observing the speed of movement of dye after splenic venography. Recently Lipiodol has been injected through the obliterated umbilical vein and the speed at which the droplets were seen to move in the portal vein have been calculated from cine-radiographic films (Reichle, 1972).

Wedged hepatic pressure

A catheter is passed through a peripheral systemic vein into the vena cava and wedged in one of the radicals of the hepatic veins. The pressure has been shown to reflect the intrahepatic sinusoidal pressure in most patients. In patients with presinusoidal block, however, there is a considerable difference between the portal pressure and the wedged hepatic pressure.

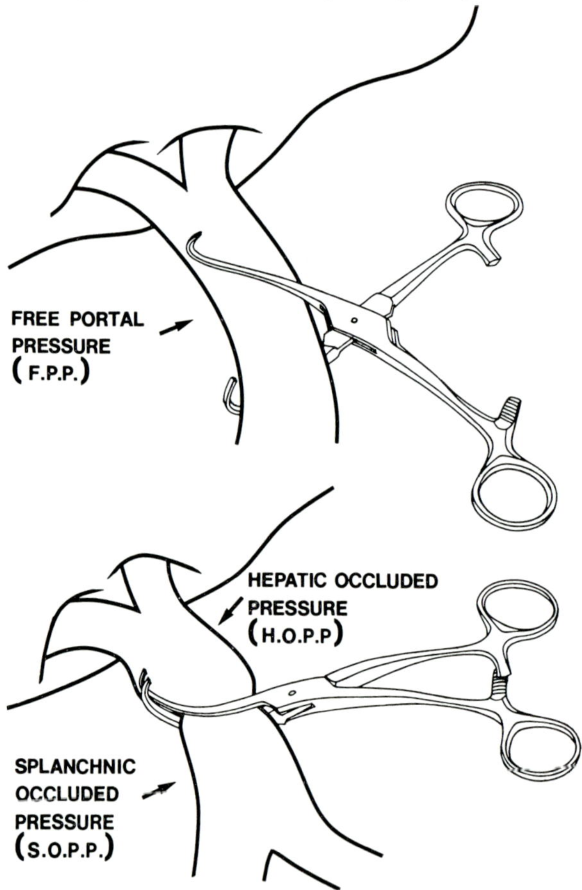

Figure 3.4   Diagram to show the measurement of free portal pressure and, following the application of an occlusion clamp to the portal vein, the hepatic occluded portal pressure and the splanchnic occluded portal pressure

Portal pressure

Portal pressure is best measured before operation by measuring the splenic pulp pressure during splenic venography. It has been shown that pressure measurements taken during operation are much less accurate as they are affected by such factors as the anaesthetic agents and the fact that the peritoneal cavity is open.

Measurements Taken at Operation

Electromagnetic flow meters
These may be placed around the hepatic artery and portal vein at operation to get direct flow measurements. However, the dissection required to place the probes may be considerable and some of the perivascular autonomic nerves are probably damaged resulting in changes of blood flow. Such flow probes are less satisfactory in measuring venous flow than arterial. The results of these measurements have usually been expressed as a ratio of hepatic artery to portal vein flow. The lower the flow in the portal vein (Stage III) the higher will this ratio be (normally it is 1:3). When measured in cirrhotics it shows a wide variation, the mean value in one series of 145 patients was 1:1.1 (Burchell et al, 1974).

Effect of occlusion on portal pressure
After the portal vein is isolated a clamp is applied (Fig. 3.4) and the pressure is measured on the splanchnic side to give the splanchnic occluded pressure (SOPP) and on the hepatic side to give the hepatic occluded pressure (HOPP). The difference between the two measurements represents the head of pressure perfusing the liver. This is known as the maximum perfusing pressure (MPP). Obviously the effect of blood loss, anaesthetic agents and dissection may all affect the absolute readings but the ratio between splanchnic occluded pressure and hepatic occluded pressure probably does not alter under such circumstances. In patients with reversed flow (Stage III) clearly the hepatic occluded pressure will exceed the splanchnic occluded pressure. However the interpretation of these pressure studies has been questioned recently and the evidence for hepatofugal flow is poor (Moreno et al, 1975).

Criteria for Shunt Operations

Patients who survive a gastrointestinal bleed and are found to have varices are candidates for operation, but before embarking on any operation the surgeon should have:

1. Accurate knowledge of the patient's liver disease including the histology and biochemical function.
2. Be satisfied the patient actually bled from oesophageal varices.
3. Have accurate radiographs of the pathological portal circulation.

Assessment of liver disease
The clinical examination and assessment of the patient is all important. Those patients who look well and feel well usually do well after surgery. Gardner Child has pioneered the idea of grading the severity of patients' liver disease into A, B and C (Child, 1964). This has been modified into a

slightly more flexible system by using points as follows (Pugh et al, 1973):

	1 Point	2 Points	3 Points
Serum bilirubin (mg/100 ml)	< 2	2–3	> 3
Serum albumin (g/100 ml)	> 3.5	3–3.5	< 3
Prothrombin time (seconds prolonged)	≤ 2	3–5	> 5
Ascites	None	Mild/moderate	Gross
Encephalopathy	None	Minimal	Moderate/severe

The points are then added and the patients classified as follows:

$$A = 5\text{--}7 \text{ points}$$
$$B = 8\text{--}9 \text{ points}$$
$$C = 10\text{--}15 \text{ points}$$

A liver biopsy is essential in assessing the presence or absence of liver disease. The type of liver disease is important, some forms of cirrhosis are comparatively inactive and progress only slowly over the years.

Patients admitted after an acute alcoholic episode may show considerable fatty change in the liver which is reversible with medical treatment. Such episodes are often associated with gross malnutrition and these patients are quite common in the United States but rare in the United Kingdom. The clinical improvement after medical treatment is often spectacular; such patients may be Grade 'C' on admission but improve to become Grade 'B' or even 'A'.

It is also important to exclude the presence of a hepatoma as this is quite a common mode of death in patients with cirrhosis (Stone et al, 1968). A liver scan using both technetium which shows liver tumours as a filling defect and selenomethionine which is taken up by the hepatoma is very useful. Some hepatomas may be associated with an elevation of the alpha-feto protein level in the blood.

The origin of bleeding

All patients should be thoroughly investigated by barium studies and fiberendoscopy. Peptic ulcer disease is more common in cirrhotics and the mere presence of varices does not necessarily mean that they are the source of an upper gastrointestinal haemorrhage. Varices are more readily displayed by using Buscopan during the examination to produce oesophageal relaxation (see Fig. 3.1).

The anatomy of the portal venous system

A venogram must be done on all patients before embarking on a shunt operation so as to exclude any secondary thrombosis in the vein which is being considered for use in the shunt. This may be done preoperatively or intraoperatively.

Preoperative methods. Providing the prothrombin time is normal and the platelet count about $100\,000/\mu l$ a preoperative splenic venogram is the most convenient method of demonstrating the portal vessels (Fig. 3.5). The superior mesenteric blood flow does produce some streaming in the portal vein which must be differentiated from portal vein thrombosis.

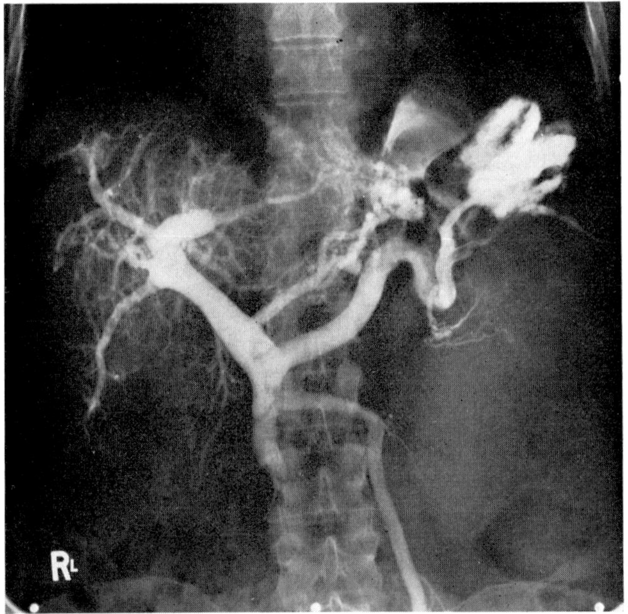

Figure 3.5 Radiograph of splenic portogram in a patient with primary biliary cirrhosis. The portal vein is patent and the oesophageal collaterals connecting with the left gastric vein are well seen

If the spleen has been removed or if haemostasis is mildly impaired, then pictures of the portal system may be obtained by an aorto-portogram, i.e. selective catheterisation of the superior mesenteric artery and examination of the venous phase films (Fig. 3.6). However, the definition on these films is at best only moderate.

Intraoperative methods. Good pictures of the portal system may be obtained by inserting a small cannula into a small jejunal vein on or close to the serosa of the bowel (use of veins in the mesentery itself should be avoided as haematoma formation is more difficult to prevent). Twenty millilitres of contrast medium is injected rapidly and serial films taken at the end of the injection.

This method is especially useful in patients with an extrahepatic block in whom the spleen has been removed. It is not uncommon for the superior mesenteric vein to be occluded and replaced by a leash of collaterals. In such patients any orthodox shunt operation is obviously impossible and the venograms may save much tedious and fruitless dissection.

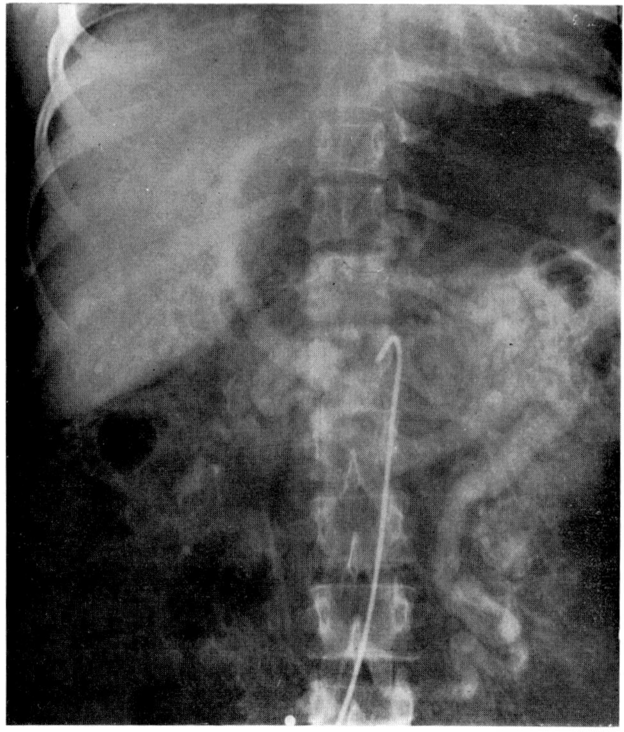

Figure 3.6   Radiograph taken during the venous phase of a selective coeliac angiogram (aortoportogram). The portal vein is seen to be patent, but the detail is not nearly so clear as that produced by a splenic venogram

Risks of Shunt Operations

Shunt operations are major operations and carry a definite risk to life. The immediate risk is directly related to the severity of the liver disease provided the patient is otherwise fit. Thus in one series the risk in category 'A' patients was 10 per cent, in 'B' patients 16 per cent and in 'C' patients 54 per cent (Turcotte, Wallin and Child, 1969). However, the risk of encephalopathy is more difficult to predict and is not so clearly related to preoperative liver function. Certain factors are associated with an increased incidence of post-shunt encephalopathy.

Age

The older the patient the greater the risk of postshunt encephalopathy. Some authors have suggested that patients over 45 years should be rejected (Hourigan et al, 1971). However, it seems that the risk is not prohibitive if patients of up to 65 years, in otherwise good health, are accepted (Shaldon, 1962; Zeegen et al, 1973).

Effect of gastrointestinal bleed

If a patient develops significant encephalopathy after a gastrointestinal haemorrhage then encephalopathy is more likely to develop after shunting than in a patient in whom haemorrhage causes no upset (Hourigan et al, 1971).

Diabetes mellitus

In some series the incidence of encephalopathy is double in those patients with diabetes mellitus who undergo a portocaval shunt (Voorhees, Price and Britton, 1970; Hourigan et al, 1971).

Type of parenchymal lesion

Certain types of hepatic lesions, e.g. schistosomiasis are known to fare badly after portosystemic shunting. Portal hypertension may develop in these patients without true cirrhosis. After the shunt operation serial hepatic arteriograms show a progressive change to the cirrhotic pattern. This process may take several years. The incidence of postshunt encephalopathy is very high, probably over 60 per cent or more (Hassab, 1967). In Egypt and South America where schistosomiasis is endemic many surgeons do not undertake shunt operations.

Haemodynamic predictions

Both preoperative and intraoperative haemodynamic studies have been used extensively in an effort to predict the outcome of shunt surgery. Theoretically it would be expected that those patients with normal or near normal forward flow to the liver (Stage I) would be more adversely affected haemodynamically by total diversion of all portal blood away from the liver than Stage III patients.

However, the only two large studies which attempt to correlate haemodynamic measurements with the clinical results cast real doubt on the validity of the concept of haemodynamic predictions.

In a series of 145 patients, no correlation was found between portal vein flow or the ratio of hepatic artery:portal vein flow in predicting the outcome of a portosystemic shunt (Burchell et al, 1974). In another series of 115 patients undergoing emergency portocaval shunts for haemorrhage, forward flow was assessed from hepatic occluded and splanchnic occluded portal pressures. Under one-third of this series had reversed or stagnant portal flow and contrary to the haemodynamic hypothesis they fared badly compared with patients with forward flow; more of them died after operation and the incidence of encephalopathy was double (Orloff et al, 1974).

In summary then an ideal patient for a shunt operation should be under 45 years, in category 'A' or 'B', have inactive liver disease and should look and feel well. If less rigid criteria are accepted then inevitably this will be reflected in a rise of both the mordibity and the mortality rate.

ELECTIVE SURGICAL TREATMENT

Oesophageal varices are dealt with either by lowering the portal pressure or some direct attack on the varices.

Shunt operations

The only reliable protection against haemorrhage from oesophageal varices is a shunt operation which permanently lowers the portal pressure. However, successful shunt operations are associated with a serious drawback; they hasten the onset of liver failure (Grace, Muench and Chalmers, 1966; Resnick et al, 1974).

Direct operations

Various procedures including oesophageal and gastric transections, devascularisations, resections and sclerotherapy have all been tried. However, all are associated with a high incidence of rebleeding in the long term. Because of the pressure gradient between the abdominal and thoracic cavity, this tendency to recurrence of varices after local operations is hardly surprising.

Portosystemic Shunt Operations

There are two types of portosystemic shunt operations, (a) end-to-side portocaval shunt in which the whole of the portal blood is diverted from the liver into the vena cava and (b) side-to-side anastomosis between the portal and systemic venous system. All portosystemic shunts, except the end-to-side portocaval, fall into this category, viz. side-to-side portocaval anastomosis, conventional (central) splenorenal anastomosis, mesentericocaval anastomosis (Marion, 1966; Clatworthy, 1974), mesentericocaval (mesocaval) jump graft (Lord et al, 1970; Drapanas, 1972), distal splenorenal shunt (Warren, Zeppa and Fomon, 1967).

In a side-to-side operation some portal blood may continue to perfuse the liver but this is open to some doubt. If the shunt created lowers the portal pressure to the normal range then it seems unlikely that any significant amount of blood flow will take place through the obstructed portal radicles when there is little or no resistance to retrograde flow through the shunt. The only shunt operation in which significant portal perfusion of the liver continues is the distal splenorenal operation (Warren et al, 1967). Evidence has been produced to show that liver function is well maintained after this selective shunt (Warren et al, 1974).

End-in-side portocaval shunt

End-in-side portocaval anastomosis is the most widely used shunt. It has the lowest incidence of occlusion probably because the stoma is large, and the whole of the portal blood flow passes through it. It is usually the easiest of the shunt operations to perform and the operative mortality rate of elective operations in good risk patients is around 5 to 10 per cent in most series. But this operation carries the highest incidence of postshunt encephalopathy, probably because it has the highest patency rate.

Side-to-side portocaval shunt

This operation is facilitated by the use of a three-bladed clamp which holds the portal vein and inferior vena cava in apposition for the vascular anastomosis. Sometimes the size of the caudate lobe is such that it is technically impossible to approximate the veins. There is no clear evidence that it is either better or worse than the end-in-side operation although in one series the mortality rate in poor risk patients (category 'C') was significantly lower than for end-in-side portocaval shunts (Turcotte et al, 1969).

Conventional splenorenal anastomosis

In this operation the spleen is removed and the end of the splenic vein anastomosed end-to-side to the left renal vein. Technically it is usually the most difficult of the conventional shunt operations and the removal of the spleen in portal hypertension may present considerable problems. The incidence of thrombosis of the anastomosis is high, probably around 25 per cent and the incidence of shunt occlusion is increased if the stoma is less than 1 cm in diameter (Hallenbeck and Adson, 1961; Voorhees et al, 1970). The proponents of this operation claim the main advantages are the correction of any effects of hypersplenism and the lower incidence of encephalopathy (Barnes et al, 1971). This latter claim may well be accounted for by the fact that many of the shunts occlude. In one series of 29 patients from England only two bled again, but 11 (that is 38 per cent) showed evidence of encephalopathy (Riddell et al, 1972). In other words if the shunt is big enough to stop oesophageal bleeding it is probably big enough to produce encephalopathy. Splenorenal anastomosis is probably the operation of choice for patients with considerable haematological changes of hypersplenism but even after portocaval shunting there is evidence to suggest that hypersplenism improves (Felix et al, 1974).

Mesentericocaval anastomosis (Marion, 1966; Clatworthy, 1974)

In this operation the inferior vena cava is mobilised by dividing the lumbar veins, the cava (or common iliac veins) is transected and the distal cava is then swung to the left and anastomosed to the superior mesenteric vein at the root of the small bowel mesentery. The operation is well tolerated in children and was designed primarily for use in young patients with extrahepatic portal obstruction. In adults, oedema of the extremities is a common sequel to division of the cava.

Interposition mesentericocaval shunt (mesocaval jump graft)

In the last few years several reports have been published concerning the mesocaval jump graft using a Dacron prosthesis (Lord et al, 1970; Drapanas, 1972; Smith et al, 1974). The patient's own internal jugular vein has also been utilised as the graft material (Stipa et al, 1973). The large majority of these grafts are reported to stay patent for at least three years. No very long term follow-up is available, but patency has been demonstrated radiologically, at autopsy and by the fact the varices regress and patients do not bleed again The Dacron graft used is 18 to 22 mm diamter, and radiopaque markers may be put on the peritoneum adjacent to the prosthesis to facilitate postoperative venograms to study patency.

It has been claimed that the operation is easier than a portocaval shunt (Drapanas, 1972) but this is certainly not so in an obese patient. Theoretically it is also claimed that the encephalopathy rate may be lower because some portal blood continues to perfuse the liver. This claim is not yet completely substantiated and certainly contested by some (Warren et al, 1974).

Distal splenorenal shunt (Warren et al, 1967, 1974)

The aim of this ingenious operation is to decompress the portal tributaries of the left upper quadrant of the abdomen while maintaining the portal flow largely undisturbed (Fig. 3.7). The left gastric vein and the right gastro-epiploic veins are divided on the wall of the stomach. The splenic vein is dissected behind the pancreas and transected. The central end is then over-sewn and the distal end anastomosed to the left renal vein. The operation is technically difficult especially in muscular or obese patients. The mortality rate in the initial series was high (58 per cent) but this has now dropped, and in a recent series of 46 patients the mortality rate was only 7 per cent. The operation is contraindicated in moderate to severe ascites as this is reported to become uncontrollable after a selective shunt. A further modification of the operation has been described in which the left renal vein is divided and anastomosed end-to-side to the splenic vein, the splenic vein is then occluded by sutures between the anastomosis and the superior mesenteric vein (Warren et al, 1974).

Makeshift shunts

Various makeshift shunts have been described especially in patients with extrahepatic obstruction. Collateral veins may enlarge grossly in this condition and reach sufficient size to be used for shunting, e.g. those in the falciform ligament or those in the peripheral part of the mesentery. Unfortunately the occlusion rate after such operations is high, up to 70 per cent in one series (Voorhees and Price, 1974).

Arteriolisation of the Portal Bed

After a portocaval shunt it has been shown that there is a reduction in the hepatic blood flow. It has been claimed that the patients who fare worst have the greatest fall in hepatic blood flow after operation (Warren et al, 1963).

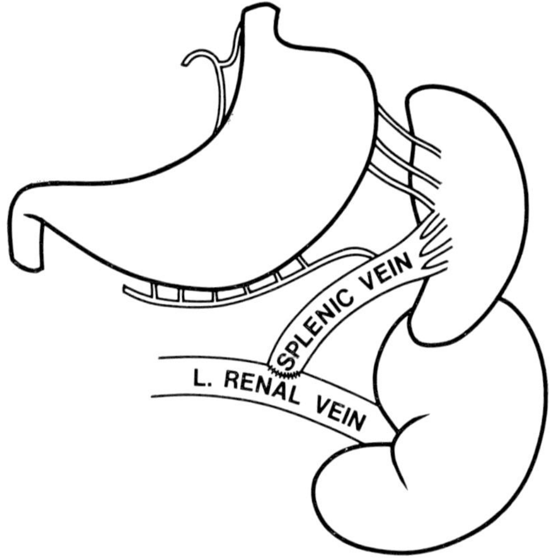

Figure 3.7 Diagram to show the essential features of the distal splenorenal shunt described by Warren et al (1967). The right gastroepiploic and the left gastric vein are ligated adjacent to the stomach in order to decompress the viscera of the left upper quadrant into the left renal vein. The central end of the splenic vein (not shown) is oversewn

Experimental work has shown that arteriolisation of the stump of the portal vein is possible and maintains hepatic perfusion. It was thought that this procedure might prevent the progressive postoperative hepatic failure but the full arterial pressure on the portal bed produced secondary adverse changes of vasculitis and thrombosis in the portal radicals of animals (Zuidema et al, 1963).

Encouraging results have been reported in man by anastomosing the right gastroepiploic artery to the umbilical vein after the latter has been opened up down to the left branch of the portal vein using dilators (Adamson and Levin, 1974). The use of such a small artery is claimed to prevent the adverse changes in the portal vein radicals (Maillard et al, 1974).

SHUNT SURGERY AND ITS RESULTS

Since the introduction of shunt surgery by Blakemore in 1948, each of the various shunt operations have at one time or another claimed to be superior to the others. The initial results have always been enthusiastically received, but when widely adopted, enthusiasm has waned. The latest operation is the distal splenorenal shunt: whether it lives up to the initial claims and becomes widely adopted remains to be seen. In the accompanying Table 3.1 the reports of two big series of elective end in side portocaval shunt are shown.

Table 3.1   Results of elective end-in-side portocaval shunts

Author	No.	Mortality (%)	Occlusion (%)	Encephalopathy (%)
Voorhees and Price (USA, 1970)	271	12	4	34
Zeegen et al (UK, 1973)	174	10	2.5	24

It will be seen that although in good risk patients the operative mortality rate is acceptable the encephalopathy rate is high. The ineffectiveness of portocaval shunting to rehabilitate the patient fully is demonstrated by a subgroup of 60 men in the Voorhees series.

> 60 male patients
> 36 survived two years
> 28 were previously fully employed
> Only 14 fit to work.

The results of splenorenal anastomosis in three different series is shown in Table 3.2. It will be seen that although conventional splenorenal anasto-

Table 3.2   Results of splenorenal anastomosis

Author	No.	Mortality (%)	Occlusion (%)	Encephalopathy (%)
Voorhees et al (1970)	48	12	19	30
Riddell et al (1972)	29	11	7	38
Zeegen et al (1973)	29	14	20	16

mosis has often been claimed to have a lower encephalopathy rate this merely probably reflects the incidence of shunt thrombosis. In the series with the lowest known occlusion rate of 7 per cent (incidence of rebleeding or persistence of unchanged varices) the encephalopathy rate was the highest at 38 per cent (Riddell et al, 1972).

The long-term results of mesocaval jump grafts are not yet known, but the initial results in this author's experience are probably not much different from other shunts (Smith et al, 1974). It would appear that if a portosystemic shunt is large enough to reduce portal pressure effectively it is large enough to produce encephalopathy. Selective distal splenorenal shunt is not applicable to all patients, it is technically difficult and the actual impact of this operation on the mortality rate and postshunt morbidity rate in an unselected group of cirrhotics who present themselves for operation is not yet clear.

Prophylactic shunt operations

After portocaval shunt operations became established, it seemed logical to operate on cirrhotic patients with varices before bleeding took place and thus avoid the serious risk to life associated with an episode of haemorrhage. However, prospective randomised controlled trials by the Boston Inter-Hospital Liver Group have shown this advice to be of dubious value (Grace et al, 1966). Patients with varices and well compensated cirrhosis were randomly allocated for either (a) prophylactic portocaval shunt or (b) medical therapy. At the end of five years there was no difference in the survival rate but the natural history of the disease was altered by operation. The shunted patients died of liver failure the onset of which was hastened by operation, but only 1.5 per cent bled. The medically treated group had a much higher incidence of death from haemorrhage (26 per cent) but the incidence of liver failure was considerably less. Thus protection from oesophageal variceal haemorrhage was countered by the hastening of hepatic failure. These findings have been confirmed by other groups (Conn and Lindenmuth, 1969).

Prospective trial of therapeutic shunt

After it was shown that prophylactic shunting was not indicated the next step was to test the value of therapeutic shunts and recently the initial results of such series have been published and the results have thrown real doubt, even on the place of therapeutic shunts. A series of 79 cirrhotic patients who had bled at least once from varices were randomised into (a) medical treatment and (b) shunt operations. Although shunted patients were protected from haemorrhage many were rendered encephalopathic and the onset of liver failure was hastened; thus at the end of five years there was no statistical difference in the survival between the two groups (Resnick et al, 1974). A shunt operation is merely a palliative procedure for most patients.

Direct Operations

A great variety of direct operations have been described and most involve dividing the vascular connections of the lower oesophagus and/or the fundus of the stomach together with some procedure which interrupts the sub-mucosal varices.

All of the direct operations are associated with a high incidence of recurrent bleeding and the longer and more complete the follow-up the greater is this incidence. The operations tend to be used in patients with extrahepatic obstruction especially when there is no suitable vein for a shunt operation.

They are often used in childhood to carry the child through to adolescence when after growth, the larger calibre veins offer a much better prospect of a successful portosystemic shunt. Among the commoner direct operations used are the following.

Oesophageal transection (Walker, 1960)

The lower left chest is opened and the oesophagus mobilised, the muscle layers of the oesophagus are split longitudinally and the mucosal tube together with the submucosal varices is dissected free for about 5 cm. The mucosa is

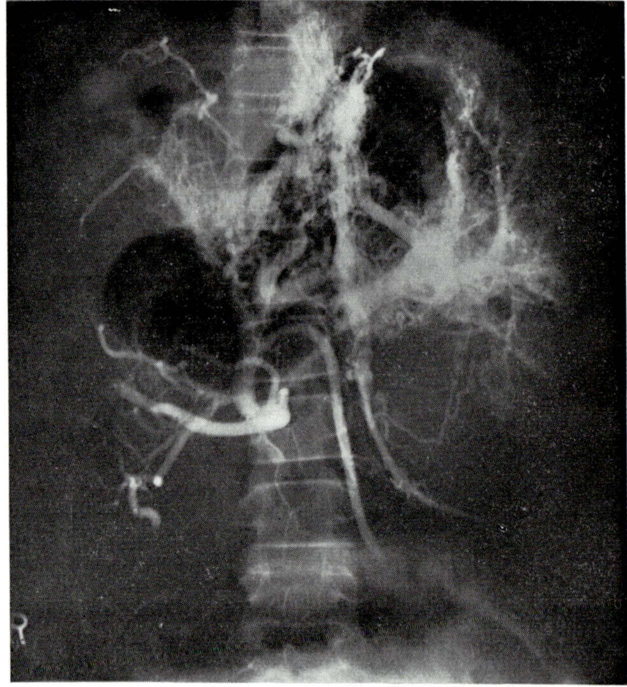

Figure 3.8   Splenic venogram taken three weeks after an emergency oesophageal transection. The portal vein is seen to be thrombosed and the oesophageal collaterals interrupted by the transection operation.

then transected as near to the cardia as possible and resutured with a continuous suture thus interrupting the submucosal varices. Leakage is uncommon as the two suture lines lie at right angles to one another (Walker, 1962; Pugh et al, 1973). The effective interruption of oesophageal collaterals may be demonstrated on splenoportography (Fig. 3.8).

Boerema–Crile operation

In this operation the oesophagus is mobilised through the left chest and the oesophagus opened longitudinally right into the lumen; the columns of varices are underrun to stop the bleeding and promote occlusion of the varices. Leakage from the oesophagotomy is common (Rothwell-Jackson and Hunt, 1971).

Portoazygos disconnection (Tanner, 1961)

In this operation the lower 5 cm of oesophagus and upper 5 cm of stomach are dissected free of all external vascular connections and the upper stomach is then transected and resutured in order to interrupt the submucosal collaterals. Both the thoracic and abdominal cavities have to be opened and the operation may be prolonged by what is sometimes a tedious dissection. Reflux oesophagitis may occur after the procedure and makes recurrent bleeding more likely. Sometimes the leakage of ascitic fluid from the abdominal cavity into the chest leads to post operative difficulties.

Gastrooesophageal decongestion (Hassab, 1967)

In this operation the spleen is removed and all of the vascular connections to the lower oesophagus and upper two-thirds of the stomach divided. No transection is done. The operation has been used extensively in Egypt because of the high incidence of postshunt encephalopathy in schistosomiasis. Recurrent haemorrhage is claimed to be rare but the completeness and the length of follow-up are not described in detail in the report.

Boerema button operation

In this operation a mechanical device, the Boerema button, is used to achieve a rapid full thickness oesophageal transection via an abdominal incision. There are no satisfactory long-term assessments of its value.

Other operations such as oesophagectomy with oesophagogastric anastomosis, jejunal interposition or colonic interposition, have all been used but the incidence of rebleeding is much higher than after shunt operation.

Portal Hypertension in Childhood

Oesophageal varices are the commonest cause of haematemesis in childhood, and they are usually secondary to extrahepatic portal vein block.

Often there is no underlying cause for the portal block but in some patients there is a clear story of umbilical sepsis at birth. Symptomless splenomegaly is often noted between the ages of three and five years. It is a disaster for the child if the spleen is removed at this stage, as a later splenorenal shunt is thereby precluded. Variceal haemorrhage often starts between seven and nine years and frequently seems to follow an upper respiratory tract infection. Some clinicians provide these patients with a course of prophylactic antibiotics to be taken when they get a cold to try to prevent the ensuing haemorrhage. As yet there is no good evidence that this has any real effect.

Operation is delayed, if possible, until such time as the child grows to a size which allows a reasonable prospect of success for a shunt operation. It has been claimed that the splenic vein should be at least 1 cm in diameter for a successful splenorenal shunt. Sometimes, however, severe persistent haemorrhage demands operation when the child is small. One of the direct operations may then be used such as an oesophageal transection or oesophagogastrectomy. However, none of these operations gives lasting protection and once operation is undertaken subsequent bleeds often seem to demand further operations (Fonkalsrud, Myers and Robinson, 1974; Voorhees and Price, 1974; Clatworthy, 1974).

As the child grows up the frequency of haemorrhage in those who have not undergone operation often seems to decrease and in some series a successful policy of non-operation has been pursued (Folkalsrud et al, 1974) especially in children in whom there was no favourable vein available for shunting. The direct operations all have a considerable morbidity and mortality rate (Clatworthy, 1974). A successful shunt is the only procedure to give lasting protection from bleeding. However, in practice this is not easy to achieve and a high recurrent bleeding rate is reported after shunts because of thrombosis, e.g. 44 per cent after splenorenal shunts in children. The most successful shunt is the mesocaval (Clatworthy, 1974). A high incidence of failure for makeshift shunts, such as anastomosing collateral veins to the cava, is reported in most series.

One disquieting feature which has come to light in recent years is that although the risk of encephalopathy in patients undergoing shunt surgery for extrahepatic block was thought to be negligible, it is now clear from long-term studies that there is a very high incidence of emotional and psychiatric problems in these patients and also a hepatic foetor has been noted after some years (Mikkelsen, 1974; Voorhees and Price, 1974). Further long-term studies are required but it seems likely that these patients will not escape encephalopathy.

In a review of the literature, 418 patients with extrahepatic portal hypertension in childhood were analysed (Clatworthy, 1974). The overall mortality rate was 12 per cent; bleeding accounted for 5 per cent of deaths, operations for 5 per cent and hepatitis for 2 per cent. If no direct operation is possible and there are no suitable veins for shunting, then injection of oesophageal varices with a sclerosant may be used with some success (Johnston and Rodgers, 1973).

Emergency Treatment of Variceal Haemorrhage

The outlook for a patient who presents with bleeding oesophageal varices is related mainly to the state of the hepatic parenchymal function.

EXTRAHEPATIC BLOCK

In those patients with an extrahepatic block and a normal liver, the risk to life in a particular episode of haemorrhage is low. One estimate was 1 per cent

(Walker, 1962) and in another series of 40 patients there was only one death in the year after the first presenting bleed (Shaldon and Sherlock, 1962). The haemorrhages are quite unpredictable and some patients may go several years between bleeds.

INTRAHEPATIC BLOCK

In the patients with cirrhosis and bleeding varices the outlook is grim for it is usually the patients with poor liver function (category 'C') in whom bleeding is persistent. In most published series the overall mortality rate is around 50 per cent. The exact risk of recurrence of bleeding in a particular patient is difficult to assess. The experience in the United Kingdom is very different from the United States, for in the latter the majority of cirrhotics are alcoholic. Bleeding is often precipitated by severe bouts of drinking associated with poor nutrition which produces fatty change and swelling in the liver, together with a rise in portal pressure. If the patient stops drinking then considerable recovery of liver function may occur, but if drinking continues the outlook is poor. In a series of 464 patients reported from Boston only 30 per cent were alive one year after presenting with a haemorrhage (Garceau and Chalmers, 1963). In a series of 120 patients seen in London, 66 per cent were alive one year after being first seen. Only a minority of patients in this series were alcoholic (Sherlock, 1964).

The *principles of management* of a patient who presents with gastrointestinal haemorrhage and oesophageal varices are as follows:

1. replace the blood loss,
2. minimise risk of coma,
3. confirm the site of bleeding, and
4. take active measure to stop the bleeding if necessary.

Replacement of blood loss

The adequate replacement of blood loss is all important. If the patient is allowed to remain in shock then further ischaemic damage to the hepatic parenchyma will occur. For the seriously ill patient with clotting difficulties, fresh blood should be used if it is available.

Prevention of coma

Encephalopathy is frequently precipitated by a haemorrhage as a result of the protein load in the gut (i.e. the blood) together with the imparied hepatocyte function occasioned by the bleeding. The gut is therefore emptied of blood by purgation using magnesium sulphate orally (or via a tube) and by enemata. Neomycin is also given, its powerful effect on gut flora interferes with the production of the toxic substances from protein breakdown and lightens the coma.

Confirmation of the site of bleeding

Despite the fact that a patient is known or shown by barium studies to have oesophageal varices it cannot be assumed that these are always the source of any massive upper intestinal haemorrhage.

The introduction of emergency fiberendoscopy has demonstrated that up to 40 per cent of patients admitted with bleeding varices the bleeding is coming from another lesion, e.g. chronic peptic ulcer or erosive gastritis (Palmer, 1969; McCray et al, 1969; Waldram et al, 1973). This fact makes much of the literature on the treatment of bleeding varices difficult to assess for until the last few years the site of bleeding was usually assumed to be from varices and no emergency endoscopy was undertaken.

Active measures to stop bleeding

The two commonest non-operative measures used to stop bleeding are the administration of pitocin and the use of balloon tamponade.

Pitocin (posterior pituitary extract)

This is infused intravenously (20 units in 100 ml saline over a 10–15 min period). The effect is to cause profound smooth muscle contraction which reduces portal inflow and hence lowers the portal pressure. The effect is short lived but may be sufficient to allow haemorrhage to stop, unfortunately further bleeding within a few days is common.

The infusion of pitocin into the superior mesenteric artery via a trans-femoral arterial cannula has been enthusiastically reported by some (Nusbaum et al, 1974) but other workers have reported poor control of haemorrhage and a high complication rate, e.g. false aneurysm in the groin (Murray-Lyon et al, 1973).

Balloon tamponade (Sengstaken–Blakemore tube)

This is probably the most effective and most widely used method of controlling bleeding from oesophageal varices. The disadvantages are the risk of aspiration pneumonia and pressure necrosis of the oesophageal mucosa. A small Ryles tube should be fixed to the commercially available tube to allow aspiration of the oesophageal lumen just proximal to the balloon. The oesophageal balloon is inflated to 30 to 50 mmHg as measured on an aneroid pressure gauge connected to the tube. The balloon is deflated after 12 to 24 h to prevent mucosal necrosis.

With good nursing and careful attention to detail, trouble-free temporary control of variceal haemorrhage can usually be achieved (Pitcher, 1971). Some 57 per cent of patients stop bleeding (Sherlock, 1964).

Operative measures to stop bleeding

These consist of either a direct attack on the varices or an emergency shunt operation.

Injection of oesophageal varices

Although the injection of sclerosants into oesophageal varices was first practised over 35 years ago (Crafoord and Frenckner, 1939) it is comparatively recently that convincing evidence has been produced to show that it stops bleeding from varices (Johnston and Rodgers, 1973). In this latter series from Belfast of over 100 patients, a 90 per cent control of bleeding was reported. The mortality rate for cirrhotic patients was 30 per cent which is considerably less than for other methods of treatment. The published results certainly warrant its more widespread use. A modification to the Negus oesophagoscope greatly facilitates the procedure (Bailey and Dawson, 1975). There is a needle attachment available for use with the flexible endoscope but it is more difficult to use especially in large varices as any bleeding rapidly obscures the distal viewing lens.

Ligation of varices

Transthoracic ligation of varices is probably the most commonly used operation in Britain. Its advantages are that it is usually quick and it controls the bleeding. However, the mortality rate in category 'C' patients is formidable (Rothwell-Jackson and Hunt, 1971; George et al, 1973; Pugh et al, 1973).

Transabdominal operations to devascularise or transect the stomach are much more difficult because the thickened vascular peritoneum is likely to make any operation difficult and tedious, and from the published data they do not seem any more effective in controlling haemorrhage than the easier transthoracic procedures.

Emergency shunt operations

Emergency shunt operations have been employed in the United States (Orloff et al, 1974). It is reported that a mortality rate is no greater than when lesser procedures are used, that is about 50 per cent. Furthermore once the patient is discharged from hospital the threat of any further haemorrhage has been removed, so that the seven year survival rate in this series was 42.5 per cent. It is unlikely that such good results could be obtained in the United Kingdom. The majority of the patients operated on in this series were alcoholic and the good long-term results after the shunt operation were possibly related to the combination of abstinence from alcohol and the great improvement in body nutrition. The situation in the United Kingdom is different. The emaciated malnourished alcoholic is a rarity and the clinical syndrome of acute alcoholic hepatitis is not often seen. It has been the experience of most surgeons in the British Isles that although they could return a mortality rate of 5 to 10 per cent for elective shunt operations once they embarked on emergency shunt procedures the mortality rate rose to 30 per cent or more, even in good risk patients. Indeed when the results from three series of patients who underwent transoesophageal ligation are examined it will be seen that the majority of the survivors were quite unsuitable for any elective shunt surgery (Rothwell-Jackson and Hunt, 1971; George et al, 1973; Pugh et al, 1973). It is difficult to imagine that had a shunt operation been applied to all of these patients, with its prolonged dissection and adverse haemodynamic effect on the liver, it could achieve a lower mortality rate than the direct operations on the gullet. Clearly a controlled trial in Britain would be required to establish the point. In one series only 12 per cent of category 'C' patients survived to be discharged from hospital (the majority dying of liver failure). All of those who survived to leave hospital died within a year of their admission (Pugh et al, 1973).

Miscellaneous methods

Various other techniques have been reported to control variceal bleeding including oesophageal and gastric cooling, thoracic duct fistula and an external portosystemic shunt via the umbilical vein which is dilated up to its connection with the left branch of the portal vein. None of these methods has found general acceptance to date.

REFERENCES

Adamson, R. J. & Levin, D. C. (1974) Hepatic encephalopathy after portasystemic shunt treated by sterilisation of intrahepatic portal vein. *Surgical Forum,* **25,** 348–351.

Bailey, M. E. & Dawson, J. L. (1975) Modified oesophagoscope for injecting oesophageal varices. *British Medical Journal,* **2,** 540–541.

Barnes, B. A., Ackroyd, F. W., Battit, G. E., Kantrowitz, P. A., Schapiro, R. H., Strole, W. E., Todd, D. P. & McDermott, W. V. (1971) Elective portasystemic shunts: morbidity and survival data. *Annals of Surgery,* **174,** 76–84.

Bradley, S. E., Macpherson, A. I., Gammeltoft, A. & Blakemore, A. H. (1951) Effect of portacaval anastomosis on hepatic oxygen extraction and estimated hepatic blood flow in patients with cirrhosis. *Journal of Clinical Investigation,* **30,** 630.

Burchell, A. R., Moreno, A. H., Panke, W. F. & Nealon, T. F. (1974) Hemodynamic variables and prognosis following portacaval shunts. *Surgery Gyneacology and Obstetrics,* **138,** 359–369.

Child, C. G. (1964) *The Liver and Portal Hypertension.* Philadelphia, PA; Saunders.

Clatworthy, H. W. (1974) Management of extrahepatic portal hypertension in children (discussion). *Annals of Surgery,* **180,** 491–492.

Crafoord, C. & Frenckner, P. (1939) New surgical treatment of varicose veins of oesophagus. *Acta Otolaryngologia,* **27,** 422–429.

Conn, H. O. & Lindenmuth, W. W. (1969) Prophylactic portacaval anastomosis in cirrhotic patients with esophageal varices and ascites. *American Journal of Surgery,* **117,** 656–661.

Drapanas, T. (1972) Interposition mesocaval shunt for treatment of portal hypertension. *Annals of Surgery,* **176,** 435–448.

Elkington, S. G. (1970) Lactulose. *Gut,* **11,** 1043–1048.

Felix, W. R., Myerson, R. M., Sigel, B., Perrin, E. B. & Jackson, F. C. (1974) The effect of portacaval shunt on hypersplenism. *Surgery Gynaecology and Obstetrics,* **139,** 899–904.

Fonkalsrud, E. W., Myers, N. A. & Robinson, M. J. (1974) Management of extrahepatic portal hypertension in children. *Annals of Surgery,* **180,** 487–493.

Garceau, A. J. & Chalmers, T. C. (1963) The natural history of cirrhosis. 1. Survival with esophageal varices. *New England Journal of Medicine,* **268,** 469–473.

George, P., Brown, C., Ridgway, G., Crofts, B. & Sherlock, S. (1973) Emergency oesophageal transection in uncontrolled variceal haemorrhage. *British Journal of Surgery,* **60,** 635–640.

Grace, N. D., Muench, H. & Chalmers, T. C. (1966) The present status of shunts for portal hypertension in cirrhosis. *Gastroenterology,* **50,** 684–691.

Hallenbeck, G. A. & Adson, M. A. (1961) Esophagogastric varices without hepatic cirrhosis. *Archives of Surgery*, **83**, 370–383.

Hassab, M. A. (1967) Gastroesophageal decongestion and splenectomy in the treatment of esophageal varices in bilharzial cirrhosis: further studies with a report of 355 operations. *Surgery*, **61**, 169–176.

Hourigan, K., Sherlock, S., George, P. & Mindel, S. (1971) Elective end-to-side portacaval shunt: results in 64 cases. *British Medical Journal*, **4**, 473–477.

Johnston, G. W. & Rodgers, H. W. (1973) A review of 15 years' experience in the use of sclerotherapy in the control of acute haemorrhage from oesophageal varices. *British Journal of Surgery*, **60**, 797–800.

Lord, J. W., Rossi, G., Daliana, M. & Rosati, L. M. (1970) Mesocaval shunt modified by the use of Teflon® prosthesis. *Surgery Gynaecology and Obstetrics*, **130**, 525–526.

McCray, R. S., Martin, F., Amir-Ahmadi, A., Sheahan, D. G. & Zamcheck, N. (1969) Erroneous diagnosis of hemorrhage from esophageal varices. *American Journal of Digestive Diseases*, **14**, 755–760.

McDermott, W. V. & Adams, R. (1954) Episodic stupor associated with an Eck fistula in the human with particular reference to the metabolism of ammonia. *Journal of Clinical Investigation*, **33**, 1–9.

McDermott, W. V. Jr (1972) Evaluation of the hemodynamics of portal hypertension in the selection of patients with shunt surgery. *Annals of Surgery*, **176**, 449–456.

Maillard, J., Rueff, B., Prandi, D. & Sicot, C. (1974) Hepatic arterialisation and portacaval shunt in hepatic cirrhosis: an assessment. *Archives of Surgery*, **108**, 315–320.

Marion, P. (1966) Mesenterico-caval anastomoses. *Journal of Cardiovascular Surgery*, Suppl. 70–81.

Mikkelsen, W. P., Edmondson, H. A., Peters, R. L., Redeker, A. G. & Reynolds, T. B. (1965) Extra- and intrahepatic portal hypertension without cirrhosis (hepatoportal sclerosis). *Annals of Surgery*, **162**, 602–620.

Mikkelsen, W. P. (1974) Management of extrahepatic portal hypertension in children (discussion). *Annals of Surgery*, **180**, 487–493.

Moreno, A. H., Burchell, A. R., Reddy, R. V., Steen, J. A., Panke, W. F. & Nealon, T. F. (1975) Spontaneous reversal of portal blood flow: the case for and against its occurrence in patients with cirrhosis of the liver. *Annals of surgery*, **181**, 346–358.

Murray-Lyon, I. M., Pugh, R. N. H., Nunnerley, H. B., Laws, J. W., Dawson, J. L. & Williams, R. (1973) Treatment of bleeding oesophageal varices by infusion of vasopressin into the superior mesenteric artery. *Gut*, **14**, 59–63.

Nusbaum, M., Younis, M. T., Baum, S. & Blakemore, W. S. (1974) Control of portal hypertension: selective mesenteric arterial infusion of vasopressin. *Archives of Surgery*, **108**, 342–347.

Orloff, M. J., Chandler, J. G., Charters, A. C., Condon, J. K., Grambort, D. E., Modafferi, R. T. & Levin, S. E. (1974) Emergency portacaval shunt treatment for bleeding esophageal varices. *Archives of Surgery*, **108**, 293–299.

Palmer, E. D. (1969) The vigorous diagnostic approach to upper-gastrointestinal tract hemorrhage. *Journal of the American Medical Association*, **207**, 1477–1480.

Pitcher, J. L. (1971) Safety and effectiveness of the modified Sengstaken–Blakemore tube: a prospective study. *Gastroenterology*, **61**, 291–298.

Pugh, R. N. H., Murray Lyon, I. M., Dawson, J. L., Pietroni, M. C. & Williams, R. (1973) Transection of the oesophagus for bleeding oesophageal varices. *British Journal of Surgery*, **60**, 646–649.

Reichle, F. A. (1972) Evaluation of the hemodynamics of portal hypertension in the selection of patients for shunt surgery (discussion). *Annals of Surgery*, **176**, 454–455.

Resnick, R. H., Ishihara, A., Chalmers, T. C. & Schimmel, E. M. (1968) A controlled trial of colon bypass in chronic hepatic encephalopathy. *Gastroenterology*, **54**, 1057–1069.

Resnick, R. H., Iber, F. L., Ishihara, A. M., Chalmers, T. C. & Simmerman, H. (1974) A controlled study of the therapeutic portacaval shunt. *Gastroenterology*, **67**, 843–857.

Rothwell-Jackson, R. L. & Hunt, A. H. (1971) The results obtained with emergency surgery in the treatment of persistent haemorrhage from gastro-oesophageal varices in the cirrhotic patient. *British Journal of Surgery*, **58**, 205–215.

Riddell, A. G., Bloor, K., Hobbs, K. E. F. & Jaquet, N. (1972) Elective splenorenal anastomosis. *British Medical Journal*, **1**, 731–732.

Shaldon, C. (1962) Dynamic aspects of portal hypertension. *Annals of the Royal College of Surgeons*, **31**, 308–329.

Shaldon, S. & Sherlock, S. (1962) Obstruction to the extrahepatic portal system in childhood. *Lancet*, **1**, 62–67.

Sherlock, S. (1964) Haematemesis in portal hypertension. *British Journal of Surgery*, **51**, 746–749.

Smith, G. W. (1974) Use of hemodynamic selection criteria in the management of cirrhotic patients with portal hypertension. *Annals of Surgery*, **179**, 782–790.

Smith, M. G. M., Tuft, R. J., Davidson, A. R., Laws, J. W., Dawson, J. L. & Williams, R. (1974) Mesentericocaval 'jump' graft in management of portal hypertension: experience with 24 cases. *British Medical Journal*, **3**, 705–708.

Stipa, S., Thau, A., Cavallaro, A. & Rossi, P. (1973) A technique for mesentericocaval shunt. *Surgery Gynaecology and Obstetrics*, **137**, 285–287.

Stone, W. D., Islam, N. R. K. & Paton, A. (1968) The natural history of cirrhosis. *Quarterly Journal of Medicine* (*New Series*), **37**, 119–132.

Tanner, N. C. (1961) The late results of porto-azygos disconnexion in the treatment of bleeding from oesophageal varices. *Annals of the Royal College of Surgeons*, **28**, 153–174.

Turcotte, J. G., Wallin, W. W. & Child, C. G. (1969) End to side versus side to side portacaval shunts in patients with hepatic cirrhosis. *American Journal of Surgery*, **117**, 108–116.

Voorhees, A. B., Price, J. B. & Britton, R. C. (1970) Portasystemic shunting procedures for portal hypertension. *American Journal of Surgery*, **119**, 501–505.

Voorhees, A. B. & Price, J. B. (1974) Extrahepatic portal hypertension. *Archives of Surgery*, **108**, 338–341.

Waldram, R., Davis, M., Nunnerley, H. & Williams, R. (1973) Emergency fibreendoscopy following acute gastrointestinal haemorrhage in patients with portal hypertension. *Gut*, **14**, 920.

Walker, R. M. (1960) Transection operations for portal hypertension. *Thorax*, **15**, 218–224.

Walker, R. M. (1962) Treatment of portal hypertension in children. *Proceedings of the Royal Society of Medicine*, **55**, 770–772.

Warren, W. D., Restrepo, J. E., Respess, J. C. & Muller, W. H. (1963) The importance of hemodynamic studies in management of portal hypertension. *Annals of Surgery*, **158**, 387–400.

Warren, W. D., Zeppa, R. & Fomon, J. J. (1967) Selective trans-splenic decompression of gastroesophageal varices by distal splenorenal shunt. *Annals of Surgery*, **166**, 437–455.

Warren, W. D., Rudman, D., Millikan, W., Galambos, J. T., Salam, A. A. & Smith, R. B. (1974) The metabolic basis of portasystemic encephalopathy and the effect of selective vs. nonselective shunts. *Annals of Surgery*, **180**, 573–579.

Warren, W. D., Salam, A. A., Hutson, D. & Zeppa, R. (1974) Selective distal splenorenal shunt: technique and results of operation. *Archives of Surgery*, **108**, 306–314.

Whipple, A. O. (1945) The problem of portal hypertension in relation to the hepatosplenopathies. *Annals of Surgery*, **122**, 449–475.

Yamamoto, S., Yokoyama, Y., Takeshige, K. & Iwatsuki, S. (1968) Budd–Chiari syndrome with obstruction of the inferior vena cava. *Gastroenterology*, **54**, 1070–1084.

Zeegen, R., Stansfeld, A. G., Dawson, A. M. & Hunt, A. H. (1970) Prolonged survival after portal decompression of patients with non-cirrhotic intrahepatic portal hypertension. *Gut*, **11**, 610–617.

Zeegen, R., Stansfeld, A. G., Dawson, A. M. & Hunt, A. H. (1973) Portal decompression for intrahepatic portal hypertension: long-term follow-up of 253 cases. *Gut*, **14**, 816.

Zuidema, G. D., Gaisford, W. D., Abell, M. R., Brody, T. M., Neill, S. A. & Child, C. G. (1963) Segmental portal arterialisation of canine liver. *Surgery*, **53**, 689–698.

4
ACUTE PANCREATITIS

L. R. J. de Jode

Acute pancreatitis continues to present a major challenge to the practising surgeon and to the research worker as witnessed by the large and rapidly growing volume of literature devoted to the subject. Recent advances in our concepts of the pathological mechanisms involved in this puzzling disease, and the introduction of new methods of treatment make a review of the subject appropriate.

This article deals with acute and acute relapsing pancreatitis in accordance with the classification adopted at Marseilles in 1963 and now widely accepted (Bockus, 1965); chronic and chronic relapsing pancreatitis characterised by the presence of permanent and progressive damage to the pancreas will not be discussed although it is recognised that the demarcation is not absolute.

Despite a great deal of experimental work, and notably investigations into the role of enzymes other than trypsin, the initiating mechanisms which trigger off the series of events leading to autodigestion of the pancreas remain obscure. Although the list of aetiological conditions associated with acute pancreatitis grows yearly, much of it iatrogenic, but including such oddities as the bite of the Trinidad scorpion, the precise link between these and the onset of the illness is uncertain. This uncertainty is compensated for by many and ingenious theories none of which explain all the facts but which, taken together, strongly suggest that the disease is multifactorial in its causation.

The high mortality remains the greatest challenge facing the clinician. The problem is, however, complicated by marked differences in mortality in reported series not only between series from different parts of the world but also between different parts of the same country, a difference not entirely explained by variations in the relative proportions of cases associated with different aetiologies, such as biliary disease or alcohol.

The importance of this lies in the fact that new drugs or other methods of treatment have often been assessed by comparing mortality rates in various series. It is clear that such comparisons are not valid and controlled trials are clearly essential for critical evaluation. A prospective multicentre trial designed to clarify the value of two recent therapeutic agents, glucagon and trasylol, has been organised by the Medical Research Council and its results are awaited with interest.

INCIDENCE AND MORTALITY

Figures for the overall yearly incidence in Great Britain are not known but Trapnell and Duncan (1975) have produced data for the Bristol clinical area of 53.8 cases of acute pancreatitis per million of population (yearly) over a seven year period. This compares with the results of a population survey in Rochester, Minnesota, which gave a yearly incidence of from 100 to 115 cases per million of population (O'Sullivan et al, 1972).

Review of published reports in the world literature show a wide variation in the composition of different series according to the aetiological factors; these almost certainly influence both the frequency of the disease and mortality, and renders comparison between series of limited value. Variations are particularly great in the proportion of cases allotted to two main subgroups; the gallstone, and alcohol group. Howard and Jordan (1960) reviewed a large number of reports of acute pancreatitis in the world literature and found that the incidence of gall stones reported varied from 13 to 96 per cent.

Biliary disease is the most commonly associated pathology in British series (Pollock, 1959; Trapnell, 1966; Gillespie, 1973), and there seems to be no change in its incidence. British series have, in the past, been notable for the small number of cases associated with alcoholism; thus, Pollock (1959) was not able to find a single case in a review of 100 cases. The pattern, however, appears to be changing and Imrie (1974) and Gillespie (1973) found 25 and 23 per cent of associated acute pancreatitis and alcoholism in the Glasgow and Edinburgh areas respectively. Steroid pancreatitis also appears to be increasing (Trapnell and Duncan, 1975) presumably because of increasing use of long-term steroid therapy.

Mortality figures in acute pancreatitis are often produced as a percentage of cases diagnosed and treated. Clearly if more cases are diagnosed the apparent mortality may fall without any change in actual mortality, especially if milder forms of the disease are discovered more frequently. These figures may then be incorrectly attributed to improvements in the treatment of the disease. An increased interest in acute pancreatitis has resulted from the introduction of new methods of treatment and this in turn leads to a greater awareness of the condition and to the wider use of serum amylase estimations in acute abdominal emergencies.

The most reliable statistic available is mortality and the overall mortality for England and Wales (Registrar General's *Statistical Review of England and Wales, 1969*) is 11.4 per million of population. It is likely that this mortality varies regionally and recent figures for the Bristol clinical area (Trapnell an Duncan, 1975) give a lower figure of 9.0 per million of the population although the difference is not significant. Of interest was the marked discrepancy between the mortality in the initial attack of acute pancreatitis and in recurrent acute pancreatitis noted by these authors. Expressed in terms of case mortality the figure was 17 per cent compared with 1.5 per cent for the recurrent attacks. As already pointed out a comparison of case mortality figures for different series is of very limited value. Such factors as age, and the type of patient admitted to different hospitals will influence the mortality markedly. Many series from the USA for instance are derived from Veteran Hospitals, or the large 'charity' hospital.

Acute pancreatitis under the age of 50 years is relatively benign (Imrie, 1974); viral pancreatitis as in mumps is also benign. High mortality occurs in the aged, in pancreatitis due to trauma (whether blunt or surgical) and in steroid pancreatitis (Trapnell et al, 1974).

Haemorrhagic pancreatitis occurs in 10 to 25 per cent of all cases, with a death rate of between 40 and 70 per cent (Barraclough and Coupland, 1972). This lethal form of pancreatitis therefore remains a challenge to the efficacy of new therapy which must be judged against the background of the proportion of cases of haemorrhagic pancreatitis in any given series.

PATHOGENESIS AND AETIOLOGY OF ACUTE PANCREATITIS

The distinction formerly made between oedematous pancreatitis, a generally benign disease, and haemorrhagic or necrotic pancreatitis which is a dangerous disease carrying a high mortality, is now considered arbitrary (Glazer, 1975), the latter merely being the result of progression from the oedematous stage in some cases. Autodigestion of the pancreas has been recognised as the basic lesion in acute pancreatitis for many years (Chiari, 1896), and much research has been carried out in attempts to identify the mechanisms involved in bringing about this process.

The question can be approached from the opposite point of view. What are the mechanisms in the pancreas which protect it from digestion by its own formidable array of proteolytic and lipolytic enzymes? Why is acute pancreatitis not an everyday occurrence? A review by Hermon-Taylor (1972) examines this question in detail and enumerates the physiological safeguards normally present. The first and most important step in protein digestion is the activation of proteolytic enzymes by enterokinase in the duodenum. Inactive trypsinogen is converted to trypsin which in turn activates the other proteolytic proenzymes.

As a result of recent experimental studies interest has shifted from trypsin to the part played by other proteolytic enzymes (Creutzfeldt and Schmidt, 1970). Elastase is able to digest elastic fibres in blood vessels and, in the experimental animal, produces changes similar to those seen in clinical haemorrhagic pancreatitis (Geokas, 1968). A high level of elastase has been found in the pancreas in fatal cases of haemorrhagic pancreatitis (Geokas et al, 1968). Kallikrein, one of a group of kinin-forming enzymes, is also activated by trypsin and may, with other substances such as histamine and prostaglandins, play a part in the hypotension and pain of pancreatitis (Ofstad, Amundsen and Hagen, 1969; Glazer and Bennet, 1974).

4

The possibility that lipolytic digestive enzymes play an important part in the pathogenesis of acute pancreatitis was suggested by the morphological appearances of coagulative necrosis. Lipolytic enzyme action depends on the presence of bile acids and this hypothesis assumes bile reflux into the pancreatic duct system. Phospholipase A, long known as a catalyst in venoms, produces lysolecithin from the lecithin in bile. It has been shown to cause pancreatic necrosis in the experimental animal and abnormally high levels of lysolecithin and low levels of lecithin have been found in the human pancreas after acute necrosis at necropsy (Schmidt and Creutzfeldt, 1969).

The difficulty lies in relating the mechanisms described above to the many aetiological factors known to be associated with acute pancreatitis. The following list is not exhaustive but emphasises the wide variety of possible causes of acute pancreatitis:

biliary disease	
alcoholism	
trauma	postoperative (including endoscopic cannulation), blunt abdominal injury
metabolic	hyperlipaemia
	hyperparathyroidism
	hypothermia
drugs	steroids azothioprine
	oestrogens phenformin
	thiazides frusemide
	opiates

pregnancy?
liver disease with fulminating liver failure (Parbhoo, Welch and Sherlock, 1973)
carcinoma of pancreas
scorpion bite (Trinidad)
Ascaris lumbricoides (Schmieden and Sebening, 1928)
mumps
blood dyscrasia (Olsen, 1973)
'idiopathic'

Is there a factor common to such diverse aetiological agents which can adequately explain the autodigestion of acute pancreatitis in the light of mechanisms put forward in the preceding paragraphs? Four main theories have been suggested.

1. Obstructive hypersecretion
2. Duodenal reflux
3. Bile reflux
4. Acinar cell derangement or injury

The evidence against the theory that acute pancreatitis results from active secretion against an obstructed duct has been convincingly summarised by

McCutcheon (1968). Experimentally, pancreatic oedema but not necrosis can be produced (Thal, Perry and Egner, 1957) and deliberate ligation of pancreatic ducts in patients with relapsing pancreatitis has not produced pancreatitis in the postoperative period (Howard and Jordan, 1960). Only in a minority of cases of carcinoma of the pancreas does acute pancreatitis occur.

Duodenal reflux

Reflux of duodenal contents into the pancreatic duct system as a cause of acute pancreatitis has been powerfully argued by McCutcheon (1968). Acute haemorrhagic pancreatitis has been produced in the dog by establishing a closed duodenal loop with reflux of duodenal contents into the duct due to over dilatation of the blind loop (Pfeffer, Stasior and Hinton, 1957). These changes were prevented by ligation of the pancreatic duct (McCutcheon and Race, 1962). Clinical support for this theory is the occurrence of pancreatitis as a complication of afferent loop obstruction after Polya gastrectomy (Wallensten, 1958) and of long arm T tube drainage which, by splinting, prevents closure of the pancreatic and bile ducts (Thompson, Howard and Vowles, 1957). A gallstone impacted at the ampulla could have a similar effect and a recent study in which the faeces of patients suffering from acute pancreatitis were sifted showed the presence of gallstones in 34 of 36 patients (Acosta and Ledesma, 1974). These authors found gallstones in the faeces of only 3 of 36 patients who did not suffer from pancreatitis but were known to have gallstones. The passage of small gallstones usually preceded the relief of pain in pancreatitis. It was concluded that this supported the obstructive theory but the splinting effect of stones holding open the ampulla is equally plausible, underlying the speculative nature of such theories.

Bile reflux

Bile reflux as a cause of acute pancreatitis has a venerable history generally associated with the name of Opie (1901) who formulated the 'common channel' theory. Operative cholangiograms frequently outline part of the pancreatic duct confirming that bile reflux can occur although under physiologically abnormal pressures.

Impaction of a stone at the ampulla of Vater is only found at autopsy in 5 per cent of cases of fatal acute pancreatitis (Wapshaw, 1955) but, as noted above, transient obstruction with the passage of stones into the duodenum is known to occur.

Acinar cell derangement

Alterations in acinar cell structure due to metabolic disturbances have been put forward as a cause of pancreatitis. Histological changes have been demonstrated in rats after prolonged alcohol feeding (Darle, Ekholm and Edlund, 1970). Acute fatty infiltration of acinar cells may be the link between hyperlipaemia and acute pancreatitis. Anoxia and ischaemia may also be a predisposing factor. Vascular damage may result from trauma, and acute pancreatitis associated with venous thrombosis has been reported after accidental hypothermia (Savides and Hoffbrand, 1974).

Some Forms of Pancreatitis of Special Interest

Drugs and pancreatitis

The number of drugs reported incriminated as possible causes of acute pancreatitis is considerable and increasing. They include opiates, steroids (Nelp, 1961), the contraceptive hormones (Davidoff, Tishler and Rosoff, 1973), phenformin (Levitan, 1973), chlorothiazides (Johnston and Cornish, 1959), chlorthalidone (Jones and Caldwell, 1962), Frusemide (Jones and Oelbaum, 1975), and Imuran (Nogueira and Freedman, 1972). Aspirin and anticholinergic drugs have been implicated in postoperative pancreatitis (Gambill, 1973). Various possible explanations for the deleterious effect of these drugs include spasm of the duodenum and sphincter of Oddi (Wapshaw, 1955), gastritis and duodenitis, an increase in gastric acid production, increased viscosity of pancreatic secretions, cellular derangement, impaired blood flow and allergic mechanisms.

Surgery and pancreatitis

The advent of peroral cholangiopancreatography has brought reports of acute pancreatitis following its use (Classen et al, 1973), and fatal cases have been reported. Nevertheless, this method of investigation has been used in relapsing pancreatitis (Cotton and Beales, 1974) and may give useful information.

Pancreatitis has been recorded after a variety of surgical operations, including procedures as remote from the pancreas and as diverse as transurethral resections (Levine, Gambill and Greene, 1962), thyroidectomy, neurosurgical operations, hemicolectomy, appendicectomy, caecostomy, colostomy, femoral embolectomy and caesarean section (Howard and Jordan, 1960). Such cases are rare, and the causes are obscure but probably multiple. Preoperative medication (e.g. morphine), drug treatment of associated disease, electrolyte disturbances and postoperative complications which may lead to capillary stasis or thrombosis, may all play a part.

Operations on the pancreas or adjacent to it are more prone to result in postoperative acute pancreatitis. The risk of this complication is well known after direct biopsy of the pancreas (Schultz and Sanders, 1963; Levine et al, 1962) and (less frequently) after gastric resection. Recent interest has been focused on the incidence of pancreatitis after biliary tract surgery and particularly after operations for common duct calculi. There is general agreement that cholecystectomy alone causes a minimal risk of postoperative pancreatitis (Thompson et al, 1957; Keighley and Graham, 1973).

The controversy centres on the choice of approach in exploration of the common duct, i.e. supraduodenal versus transduodenal. Estimates of the incidence of this complication after exploration of the common bile duct depend on the frequency with which postoperative serum amylase levels are done. Keighley and Graham (1973) showed, in a prospective study, evidence of biochemical pancreatitis in over a third of choledochotomies. They also found clinical pancreatitis with raised serum amylase levels in every case in which sphincterotomy was done at the same time as supraduodenal chole-dochotomy, and recommended that sphincterotomy should be avoided wherever possible. The converse view has been put forward by Peel et al (1975) from the London Hospital who found no case after transduodenal sphincterectomy in 82 patients but recorded one case after supraduodenal exploration (101 patients) and one after the combined approach (26 patients).

The problem is far from academic because the mortality of pancreatitis when it complicates choledochotomy is of the order of 80 per cent (Thompson et al, 1957). Clearly the question remains open but unnecessary exploration and instrumentation of the common bile duct should be avoided and the routine use of operative cholangiograms is helpful in this respect. The exploration should be done with utmost gentleness, long-arm T-tubes should be avoided, and care taken to avoid encroaching on the orifice of the pancreatic duct with sutures.

Hyperlipaemia and pancreatitis

The association of hyperlipaemia and pancreatitis is well established but controversy has surrounded the relationship of one to the other. The classification of hyperlipoproteinaemias (Frederickson, Levy and Lees, 1967) has helped to clarify the significance of hyperlipaemia. Recent prospective studies (Cameron et al, 1973; Farmer et al, 1973) have shed further light on the problem. The latter workers studied 10 patients who suffered from relapsing acute pancreatitis not associated with gallstones or alcohol consumption, and who were found to have hyperlipoproteinaemia (Type V of Frederickson) and chylomicronaemia during the acute attacks. These attacks usually occurred when the serum triglyceride levels were greater than 1000 mg/100 ml. Dietary fat reduction reduced serum lipids to normal levels in five cases and no further attacks of pain occurred, while three other patients were improved. This condition probably occurs more frequently than has been realised and the response to dietary treatment is important. A possible link between alcohol intake and acute pancreatitis is its effect in raising serum triglycerides.

Acute Pancreatitis in Children

Acute pancreatitis in children is rare. The aetiology differs from the condition in adults and cholelithiasis is a rare cause (Moossa, 1972). The commonest variety is the 'idiopathic' group but other predisposing factors include cystic fibrosis, congenital obstruction of the pancreatic or biliary duct, trauma, viral infections such as mumps, hyperlipoproteinaemia, obstruction of pancreatic ducts by worm infestation, drugs notably steroids and the recently described hereditary pancreatitis (Moossa, 1972; Kattwinkel et al, 1973). The latter is an autosomal dominant disorder which tends to run a relapsing course and to be associated with complications such as pseudocyst and calcification. Haemorrhagic pancreatitis is unusual.

Acute pancreatitis must be borne in mind in the differential diagnosis of abdominal pain in children. Mumps pancreatitis presents the special problem that the serum amylase is elevated in some 70 per cent of cases of acute parotitis (Zelman, 1944) and the clinician must not miss other surgical emergencies such as appendicitis by misinterpreting a raised amylase.

Abdominal pain and tenderness in mumps pancreatitis improves within 24 h and laparotomy can thus be avoided (Moossa, 1972). Fortunately the overall mortality of acute pancreatitis in children is low, even in the presence of complications. Recurrence is rare but it is important to investigate the aetiology in order to eliminate any predisposing factors such as hyperlipaemia, or an obstructive lesion.

DIAGNOSIS

In areas of the world where acute pancreatitis is frequent the index of suspicion is high, the clinical picture well known and the diagnosis readily made. The King's County Hospital Centre in New York State, for example, admitted an average of 159 patients per year (Gliedman, Bolooki and Rosen, 1970) suffering from acute pancreatitis and this diagnosis was one of the most common surgical admission diagnoses.

Failure to think of the diagnosis is often due to lack of appreciation of the very variable clinical picture and yet it is this variability which is itself characteristic of acute pancreatitis. No age group is immune and although uncommon in children the diagnosis should be kept in mind.

Acute pancreatitis is generally thought of as a painful surgical emergency but the occasional case presents with little or no pain (Gambill, 1973). The unpredictable site, severity and duration of pain and the inconstant physical signs may suggest common abdominal emergencies such as biliary or renal colic, perforated peptic ulcer, peritonitis or intestinal obstruction or less common conditions such as mesenteric vascular occlusion and ruptured or dissecting aortic aneurisms.

The presence of fever, tachycardia, vomiting, jaundice, rigidity, distension or hypotension are compatible with one or more of these diagnoses. Grey Turner's sign though frequently quoted is rare and late to develop, whilst extensive and early skin bruising is more often seen in ruptured aortic aneurisms (Glazer, 1975).

Extra-abdominal emergencies notably cardiac infarction and pulmonary embolism may be simulated. The latter diagnosis is particularly likely to be made in patients presenting with marked dyspnoea, a feature which has not been sufficiently emphasised in descriptions of the clinical picture.

Postoperative pancreatitis often presents difficulty in diagnosis. The hypovolaemic shock so often seen in such cases may be confused with post-operative peritonitis or haemorrhage or with pulmonary embolism.

Toxic psychosis developing in haemorrhagic pancreatitis during the first or second day of the illness (Gliedman et al, 1970) may be misleading but tends to clear paripassu with improvement in the patient's general condition.

A clinical picture which does not fit the pattern of other abdominal emergencies must alert the clinician to the diagnosis. Fortunately the use of serum amylase as a screening test on admission is becoming acceptable surgical practice.

This and other laboratory tests are discussed more fully below. Many radiological signs have been described but none is diagnostic. The presence of localised ileus adjacent to the inflamed pancreas, the so-called 'sentinel loop' seen in the left mid-abdomen or left upper quadrant is helpful when present, but may be seen in other conditions.

Pancreatic calcification is very uncommon at the first attack of acute pancreatitis. The chest radiograph not infrequently shows basal atelectasis, and a small pleural effusion more commonly on the left side. Radiology is a valuable help in the management of the complications of pancreatitis and the investigation of its aetiology.

From time to time the clinical picture may give serious doubts as to the correct diagnosis even with serum amylase values in excess of 1000 Somogyi units (1800 international units), and conversely acute pancreatitis may not always be accompanied by a raised serum amylase. Laparotomy in these circumstances is the only way of confirming or excluding the diagnosis. Failure to do so and perhaps to miss a strangulating obstruction may cost the patient's life.

Enzyme Tests

Serum amylase

The serum amylase estimation remains the most widely used confirmatory test in the diagnosis of acute pancreatitis but its limitations must be clearly understood. The method has the advantage of being simple and quick to perform and may therefore be carried out as an emergency procedure. Serial estimations are essential and usually the highest concentration is found in the first specimen, the values generally returning to normal from one to six days after the onset. A normal value does not exclude the diagnosis (Janowitz and Dreiling, 1959) and may occasionally be found very early in the course of the disease, or more commonly when there is a delay of 48 h or more in requesting the test. Pancreatic necrosis, severe enough to result in a slough of the whole pancreas has also been associated with almost complete disappearance of amylase activity (Howard and Jordan, 1960).

There is no precise diagnostic level of amylase activity but values greater than five times the upper limit of normal, i.e. 1000 Somogyi units or 1800 international units per litre when taken in conjunction with the clinical picture are regarded as diagnostic, although lower levels are compatible with the diagnosis. The height of the serum amylase level does not correlate well with the severity of the attack nor does it help to distinguish between pancreatic oedema or necrosis (Probstein and Pareira, 1952). The duration of the elevation is of limited value as a guide to progress of the illness. Persistently elevated values in patients with normal renal function may, on the other hand, suggest progressive necrosis or the development of pancreatic collections (Howard and Jordan, 1960).

Elevation of the serum amylase occurs in many conditions other than acute pancreatitis. Acute abdominal emergencies constitute the most important of these in relation to differential diagnosis. Acute cholecystitis, biliary peritonitis, perforated peptic ulcer, intestinal obstruction with strangulation, and afferent loop obstruction after partial gastrectomy may all be associated with elevated serum amylase even reaching values of 1000 Somogyi units (1800 iu/litre) in some cases. High levels giving rise to diagnostic difficulty are most likely to occur in perforated peptic ulcer, biliary peritonitis and afferent loop obstruction. McGowan and Wills (1964) reviewed 119 patients with acute abdominal symptoms and a plasma amylase level of more than 1000 (Somogyi) units per cent, and found that 22 of these (19 per cent) had an acute surgical condition requiring laparotomy. A little over half of these patients had a history of previous gastrectomy and the usual complication was afferent loop obstruction, a condition carrying a high mortality if treated conservatively.

High amylase values have also been found in such diverse conditions as mesenteric arterial thrombosis, ruptured aortic aneurism, acute parotitis and the administration of codein and other opiates in sensitive individuals (Wapshaw, 1955). Mention must also be made of macroamylasaemia (Wilding, Cooke and Nicholson, 1964) a condition in which the amylase, bound to a globulin, produces persistently high serum amylase and low urine amylase levels in the presence of normal renal function (Berk et al, 1967).

Serum lipase

The diagnostic value of elevated serum lipase in acute pancreatitis has been recognised for many years (Comfort, 1937), but has been less widely used than serum amylase determinations because the test has been more complicated to perform. Recent simplified laboratory estimations using a 5 min turbidimetric method have been employed to re-evaluate the place of serum lipase in diagnosis and particularly in comparison with serum amylase (Lifton et al, 1974). These workers carried out simultaneous determinations of serum lipase and amylase in 30 patients suffering from acute pancreatitis; they found that 70 per cent had increased amylase levels, 63 per cent had increased lipase levels, and that 83 per cent had an elevation of one or both. All patients were found to have elevations of either amylase or lipase at some time in the course of the illness. Lipase elevations on the whole ran parallel to the amylase levels though occasionally preceding them. The generally held belief that lipase levels were elevated after serum amylase and that the elevation persisted after the amylase levels had fallen to normal was not found to be true. Serum catalase although not specific, is also elevated in acute pancreatitis (Meszaros, Goth and Vattay, 1973).

Peritoneal tap

The peritoneal exudate which occurs in acute pancreatitis contains pancreatic enzymes in high concentration. Aspiration of this fluid allows examination of its characteristics and the enzyme content can be measured. Red or rusty fluid is obtained in haemorrhagic necrosis and clear, yellow or turbid fluid in oedematous pancreatitis. Pus cells are absent. A refinement of needle aspiration is the use of a dialysis catheter. The raised amylase levels in peritoneal aspirate may persist two or three days after the serum levels have returned to normal (Keith et al, 1950).

Perforated peptic ulcers may also be associated with high peritoneal amylase levels (Amerson et al, 1958) but the fluid is typically bile stained. High amylase values have also been noted in pleural effusions (Coffey, 1952) in acute pancreatitis.

Serum Methaemalbumin

The presence of methaemalbumin in the serum of patients suffering from acute pancreatitis is of value in the differentiation of the haemorrhagic from the oedematous forms of the disease (Northam, Rowe and Winstone, 1963). Ferric haem (methaem or haematin), a breakdown product of haemoglobin, combines with albumin to form methaemalbumin. The latter is also present in the serum in severe intravascular haemolytic states when haemoglobin is liberated in greater quantity than can be absorbed by serum haptoglobin and under these conditions no haptoglobin is present. Methaemalbumin is present in acute haemorrhagic pancreatitis with haptoglobin and in the absence of intravascular haemolysis. It is postulated that the high concentration of locally liberated pancreatic enzymes act on extravasated blood to split haem from the globin and oxidise haem to form ferric haematin which is absorbed into the circulation where it combines with albumin to form methaemalbumin (MHA). The serum of patients suffering from gastrointestinal haemorrhage, haemoperitoneum and retroperitoneal haematoma as well as bowel strangulation has, however, also been found to contain MHA (Battersby and Green, 1971). Bowel strangulation may be confused with acute pancreatitis and in cases of doubt laparotomy may be required. It must be emphasised that the MHA level is not elevated in every case of haemorrhagic pancreatitis.

The estimation of MHA can be done by a non-quantitative method (Schumm's reagent) a spectrometric method if the serum is heavily stained (brown) or an electrophoretic method if the level of MHA is lower. A positive test in acute pancreatitis is associated with an increased mortality (Winstone, 1965).

Other Laboratory Tests

The haemoglobin level and haematocrit are often raised at the onset of the attack as a result of dehydration due to vomiting and ileus. The haemoglobin level may fall during the course of a severe attack because of intrapancreatic and retroperitoneal haemorrhage, sepsis, or less commonly from gastro-intestinal bleeding caused by peptic ulcer, concomitant varices or gastritis. The white cell count follows a similar pattern; an initial high count settles to normal but may rise to 20000 or more in the presence of continued pancreatic necrosis or abscess formation.

Serum bilirubin levels are raised in around a quarter of patients with acute pancreatitis. The elevation is usually modest (4–8 mg/100 ml) and transient. Marked clinical jaundice is more often seen in severe disease and is not necessarily due to stone in the common bile duct. Liver function tests including alkaline phosphatase, enzyme studies and prothrombin time are indicated. The possibility of hepatic cirrhosis in alcoholic pancreatitis must be borne in mind.

The serum fibrinogen level, normal at the onset, rises to a maximum from the fifth to the eighth day of the illness, and returns to normal by the end of the second week in the uncomplicated case (Trapnell, 1966). Persistent elevation after the fourteenth day indicates a severe illness or the onset of complications.

Serum sodium, potassium, chloride, bicarbonate and urea are necessary in the management of the electrolyte disturbances which result from prolonged ileus especially if the illness is complicated by renal failure. Blood-gas analysis and pH estimations are necessary in treating respiratory failure and acid base disturbance. The blood sugar may be moderately or markedly raised in severe acute pancreatitis and fasting blood sugar tests should be done.

Serum calcium

Serum calcium is of particular value as a guide to the severity of acute pancreatitis. The level tends to fall in the course of the illness (Hayes, 1955) but remains above the lower limit of the normal range in the majority of cases. A fall below 8 mg/100 ml is associated with a severe illness and below 7 mg/100 ml the prognosis is very grave (Lilljekvist, 1958). The drop in serum calcium may be diagnostic when serum amylase is not elevated in patients with complete destruction of the pancreas or in those cases seen late in the course of the disease (Edmondson et al, 1952). It is maximal towards the end of the first week (Lipp and Hubbard, 1950).

The association of hyperparathyroidism with acute pancreatitis is well recognised (Mixter, Keynes and Cope, 1962) but the view that hyperparathyroidism precedes pancreatitis has been challenged (Cortes, 1971). In practice serum calcium levels should be estimated after the pancreatitis has subsided to exclude hyperparathyroidism.

The mechanisms concerned in the depression of serum calcium were formerly accepted as resulting from the combination of fatty acids, released by lipolysis, with calcium to form calcium soaps in fat necrosis (Langerhans, 1890). The quantities involved are considerable. The normal pancreas and surrounding fat have been estimated by semiquantitative measurement to contain less than 100 mg of calcium; as a result of acute pancreatitis the amount of calcium deposited (over 1.5 g) may, on occasion, equal or exceed the normal 'circulating' calcium (Edmondson and Fields, 1942).

Hayes (1955) carried out detailed metabolic studies in two patients who developed tetany in the early phase of acute pancreatitis. Both patients, who had serum calcium levels within the normal range, did not respond to intravenous calcium salts but improved at once after treatment with parathyroid hormone. Binding of ionic calcium by fatty acids was suggested by the finding of increased serum levels of fatty acids in both cases. The value of parathyroid hormone was confirmed by Hernandez, Powers and Frawley (1961) and supported by experimental work in dogs.

Glucagon has also been put forward as a factor in the hypocalcaemia of acute pancreatitis (Paloyan et al, 1966). Glucagon may lower the serum calcium either by releasing calcitonin (Pickleman et al, 1969) or directly by inhibiting bone resorption (Stern and Bell, 1970).

Serum magnesium

The serum magnesium level is depressed in some cases of severe acute pancreatitis although much less commonly than the serum calcium (Edmondson et al, 1952). The fall tends to occur in the first four or five days of the disease, to last for only 24 to 48 h, and to bear no relation to the fall in serum calcium.

CLINICAL METHODS

Assessment of severity of illness

The variable clinical presentation of acute pancreatitis is paralleled by similar uncertainty with regard to the outcome of the individual case. Because pain is usually the outstanding feature of the illness its intensity has often been used as the yardstick by which to judge both the severity of the attack and its response to treatment. Unfortunately, in a minority of cases pain does not consistently reflect the progress of the illness and may disappear completely at the same time as the patient's condition deteriorates.

It is also recognised that the degree of the elevation of serum amylase is no criterion of severity of the illness (Howard and Jordan, 1960) neither is the rate of decline an index of improvement.

Trapnell et al (1974) graded the initial severity of the illness according to the presence or absence of vomiting in addition to pain, to the degree and extent of abdominal physical signs, and to the presence or absence of shock, in an attempt to obtain a more accurate guide as to the outcome of the disease. He was forced to conclude, however, 'that the initial estimate of a patient's condition does not give any definite guidance as to the immediate prognosis in an individual case'.

Assessment of the severity of the illness must be based on a number of factors both clinical and laboratory and include duration of paralytic ileus, persistent severe pain, refractory shock, respiratory and renal failure, and septic complications, as well as fall in serum calcium, a low arterial Po_2 and elevated serum methaemalbumin. The presence of one or more of these features usually indicates haemorrhagic or necrotising pancreatitis.

Local complications

The initial local lesion is a large loss of plasma and, in haemorrhagic pancreatitis, of red blood cells. This takes place around the pancreas and in the retroperitoneal tissues and is comparable to the situation in an extensive burn. Management is made difficult by the impossibility of calculating the loss precisely and replacement of the loss will tend to 'leak out' through the damaged capillary bed. Added to this is injury, caused by the enzyme-rich exudate to the neighbouring structures, such as major blood vessels, duodenum, colon and spleen. These lesions account for some of the well-known complications. Thus secondary haemorrhage may occur later and is a common cause of late death in pancreatitis (Howard and Jordan, 1960).

Duodenal obstruction may develop in the third or fourth week as a result of involvement of the duodenum in the inflammatory or necrotic mass and should be suspected in patients, who having recovered from an earlier ileus proceed to develop high intestinal obstruction (Trapnell, 1966). Necrosis of the transverse colon occasionally occurs (Katz, Dorman and Aufses, 1974). Damage to the bowel wall short of necrosis is more frequent and allows bacteria to cross the gut wall leading to endotoxaemia (Fine, 1975). The endotoxaemia in turn contributes to the deterioration in the patient's condition and may lead to further vascular collapse, hypoxia, disseminated intravascular coagulation and haemorrhagic ulceration of the intestinal mucosa.

Jaundice may result from oedema of the pancreatic head compressing the intrapancreatic common bile duct or from a stone in the common bile duct.

Pancreatic fluid collections of greater or lesser extent commonly develop during the first or second weeks in severe pancreatitis and are due to rupture of a pancreatic duct or peritoneal irritation associated with miliary areas of fat necrosis. A high amylase content is present in the fluid.

Pancreatic necrosis may be slow, insidious, but relentlessly progressive over a period of weeks, a smouldering bonfire which consumes not only the major part of the pancreas but wide areas of retroperitoneal tissues and even the mediastinum. Masses of partly digested and necrotic tissue form an excellent nidus for infection. Abscesses may occur anywhere in the upper abdomen and subphrenic regions but especially in the lesser sac and they are often multiple.

Pseudocyst is a well-known complication which appears to be more commonly seen in the alcoholic group (Louw, Marks and Bank, 1967; Sankaran and Walt, 1975). This may lead to further complications such as obstruction, rupture and haemorrhage occurring early in the development of the pseudocyst. Small cysts may be impalpable and yet cause severe symptoms. On the other hand spontaneous regression occurred in 8 per cent in one series (Sankarand and Walt, 1975). Pseudocysts may be multiple.

SYSTEMIC COMPLICATIONS

The shock state of pancreatitis does not always respond to replacement therapy despite large volumes of fluid, electrolyte, plasma, plasma substitute and blood. This has been attributed to the release into the blood stream of vasoactive substances, such as kallikrein and bradykinin, and experimental work has shown beneficial effects of the trypsin and kallikrein inhibitor Trasylol (Kune, 1968). The clinical applications are discussed later.

Recent studies have focused on respiratory failure in acute pancreatitis. Ransom, Roses and Fink (1973) found arterial hypoxia (with a Po_2 below 77 mmHg) in more than half of a group of 40 unselected patients suffering from acute pancreatitis. The fall tended to occur within the first few days of the illness, with lowest levels of arterial oxygen occurring between the second and fourth days.

In the course of a prospective study Imrie and his coworkers (1975) found that 67 of 84 patients with acute pancreatitis developed arterial Po_2 levels of less than 70 mmHg during the first five days of admission without operation. All six deaths occurred in this group. Matched controls not suffering from acute pancreatitis were found to have a significantly lower incidence of arterial hypoxia (41 per cent). They suggest that measurement of the arterial Po_2 is of prognostic significance and were able to show that treatment with humidified oxygen reversed the hypoxia and was associated with a downward trend in mortality, particularly in the older patients.

The causes of this hypoxia appear to be multiple and include pleural effusion (more often left sided), atelectasis, diaphragmatic elevation and 'splinting', pulmonary oedema and microembolism, loss of pulmonary surfactant (which may be associated with elevated levels of serum lecithinase (Zieve and Vogel, 1960)) and intravascular coagulation. Imrie and his associates showed a high incidence of abnormalities on chest x-ray, of ventilation perfusion defects with right to left shunts and elevated levels of fibrin degradation products.

Renal failure is another important factor contributing to the mortality of acute pancreatitis (Gliedman et al, 1970; Gordon and Calne, 1972). Loss of fluid and electrolytes and associated hypovolaemic shock are perhaps only part of the story and Thal et al (1957) noted 10 deaths with anuria but without preceding shock in a study of 42 fatal cases.

The toxic products of pancreatic autodigestion such as vasoactive polypeptides may play an important part.

Other systemic complications

Cardiopathy. Severe upper abdominal or retrosternal pain, shock and changes in the electrocardiogram simulating coronary artery occlusion are seen in some patients (Gottesman, Casten and Beller, 1943). The electrocardiogram reverts to normal as the patient improves. The picture can be explained on the basis of a toxic myocarditis (Gliedman et al, 1970).

Encephalopathy. Toxic encephalopathy manifested by agitation or stupor must be differentiated from delirium tremens in alcoholic patients. It is usually the result of cerebral anoxia and this diagnosis must be supported by blood gas analysis.

Diabetes. Although relatively common in chronic pancreatitis this complication is rarer in acute pancreatitis and usually takes the form of transient hyperglycaemia and glycosuria which subsides often without the need to use insulin.

Metastatic fat necrosis is unusual but is occasionally found in such sites as subcutaneous fat, usually of the lower anterior shin, and also in bone (Louw et al, 1967).

THE MANAGEMENT OF ACUTE PANCREATITIS

The initial management of acute pancreatitis is directed towards the treatment of shock, the inhibition of vasoactive materials and the prevention and treatment of respiratory, renal and metabolic complications. Later, the emphasis shifts to the treatment of sepsis and its complications and to the effects of destruction of pancreatic tissue, including the treatment of pseudocysts; the latter subjects relate more often to cases of chronic pancreatitis. Equally important is the investigation of the aetiology of the individual attack with a view to the elimination of any predisposing causes of further attacks.

Medical Measures

Shock

Shock is an index (inter alia) of a severe attack of pancreatitis and, even if absent initially, its onset may be anticipated by a raised haematocrit (Louw et al, 1967). Thirty to forty per cent of the blood volume may be lost and considerable red blood cell destruction may also occur. Fluid, electrolyte and plasma expanders will be required in considerable quantities. Ringer lactate or sodium bicarbonate may be necessary to counteract metabolic acidosis. Blood should form up to half the total replacement fluid volume in haemorrhagic pancreatitis.

The effect of these measures is assessed by serial recordings of the central venous pressure, the systemic blood pressure, urine volume and specific gravity, haematocrit, haemoglobin, electrolytes and acid-base studies. Persistent hypotension in the presence of a rising or elevated central venous pressure indicates cardiac failure and should be treated by digitalisation.

Isoprenaline (monitored by continuous ECG tracing) may be of value (Louw et al, 1967). The use of corticosteroids is controversial and, in view of the fact that pancreatitis may be the result of steroid therapy (Nelp, 1961), not without risk.

Respiratory failure

The presence of cyanosis, or increase in the respiratory effort or rate may be obvious. These signs may not be present and hypoxia may result in psychosis and mislead the clinician. The early detection of respiratory failure requires blood-gas analysis. Humidified oxygen is administered if the Po_2 falls below 70 mmHg in younger patients and is recommended in all patients over 60 years of age (Imrie et al, 1975). Atelectasis is treated by energetic physiotherapy aided by bronchoscopic suction if necessary. Diuretics are given for pulmonary oedema and pleural effusions are aspirated. The most severe cases are characterised by enormous increases in respiratory work and consequent oxygen requirements, and these patients require positive pressure respiration and tracheostomy (Gliedman et al, 1970).

Renal failure

Careful records of urinary output are essential and any suspicion of oliguria suggests the need for catheterisation. Should the hourly urine flow fall below 30 ml/h, despite adequate fluid replacement as judged by central venous pressure, mannitol or frusemide is given. Failure to respond to these measures and a rise in blood urea above 100 mg/100 ml, indicate the need for dialysis (Gordon and Calne, 1972).

Haemodialysis, although more efficient in the treatment of renal failure is potentially hazardous, and haemorrhage may result from the heparin used.

Peritoneal dialysis has the merit of 'washing out' pancreatic enzymes and vasoactive substances, produced by autodigestion of the pancreas and neighbouring tissues, from the peritoneal cavity (Wall, 1965). It is safer, simpler and more generally available than haemodialysis, and has been advocated in severe pancreatitis unresponsive to therapy, even in the absence of renal failure (Gliedman et al, 1970).

Other complications

Ileus is treated by nasogastric suction and intravenous infusion, with parenteral feeding if it is prolonged.

Hypocalcaemia is treated with 10 per cent calcium gluconate intravenously. Parathyroid hormone is given in the rare patient who does not respond to calcium gluconate. Hypomagnesaemia is rarely seen and is treated with 25 per cent magnesium sulphate intramuscularly. Persistent hyperglycaemia or ketosis, a rare event, requires insulin (Glazer, 1975).

Coagulation abnormalities possibly due to antithrombins or increased fibrinolysis may develop and contribute to haemorrhage in the retroperitoneal tissues or from the gastrointestinal tract. Disseminated intravascular coagulation is occasionally seen. Treatment including vitamin K, fibrinogen, epsicapron, trasylol, fresh-frozen plasma or fresh blood may be required depending on the specific haematological defect.

Trasylol

The difficulties inherent in evaluating the efficacy of treatment in acute pancreatitis are well shown by the history of the drug Trasylol. A polypeptide of low molecular weight isolated from the parotid glands of cattle, Trasylol was introduced by Frey, Kraut and Werle (1950) as a proteolytic enzyme inhibitor active against trypsin and kallikrein. Since the late 1950s there have been many reports of its use in clinical acute pancreatitis. Evidence of benefit in experimental pancreatitis contrasts, however, with variable clinical results. Much of this work has been criticised (Trapnell et al, 1974) because numbers were small (Almgren et al, 1965; Skyring, Singer and Tornya, 1965), the clinical material was variable (Bachrach and Schild, 1968) and included recurrent pancreatitis; and treatment schedules were not comparable as variable doses of Trasylol were used. The work of Moshal et al (1963) and Goldberg and Roy (1965) suggested that many previous results were likely to be invalid because the dose of Trasylol used had been too low.

A recent strictly controlled double blind trial (Trapnell et al, 1974) has aimed at overcoming these difficulties, and has renewed interest in Trasylol. There were 105 patients with idiopathic or gall bladder pancreatitis in their first attack. The treatment schedule consisted of Trasylol 200000 units initially, followed by 200000 units six-hourly intravenously given for five days. Objective criteria were used to classify the severity of the illness and treatment schedules were uniform, except that patients received either Trasylol or a placebo. A statistically significant difference in mortality was found between the Trasylol treated group (7.5 per cent) and the controls (25 per cent). This was largely due to reduction in the raised mortality usually found in patients above 50 years of age.

Glucagon

A more recent addition to the drug treatment of acute pancreatitis, glucagon was introduced as a result of observations on its effect in pancreatic fistulae (Knight, Condon and Smith, 1971). Isolated from crude preparations of insulin (Kimball and Murlin, 1924) and purified in 1953 (Staub, Sinn and Behrens), its role in human physiology is still not clear (Bloom, 1975) although a good deal is known of its pharmacology (Lefebvre and Unger, 1972). Experimental work in dogs with pancreatic fistulae has shown that it depresses the rate of flow, volume, and enzyme concentration in the pancreozymin/secretin stimulated pancreas (Dyck et al, 1969; Nakajima and Magee, 1970). Similar observations have been made in human subjects by Dyck et al (1970) who postulated a regulatory role for glucagon in the control of pancreatic exocrine secretion. Other gastrointestinal actions some of which could be indirectly beneficial in acute pancreatitis include suppression of gastric secretion in man (Dreiling and Janowitz, 1959), inhibition of gastric and jejunal mobility (Stunkard, Van Itallie and Reis, 1955), and relaxation of duodenal musculature (Chernish, Miller and Rosenak, 1972). Blood flow in the coeliac axis is also greatly increased.

The most important metabolic effect is the release of liver glycogen to raise blood glucose but pituitary hormones and catechol amines are also released and the force of cardiac contraction is increased (Bloom, 1975). Endogenous glucagon is released in conditions of stress by the sympathetic nervous system (Bloom, Edwards and Vaughan, 1973) and elevated levels have been found during and until the fourth day after laparotomy (Walker, Russell and Bloom, 1974). Experimental non-fatal pancreatitis is accompanied by raised glucagon levels (Paloyan et al, 1966) which falls during the progression to fatal haemorrhagic pancreatitis (Knight, Condon and Day, 1972). The last named workers also found a relative hyperglucagonaemia in mild clinical acute pancreatitis but low plasma glucagon levels in severe haemorrhagic pancreatitis. They speculated that endogenous glucagon might, by inhibiting pancreatic exocrine secretion, retard or prevent progression from mild to haemorrhagic pancreatitis. Failure of this mechanism as shown by low plasma glucagon levels would allow pancreatitis to progress.

The evidence that glucagon is effective in the treatment of clinical acute pancreatitis is still scanty although relief of pain and clinical improvement was noted in 30 patients by Condon, Knight and Day (1973). Only two patients died in this small series but firm proof of efficacy in lowering mortality awaits a controlled trial which is currently under way. Relief of pain is often rapid and dramatic and has been studied in some detail by Waterworth and

Bevan (1975). They obtained complete relief of pain in 21 of 30 patients given glucagon with marked reduction in a further six. Formal analgesia was only required in eight patients.

The glucagon regime consists in 1 mg intravenously followed by an intravenous infusion of 1 to 1.5 mgs every 4 h in 5 per cent dextrose or normal saline given for 24 to 96 h (Condon et al, 1973). Side effects are few though nausea or vomiting may occur with large doses and hypocalcaemia has been reported (Paloyan, Paloyan and Harper, 1967).

Other drugs

Suppression of pancreatic secretion is theoretically desirable in acute pancreatitis but little data is available on secretion during the attack and it is possible that the pancreas is 'shut down'. The traditional drugs used are anticholinergics. They have not been shown to be of benefit (Trapnell, 1966) and tend to accentuate paralytic ileus, aggravate hypotension and precipitate urinary retention in the elderly. Propylthiouracil and acetazolamide have also been advocated (Welch and Montanez, 1965) but their value is not established.

Pethidine should be used to control pain but morphia and its derivatives are contraindicated (Wapshaw, 1955).

Antibiotics are logical in the treatment of associated biliary tract or respiratory infection but Trapnell (1966) did not find that they prevented the late septic complications.

THE PLACE OF SURGERY

Laparotomy

Laparotomy may precede or follow the diagnosis of acute pancreatitis. At the present time the increased interest in, and awareness of, pancreatitis and the more frequent use of enzyme tests and of peritoneal fluid aspiration should reduce to a minimum the number of occasions on which pancreatitis is a totally unexpected finding.

There remain, however, instances where the diagnosis is suspected but to avoid laparotomy would expose the patient to the unacceptable risk of missing, for example, a strangulated intestinal obstruction. The widely held view that diagnostic laparotomy, though undesirable, does not materially add to the mortality of acute pancreatitis (Trapnell, 1966; Louw et al, 1967) has recently been challenged (Imrie and Whyte, 1975). They report a 46 per cent mortality in patients subjected to laparotomy compared with 6 per cent for patients managed conservatively, and suggest as a possible explanation the increase in respiratory complications leading to hypoxia. These factors are particularly important in the elderly whose respiratory function may be impaired as a result of bronchitis or emphysema. It must, however, be recognised that the more severe case of acute pancreatitis, who already has a poorer prognosis, is more likely to undergo laparotomy and so to swell the mortality in this group. Morbidity of the procedure includes a high incidence of burst abdomen (Trapnell, 1972).

The findings at laparotomy determine the further measures to be adopted. Haemorrhagic pancreatitis without necrosis requires only peritoneal toilet but it is reasonable to leave catheters in situ to enable peritoneal lavage to be continued postoperatively (Rosato, Mullis and Rosato, 1973).

Fine judgement is called for in the presence of biliary disease. The need for dealing with the biliary pathology must be weighed against the hazards of a more prolonged procedure in an ill patient. The severity of the local changes in the pancreas and the general condition of the patient must be carefully assessed. In the one case biliary tract disease may predominate, with acute inflammation or obstruction and yet a mild oedematous pancreatitis, whilst in another severe haemorrhagic pancreatitis may be associated with long-standing stones in an uninflamed gall bladder.

An acutely inflamed gall bladder will require cholecystostomy with, if possible, removal of stones within the gall bladder, or cholecystectomy if conditions are favourable. Gallstones in an uninflamed gall bladder are best left and definitive cholecystectomy postponed until recovery from the acute pancreatitis. Should stones be present in the common bile duct, particularly in the presence of jaundice, cautious exploration of the common bile duct is reasonable with removal of mobile stones where the patient's condition permits. Instrumentation of the ampulla is, however, fraught with danger and any procedures in this area should be avoided (Louw et al, 1967; Trapnell, 1972).

A recent case seen by the author illustrates some of the problems. An elderly lady suffering from biliary colic due to gallstones was found at operation to have several stones in the common bile duct and also to have fat necrosis due to pancreatitis.

Gentle exploration of the common bile duct and removal of several gallstones was performed but no instruments were passed into the ampullary region for fear of reactivating her pancreatitis.

Postoperation T-tube cholangiogram showed, not unexpectedly, at least three small residual stones in the lower end of the common bile duct.

Dissolution of the stones was attempted using sodium cholate (Way, Admirand and Dunphy, 1972). Her serum amylase, however, rose to 2000 Somogyi units (3600 iu/litre) at the onset of treatment; further instillation of sodium cholate was then accompanied by glucagon and the amylase level fell to normal level. She did not complain of pain during this procedure, and the final T-tube cholangiogram showed complete disappearance of the stones.

The failure to respond to conservative treatment and the progressive unremitting deterioration seen in a minority of cases of severe pancreatitis have prompted a few surgeons, particularly on the continent, to adopt a more radical approach. A French group, Guivarch, et al (1972) reported 20 cases of necrotising pancreatitis treated by excision. The majority were subjected to subtotal, left to right pancreatectomy preserving a remnant of the head adjacent to the duodenum and termination of the common bile duct. Other cases were treated by partial excision of the body and tail, the head, or by total pancreatectomy, according to the site and extent of necrosis. The mortality in the whole group was 50 per cent and the formidable list of complications included further necrosis of the pancreatic remnant, abscess formation in the remaining pancreas, left upper abdomen or abdominal wall external pancreatic fistulae, gastric or intestinal fistulae, septicaemia and haemorrhage, the latter complication causing death in seven patients.

In this country Watts (1963) reported recovery after total pancreatectomy for a case of fulminant pancreatitis, and commented on the rapid recovery after operation. However, the grave clinical condition of these patients and

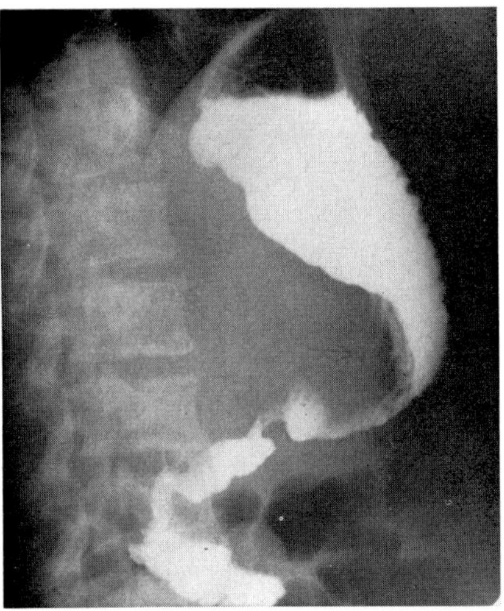

Figure 4.1   A pancreatic abscess. The stomach is displaced forward and there is indentation of the posterior wall and of the antrum by a soft tissue swelling

the extent of the surgical procedure required are likely to deter most surgeons.

Abscess formation, the result of progressive necrosis of the pancreas and adjacent retroperitoneal tissues, presents as a mass, with persistent or recurrent fever towards the end of the second week of the illness or later. The patient's condition fails to improve or deteriorates after an interval and leucocytosis is often found. Radiography of the abdomen supplemented by barium contrast studies show forward displacement of the stomach, an increased distance between stomach and transverse colon or widening of the duodenal loop (Fig. 4.1). Multiple gas bubbles may be seen in the area of the lesser sac. Surgical drainage is required with emphasis on careful exploration, thorough débridement and wide drainage, because of the extent of necrosis often found. Abscess cavities burrow deep to the small bowel mesentery or above the diaphragm and into the mediastinum. Large areas or even the whole pancreas may be totally necrotic. Exposure is facilitated by mobilisation of the hepatic and splenic flexures. Small abscesses or ascitic fluid collections are drained by separate stab wounds using rubber tube or corrugated drains, but larger collections are best marsupialised and packed (Gliedman et al, 1970).

Pancreatic pseudocysts generally require surgical treatment; although spontaneous regression occurs in a minority of cases, complications such as rupture, obstruction of adjacent structures and haemorrhage are relatively frequent, dangerous and unpredictable (Sankaran and Walt, 1975). Surgical intervention should be delayed in order to allow the cyst wall to become thick enough to permit internal drainage. The cyst may be drained into the stomach, duodenum or jejunum depending on the location of the cyst.

Pancreatography either preoperatively by fibreoptic endoscopy or at operation, is of value where localisation of the cyst is uncertain particularly in the presence of pancreatic ascites, and in the demonstration of abnormalities in the duct system. (Sankaran and Walt, 1975). Multiple pseudocysts may also be found (Anderson, 1972). Ultrasound scans are also being employed to localise pseudocysts and are likely to find increasing application in the future as the accuracy of the technique improves.

RECURRENT ACUTE PANCREATITIS

Detailed evidence on the risk of recurrence facing patients who recover from an initial attack of acute pancreatitis is presented by Trapnell and Duncan (1975) from their review of 590 cases in the Bristol clinical area over a 20 year period. Of 430 survivors traced (eight were lost to follow-up), 133 had a total of 261 recurrent attacks, but only four of these died.

Eighty-eight patients in the gallstone group (which comprised 232 patients) had recurrent attacks and 36 of these were awaiting cholecystectomy. Several patients had long gaps of 10 to 15 years between attacks with no symptoms during the interval.

The idiopathic group, which comprised 148 patients, had a 10 per cent likelihood of recurrence within the first year after the initial attack, and a 25 per cent chance of a second attack within six years.

Alcoholic pancreatitis tends to progress to the chronic forms of the disease unless the patient is able to stop drinking, but Trapnell and Duncan (1975) describe 10 patients who appeared to be suffering from recurrent acute pancreatitis.

Prevention of further attacks

Iatrogenic disease is on the increase in many fields of medicine and pancreatitis is no exception. A careful history of drug taking will discover or eliminate drugs known to be associated with acute pancreatitis; the most widely used are the steroid group, the contraceptive hormones and thiazide diuretics. Alcohol intake may not be admitted by the patient but may be suspected from clinical appearances or from the occupational or social circumstances.

Biochemical investigations after recovery from the initial attack should include the serum lipoprotein and lipid pattern, serum calcium and phosphorus and, where indicated, further investigations to exclude the rare case of hyperparathyroidism.

The diagnosis of gallstones in relapsing pancreatitis by oral cholecystography generally presents no difficulty. The exception is the patient with a doubtful small stone at the lower end of the common bile duct and a normal gall bladder. Intravenous cholangiography aided by tomography usually resolve the difficulty but in equivocal cases endoscopic retrograde cholangiography may help (Cotton and Beales, 1974).

Where further attacks of acute pancreatitis occur and all investigations are negative endoscopic cannulation of the pancreatic duct (ERCP) should be considered; in experienced centres the success rate of this manoeuvre is around 90 per cent. Obstruction, stricture or pseudocyst have been found in approximately half the cases investigated (Cotton and Beales, 1974). Failure to obtain pancreatograms may be due to obstruction of the pancreatic duct close to the papilla. Surgery may be planned on the results but further follow-up will be needed to assess the results. The procedure is contraindicated during an attack of acute pancreatitis and is not free of risk of precipitating a further attack particularly in patients with pseudocyst.

REFERENCES

Acosta, J. M. & Ledesma, C. L. (1974) Gallstone migration as a cause of acute pancreatitis. *New England Journal of Medicine*, **290**, 484–487.

Almgren, K. G., Edlund, Y., Norback, B. & Gelin, L. E. (1965) Trypsin-inhibitor (Trasylol) in acute pancreatitis—a double blind study. *Bulletin International de la Société des Chirurgiens*, **14**, 356–365.

Amerson, R., Howard, J. M. & Vowles, K. D. J. (1958) Amylase concentration in serum and peritoneal fluid in patients with acute perforations of gastroduodenal ulcers. *Annals of Surgery*, **147**, 245–250.

Anderson, M. D. (1972) Management of pancreatic pseudocysts. *American Journal of Surgery*, **123**, 209–221.

Bachrach, W. H. & Schild, P. D. (1968) A double blind study of Trasylol in the treatment of pancreatitis. *Annals of the New York Academy of Science*, **146**, 540–549.

Barraclough, B. H. & Coupland, G. A. E. (1972) Acute pancreatitis; a review. *Australian and New Zealand Journal of Surgery*, **41**, 211–218.

Battersby, C. & Green, M. K. (1971) The surgical significance of methaemalbuminaemia. *Gut*, **12**, 995–1000.

Berk, J. E., Kizu, H., Wilding, P. & Searcy, R. L. (1967) Macro-amylasemia—a newly recognised cause for elevated serum amylase activity. *New England Journal of Medicine*, **277**, 941–946.

Bloom, S. R. (1975) Glucagon. *British Journal of Hospital Medicine*, **13**, 150–158.

Bloom, S. R., Edwards, A. V. & Vaughan, N. J. A. (1973) The role of the sympathetic innervation in the control of plasma glucagon concentration in the calf. *Journal of Physiology*, **233**, 457–466.

Bockus, H. L. (1965) In *Gastroenterology* 2nd edn, Vol. 3, p. 999. Philadelphia and London: W. B. Saunders Company.

Cameron, J. L., Capuzzi, D. M., Zuidema, G. D. & Margolis, S. (1973) Acute pancreatitis with hyperlipaemia. *Annals of Surgery*, **177**, 483–489.

Chernish, S. M., Miller, R. E. & Rosenak, B. D. (1972) Hypotonic duodenography with the use of glucagon. *Gastroenterology*, **63**, 392–398.

Chiari, H. (1896) Uber die Selbst verdauung des menschlichen Pankreas. *Zeitschrift für Heilkunde*, **17**, 69–96.

Classen, M., Koch, H., Ruskin, H., Pesch, H. J. & Demling, L. (1973) Pancreatitis after endoscopic retrograde pancreatography. *Gut*, **14**, 431.

Coffey, R. J. (1952) Unusual features of acute pancreatic disease. *Annals of Surgery*, **135**, 715–720.

Comfort, M. W. (1937) Serum lipase: its diagnostic value. *American Journal of Digestive Disease*, **3**, 817–821.

Condon, J. R., Knight, M. J. & Day, J. L. (1973) Glucagon therapy in acute pancreatitis. *British Journal of Surgery*, **60**, 509–511.

Condon, J. R., Ives, D., Knight, M. J. & Day, J. (1975) The aetiology of hypocalcaemia in acute pancreatitis. *British Journal of Surgery*, **62**, 115–118.

Cortes, E. P. (1971) Pancreatitis and calcium metabolism. *Annals of Internal Medicine*, **74**, 1014.

Cotton, P. B. & Beales, J. S. M. (1974) Endoscopic pancreatography in management of relapsing acute pancreatitis. *British Medical Journal*, **1**, 608–611.

Creutzfeldt, W. & Schmidt, H. (1970) Aetiology and pathogenesis of pancreatitis (current concepts) *Scandinavian Journal of Gastro-enterology*, Suppl. **6**, 47–62.

Darle, N., Ekholm, R. & Edlund, Y. (1970) Ultrastructure of the rat exocrine pancreas after a long-term intake of ethanol. *Gastroenterology*, **58**, 62–72.

Davidoff, F., Tishler, S. & Rosoff, C. (1973) Marked hyperlipidaemia and pancreatitis associated with oral contraceptive therapy. *New England Journal of Medicine*, **289**, 552–555.

Dreiling, D. A. & Janowitz, H. D. (1959) The effect of glucagon on gastric secretion in man. *Gastroenterology*, **36**, 580–581.

Dyck, W. P., Rudick, J., Hoexter, B. & Janowitz, H. D. (1969) Influence of glucagon on pancreatic exocrine secretion. *Gastroenterology*, **56**, 531–537.

Dyck, W. P., Texter, E. C., Lasater, J. M. & Hightower, N. C. (1970) Influence of glucagon on pancreatic exocrine secretion in man. *Gastroenterology*, **58**, 532–539.

Edmondson, H. A. & Fields, I. (1942) Relation of calcium and lipids to acute pancreatic necrosis. *Archives of Internal Medicine*, **69**, 177–190.

Edmondson, H. A., Berne, C. J., Homann, R. E. & Wertman, M. (1952) Calcium, potassium, magnesium and amylase disturbances in acute pancreatitis. *American Journal of Medicine*, **12**, 34–42.

Farmer, R. G., Winkelman, E. I., Brown, H. B. & Lewis, L. A. (1973) Hyperlipoproteinaemia and pancreatitis. *American Journal of Medicine*, **54**, 161–165.

Fine, J. (1975) Acute pancreatitis. *Lancet*, **1**, 1092.

Frederickson, D. S., Levy, R. I. & Lees, R. S. (1967) Fat transport in lipoproteins: an integrated approach to mechanisms and disorders. *New England Journal of Medicine*, **276**, 34, 94, 148, 215 and 273.

Frey, E. K., Kraut, H. & Werle, E. (1950) *Kallikrein* (*Glumorin*). Stuttgart: Ferd. Enke.

Gambill, E. E. (1973) Etiology and mechanisms of pancreatitis. In *Pancreatitis*, p. 63. St Louis: C. V. Mosby Co.

Geokas, M. C. (1968) The role of elastase in acute pancreatic tissue in vivo and in vitro. *Archives of Pathology*, **86**, 135–141.

Geokas, M. C., Rinderknecht, H., Swanson, V. & Haverback, B. (1968) The role of elastase in acute haemorrhagic pancreatitis in man. *Laboratory Investigation*, **19**, 235–239.

Gillespie, W. J. (1973) Observations on acute pancreatitis. *British Journal of Surgery*, **60**, 63–65.

Glazer, G. (1975) Haemorrhagic and necrotising pancreatitis. *British Journal of Surgery*, **62**, 169–176.

Glazer, G. & Bennet, A. (1974) Elevation of prostaglandin-like activity in the blood and peritoneal exudate of dogs with acute pancreatitis. *British Journal of Surgery*, **61**, 922.

Gliedman, M. L., Bolooki, H. & Rosen, R. G. (1970) Acute pancreatitis. *Current Problems in Surgery*, August. Chicago: Year Book Medical Publishers.

Goldberg, D. M. & Roy, A. D. (1965) Trasylol and acute pancreatitis. *British Medical Journal*, **2**, 943–944.

Gordon, D. & Calne, R. Y. (1972) Renal failure in acute pancreatitis. *British Medical Journal*, **2**, 801–802.

Gottesman, J., Casten, D. & Beller, A. J. (1943) Changes in electrocardiogram induced by acute pancreatitis: clinical and experimental study. *Journal of the American Medical Association*, **123**, 892–894.

Guivarch, M., Beaufils, F., Neury, N., Marquand, J. & Mouchet, A. (1972) Excisional surgery in necrotic pancreatitis. *Journal de Chirurgie (Paris)*, **103**, 479–492.

Hayes, M. A. (1955) A disturbance in calcium metabolism leading to tetany occurring early in acute pancreatitis. *Annals of Surgery*, **142**, 346–350.

Hermon-Taylor, J. (1972) The exocrine pancreas. In *The Scientific Basis of Surgery* 2nd edn, ed. Irvine, W. T., pp. 135–157. Edinburgh: Churchill Livingstone.

Hernandez, I. A., Powers, S. R. & Frawley, T. F. (1961) The role of the parathyroid glands in calcium and magnesium metabolism in acute haemorrhagic pancreatitis. *Surgery*, **50**, 143–150.

Howard, J. M. & Jordan, G. L. (1960) *Surgical Diseases of the Pancreas*. Philadelphia: Lippincott.

Imrie, C. W. (1974) Observations on acute pancreatitis. *British Journal of Surgery*, **61**, 539–544.

Imrie, C. W. & Whyte, A. S. (1975) A prospective study of acute pancreatitis. *British Journal of Surgery*, **62**, 490–494.

Imrie, C. W., Murphy, D., Ferguson, J. C. & Blumgart, L. H. (1975) Arterial hympoxia in acute pancreatitis. Inaugural meeting of the Pancreatic Society of Great Britain and Ireland.

Janowitz, H. D. & Dreiling, D. A. (1959) The plasma amylase. Source, regulation and diagnostic significance. *American Journal of Medicine*, **27**, 924–935.

Johnston, D. H. & Cornish, A. L. (1959) Acute pancreatitis in patients receiving chlorothiazide. *Journal of the American Medical Association*, **170**, 2054.

Jones, M. F. & Caldwell, J. R. (1962) Acute haemorrhagic pancreatitis associated with administration of chlorthalidone. *New England Journal of Medicine*, **267**, 1029–1031.

Jones, P. E. & Oelbaum, M. H. (1975) Frusemide-induced pancreatitis. *British Medical Journal*, **1**, 133–134.

Kattwinkel, J., Lapey, A., di Sant' Agnese, P. A., Edwards, W. A., & Hufty, M. P. (1973) Hereditary pancreatitis. Review article, *Paediatrics*, **51**, 55–69.

Katz, P., Dorman, M. J. & Aufses, A. H. (1974) Colonic necrosis complicating post-operative pancreatitis. *Annals of Surgery*, **179**, 403–405.

Keighley, M. R. B. & Graham, N. G. (1973) The aetiology and prevention of pancreatitis following biliary-tract operations. *British Journal of Surgery*, **60**, 149–152.

Keith, L. M., Zollinger, R. N. & McCleary, R. S. (1950) Peritoneal fluid amylase determinations as an aid in diagnosis of acute pancreatitis. *Archives of Surgery*, **61**, 930–936.

Kimball, C. P. & Murlin, J. R. (1924) Aquious extracts of pancreas. *Journal of Biological Chemistry*, **58**, 337–346.

Knight, M. J., Condon, J. R. & Smith, R. (1971) Possible use of glucagon in the treatment of pancreatitis. *British Medical Journal*, **1**, 440–442.

Knight, M. J., Condon, J. R. & Day, J. L. (1972) Possible role of glucagon in pathogenesis of acute pancreatitis. *Lancet*, **1**, 1097–1099.

Kune, G. A. (1968) The treatment of experimentally induced acute pancreatitis. *Australian and New Zealand Journal of Surgery*, **38**, 150–153.

Langerhans, R. (1890) Uber multiple fettgewebsnekrose. *Virchows Archiv für pathologische anatomie*, **122**, 252–270.

Lefebvre, P. J. & Unger, R. H. (1972) *Glucagon*. Oxford: Pergamon Press.

Levine, S. R., Gambill, E. E. & Greene, L. F. (1962) Acute pancreatitis following trans-urethral prostatic resection: report of six cases. *Journal of Urology*, **88**, 657–663.

Levitan, A. A. (1973) Phenformin and pancreatitis. *Annals of Internal Medicine*, **78**, 306–307.

Levitt, M. D., Rapoport, M. & Cooperband, S. R. (1969) The renal clearance of amylase in renal insufficiency, acute pancreatitis and macroamylasemia. *Annals of Internal Medicine*, **71**, 919–925.

Lifton, L. J., Slickers, K. A., Pragay, D. A. & Katz, L. A. (1974) Pancreatitis and lipase. A re-evaluation with a five minute turbimetric determination. *Journal of the American Medical Association*, **229**, 47–50.

Lilljekvist, R. E. (1958) Hypocalcemia and the diagnosis of acute pancreatitis. *Acta chirurgica scandinavica*, **115**, 433–446.

Lipp, W. F. & Hubbard, R., (1950) The serum calcium in acute pancreatitis. *Gastroenterology*, **16**, 726–730.

Louw, J. H., Marks, I. N. & Bank, S. (1967) The management of severe acute pancreatitis. *Post-graduate Medical Journal*, **43**, 31–44.

McCutcheon, A. D. (1968) A fresh approach to the pathogenesis of pancreatitis. *Gut*, **9**, 296–310.

McCutcheon, A. D. & Race, D. (1962) Experimental pancreatitis: a possible aetiology of post-operative pancreatitis. *Annals of Surgery*, **155**, 523–531.

McGowan, G. K. & Wills, M. R. (1964) Diagnostic value of plasma amylase, especially after gastrectomy. *British Medical Journal*, **1**, 160–162.

Meszaros, I., Goth, L. & Vattay, G. Y. (1973) The value of scrum catalase activity determina-tions in acute pancreatitis. *American Journal of Digestive Disease*, **18**, 1035–1041.

Mixter, C. G., Keynes, W. M. & Cope, O. (1962) Further experience with pancreatitis as a diagnostic clue to hyperparathyroidism. *New England Journal of Medicine*, **266**, 265–272.

Moossa, A. R. (1972) Acute pancreatitis in childhood. In *Progress in Paediatric Surgery*, **4**, 111–127.

Moshal, M. C., Marks, I. N., Bank, S. & Ford, D. A. (1963) A trial of Trasylol in the treat-ment of acute pancreatitis. *South African Medical Journal*, **37**, 1072–1076.

Nakajima, S. & Magee, D. F. (1970) Inhibition of exocrine pancreatic secretion by glucagon and D glucose given intra-venously. *Canadian Journal of Physiology and Parmacology*, **48**, 299–305.

Nelp, W. B. (1961) Acute pancreatitis associated with steroid therapy. *Archives of Internal Medicine*, **108**, 702–710.

Nogueira, J. R. & Freedman, M. A. (1972) Acute pancreatitis as a complication of Imuran therapy in regional enteritis. *Gastroenterology*, **62**, 1040–1041.

Northam, B. E., Rowe, D. S. & Winstone, N. E. (1963) Methaemalbumin in the differential diagnosis of acute haemorrhagic and oedematous pancreatitis. *Lancet*, **1**, 348–351.

Ofstad, E., Amundsen, E. & Hagen, P. O. (1969) Experimental acute pancreatitis in dogs. Histamine release induced by pancreatic exudate. *Scandinavian Journal of Gastro-enterology*, **4**, 75–79.

Olsen, H. (1973) Thrombotic thromocytopenic purpura as a cause of pancreatitis. Report of a case and review of the literature. *American Journal of Digestive Diseases*, **18**, 238–244.

Opie, E. L. (1901) The aetiology of acute haemorrhagic pancreatitis. *Bulletin of Johns Hopkins Hospital*, **12**, 182–188.

O'Sullivan, J. N., Nobrega, F. T., Morlock, C. G., Brown, A. L. & Bartholomew, L. G. (1972) Acute and chronic pancreatitis in Rochester, Minnesota, 1940–1969. *Gastro-enterology*, **62**, 373–379.

Paloyan, D., Paloyan, E. & Harper, P. V. (1967) Glucagon induced hypocalcaemia. *Metabolism*, **16**, 35–39.

Paloyan, D., Paloyan, E., Worobec, R., Ernst, K., Deininger, E. & Harper, P. V. (1966) Serum glucagon levels in experimental acute pancreatitis in the dog. *Surgical Forum*, **17**, 348–349.

Parbhoo, S. P., Welch, J. & Sherlock, S. (1973) Acute pancreatitis in patients with fulminant hepatic failure. *Gut*, **14**, 428.

Peel, A. L. G., Bourke, J. B., Hermon-Taylor, J., MacLean, A. D. W., Mann, C. V. & Ritchie, H. D. (1975) *Annals of the Royal College of Surgeons of England*, **56**, 124–134.

Pfeffer, R. B., Stasior, O. & Hinton, J. W. (1957) The clinical picture of the sequential development of acute haemorrhagic pancreatitis in the dog. *Surgical Forum*, **8**, 248–251.

Pickleman, J. R., Ernst, K., Brown, S. & Paloyan, E. (1969) Glucagon induced hypocalcaemia: effect of the thyroid gland. *Surgical Forum*, **20**, 85–87.

Pollock, A. V. (1959) Acute pancreatitis—a review of one hundred cases. *British Medical Journal*, **1**, 6–10.

Probstein, J. G. & Pareira, M. D. (1952) Pancreatitis: current concepts. *American Surgeon*, **18**, 497–503.

Ranson, J. H. C., Roses, D. F. & Fink, S. D. (1973) Early respiratory insufficiency in acute pancreatitis. *Annals of Surgery*, **178**, 75–79.

Rosato, E. F., Mullis, F. W. & Rosato, F. E. (1973) Peritoneal lavage therapy in haemorrhagic pancreatitis. *Surgery*, **74**, 106–115.

Sankaran, S. & Walt, A. J. (1975) The natural and unnatural history of pancreatic pseudo-cysts. *British Journal of Surgery*, **62**, 37–44.

Savides, E. P. & Hoffbrand, B. I. (1974) Hypothermia, thrombosis and acute pancreatitis. *British Medical Journal*, **1**, 614.

Schmidt, H. & Creutzfeldt, W. (1969) The possible role of phospholipase A in the pathogenesis of acute pancreatitis. *Scandinavian Journal of Gastroenterology*, **4**, 39–48.

Schmieden, V. & Sebening, W. (1928) Surgery of the pancreas: with especial consideration of acute pancreatic necrosis. *Surgery, Gynecology and Obstetrics*, **46**, 735–751.

Schultz, N. J. & Sanders, R. J. (1963) Evaluation of pancreatic biopsy. *Annals of Surgery*, **1958**, 1053–1057.

Skyring, A., Singer, A. & Tornya, P. (1965) Treatment of acute pancreatitis with Trasylol: report of a controlled therapeutic trial. *British Medical Journal*, **2**, 627–629.

Staub, A., Sinn, L. & Behrens, O. K. (1953) Purification and crystallisation of hyperglycemic glycogenolytic factor. *Science*, **117**, 628–629.

Stern, P. H. & Bell, N. N. (1970) Effect of glucagon on serum calcium in the rat and on bone resorption in tissue culture. *Endocrinology*, **87**, 111–117.

Stunkard, A. J., Van Itallie, T. B. & Reis, B. B. (1955) The mechanism of satiety. Effect of glucagon on gastric hunger contractions in man. *Proceedings of the Society for Experimental Biology and Medicine*, **89**, 258–261.

Thal, A. P., Perry, J. F. & Egner, W. (1957) A clinical and morphological study of 42 cases of fatal acute pancreatitis. *Surgery, Gynecology and Obstetrics*, **105**, 191–202.

Thompson, A. G. (1968) Proteinase inhibitors in experimental and clinical pancreatitis. *Annals of the New York Academy of Science*, **146**, 540–543.

Thompson, J. A., Howard, J. M. & Vowles, K. D. J. (1957) Acute pancreatitis following choledochotomy. *Surgery, Gynecology and Obstetrics*, **105**, 706–710.

Trapnell, J. E. (1966) The natural history and prognosis of acute pancreatitis. *Annals of The Royal College of Surgeons of England*, **38**, 265–287.

Trapnell, J. E. (1972) The natural history and management of acute pancreatitis. *Clinical Gastroenterology*, **1**, 147–166.

Trapnell, J. E. & Duncan, F. H. (1975) Patterns of incidence in acute pancreatitis. *British Medical Journal*, **1**, 179–183.

Trapnell, J. E., Rigby, C. C., Talbot, C. H. & Duncan, E. H. L. (1974) A controlled trial of Trasylol in the treatment of acute pancreatitis. *British Journal of Surgery*, **61**, 177–182.

Walker, C., Russell, R. C. G. & Bloom, S. R. (1974) The effects of surgical operations on levels of pancreatic glucagon in plasma. *British Journal of Surgery*, **61**, 923.

Wall, A. J. (1965) Peritoneal dialysis in the treatment of severe acute pancreatitis. *Medical Journal of Australia*, **2**, 281–283.

Wallensten, S. (1958) Acute pancreatitis and diastasuria after partial gastrectomy. *Acta chirurgica scandinavica*, **115**, 182–188.

Waller, S. L. & Ralston, A. J. (1971) The hourly rate of urinary amylase excretion, serum amylase and serum lipase. *Gut*, **12**, 878–890.

Wapshaw, H. (1955) The pathogenesis of acute pancreatitis, with particular reference to the bile and obstructive factors. *Glasgow Medical Journal*, **36**, 76–101.

Waterworth, T. A. & Bevan, P. G. (1975) The effect of glucagon on pain in acute pancreatitis. Inaugural Meeting of the Pancreatic Society of Great Britain and Ireland.

Watts, G. T. (1963) Total pancreatectomy for fulminant pancreatitis. *Lancet*, **2**, 384.

Way, L. W., Admirand, W. H. & Dunphy, J. E. (1972) Management of choledocholithiasis. *Annals of Surgery*, **176**, 347–359.

Welch, G. E. & Montanez, C. (1965) Treatment of acute pancreatitis and its complications. In *Modern Treatment*, **2**, 443. New York: Harper & Row.

Wilding, P. W., Cooke, W. T. & Nicholson, G. I. (1964) Globulin bound amylase—a cause of persistently elevated levels in serum. *Annals of Internal Medicine*, **60**, 1053–1059.

Winstone, N. E. (1965) Methaemalbumin in acute pancreatitis. *British Journal of Surgery*, **52**, 804–808.

Zelman, S. (1944) Blood diatase values in mumps and mumps pancreatitis. *American Journal of Medical Science*, **207**, 461–464.

Zieve, L. & Vogel, W. C. (1960) Measurement of lecithurase A in serum and other body fluids. *Journal of Laboratory and Clinical Medicine*, **57**, 586–599.

5
THE SURGICAL MANAGEMENT OF OBESITY

R. M. Baddeley

The strong impression, long held by clinicians, that obesity shortens longevity and increases the risk of sudden death has been well confirmed by actuarial statistics and the findings of the well-known Framingham study (Kannel, Troy and McNamara, 1967). A 15 per cent rise in mortality rate with an excess of 20 per cent above standard weight for age, height and sex, rises to 250 per cent when the excess reaches 90 per cent. This is due largely to cardiovascular disease, accident and suicide. Obesity of this massive dimension is also associated with high morbidity due to such complications as diabetes, osteroarthritis, gravitational oedema, varicose veins and ulceration, bronchitis, hiatus hernia, gallstones, subfertility and thromboembolic disease. There is greater difficulty in establishing diagnoses on the basis of physical signs as these may be obscured. There is a greater risk of surgical complications and consequently higher surgical mortality and morbidity.

The management of choice in the large majority of cases of simple obesity is by long-term dietary restriction. Unfortunately, the late results indicate an 80 to 90 per cent failure rate, most spending their lives swinging from one peak of weight to another. Even more unsuccessful has been therapeutic starvation under close medical supervision in hospital. Not only is this expensive but is usually followed by regain of much or all of the weight lost upon return home and is not without hazard (Innes et al, 1974). Equally unsuccessful has been the use of psychotherapy, hypnosis and group therapy.

When massively obese patients have failed such conventional conservative regimes and have reached a magnitude which makes them prone to significant mortality and morbidity, resort to more radical surgical measures may be necessary. These have been evolved during the past 20 years and include:

Dietary restriction enforced by dental splintage.
Gastric bypass.
Small bowel bypass.

DENTAL SPLINTAGE

Satisfactory weight reduction during all forms of dietary restriction is often frustrated by depressive mood change which results in compulsive or episodic overeating. This not only reverses the weight reduction which has been achieved but destroys the morale and will to continue. Dental splintage offers a means of preventing overeating when the stresses, which provoke it, occur. Garrow (1974) reported two patients so treated who were able to lose over 40 kg in five months.

At Birmingham General and Dental Hospitals, Wood and Baddeley (1976) have managed 20 patients by dental splintage and dietary restriction. All were at least 50 kg above standard weight for age, height and sex and had satisfactory natural dentition. They were unacceptable for small bowel bypass not having undergone supervised dietary restriction for a minimum of five years or were considered psychologically unsuitable. Cap splints or interdental wiring were released at monthly intervals for two to three days to allow jaw movements and prevent the trismus which is liable to occur with more prolonged fixation. They were removed entirely at three months for dental hygiene purposes. A fluid diet based on milk or soups with iron and vitamin supplements was continued throughout.

Half the patients were considered early failures as they could not tolerate the splints, cut the interdental wires or broke the splints in order to eat solid foods. One case was abandoned because of pregnancy. Ten patients cooperated well and lost 12 to 60 kg in the first three months.

Whether the long-term results of this method will be an improvement upon those of other conservative measures is doubtful. Much depends upon the motivation of the patient, which thus renders many unsuitable, and upon strenuous efforts in re-education of eating habits during and following the period of restraint. In the short term dental splintage undoubtedly can achieve good results. It is considerably less expensive than therapeutic starvation as inpatient care is avoided and the patient is able to continue her or his occupation.

GASTRIC BYPASS

Extensive Billroth II partial gastrectomy can cause substantial weight loss by creating a small gastric reservoir and by provoking dumping symptoms. In 1973, Printen and Mason reported the early results of a large series in which these side effects were utilised to treat patients suffering from gross refractory obesity.

The gastric reservoir was reduced to 10 per cent of its original size using the techniques of gastric transection or of gastroplasty. In the former, continuity of the gastrointestinal tract was restored by retrocolic gastrojejunostomy, the bypassed 90 per cent of the stomach being closed and left in situ. In gastroplasty, the transection was incomplete, a narrow tube of greater curvature being preserved to retain continuity between the fundic pouch and the body of the stomach. This technique avoided both an anastomosis and dumping symptoms.

The results in 130 gastric bypasses and 56 gastroplasties revealed satisfactory weight reduction and an overall 3.8 per cent mortality. The bypass technique was more effective than gastroplasty as the latter required more frequent revision to achieve the desired effect. The proximal gastric pouch and the connecting channel was prone to stretch and thus defeat the main objective of the procedure. Thus its use has now been discontinued.

Bypass of 90 per cent of the stomach was not associated with stomal ulceration (Mason and Ito, 1967) and the incidence of diarrhoea was negligible. Stomal revision was necessary in seven patients but there was only one instance of anastomotic leak. Its attraction as compared with small bowel bypass was the avoidance of many of the potential metabolic sequelae of the latter. Increased fatty infiltration in the liver was not seen and in this series the risks of fluid and electrolyte imbalance were less due to the absence of diarrhoea. The authors accepted dumping symptoms as an asset which curtailed the high carbohydrate dietary habits of their obese patients. As with small bowel bypass the procedure could be reversed if side effects became excessive.

The main disadvantage appears to be the technical difficulties likely to be encountered. It is a lengthy procedure which requires meticulous operative technique and careful postoperative management. It is probably not surprising that to date no other comparable report has been published.

SMALL BOWEL BYPASS

The absorption of fat, protein, carbohydrates and the constitutents of the normal diet depend upon the surface area of the intestinal mucosa and the time they are in contact with it. Preferential absorption of iron and folate occurs in the duodenum and upper jejunum and of bile salts and vitamin B_{12} in the lower ileum. Otherwise all food substances can be absorbed throughout the length of the small bowel, though that of fat is maximal in the upper ileum as compared with carbohydrate and protein which are readily absorbed in the upper jejunum.

Following the realisation that many patients have survived massive bowel resections for infarction or regional ileitis and sustained an adequate though reduced weight, surgeons have endeavoured to apply the physiology of absorption in the small bowel to the management of massive refractory obesity.

Techniques of Small Bowel Bypass

This field of bowel surgery was pioneered by Payne and colleagues in Los Angeles in the late 1950s and early 1960s. Their initial technique was jejunocolostomy in which the upper jejunum was divided 37 cm from the duodenojejunal flexure and anastomosed end-to-side to the mid transverse colon. The free end of the jejunum was anchored to the mesocolon or mesentery to prevent intussusception (Payne, DeWind and Commons, 1963). Metabolic difficulties, chiefly related to fluid, electrolyte and hepatic disturbances consequent upon the profuse diarrhoea which often ensued, necessitated reversal of the bypass in some cases. Because this was usually followed by regain of the weight loss, they and others subsequently abandoned this technique in favour of the less radical jejuno-ileal bypass.

By trial and elimination, Payne and DeWind (1963) reported that satisfactory and consistent weight reduction was achieved when the small bowel was short circuited to 35 cm of jejunum and 10 cm of ileum. Longer lengths of bowel in circuit were less effective and less reliable. Retention of ileocaecal valve function reduced the hazard of uncontrollable diarrhoea and consequent fluid, electrolyte and liver disturbances.

In a few patients the Payne technique of end-to-side jejuno-ileostomy failed to achieve adequate weight reduction (Payne et al, 1973). Others who experienced similar disappointment (Scott et al, 1971; Salmon, 1971; Buchwald and Varco, 1971) attributed failure to increased absorption through reflux into the excluded ileum. To overcome this they performed end-to-end jejuno-ileostomy implanting the free end of the divided ileum into the caecum, transverse colon or sigmoid.

The large majority of reports in the literature of jejuno-ileal bypass surgery have utilised the bowel measurements originally advocated by Payne and his colleagues. Others who have varied these measurements include Salmon (1971) (25 cm jejunum, 50 cm of ileum), Scott et al (1973) (30 cm each of jejunum and ileum), Schwartz, Varco and Buchwald (1973) (40 cm of jejunum, 4 cm of ileum), Gazet et al (1974) (10 cm jejunum, 25 cm of ileum) and Corso and Joseph (1974) (30 cm jejunum, 25–30 cm of ileum). Most of these authors have found satisfaction with the weight loss achieved but Scott and colleagues felt that the $30+15$ cm jejuno-ileostomy was more reliable. The author's preference has been the end-to-side bypass technique of Payne and DeWind (1963) (Figure 5.1) as it is simpler and quicker than the end-to-end procedure. Only one anastomosis is involved and potential late vitamin B_{12} deficiency is less likely to occur.

Through a midabdominal midline incision which skirts the umbilicus, the wound is held open with a modified self-retaining retractor in which the blades have been deepened to 12 cm length (the 'fattichetto'). The jejunum is measured from the ligament of Treitz, along its antimesenteric border for a length of 35 cm using sterile silk ligature material previously prepared. This measurement is twice checked. The jejunum is divided after the creation of a 4 cm window in the mesentery. The free end of jejunum is closed with catgut in two layers and anchored with silk sutures to the mesentery to prevent late intussusception by peristatic movement.

The terminal ileum is then mobilised, if necessary, and a marker stitch inserted 10 cm from the ileocaecal valve again measured along the antimesenteric border. At this site the end-to-end jejuno-ileostomy is fashioned and completed with two layers of sutures. The mesenteric defect thus created is closed to prevent herniation and volvulus. The abdomen is now closed with looped O monofilament nylon and as many layers of fat stitches as are required to close the subcutaneous tissues. Silk has been used for skin closure.

Some authors have performed abdominal apronectomy at the same operating session. This is probably not good practice as it may increase the already

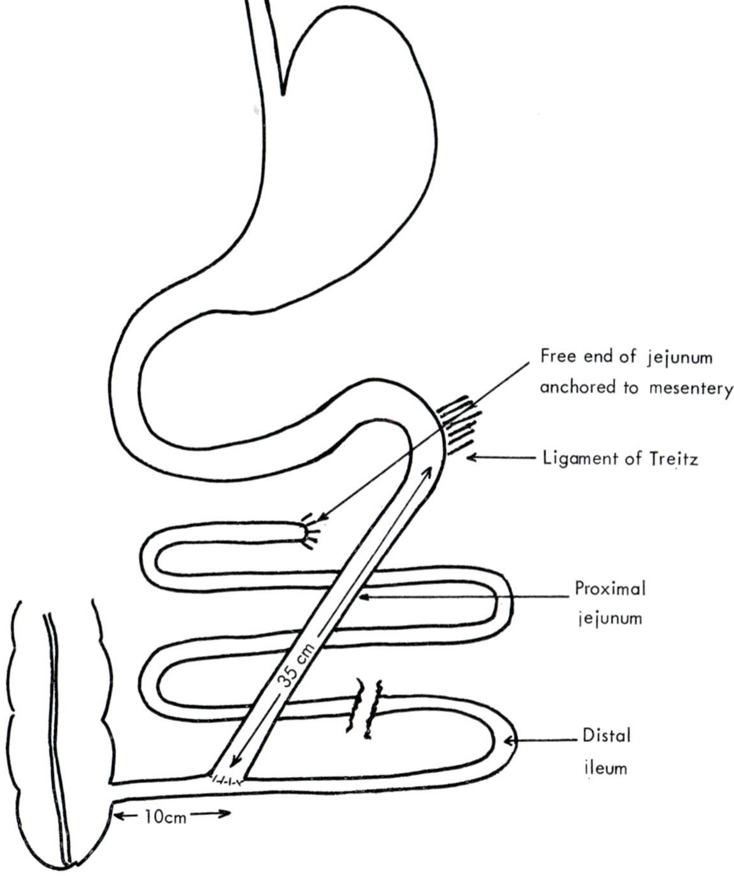

Figure 5.1   End-to-side jejuno-ileostomy

high infection rate and thereby the risk of incisional hernia, as well as adding to the general hazards of long operations in poor risk patients. Furthermore, it is unlikely to be as cosmetically satisfactory as if delayed for two years or so when weight reduction has ceased.

Routine postoperative intravenous infusions and nasogastric aspiration are continued for about three days. Diphenoxylate hydrochloride with atropine (Lomotil) is usually commenced with the onset of diarrhoea. It may be neces-

5

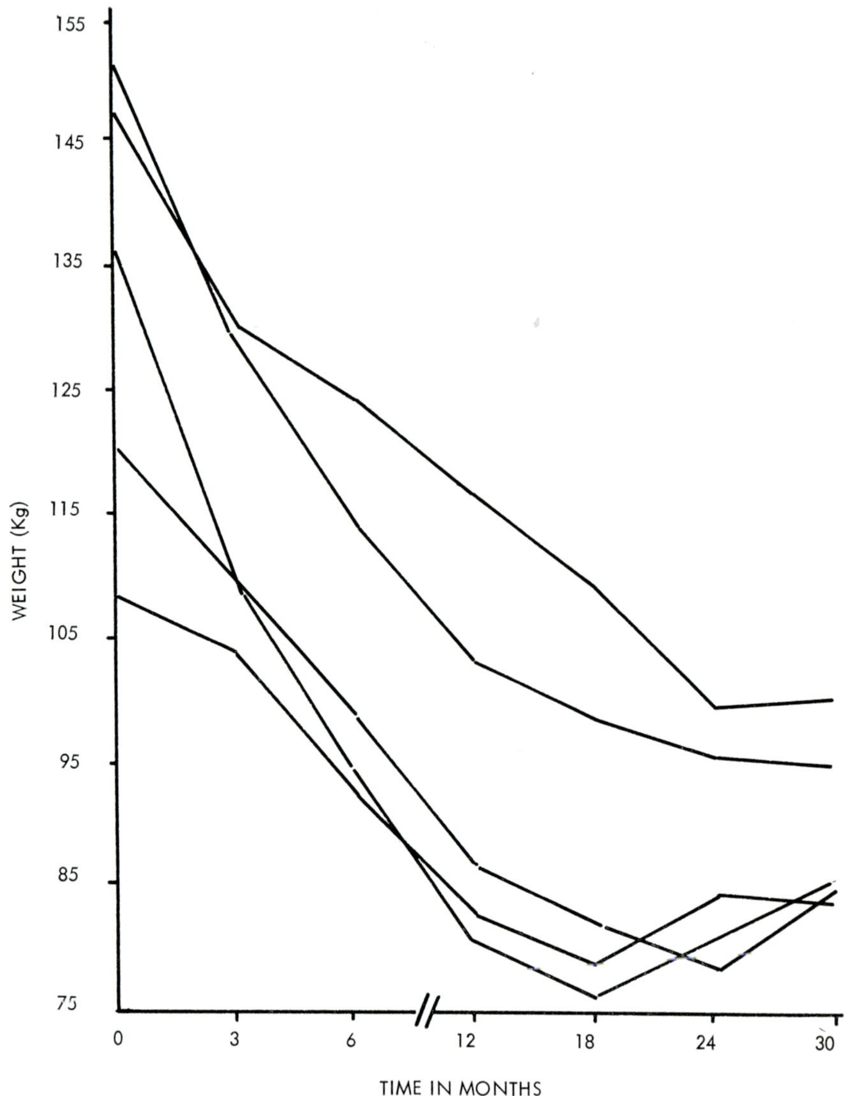

Figure 5.2   Pattern of weight loss after jejuno-ileostomy in five patients

sary to supplement this with codeine phosphate if the diarrhoea is excessive. It is also wise to give an oral potassium supplement to replace loss of this ion whilst diarrhoea persists.

Patients are seen at monthly intervals during the first six postoperative months and at lengthening intervals thereafter for an indefinite period. At these follow-up examinations, full haematological and serum biochemical assessments are repeated.

Results of Jejuno-ileostomy

Weight loss

Most series have reported acceptable and sustained weight reduction in the large majority of patients. The average loss has varied but has usually been about 20 kg by three months, 30 kg by six months, 41 kg by one year, 49 kg by 18 months and 53 kg by two years (Baddeley, 1975). Figure 5.2 reveals that most of the reduction occurs in the first year and slows down the period up to two years. Thereafter fluctuations of 5 to 6 kg and occasionally more, have occurred but there has been no instance when the original weight has been largely regained.

Because of individual variations from one report to another, comparisons are difficult unless weight reduction is assessed as a percentage of the mean of the initial weights. On this basis, Chandler (1974) compiled data from six well-documented series and demonstrated consistent loss of about one-fifth of the original weight at six months and about one-third at the end of the first year. In most the ultimate plateau has occurred somewhat above the standard weight for individual patients but usually relief of symptoms and of complications of obesity has been achieved.

There is a low but definite incidence of failure to lose an adequate amount of weight and several authors have revealed cases which have required further operation. In these, to obtain greater weight reduction, the shunt has been converted from end-to-side to end-to-end jejuno-ileostomy or further shortening of the functioning bowel has been performed. Others have achieved additional weight loss with conventional dietary restrictions. The failure rate, which is probably of the order of 3 to 4 per cent, has been attributed to reflux of bowel contents into the excluded ileum thereby increasing the absorptive surface. Quaade et al (1971), however, doubted this explanation invoking slow gastrointestinal transit time as a more likely alternative. Both explanations are probably valid but the fact that barium meal and follow-through examinations often reveal ileal reflux in many successful cases, adds further support for Quaade's contention. Furthermore, the conversion to end-to-end jejuno-ileostomy has not always achieved the desired additional weight reduction.

Symptomatic and socioeconomic benefits

The loss of large amounts of adipose tissue has been of considerable physical benefit in the reversal of symptoms and complications caused by massive obesity. Blood pressure levels have been reduced. Backache and the pain of osteoarthritis in the hips, knees and feet, have been palliated. Respiratory impairment associated with the Pickwickian syndrome, bronchitis and asthma have been eliminated or much improved. Chronic gravitational ulceration, some having been present for several years, may heal even though varicose veins may persist to a grotesque degree. Severe ankle oedema which is some-

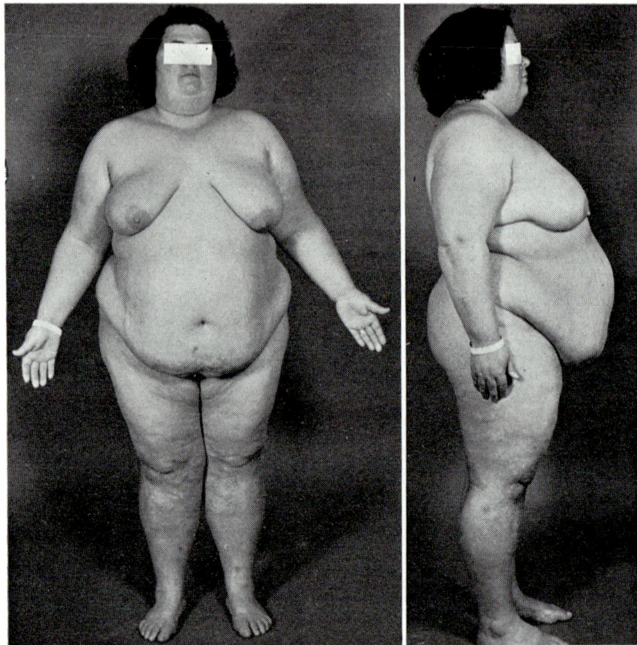

Figure 5.3A   A case of gross simple obesity weighing 135.6 kg immediately before end-to-side jejuno-ileostomy

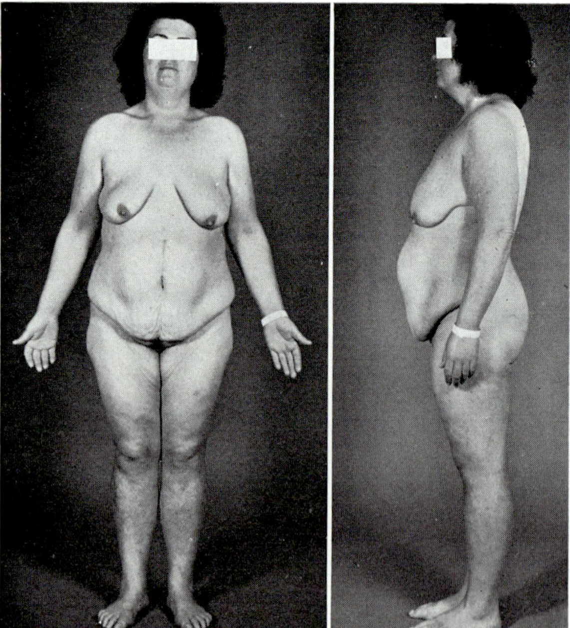

Figure 5.3B   The same patient 14 months later having lost 57 kg in weight

times present in obese patients, whether or not varicose veins are present, may resolve though sometimes the need for a non-kaluretic diuretic may persist. An example of the improvement in physical appearance can be readily seen in Figures 5.3A and B.

Striking socioeconomic benefits can be achieved. Many patients return to or start work previously abandoned or not open to them because of their size. Thus income is improved and the expense of special clothing, shoes and diet reduced. Marital and family disharmony has often improved although the benefits of the operation are sometimes too late to avoid divorce. Overall the quality and pattern of life is much enhanced.

Biochemical benefits

Early and significant flattening of glucose tolerance curves which were noted by Payne and DeWind (1963) have been confirmed by most subsequent authors. The need for insulin or hypoglycaemic agents may be reduced or eliminated.

Table 5.1   Fall in serum cholesterol after jejuno-ileostomy

Time (months)	Mean value (mmol/litre)	No. patients
0	5.88	118
3	3.85	96
6	3.66	84
12	3.53	68
18	3.65	51
24	3.66	29

Serum cholesterol values (Table 5.1) fall early after small bowel bypass by as much as 40 per cent and appear to remain low for at least two to five years. Serum triglycerides follow a similar pattern and the fall in serum carotene to very low levels indicates the efficiency of the bowel bypass in reducing fat absorption.

Serum uric acid levels on average are higher than normal in obese patients and may rise sharply during the first postoperative month. They then slowly return to preoperative values or even to normal (Weismann, 1973). There appears to be only a low incidence of symptomatic gout during this time.

Psychological benefits

Considerable psychological change and benefit accrues from the marked weight loss which follows jejuno-ileostomy. Although the patients continue to overestimate their body size (Gazet et al, 1974) there is a marked improvement in mood and self esteem. The feeling of entrapment, helplessness and failure is lost (Solow, Silberfarb and Swift, 1974). Eating habits are often modified. The compulsive or episodic overeating associated with depressive disturbances is largely lost (Brewer, White and Baddeley, 1974). Symptom substitution does not appear to occur as psychiatric symptoms disappear or are improved. It seems that the obesity rather than a psychiatric disorder is normally the main cause of personality disturbance which is so often ascribed to these patients.

Short-term irritability, depression, tiredness and anxiety are not uncommon during the period of rapid weight loss, possibly due to overestimation of the benefits which accrue from the operation. The replacement of gross rolls of fat with thin folds of wrinkled stretched skin sometimes causes more apparent embarrassment than the original obesity. It may be desirable to restore the patient's confidence by panniculectomy of the abdomen (apronectomy), thighs and arms, but this is best deferred until weight reduction has ceased when the extent of the resections required can be better assessed.

Table 5.2   Mortality after small bowel bypass

Author	Number of cases	Hospital mortality		Late mortality		Overall mortality (%)
		No.	%	No.	%	
Payne et al (1973)	165	6	3.6	10	6.1	9.7
Salmon (1971)	120	5	4.1	0	0	4.1
Wills (1972)	259	9	3.5	8	3.1	6.6
Weismann (1973)	123	2	1.6	1	0.8	2.4
Baddeley (1975)	170	2	1.2	8	4.7	5.9
Backman and Hallberg (1976)	103	1	1.0	3	2.9	3.9
Average			2.5		2.9	5.4

Mortality

The early, late and overall mortalities in six large series, each involving over 100 cases, are shown in Table 5.2. The hospital mortality rate of the range 2 to 3 per cent, is in keeping with that of major bowel surgery in the non-obese. Late mortality of a further 3 per cent is probably acceptable when contrasted with the hazards of sustained massive obesity as exhibited by the patients selected for such surgery.

The common causes of death have included myocardial infarction, pulmonary embolism, cardiac failure, septicaemia, electrolyte imbalance and liver failure. The last two are specifically attributable to the effects of small bowel bypass but constitute a minority of the total. This is illustrated by Payne's (1973) large pioneering series in which there were 16 deaths, three due to myocardial infarction and cardiac failure, three to pulmonary embolism, one to pancreatitis and one to mammary carcinoma, one to myasthenia gravis, one to renal tubular acidosis, five to hepatic jaundice and one to electrolyte imbalance. Of their overall figure of 9.7 per cent, the mortality attributable to intestinal bypass was 6 per cent. Of the author's 10 deaths (5.9 per cent) half were due directly to the effects of the shunt. In other series this figure is even lower.

Clearly, when surgery is performed in these massive and unhealthy people a mortality rate is inevitable. The greater the obesity the greater the risk.

Morbidity

After small bowel bypass most patients experience considerable discomfort caused by side effects which vary in severity and duration and which are attributable either to the nature of the operation or to the hazards of obesity. These include diarrhoea and its associated anal soreness or pain due to haemorrhoids, fissure or excoriation, polyarthralgia and polymyalgia, fatty liver, fluid and electrolyte disturbances, transient thinning of the hair and postprandial bloating. The latter is normally relieved by the passage of large quantities of

Table 5.3   Stool frequency after jejuno-ileostomy

Time (months)	Average daily stool frequency	Total number of patients	Number of patients with > 5 stools daily
3	4.6	131	36
6	4.0	121	14
12	3.6	99	12
18	2.9	71	2
24	2.8	47	1

foul flatus and may be a nuisance and, or embarrassment. There are potential haematological problems and a suggestion of increased calculus formation. Due to obesity itself, there is proneness to sepsis, chest infections, deep vein thrombosis, pulmonary embolism and incisional hernia.

Diarrhoea

With such drastic shortening of the functioning jejuno-ileum, it is not surprising that diarrhoea is initially severe. Satisfactory control of stool frequency is usually achieved by routine use of diphenoxylate hydrochloride with atropine (Lomotil) and/or codeine phosphate. The problem may be compounded by the cathartic effect of unabsorbed bile acids in the colon but this may be minimised by cholestyramine. Occasionally underlying depression or anxiety may cause persisting diarrhoea and be resolved by amitriptyline or other tranquilliser.

As can be seen in Table 5.3, stool frequency, on average, is not excessive by the time three months have elapsed and further improvement thereafter occurs as the functioning bowel dilates and hypertrophies. Ultimately, anti-diarrhoea medication can be discontinued. In a few patients the diarrhoea persists despite all medication and the potential threat of fluid and electrolyte disturbance may justify removal of the shunt and restoration to normal anatomy. This was necessary in one patient in the author's series, 14 months after the original operation.

Polyarthralgia and polymyalgia

A small proportion of patients experience pain in joints and muscles which vary in severity and duration. In most it is usually transient and responsive to conventional analgesic medication. Others exhibit incapacitating pain and swelling of multiple small and large joints which may mimic closely the features of rheumatoid arthritis. Routine investigations have usually excluded this cause. Gout occasionally occurs but applies to only a minority as hyperuricaemia, commonly present preoperatively, has not been consistently present in affected patients.

These side effects appear to have been more frequent in jejunocolostomy cases. Seven of 22 patients who underwent this operation in the series of Shagrin, Frame and Duncan (1971) developed articular complications and one required reversal of the bypass for this reason. Mir Madjlessi, Mackenzie and Winkelman (1974) has similar experience in 8 of 27 cases, 3 to 23 months after the operation. The incidence appears to be lower after jejuno-ileostomy. The author has 13 affected, plus two cases of gout, in the first 150 patients followed up for a minimum of six months. The onset has varied from 6 to 40 months postoperation. Most were troubled for a few weeks only but one was sufficiently severe and persistent to necessitate reversal of the operation. This brought about instant relief.

Various explanations have been proposed for this complication. Analogy has been drawn with the arthritic complications of chronic inflammatory bowel conditions such as Crohn's disease, ulcerative colitis and Whipple's disease (Shagrin et al, 1971). However, in the case mentioned where reversal of the bypass became necessary, no inflammatory change or significant bacteriological abnormality was found in the upper jejunal segment of the excluded bowel. Mir Madjlessi et al (1974) drew attention to the occurrence of joint symptoms in patients with acute and chronic liver disease. This may be relevant to the cases affected during the weight reduction phase but is unlikely to be appropriate in later ones as liver function has usually returned to normal by such time. Obscure arthritides have also been observed in certain malignancies. The catabolic state existing after small bowel bypass may present a comparable state of debility in which the patient is unable to metabolise or detoxify the products of tissue breakdown.

Fatty liver and liver failure

Abnormalities of liver structure and function following small bowel bypass are well recognised and are the source of greatest concern to clinicians. Herein lies the most worrying cause of morbidity and mortality.

It is common to find mild to severe fatty infiltration in liver biopsies of massively obese patients. Juhl et al (1971) observed it in six of eight patients, Salmon (1971) in 61 per cent of 33 patients, Weismann (1973) in 72 per cent of 123 patients, Kern et al (1973) in 94 per cent of 151 patients and Buchwald, Lober and Varco (1974) in 64 per cent of 77 patients. Most are agreed that this fatty change is greatest in the heavier patients though Weissman (1973) and Holzback et al (1974) have found no correlation with the degree of obesity.

After jejuno-ileostomy there is a tendency for the fatty infiltration to increase during the period of weight reduction but this is usually followed by reversal of the change when it has ceased (Weismann, 1973). In the author's experience, of 61 patients undergoing liver biopsy one year after the bypass operation, 49 per cent displayed increased fatty infiltration as compared with intra-operative biopsies. This fell to 36 per cent after two years. In two patients, definite cirrhotic change has developed, one probably being related to high alcohol intake. Of the 170 patients in the series, eight have developed symptoms of hepatic insufficiency, one of them has died.

Fibrotic change or lobular deformity has only occasionally been seen preoperatively but a mild degree of inflammatory cell infiltration is common. Kern et al (1973), however, found that six of their cases displayed either definite cirrhosis or portal fibrosis suggestive of early cirrhosis, from which they concluded that fatty infiltration may lead to cirrhosis following jejuno-ileostomy.

Death due to cirrhosis after jejuno-ileostomy was reported in one patient by McGill et al (1972). From the literature, they collected a further seven deaths from a total of 63 jejunocolostomies. Brown, O'Leary and Woodward (1974) reported six cases of severe liver failure with one death and eight of mild liver abnormality in 36 jejuno-ileostomies. Five of the 16 deaths in Payne et al (1973) series of 165 patients were due to hepatic failure.

Thus, though common, fatty metamorphosis is probably harmful in only a small proportion of cases. This minority is, however, of great concern as it is not possible to predict accurately at the present time which patients will be so seriously affected. Clearly it is more likely in those with preoperative signs of impairment of liver function; these are mainly, but not exclusively, the heavier subjects and those with a history of alcoholism.

The cause of liver injury after small bowel short circuit remains unclear. That it should occur at all is surprising as extensive and rapid weight reduction, by dieting or fasting, is uniformly accompanied by a progressive diminution in the amount of fatty infiltration and, occasionally, by diminution of periportal fibrous tissue (Drenick, Simmons and Murphy, 1970). It seems reasonable to assume that amino acid deficiency, particularly of lipotropic factors, is partly responsible. White et al (1974) demonstrated significant depression of fasting serum values of most essential and non-essential amino acids during the phase of weight reduction. They drew comparisons with the morphological changes seen in the livers of kwashiorkor patients and laboratory animals rendered protein deficient. These changes were seen to reverse when weight stability occurred and the hepatic fatty change diminished. At this stage, corresponding improvement in protein absorption was observed. Thus if protein deficiency is a valid explanation, a high protein diet during the first postoperative year should be encouraged. Occasionally this is difficult due to prolonged postoperative anorexia or vomiting which in themselves may be early symptoms of liver injury.

An alternative explanation is that of Drenick et al (1970), who incriminated lithocholic acid, the product of bacterial action upon chenodeoxycholic acid in the colon, as a causative factor. This bile acid is normally absorbed in the terminal ileum but in the shortened small bowel situation its absorption is incomplete. On this basis, it is worth a trial of cholestyramine to reduce potential absorption of this hepatotoxic agent.

Toxic injury from bacterial colonisation of the excluded small bowel has been offered as a further explanation (Brown et al, 1974) but there is limited factual supporting evidence. It is noteworthy, however, that McClelland et al (1970) in an animal study, were able to prevent liver damage and prolong life without impairment of weight reduction, by infusing medium chain triglycerides through feeding jejunostomies in the excluded bowel. The benefits thus obtained could be due to the provision of essential nutrient or alternatively to the prevention of absorption of some toxic agent elaborated in the excluded segment. In the author's experience seven patients who subsequently underwent reversal of their jejuno-ileostomies or other abdominal operation, yielded no significant bacterial colonisation in the upper end of the excluded segment. Two other patients suffering from severe liver injury undoubtedly benefited from repletion through feeding jejunostomy in the excluded bowel.

Electrolyte disturbances

When diarrhoea is profuse or prolonged, or when associated with vomiting, fluid and electrolyte depletion is a hazard. Small bowel bypass patients also appear to tolerate enteric infections badly. It is routine practice to administer oral supplements of potassium from the outset but these may be passed unchanged or vomited. Thus most surgeons have experienced significant hypokalaemic problems in a small proportion of cases. In the early jejuno-colostomy cases these difficulties were sufficiently severe and frequent as to cause abandonment of the technique.

Rapid improvement in the patient's condition has normally been achieved by admission to hospital and intravenous repletion. At such times low magnesium and calcium levels can also be corrected. Hypocalcaemia associated with tetany has occurred in a very small proportion of cases where diarrhoea has been particularly troublesome. Clearly better control of the diarrhoea rectifies this problem but it may be necessary to add oral supplements of calcium and vitamin D preparations until a steady state has been achieved.

Haematopoietic deficiencies

The importance of preoperative assessment of all patients is emphasised by the observation of low serum iron and folate values in a small proportion of women (Tables 5.4 and 5.5) who present with massive obesity. Following small bowel bypass further lowering of serum iron may occur during the first six months and require prophylactic oral supplementation. Similarly, serum folate values fall to subnormal levels in approximately one-third of patients during the first two years (Table 5.5). This is particularly so in those with low

Table 5.4   Incidence of low serum iron values after jejuno-ileostomy

Time (months)	Number of patients with abnormalities	Total number of patients
Preoperation	6	139
3	19	126
6	10	109
12	10	95
18	9	70
24	4	50

Normal value: 9 to 32 mmol/litre

Table 5.5   Incidence of low serum folate values after jejuno-ileostomy

Time (months)	Number of patients with low values	Total number of patients
Preoperation	26	139
3	30	124
6	32	117
12	12	98
18	9	73
24	5	51

Normal value: 3.0 to 20.0 ng/ml

or low normal preoperative levels. Again prophylactic oral supplementation during this period prevents haemopoietic abnormalities.

There is a surprisingly low incidence of vitamin B_{12} deficiency after end-to-side jejuno-ileostomy possibly due to reflux into the bypassed ileum (Payne et al, 1973), but it is to be expected to be higher after jejunocolostomy and end-to-end jejuno-ileostomy.

Impaired vitamin K absorption resulting in raised prothrombin time has been seen by the author in five of 155 cases during the first 18 postoperative months. Three were severe enough as to present with bleeding but all have responded rapidly to temporary oral repletion.

Urinary and biliary calculus formation

Urinary urate and calcium oxalate calculi are not uncommon in sufferers from chronic diarrhoea due to inflammatory bowel disease, ileostomy or extensive bowel resection. This is possibly due to low urine flow. An increased incidence of urinary oxalate calculi was also recorded by Dickstein and Frame (1973) in patients who had undergone mainly jejunocolostomies. The incidence was lower after jejuno-ileostomy and the author has had only one case in 170 patients.

Although hyperuricaemia is common in obese patients, the incidence of gout and of uric acid calculi does not appear to be increased following small bowel bypass.

Reduction of the bile salt pool after jejuno-ileostomy might be expected to result in an increased incidence of gallstones. Massively obese patients, however, are quite likely to be candidates for this problem (Salmon, 1971; Backman and Hallberg, 1975) but there is no statistical evidence available at present which indicates that small bowel bypass compounds the hazard. A technical difficulty which arises in the diagnosis of gall-bladder disease in these patients is non-absorption by the shortened bowel of the contrast medium used in cholecystography. Intravenous cholangiography under these circumstances is more reliable.

Conclusions

In assessing the management of any clinical problem it is pertinent to weigh the hazards of the treatment proposed against the risks of the condition untreated. The mortality of obesity 100 per cent above standard body weight is probably greater than that of small bowel bypass and thus this surgical approach could be justified. On the other hand, with obesity of less than 70 per cent above standard body weight it may not be so and dietary measures with or without dental splintage should be pursued.

The large majority of patients submitted to jejuno-ileal bypass have yielded excellent results. The physical, psychological and social benefits have been gratifying to both the patients and the surgeons involved. A small minority, however, have presented difficult problems of management which constituted a hard core of morbidity and mortality. It is difficult to judge pre-operatively which cases will subsequently be afflicted by persisting excessive diarrhoea, vomiting and the associated fluid and electrolyte disturbances, polyarthralgia, polymyalgia and liver injury, some of which contribute to the overall mortality of 4 to 5 per cent.

Case selection is thus particularly important. Most reports have mentioned the minimum acceptance weight of 100 lb or 45 kg above standard weight, this figure representing a level above which non-surgical measures have an abysmal long-term success rate. Some patients seem incapable of coping adequately with the difficulties of the early post-operative period when diarrhoea and its associated anal discomforts, nausea and vomiting may occur. Some fail to keep to their prescribed supplement medication and others have not attended for follow-up examinations. Thus it is important that selected patients should be of reasonable intelligence and reliable enough to follow the instructions given. A preoperative psychiatric opinion is, therefore, important in the general assessment of suitability for surgical treatment.

Payne et al (1973) commented that patients with known cardiac disease do badly after jejuno-ileostomy. It is clear that pulmonary embolism is a significant cause of early and late death and thus a known history of deep vein thrombosis or pulmonary embolism should be viewed with some trepidation. Even those without such history should receive some form of prophylaxis against deep vein thrombosis during the operative and early postoperative period. In view of the incidence of fatty liver a history of alcoholism should exclude selection. A summary of indications and contraindications are displayed in Table 5.6.

Table 5.6 Case selection for small bowel bypass

Indications	Contraindications
1. Failed dietary treatment of five years duration	1. Insufficient supervised dietary management
2. 100 per cent above standard body weight	2. Less than 100 lb (45 kg) or 100 per cent obesity
3. 100 lb (45 kg) above standard body weight in presence of obesity complications (diabetes, hypertension, osteoarthritis, gravitational ulceration, hyperlipidaemia, etc).	3. Known heart disease
	4. Alcoholism
	5. Severe primary psychiatric abnormality
	6. Low intelligence

The recognition of dangerous liver impairment requires regular and frequent follow-up examinations in the first year. During this period the patients should be encouraged to take a high protein, high calorie diet possibly including dietary supplements. Unfortunately, routine biochemical liver function tests have not always been helpful in recognising early cases as they are often abnormal during the first six months even in those patients who are seemingly progressing satisfactorily. The earliest indications of severe liver injury are symptomatic: anorexia, nausea and vomiting, marked lethargy and a generally unwell appearance. They demand immediate hospitalisation for parenteral nutrition and electrolyte repletion. Serious consideration has to be given to reversal of the intestinal shunt in those who respond poorly to such resuscitation. It may be necessary to create a feeding jejunostomy in the excluded bowel before the patient's condition can be improved sufficiently to proceed with the reversal operation.

Surgeons who undertake the surgical management of obesity must be prepared for a considerable clinical burden involving detailed case selection and continuous follow-up. As the technique is still not yet fully evaluated it is important that patients should not be discharged from observation. It also beholds the surgeon to recognise and treat the small minority of patients at serious risk from undesirable side effects and to reverse the intestinal shunt before severe deterioration can occur.

REFERENCES

Baddeley, R. M. (1976) *British Journal of Surgery*, in press.

Backman, L. & Hallberg, D. (1976) Some somatic complications after small intestinal bypass operations for obesity. *Acta chirugica scandinavica* (in press).

Brewer, C., White, H. & Baddeley, R. M. (1974) Beneficial effects of jejuno-ileostomy on compulsive eating and associated psychiatric symptoms. *British Medical Journal*, **4**, 314–316.

Brown, R. G., O'Leary, P. J. & Woodward, E. R. (1974) Hepatic effects of jejuno-ileal bypass for morbid obesity. *American Journal of Surgery*, **127**, 53–58.

Buchwald, H. & Varco, R. L. (1971) Bypass operation for obese hyperlipidaemic patients. *Surgery*, **70**, 62–70.

Buchwald, H., Lober, P. M. & Varco, R. L. (1974) Liver biopsy findings in seventy-seven consecutive patients undergoing jejuno-ileal bypass for morbid obesity. *American Journal of Surgery*, **127**, 48–52.

Chandler, J. G. (1974) Surgical treatment of massive obesity. *Postgraduate Medicine*, **56**, 124–133.

Corso, P. J. & Joseph, W. L. (1974) Intestinal bypass in morbid obesity. *Surgery, Gynecology and Obstetrics*, **138**, 1–5.

Dickstein, S. S. & Frame, B. (1973) Urinary tract calculi after intestinal shunt operation for the treatment of obesity. *Surgery, Gynecology and Obstetrics*, **136**, 257–260.

Drenick, E. J., Simmons, F. & Murphy, J. F. (1970) Effect on hepatic morphology of treatment of obesity by fasting, reducing diets and small bowel bypass. *New England Journal of Medicine*, **282**, 829–834.

Garrow, J. S. (1974) Dental splinting in the treatment of hyperphagic obesity. *Proceedings of the Nutrition Society*, **33**, A29.

Gazet, J. C., Pilkington, T. R. E., Kalucy, R. S., Crisp, A. H. & Day, S. (1974) Treatment of gross obesity by jejunal bypass. *British Medical Journal*, **4**, 311–314.

Holzback, R. T., Wieland, R. G., Lieber, C. S., DeCarli, L. M., Koepke, K. R. & Green, S. E. (1974) Hepatic lipid in morbid obesity. *New England Journal of Medicine*, **290**, 296.

Innes, J. A., Campbell, J. W., Campbell, C. J., Needle, A. L. & Munro, J. F. (1974) Long term follow-up of therapeutic starvation. *British Medical Journal*, **2**, 356–359.

Juhl, E., Christofferson, P., Baden, H. & Quaade, F. (1971) Liver morphology and biochemistry in eight obese patients treated with jejuno-ileal anastomosis. *New England Journal of Medicine*, **285**, 543–547.

Kannel, W. B., Troy, B. L. & McNamara, P. M. (1967) Relation of body weight to development of coronary heart disease; the Framingham Study. *Circulation*, **35**, 734–744.

Kern, W. H., Heger, A. H., Payne, J. H. & DeWind, L. T. (1973) Fatty metamorphosis of the liver in morbid obesity. *Archives of Pathology*, **96**, 342–346.

McClelland, R. N., DeShazo, C. W., Heimbach, D. M., Eigenbrodt, E. H. & Dowdy, A. B. C. (1970) Prevention of hepatic injury after jejuno-ileal bypass by supplemental jejunostomy feedings. *Surgical Forum*, **21**, 368–370.

McGill, D. B., Humphreys, S. R., Baggenstoss, A. H. & Dickson, E. R. (1972) Cirrhosis and death after jejuno-ileal shunt. *Gastroenterology*, **63**, 872–877.

Mason, E. E. & Ito, C. (1967) Gastric bypass in obesity. *Surgical Clinicals of North America*, **47**, 1345–1351.

Mir-Madjlessi, S. H., Mackenzie, A. H. & Winkelman, E. J. (1974) Articular complications in obese patients after jejunocolic bypass. *Cleveland Clinic Quarterly*, **41**, 119–125.

Payne, J. H. & DeWind, L. T. (1963) Surgical treatment of obesity. *American Journal of Surgery*, **118**, 141–147.

Payne, J. H., DeWind, L. T. & Commons, R. R. (1963) Metabolic observations in patients with jejunocolic shunts. *American Journal of Surgery*, **106**, 273.

Payne, J. H., DeWind, L., Schwab, C. E. & Kern, W. H. (1973) Surgical treatment of morbid obesity. *Archives of Surgery*, **106**, 432–437.

Printen, K. J. & Mason, E. E. (1973) Gastric surgery for relief of morbid obesity. *Archives of Surgery*, **106**, 428–431.

Quaade, F., Juhl, E., Feldt-Rasmussen, K. & Baden, H. (1971) Blind loop reflux in relation to weight loss in obese patients treated with jejuno-ileal anastomosis. *Scandinavian Journal of Gastroenterology*, **6**, 537–541.

Salmon, P. A. (1971) The results of small intestine bypass operations for the treatment of obesity. *Surgery, Gynecology and Obstetrics*, **132**, 965–979.

Schwartz, M. Z., Varco, R. L. & Buckwald, H. (1973) Pre-operative preparation, operative technique, and post-operative care of patients undergoing jejuno-ileal bypass for massive exogenous obesity. *Journal of Surgical Research*, **14**, 147–150.

Scott, W. H., Dean, R., Shull, H. J., Abram, H. S., Webb, W., Younger, R. K. & Brill, A. B. (1973) New considerations in use of jejuno-ileal bypass in patients with morbid obesity. *Annals of Surgery*, **177**, 723–735.

Scott, H. W., Sandstead, H. H., Brill, A. B., Burko, H. & Younger, R. K. (1971) Experience with a new technique of intestinal bypass in the treatment of morbid obesity. *Annals of Surgery*, **174**, 560.

Shagrin, J. W., Frame, B. & Duncan, H. (1971) Polyarthritis in obese patients with intestinal bypass. *Annals of Internal Medicine*, **75**, 377–380.

Solow, C., Silberfarb, P. M. & Swift, K. (1974) Psychosocial effects of intestinal bypass surgery for severe obesity. *New England Journal of Medicine*, **290**, 300–304.

Weismann, R. E. (1973) Surgical palliation of massive and severe obesity. *American Journal of Surgery*, **125**, 437–446.

White, J. J., Maxley, R. T., Pozefsky, T. & Lockwood, D. H. (1974) Transient kashiorkor; a cause of fatty liver following small bowel bypass. *Surgery*, **75**, 829–840.

Wills, C. E. (1972) Small bowel bypass for obesity. A discussion of four different procedures. *Journal of the Medical Assocation of Georgia*, **61**, 322.

Wood, G. D. & Baddeley, R. M. (1976) In preparation.

6
PARENTERAL NUTRITION

I. D. A. Johnston

Intravenous feeding is required to meet the energy requirements of the body when the alimentary canal is unavailable for either long or short periods of time. Intravenous feeding is an old concept, milk was given intravenously to combat the wasting in cholera by Hodder in Toronto in 1873. Henriques and Anderson (1913) carried out the first successful intravenous feeding using goat muscle digested with pancreatic extract and combined with glucose, sodium and potassium. This mixture maintained dogs in positive nitrogen balance for 16 days. Surgical patients who have suffered starvation and are nutritionally depleted will gain body weight and increase their muscle mass and subcutaneous fat during adequate intravenous feeding provided they are not acutely stressed or septic (Dudrick, Wilmore and Vars, 1967). Tissue synthesis during total intravenous nutrition is certainly one of the most significant therapeutic developments of recent years.

Many patients have benefited greatly from careful intravenous feeding while others have developed complications during treatment. A number of questions, however, remain to be answered in connection with parenteral nutrition. What patients are likely to gain most from this form of treatment? When is intravenous feeding both meddlesome and unnecessary? What are the exact calorie and nutrient requirements in various acute and chronic situations? What is the most effective technique for long-term intravenous feeding? How can the biochemical complications be detected, managed and even prevented? There have been a number of advances made in the search for answers to the questions which have been posed and these form the basis of this review.

INDICATIONS FOR INTRAVENOUS FEEDING

The number of patients who require complete intravenous feeding while in hospital is less than 5 per cent of all admissions. It is not intended to provide a list of situations requiring intravenous nutrition but it should always be considered in the management of any patient when normal requirements cannot be met after three days. It must also be emphasised that intravenous feeding is never a substitute for oral feeding in any form and recent developments with elemental diets allow even greater use to be made of the alimentary route. Each gram of nitrogen lost by the body during a period of negative nitrogen balance represents a deficit of 6.25 g of protein and intravenous feeding can often restore a positive nitrogen balance or reduce the extent of a negative balance.

The importance of intravenous feeding following uncomplicated abdominal surgery in well-nourished patients has been the subject of much debate. The modest negative balance of nitrogen and weight loss which follow operation are due to a combination of starvation for a few days and the metabolic response to injury. Patients can be maintained in positive nitrogen balance after surgery (Johnston, Marino and Stevens, 1966), but there is no evidence that this expensive management results in any measurable clinical benefit such as accelerated wound healing or more rapid convalescence. The loss of a few kilograms of body weight is of little consequence in normally nourished patients and is soon regained in the anabolic phase.

The extent of the catabolic response to injury with loss of lean body mass is related directly to the severity of the trauma. Severe injury such as major burns or multiple fractures along with associated starvation and major endocrine activity constitute a maximum stimulus to muscle catabolism. The nitrogen deficit after such major stress may be around 20 g per day usually being excreted as urea, creatinine and creatine. The losses of nitrogen at this time are three times greater than those seen in starvation. Energy expenditure by the body after major injury or during major sepsis may be increased by 50 to 60 per cent (Kinney, 1960).

Large and persistent losses of nitrogen soon become evident as muscle wasting and crippling debility. It is difficult to overcome the catabolic response to major injury even without sepsis, but any contribution to the nutritional requirements by intravenous feeding is clearly going to be of considerable advantage to the patient.

Patients with granulomatous disease of the bowel frequently lose large amounts of protein into the intestine and may require intravenous supplementation.

Many patients with carcinoma of the upper gastrointestinal tract are debilitated when first seen and some require multiple operations. Mortality after major surgery increases sharply in patients who have lost 30 per cent or more of their normal body weight. Intravenous feeding is of considerable importance in the management of these patients both before and after operation.

Parenteral nutrition has proved particularly valuable in patients with enterocutaneous fistula allowing oral feeding to be stopped with a reduction in the amount lost from the fistula. There are many reports of successful prolonged intravenous feeding during intensive care. Bergstrom, Blomstrand and Jacobson (1972) describe a 43 year old woman whose nutrition was improved by a weight gain of 10 kg during seven months of total intravenous nutrition. There are many reports of dramatic gains of weight during intravenous feeding.

Patients who have had major resections of the small intestine require both oral and intravenous nutrition in the early critical weeks when the function of the residual bowel is being assessed and the need for long-term intravenous support examined. It is always easier to maintain the nutritional state than to seek to restore lost lean body mass quickly by intravenous means.

The role of intravenous feeding in either the maintenance or restoration of immunological competence in patients with malignant disease has yet to be defined (Blackburn et al, 1973). There is evidence that intravenous feeding may accelerate the growth of some neoplasms (Watkins and Stanfield, 1965) while other workers have found that improving the nutrition of the patient and altering cellular immunity leads to remission of malignant disease.

PLANNING INTRAVENOUS FEEDING

The first step is to weigh the patient and estimate the fluid requirements for a given 24 h period. Calorie and nitrogen intake should be calculated on a body weight basis.

Table 6.1   Daily nitrogen and calorie requirements

	Postoperative	Hypercatabolic states
Nitrogen (g/kg)	0.20	0.25–0.30
kcal/kg	35	45–55
kcal/g N_2	180	200–250

Ill surgical patients with sepsis or patients with severe burns have calorie demands around 30 to 40 per cent above resting requirements. A figure of 40 kcal/kg (168 J) and 0.2 g nitrogen/kg per day is a reasonable figure (Table 6.1).

About 50 per cent of the calories should come from a carbohydrate source, the concentration of glucose used depending on the fluid requirements. Fat emulsion should provide 30 to 40 per cent of the daily calorie intake with protein from amino acid solutions providing 10 to 15 per cent. When a patient has a low serum alubmin this should be corrected and intravenous feeding with crystalloids introduced only when the tissues are well perfused. The extent to which fat is used in any programme depends on the adequacy of liver function. The main attraction of fat emulsion is the large number of calories which can be given without adding an osmotic load to the body.

Amino Acids

Amino acids are essential for complete intravenous feeding (Table 6.2).

Casein hydrolysates have been the principal amino acid mixture in use since they were introduced by Elman in 1939. There is, however, a small incidence of side effects due possibly to peptide fragments in hydrolysate solutions. It is, therefore, desirable to infuse mixtures of pure amino acids if at all possible and there are now a number of synthetic amino acid mixtures available. The body can utilise only the L isomers of amino acids with the exception of small amounts of D-methionine and D-phenylalanine.

Tweedle, Spivey and Johnston (1972) compared the utilisation of five amino acid preparations after elective abdominal surgery (Fig. 6.1). The casein hydrolysate (Aminosol) and a synthetic crystalline L-amino acid solution Vamin produced the most significant improvement in nitrogen balance. Solutions which had least effect on nitrogen balance had a high concentration of non-essential amino acids particularly glycine. The adjustment of the non-essential amino acid content towards the pattern in egg protein produced solutions which were similar to Vamin and Aminosol in their effect on nitrogen balance.

Amino acid solutions do not provide energy in a readily usable form and energy substrates are required so that the principal objective of intravenous

Table 6.2   Amino acid solutions in current use

	Volume (ml)	Calories	Nitrogen (g)	Sodium (mEq)	Potassium (mmol)
Aminosol (10%)	1000	320	12.7	160	0.5
Trophysan (10%)	1000	564 (Sorbitol)	6.7	6	8
Vamin (7%)	1000	650 (Fructose)	9.4	50	20
Aminofusin (10%)	1000	200	8.8	35	25

feeding is the infusion of amino acids with an appropriate source of energy. Brunschwig in 1942 demonstrated a significant improvement in nitrogen sparing when carbohydrate was given simultaneously with amino acids. It has been suggested that the optimum calorie nitrogen ratio for utilisation of infused amino acids is 200 calories for each gram of nitrogen. The relative value of carbohydrate solutions and fat emulsions in protein sparing in different clinical situations is still uncertain.

The role of plasma insulin in the utilisation of amino acid solutions has been stressed. Carbohydrate solutions infused along with amino acids produce a brisk insulin response. Blackburn et al (1973) claim that protein anabolism can be maintained effectively by the infusion of isotonic amino acid solutions alone and the insulin response to such a regimen is minimal and endogenous fat mobilisation occurs with ketone body formation to provide the necessary calories. During starvation the urinary excretion of nitrogen falls progressively and ketone bodies are used as energy sources by nervous tissue in particular. Amino acids infused alone in starvation would certainly be used effectively. However, it is claimed that significant nitrogen retention follows the peripheral infusion of isotonic amino acids and in a variety of situations including the postoperative period. Recent evidence suggests that maximum protein sparing with amino acid solutions alone occurs only after many days of starvation but more work is required on the value of only giving amino solutions in nutritional support.

None of the commercial solutions at present available contain sufficient quantities of energy substrates even allowing for the use of alcohol. Joyeux et al (1974) in Montpellier have prepared single solutions of amino acids, lipids, electrolytes, vitamins and trace elements which have remained stable for as long as six months.

However, it is not certain that the relative amount of energy required for each gram of nitrogen infused remains constant. It is claimed that 200 kcal (840 J) of energy are required for each gram of nitrogen infused but this may

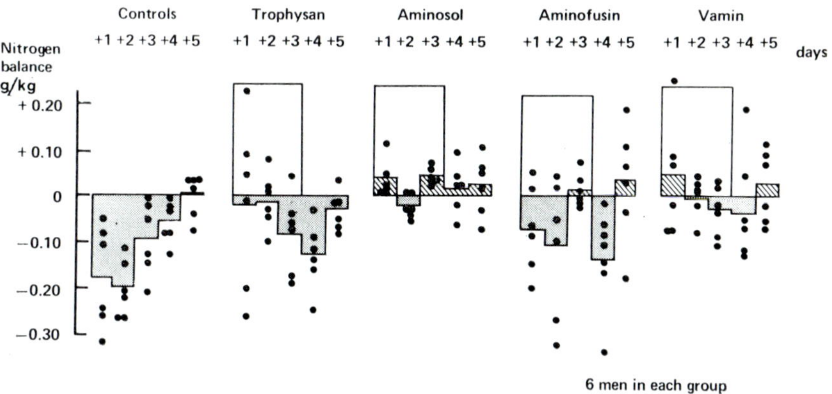

Figure 6.1   The effect of various amino acid solutions on nitrogen balance after elective abdominal operations of moderate severity

be as high as 300, for example in renal failure with excess catabolism. Johnston and Clark (1972) have shown in surgical patients that nitrogen utilisation was related to the energy provided and appeared optimum at around 220 kcal/g nitrogen (880 J). The use of single solution of amino acids containing a fixed energy content is attractive for routine use in busy understaffed wards but is not ideal compared to the separate choice of amino acids and energy substrates related to the exact metabolic requirements of each individual patient (Tweedle 1975).

The electrolyte content of amino acid solutions can often be important. The sodium content of casein hydrolysate (Aminosol) is very high (Table 6.2) and fluid retention may occur. Potassium is present in most of the solutions available today but usually in inadequate amounts as 5 mEq of potassium is required for each gram of nitrogen infused (Frost and Smith, 1953). The ammonium content of Aminosol is very high and hyperammonaemia can follow the use of solutions containing large amounts of glycine so that Aminosol and Trophysan should not be used in patients with impaired liver function.

Metabolic acidosis has been recorded during amino acid infusion. It has been suggested that some preparations have excessive amounts of the cationic amino acids lysine, arginine and histidine (Heird et al, 1972). Amino acids however are amphoteric and depending upon the pH of the plasma some amino acids will behave either as anions or cations.

Carbohydrate

Glucose has always been a principal source of calories in intravenous feeding and its position remains unchallenged (Table 6.3). Glucose can be metabolised by all the tissues of the body and is essential for protein anabolism. One litre of 5 per cent glucose, however, only provides 200 cal so there is clearly a limit to the number of calories which can be provided conveniently

Table 6.3   Carbohydrate solutions in current use

	Volume	Calories
Glucose (5%)	1000	200
Fructose (20%)	1000	800
Sorbitol (30%)	1000	1200
Ethanol[a] (5%)	1000	350

[a] Infusion limited to 10 g or 70 cal/h

by glucose. Twenty and even 50 per cent glucose solutions can be given but only through catheters inserted into major central veins.

Fructose has some theoretical advantages over glucose and has been used extensively with few problems. The liver cell is more or less freely permeable to fructose which is phosphorylated by a specific fructokinase. It is claimed that fructose is metabolised independently of insulin but recent studies show clearly that the term 'insulin independence' is misleading and only the first few metabolic steps of hepatic metabolism do not require insulin. Fructose infusions in nutritionally depleted patients or infants may lead to an accumulation of lactate and a severe lactic acidosis. Fructose should not be used in hypoxaemia, uraemia or after shock when the blood lactate level is liable to be raised. Sodium and potassium losses from the body are greater during fructose infusion than with corresponding amounts of glucose.

Sorbitol is a sugar alcohol which has been used widely in intravenous feeding as either a 10 or 20 per cent solution. Sorbitol is poorly absorbed in the renal tubules and has osmotic diuretic properties which can be a disadvantage. Sorbitol is converted to fructose and glucose and apart from a slightly higher calorie yield it provides no metabolic advantages over glucose.

A pentose sugar xylitol has also been used as a calorie source. The body can undoubtedly utilise this sugar using a different metabolic pathway to glucose. Liver toxicity, however, has been reported with this substance which is in no way superior to glucose.

Glucose remains then the carbohydrate of choice in intravenous feeding. It can be metabolised by all the tissues of the body provided insulin is available. A normal adult can utilise about 600 g of glucose daily without exogenous insulin. Patients who are severely stressed after burns, major surgery or during severe sepsis will have high glucose levels in the serum in the presence of very low concentrations of insulin. The administration of exogenous insulin under carefully controlled conditions can be of benefit to these patients (Hinton et al, 1971).

Alcohol has been included in some intravenous feeding regimens for many years and it is metabolised rapidly with an energy value greater than carbohydrate (1 g yielding 7.1 calories).

The amount of alcohol infused must be limited and should not exceed 10 g (70 cal)/h. Patients with liver dysfunction or severe protein calorie

Table 6.4 Intravenous fat emulsions in current use

	Volume (ml)	Calories	Glycerol (g)
Soya bean oil emulsion			
Intralipid (10%)	1000	1100	25
Intralipid (20%)	1000	2000	25

Emulsified with egg yolk phosphatide particle size <0.5 μm

malnutrition should not be given alcohol. A number of amino acid solutions contain alcohol and the rapid infusion of these can lead to confusion, flushing and tachycardia, the whole picture being very suggestive of a septicaemic episode.

There is now really no need to include alcohol in intravenous feeding as a calorie source and its continued use in amino acid mixtures should be discouraged.

Fat

The preparation of stable and safe fat emulsions for intravenous use has been the single most important development in intravenous feeding (Table 6.4). Early preparations of intravenous fat did produce side effects but the soya bean oil emulsion in current use (Intralipid) does not have the toxicity associated with earlier preparations. One gram of fat provides 9.3 cal and the osmotic load on the body during the delivery of large numbers of calories is negligible. The emulsions of fat particles about 0.5 μm in diameter are stabilised with glycerol. Intravenous fat is cleared as rapidly from the circulation as chylomicrons in the intestinal villi. The rate of disappearance can be measured easily and is increased after injury or in situations where energy demands are high (Feggetter, Davidson and Johnston, 1974).

The metabolism of infused fat can be followed by measuring the rate at which ^{14}C is exhaled as carbon dioxide following an injection of fat labelled with ^{14}C-oleate. There is a close correlation between clearance rates and the production of carbon dioxide in the breath indicating that intravenous fat is a readily utilised form of energy and only a proportion of the fat particles enter the reticulo-endothelial system.

Fat and glucose are interchangeable as sources of calories in most programmes. Fat, however, is necessary in any prolonged intravenous feeding in order to prevent essential fatty acid deficiency (Coats and Maynard, 1970). Heparin was added frequently to fat emulsions to enhance clearance of the fat but there is little evidence that heparin is essential for the optimal utilisation of fat.

A rise in the serum triglyceride and serum-free fatty level is the usual immediate response to intravenous fat but prolonged hyperlipidaemia after their use has not been recorded. It must be remembered that intravenous fat must be discontinued some hours before withdrawing blood for routine biochemical estimations.

BIOCHEMICAL PROBLEMS

Careful and repeated biochemical measurements are required during any prolonged infusion of hypertonic energy solutions or fat.

The infusion of phosphate-free nutrient solutions such as crystalline amino acids and glucose have a marked effect on plasma inorganic phosphate levels. Hypophosphataemia may occur within 12 to 24 h in nutritionally depleted patients given high energy phosphate-free infusions, the red cell concentration of 2,3-diphosphoglycerate falls and the oxyhaemoglobin dissociation curve shifts to the left. Hypophosphataemia is associated with a clinical syndrome of neuromuscular incoordination, dysarthria, etc. Casein hydrolysate solutions and intralipid both contain phosphate so that this complication has been prevented on many occasions.

Apart from blood glucose the plasma levels of sodium and potassium require to be followed carefully when hypertonic solutions are being given if hyperosmolar coma is to be avoided. The levels of phosphate, calcium, magnesium and zinc must also be measured regularly. Trace elements cobalt, chromium and copper are also required during prolonged intravenous feeding although the exact role of these elements in nutrition of the surgical patient remains difficult to define.

Haemoglobin concentration must be maintained during prolonged support and whole blood provides protein, minerals and also helps to prevent fatty acid deficiency (Coats and Maynard, 1970), a syndrome characterised by scaling of the skin. Plasma protein fraction or albumin may also be given during prolonged feeding.

Folic acid deficiency has also been reported as early as four weeks after starting intravenous feeding and can be dangerous.

The use of hormones to improve the utilisation of intravenous nutrients has been studied extensively. Anabolic steroids and growth hormone while of little value in the catabolic period may have a role in the anabolic or recovery period after major injury (Johnston, 1972).

Insulin has been used in quite large doses during intravenous feeding with improvement in nitrogen balance (Allison, 1974). Insulin must be given after a hypertonic glucose solution (50 per cent) has been running for some time, care being taken to monitor urine and blood glucose. The infusion of insulin and glucose must be even if rebound hypoglycaemia is to be avoided. Plasma and urinary urea fall during insulin therapy, serum potassium levels also fall as potassium passes into the cells but the sodium level frequently rises.

Insulin glucose infusions in some ill patients have been followed by evidence of cellular overhydration and cerebral oedema.

The careful use of insulin with glucose particularly during hypercatabolic situations can be a valuable adjunct, but extremely careful monitoring is required throughout insulin administration.

TECHNIQUES

The success of intravenous feeding depends on easy and safe access to the circulation for as long as is required. Thrombophlebitis and septicaemia are serious problems which still occur and in many cases are due to poor technique in inserting the intravenous catheter or maintaining the infusion.

Peripheral veins can be used when isotonic solutions of amino acids and fat emulsions are being infused simultaneously but the use of concentrated carbohydrate solutions requires the tip of the catheter to be in the subclavian vein.

A strict aseptic technique must always be observed when setting up the intravenous infusion. The position of the tip of the catheter must be checked radiologically to ensure that it has not entered the jugular veins. Povidine iodine cream or an antibiotic spray (Polybactrin) applied to the puncture site have been shown to be of value. It is advisable to change the tubing in the infusion system at least every 48 h.

Bacterial contamination can occur when adding electrolytes or trace elements to bottles of nutrients and such additions should be kept to the minimum. Evidence that the incidence of infection and thrombophlebitis is reduced by inserting a millipore filter in the infusion line is conflicting. Collin et al (1974) were unable to find any reduction in complications in a controlled trial using millipore filters. The increase in resistance to flow with millipore filters is a distinct disadvantage and roller pumps are often required to maintain the infusion rate.

Patients may develop septicaemia without any local signs of thrombo-phlebitis. A swinging temperature and positive blood cultures are suggestive of an infected thrombus around the tip of the catheter. A search should be made for obvious causes of infection and if none is found then the catheter should be removed and the clot cultured.

Many organisms have been implicated but infection with *Candida albicans* has been the most serious. Some amino acid solutions are known at body temperature to support the growth of this organism. While blood-borne organisms from infected foci in the patient will undoubtedly settle on a catheter lying in a large vein, careless aseptic techniques by medical and nursing staff add to the hazards. Candida septicaemia should be treated with intravenous Ancotyl.

Many of the problems of infection seem to have been overcome by a number of techniques. Several groups have used indwelling 'silastic' catheters placed in the right atrium for periods up to three years and some patients have been able to infuse themselves intravenously at home (Jeejeebhoy, 1973). It is possible to give the daily requirements during a period of 8 h of night-time support thus enabling the patient to be completely mobile during the day.

CONCLUSIONS

Intravenous feeding like other aspects of intensive care is costly but the day to day cost must be weighed against obvious clinical benefit and a reduced stay in hospital.

Parenteral nutrition should never be given casually or intermittently. Ill-considered and inadequate intravenous feeding has its own special morbidity but the metabolic rewards of properly controlled and administered parenteral feeding can be considerable.

Constant daily supervision and assessment are necessary to obtain the maximum benefit and a nutritional care team in a large hospital has an important role in advising on the constant and safe administration of an intravenous diet.

REFERENCES

Allison, S. P. (1974) *Carbohydrate and Fat Metabolism in Parenteral Nutrition in Acute Metabolic Illness*, ed. Lee, H. A., pp. 167–175. New York: Academic Press.

Bergstrom, K., Blomstrand, R. & Jacobson, S. (1972) Long-term complete intravenous nutrition. *Nutrition and Metabolism*, Suppl. I, 118–130.

Blackburn, G. L., Flatt, J. P., Clover, G. H. A. & O'Donnell, T. F. (1973) Peripheral intravenous feeding with isotonic amino acid solutions. *American Journal of Surgery*, **125**, 447–454.

Bistrium, D. R. & Blackburn, G. L. (1974) Role of nutrition on cellular immunity in hospitalised patients. *Federation Proceedings*, **33**, 691–693.

Coats, D. A. & Maynard, A. I. (1970) *Long-term Parenteral Nutrition in 'Parenteral Nutrition'*, ed. Mang, H. C. & Law, D. H. Springfield: Charles C. Thomas.

Collin, J., Tweedle, D. E. F., Venables, C. W., Constable, F. L. & Johnston, I. D. A. (1973) Effect of a millipore filter on complications of intravenous infusions. *British Medical Journal*, **1**, 456–459.

Dudrick, S. J., Wilmore, D. W. & Vars, H. M. (1967) Long-term parenteral nutrition with growth in puppies and positive nitrogen balance in patients. *Surgical Forum*, **18**, 356–357.

Elman, R. (1939) Time factor in retention of nitrogen after intravenous injection of mixtures of amino acids. *Proceedings of the Society for Experimental Biology and Medicine*, **40**, 484–490.

Feggetter, J. G. W., Davidson, H. A. & Johnston, I. D. A. (1974) Fat as a calorie source in the post-operative patient. *Proceedings of the International Society for Parenteral Nutrition*, Montepllier, p. 44.

Frost, P. M. & Smith, J. C. (1953) Influence of potassium salts on the efficiency of parenteral protein utilisation in the surgical patient. *Metabolism*, **2**, 529–540.

Henriques, V. & Anderson, A. C. (1913) Uber parenterale ernchrung durch. Intravenose injecktion. *Hoppe-Seylers Zeitschrift für physiologische Chemie*, **42**, 357–362.

Heird, W. C., Dell, R. D., Driscoll, J. M., Grebin, B. & Winters, W. R. (1972) Metabolic acidosis resulting from intravenous alimentation with mixtures of synthetic amino acids. *New England Journal of Medicine*, **287**, 943–950.

Hinton, P., Littlejohn, S., Allison, S. P. & Lloyd, J. (1971) Insulin and glucose to reduce the catabolic response to injury in burnt patients. *Lancet*, **1**, 767–769.

Jeejeebhoy, K. N. (1973) Long-term intravenous feeding. *Gastroenterology*, **65**, 811–816.

Johnston, A. O. B. & Clark, R. G. (1972) The effect of various calorie nitrogen ratios on nitrogen balance during intravenous feeding. *British Journal of Surgery*, **59**, 897–900.

Johnston, I. D. A., Marino, J. D. & Stevens, J. Z. (1966) The effect of intravenous feeding on the balances of nitrogen, sodium and potassium after operation. *British Journal of Surgery*, **53**, 885–889.

Johnston, I. D. A. (1972) The endocrine response to trauma. *Advances in Clinical Chemistry*, **15**, 256–285.

Joyeux, H., Abstruc, B., Yakoun, M. & Solassol, C. (1974) Eusrbm, **6**, Suppl. 1, 76–80.

Kinney, J. M. (1960) A consideration of energy exchange in human trauma. *New York Academy of Medicine*, **36**, 617–623.

Tweedle, D. E. F., Spivey, J. & Johnston, I. D. A. (1972) Choice of intravenous amino acid solutions for use after surgical operation. *Metabolism*, **22**, 173–178.

Tweedle, D. E. F. (1975) Intravenous amino acid solutions. *British Journal Hospital Medicine*, 81–92.

Watkins, D. M. & Stanfield, J. T. (1965) Nutrition and energy metabolism in patients with and without cancer given intravenous fat. *American Journal of Parenteral Nutrition*, **16**, 205–211.

7
DISORDERS OF HAEMOSTASIS IN SURGERY

Milica Brozović   R. S. Mibashan

NORMAL HAEMOSTASIS

Haemostasis is the process by which bleeding from an injured blood vessel is arrested. It is achieved by initial vasoconstriction followed by formation of a haemostatic plug consisting of platelets, which is soon reinforced by fibrin, red cells and granulocytes (Fig. 7.1). Blood flow, plasma inhibitors and fibrinolysis prevent uncontrolled growth of a haemostatic plug; fibrinolysis also ensures its dissolution by lysing the fibrin strands during tissue repair. In small blood vessels platelets play the central role, whereas in large vessels coagulation of blood assumes major importance.

Blood Vessel

The intima consists of flat endothelial cells and a subendothelial layer. In capillaries and veins endothelial cells can release an enzyme, plasminogen activator, which initiates fibrinolysis. The next layer, the media, contains collagen fibres, smooth muscle cells and fibroblasts (Stemerman, 1974). Intimal damage exposes collagen in the media, thus attracting platelets and activating coagulation through factor XII.

The initial arrest of bleeding is due to vasoconstriction: in larger vessels this takes place through contraction of smooth muscle cells in the media, whereas in smaller blood vessels it may occur through endothelial adhesion or closure of a precapillary sphincter.

Platelets

Platelets participate in the arrest of bleeding by plugging the disrupted vessel wall and providing components essential for coagulation. These functions are closely interrelated.

Circulating platelets are small discoid particles of an average volume of 7 to 8 pl. When exposed to collagen or to a foreign surface such as glass they will adhere to it. They will also clump together, or aggregate, in the presence of many substances such as thrombin, ADP, adrenaline, free fatty acids, serotonin and immune complexes. Adherent or aggregated platelets lose their discoid shape, become more spherical and form pseudopodia on their surface.

Granules present in the cytoplasm move into the centre of the platelet and are finally discharged through minute channels into the surrounding plasma. This reaction is called platelet release or secretion (Holmsen, Day and Stormorken, 1969; White, 1974). The granules contain ADP, ATP, vasoactive amines, serotonin, platelet factor 4, potassium, calcium and lysosomal enzymes. All these substances play an important part in haemostasis. ADP causes further platelet aggregation and exposes on the platelet surface a phospholipid essential for coagulation called platelet factor 3; ADP also activates factor XII on the platelet surface and thus initiates coagulation (Walsh, 1972). Serotonin causes vasoconstriction and activation of fibrinolysis. Platelet factor 4 is the heparin neutralising factor: it inactivates trace amounts

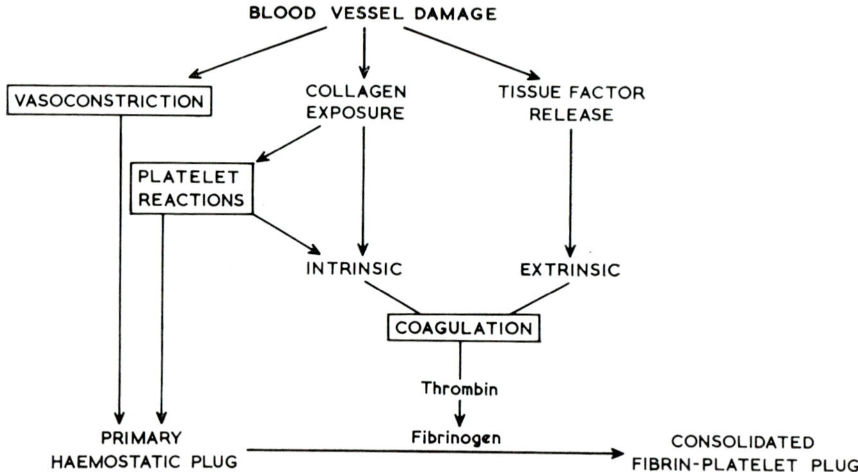

Figure 7.1 Vascular, platelet and coagulation components of haemostasis (adapted from Owen et al, 1975)

of heparin naturally present in plasma and removes its inhibitory effect on the coagulation sequence (Walsh and Biggs, 1972).

Blood Coagulation

The coagulation sequence is a chain of reactions that leads to the formation of fibrin clot. Eight proteins are involved in the generation of thrombin, an enzyme which rapidly converts soluble fibrinogen to fibrin gel. Six of these proteins circulate as inactive enzyme precursors; each is activated in turn when a bond is split to release a proteolytic enzyme, the last of which is thrombin. The remaining two factors (V and VIII) are cofactors of activation. The entire process is conceived as a biological amplification system or enzyme 'cascade' (Macfarlane, 1964, 1972) which proceeds sequentially from a relatively small vascular stimulus activating a few initial molecules, through a succession of enzyme activations which culminate in the explosive generation of thrombin.

Coagulation occurs via two alternative pathways. In the first or *intrinsic* pathway, injury to vascular intima exposes collagen which activates factor XII (Fig. 7.2). Activated factor XII activates factor XI to XIa, which in turn activates factor IX. Together with platelets, factor VIII and ionised calcium, activated factor IX converts factor X to Xa. This phase of coagulation lasts 5 to 10 min, and when it is impaired the whole blood clotting time, partial

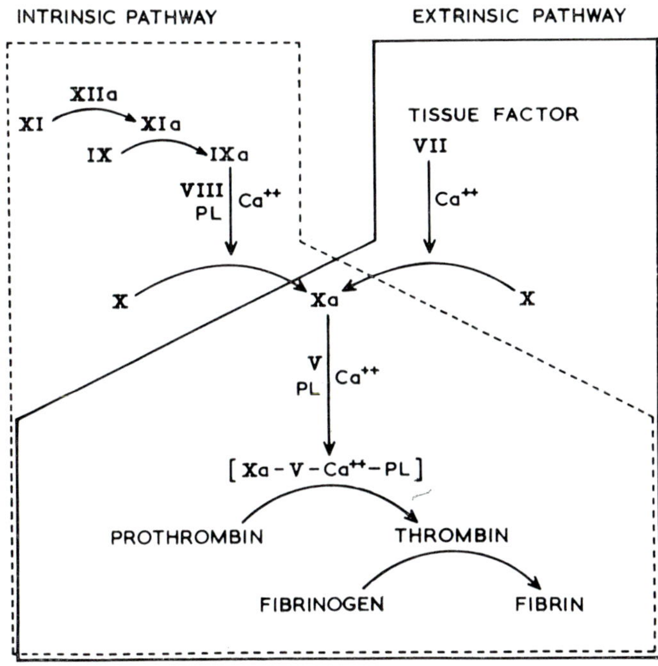

Figure 7.2 Coagulation pathways, showing their overlap after activation of factor X. The *prothrombin time* test reflects all factors enclosed in the continuous line; the *partial thromboplastin time* and other intrinsic pathway tests include all plasma factors except VII. The *thrombin clotting time* tests solely the last step in fibrin formation (PL = platelet phospholipid)

thromboplastin time and a number of other coagulation tests are prolonged. Some characteristics of coagulation factors of the intrinsic pathway are shown in Table 7.1.

In the second or *extrinsic* pathway, injury to the endothelial cell exposes tissue factor which activates or complexes with plasma factor VII to convert X into Xa. This sequence is very rapid (less than 20 s) and its defects prolong the one-stage prothrombin time.

Once activated by either the intrinsic or the extrinsic pathway, factor X forms a complex with phospholipid (from platelets or tissue), calcium ions and factor V. This complex, called variously prothrombin converting principle or prothrombinase, converts prothrombin into thrombin, which clots fibrinogen. A common pathway thus forms beyond the activation of factor X, and its defects prolong both the one-stage prothrombin and the partial thromboplastin times. Some characteristics of the extrinsic and common pathway factors are shown in Table 7.1.

Formation of Fibrin

The fibrinogen molecule is a dimer, each monomer being composed of three chains linked by disulphide bonds (Blombäck and Blombäck, 1972).

Table 7.1   Names and properties of plasma coagulation factors

Factor[a]	Synonym	Approx. mol. wt	Approx. plasma $T_{\frac{1}{2}}$	Synthesis in liver	Vitamin K-dependent
I	Fibrinogen	340 000	4 d	Yes	No
II	Prothrombin	70 000	3 d	Yes	Yes
V	Proaccelerin; labile factor	290 000	15 h	Yes	No
VII	Proconvertin; stable factor	60 000	3–6 h	Yes	Yes
VIII	Antihaemophilic factor	2×10^6	12 h	?	No
IX	Christmas factor; plasma thromboplastin component	70 000	24 h	Yes	Yes
X	Stuart-Prower factor	70 000	2 d	Yes	Yes
XI	Plasma thromboplastin antecedent	165 000	$2\frac{1}{2}$ d	Yes	No
XII	Hageman factor	80 000	$2\frac{1}{2}$ d	?Yes	No
XIII	Fibrin stabilising factor	350 000	3–7 d	Yes	No

[a] Factor III is tissue factor; factor IV is ionised calcium. These Roman numerals are not in use. Factor VI is no longer used. Platelets are not listed but contribute crucial procoagulants

Thrombin cleaves two pairs of small peptides called fibrinopeptides A and B from each fibrinogen molecule. The remaining structure is fibrin monomer. Fibrin monomers link end-to-end and side-to-side into fibrin polymers, long strands of 'unstable' fibrin, that is fibrin easily lysed by plasmin in vivo and soluble in urea and monochloracetic acid in vitro. Fibrin is stabilised through the action of thrombin-activated factor XIII which catalyses the formation of firm covalent bonds between adjacent fibrin polymers (Fig. 7.3) (Lorand, 1972). The action of thrombin on fibrinogen is instantaneous, but the stabilisation of fibrin continues for many hours. Defects in the thrombin fibrinogen reaction are reflected to varying degrees in all tests of coagulation, whereas abnormalities of factor XIII are detected only in clot solubility tests.

The overall scheme of coagulation is depicted in Figures 7.1, 7.2 and 7.3.

Inhibitors

The uncontrolled action of activated coagulation factors with consequent generalised intravascular clotting is prevented by plasma protease inhibitors, that is plasma proteins that neutralise proteolytic enzymes. Four of them play an important role in regulating haemostasis: α_2-macroglobulin, antithrombin III, α_1-antitrypsin, C_1-inactivator. Antithrombin III is also called heparin cofactor or anti-Xa, and its neutralising action on coagulation enzymes, in particular on factor Xa is greatly potentiated and accelerated in the presence of even very small amounts of heparin. This interaction between heparin and antithrombin III forms the basis of the low dose heparin prophylaxis for venous thrombosis (Rosenberg, 1975).

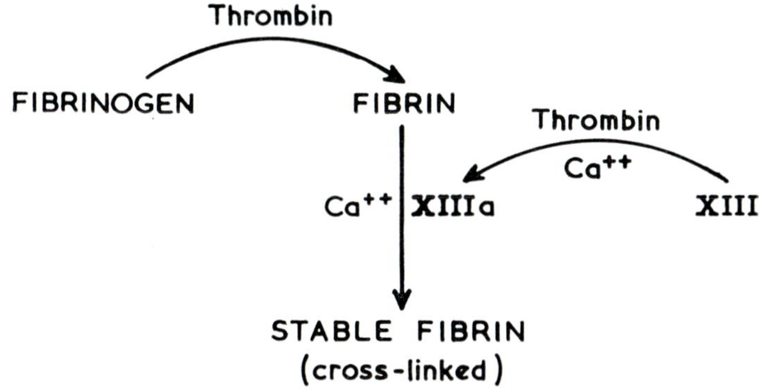

Figure 7.3   Formation and stabilisation of fibrin

Fibrinolysis

The dissolution of fibrin clots in vitro and fibrin deposits in vivo is called *fibrinolysis*. It is effected through the action of yet another proteolytic enzyme, plasmin (Nilsson, 1974). The generation of plasmin and its effects on fibrinogen and fibrin are shown in Figure 7.4.

Plasminogen is a protein produced by the liver which is converted into plasmin by activators. Plasminogen activators are enzymes present in most tissues, plasma, urine and other body fluids. Plasminogen can also be activated by exogenous activators such as streptokinase, a peptide produced by certain haemolytic streptococci.

Plasmin splits many peptide bonds in fibrin and fibrinogen, and many different fragments are formed. The larger molecular weight fragments comprise several groups named fragments X, Y, D and E (Marder, 1971). The largest fragments, X, can be clotted by thrombin and are incorporated into fibrin clots. The Y fragments have marked anticoagulant effects due to interference with normal fibrin polymerisation. The smaller fragments D and E are the derivatives commonly found in the plasma of patients with disseminated intravascular coagulation and attendant fibrinolysis. Fibrin–fibrinogen degradation products are rapidly cleared from circulation by the mononuclear phagocytic system, especially the liver.

An increase in plasma levels of plasminogen activators is often found on laboratory testing, but a measurable increase in free plasmin rarely follows because it is neutralised by inhibitory antiplasmin systems in plasma (Nilsson 1974). In contrast, plasmin readily arises from plasminogen incorporated in thrombi. To explain this, two hypotheses are proposed: one, that in the thrombus plasminogen is activated in close proximity to fibrin and acts before the inhibitors can interfere (Sherry, Fletcher and Alkjaersig, 1959).

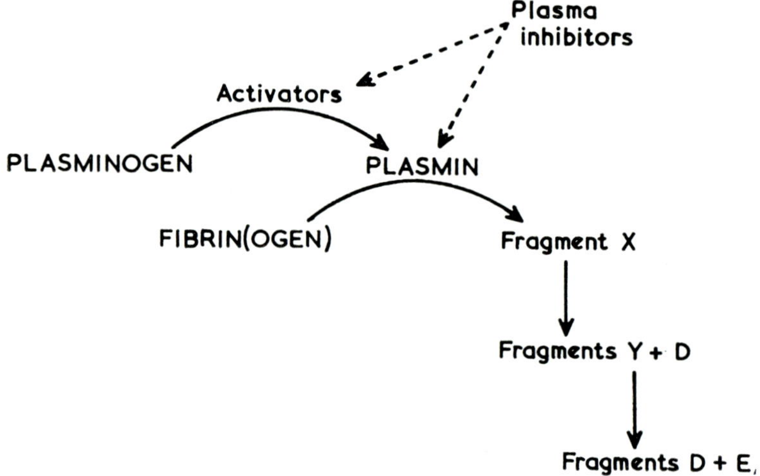

Figure 7.4   Formation of plasmin and products of fibrinolysis

The other hypothesis suggests that the plasmin formed in the circulation is rapidly complexed with inhibitors, mainly α_2-macroglobulin (Ambrus and Markus, 1960). When these complexes come into contact with thrombus, plasmin is dissociated and acts on fibrin, whereas α_2-macroglogulin is excluded due to its high molecular weight. The two hypotheses are not mutually exclusive.

LABORATORY INVESTIGATION OF HAEMOSTASIS

There is no single test which identifies all patients likely to have pathological bleeding. A relatively simple screening programme is valuable in complementing the history and examination. It must be emphasised that routine 'bleeding and clotting times' alone are not an adequate substitute for pertinent clinical and laboratory data.

Haemostatic Plug Formation

These tests examine platelet and vascular function.

Inspection of a well-stained *blood film* for normal platelet numbers and morphology will suffice in the laboratory if history and examination are entirely negative. White or red cell precursors may indicate a marrow disorder, irregular or fragmented erythrocytes may point to intravascular fibrin deposition, and rouleaux formation will prompt search for an abnormal protein with its dangers of bleeding at surgery.

A *platelet count* is often desirable, but a film should still be inspected to see if they are unduly large as in increased or abnormal platelet production.

The *bleeding time* is of special value when defective haemostasis is suspected and the platelets are normal in number. Though subject to variables of technique (which are least with a standardised Ivy method), it is the most useful test of vascular and platelet function but does not distinguish these two haemostatic components. Platelet function can be further assessed by measuring their response to aggregating agents, their retention in a glass bead column ('adhesiveness'), their release of platelet factor 3 on exposure to kaolin or in the prothrombin consumption test, and their ability to effect retraction of a whole blood clot.

Tests of Coagulation

Screening tests (Dacie and Lewis, 1975) give information about the extrinsic and intrinsic pathways of thrombin generation and the later steps in coagulation.

The *whole blood clotting time* alone is inadequate because it is insensitive, being commonly normal in defects sufficiently serious to cause dangerous surgical bleeding.

The *one-stage prothrombin time,* in which tissue thromboplastin is added to recalcified plasma, reflects the adequacy of the whole extrinsic clotting system, that is factors VII, X, V, prothrombin and fibrinogen (Fig. 7.2).

By also doing the *activated partial thromboplastin time* (PTT), in which the added phospholipid is equivalent to platelet factor 3 and the contact factors are also triggered, it is possible to screen for deficiency of all the plasma coagulation factors (Fig. 7.2). However, elevated levels of one or more individual factors, or the presence of activated clotting factors, may mask deficiency of another, and in patients with clinical evidence of bleeding further investigation is essential even if this test is within the normal range.

The *thrombin or calcium thrombin time test* is carried out by adding a dilute solution of thrombin (sometimes with calcium) to the patient's plasma and comparing the clotting time with a normal control. The test reflects the thrombin–fibrinogen reaction and is prolonged when plasma fibrinogen is unduly low or structurally abnormal, or when anticoagulants such as heparin, or FDP in high concentrations, are present.

Further investigation consists in performing individual coagulation factor assays, fibrinogen estimation, clot solubility testing and measurement of inhibitors, by clotting, chemical and immunological techniques. These tests can detect even a minor deficiency of a single factor when used with suitable standards and technical expertise.

Tests of Fibrinolysis

Tests of fibrinolytic activity are mostly qualitative and much less is known about the significance of minor changes than is the case with coagulation. No congenital abnormalities of fibrinolysis have been recognised.

Plasminogen activator. The levels of plasminogen activator are measured by the dilute whole blood clot lysis time, or by lysis of fibrin in tubes, or on a fibrin plate, produced by the euglobulin fraction of plasma. The principle of such tests is to remove natural inhibitors of plasminogen activation by dilution (whole blood clot lysis time) (Fearnley, Revill and Tweed, 1952) or dilution and acidification (euglobulin clot lysis) (Chakrabarti et al, 1968) and to record the time taken to lyse the blood or plasma clot. Very short lysis times occur in the presence of brisk fibrinolysis either therapeutically induced or as a response to stress, strenuous exercise or disseminated intravascular fibrin deposition. Prolonged lysis times are found in patients with vascular disease, obesity, renal disease, often in the aftermath of surgery and tissue damage and during pregnancy.

Fibrin–fibrinogen degradation products (FDP) can be measured by a variety of techniques, mostly immunological (Denson, 1972). Fragments X, Y, D and E have antigenic determinants common to fibrinogen and thus react when incubated with fibrinogen antisera. If the serum sample tested contains FDP the fibrinogen antiserum will be neutralised and fibrinogen-coated latex particles or tanned red cells will not agglutinate when added. FDP concentration is expressed as μg/ml (normal less than 10), or as a titre whose normal value varies with the test system. Slightly increased values are commonly found in a wide variety of conditions including liver disease, septicaemia, eclampsia, thromboembolic disease, myeloproliferative disorders and after surgery. Very high levels of FDP are usually found in fulminant disseminated intravascular coagulation.

Paracoagulation tests (Godal and Abildgaard, 1966). Plasma containing soluble complexes of fibrin monomers with fibrinogen or FDP forms a transparent gel when ethanol or protamine sulphate is added. This phenomenon is called paracoagulation. Positive paracoagulation tests are found in several diseases, particularly pneumonia and septicaemia. They may be a useful clue to disseminated intravascular coagulation in early or compensated cases when no other abnormalities may yet be discerned; elevated levels of plasma fibrinogen diminish their significance.

SURGICAL BLEEDING DUE TO EXISTING HAEMOSTATIC DEFECTS

Abnormal bleeding during or after a surgical procedure may result when any component of the haemostatic mechanism is severely impaired. While such derangements may be related to the operation itself, some precede it either as inborn defects or as acquired features possibly of the very illness leading to surgery. Awareness of this hazard enables the timely recognition of these haemorrhagic states and the control necessary to successful surgery.

Vascular Disorders

A group of conditions exists marked by spontaneous bleeding from small blood vessels without thrombocytopenia or coagulation defects. Vascular purpura results from weakness of the walls of arterioles, venules and capillaries, or of their supporting structures. Like the bleeding in platelet disorders, with which it is sometimes associated, it is characteristically seen as petechiae or ecchymoses in poorly supported skin and in mucous membranes. Vascular purpura is frequently palpable. Certain forms, notably haemorrhagic telangiectases and pseudoxanthoma elasticum among the rare hereditary anomalies, may cause serious blood loss requiring surgical intervention. Others are quite harmless (simple purpura, senile purpura), while some—like the dominant Ehlers–Danlos (lax skin) syndrome—cause poor haemostasis and defective wound healing.

Hereditary haemorrhagic telangiectases (Rendu–Osler–Weber disease), an autosomal dominant disorder, is characterised by thin-walled, non-contractile, vascular lesions which may bleed torrentially from various sites. Usually seen on the tongue, lips and extremities, the haemostatic defect is confined to the friable lesions themselves. When recurrent or dangerous haemorrhage occurs from the nose, stomach or bowel, urinary tract, bonchial tree or nervous system, surgical resection may be safely undertaken. Naso-septal dermoplasty (Hardisty, 1968; Owen, Bowie and Thompson, 1975) is particularly successful, but recurrence may mar any operative treatment.

Acquired vascular purpura is encountered in anaphylactoid, infectious, metabolic and psychiatric disturbances. Occasional surgical intervention requires awareness of its existence. *Anaphylactoid (Henoch–Schönlein) purpura* is an allergic vasculitis, often bacterial or drug-related, affecting skin, bowel, joints, kidneys and heart, the skin lesions commonly being palpable. Platelet counts and other tests of haemostasis are normal. Emergency surgery may be indicated for intussusception or uncontrolled bowel bleeding. Prognosis is determined by the severity of renal involvement.

Scurvy still occurs in the very young and old among the deprived, and may contribute to impaired haemostasis and healing. As in *amyloidosis* and some *paraproteinaemias*, both capillaries and platelet function are affected

(Hardisty, 1968; Owen et al, 1975). In *corticosteroid purpura*, sometimes of iatrogenic origin, systemic haemostasis is normal; but operative steroid cover and reassessment of dosage (or diagnosis) are indicated.

Platelet Disorders

Thrombocytopenia

In health, normal platelet numbers (150 000 to 400 000/μl of blood) reflect the balance between production by the megakaryocytes in the bone marrow and utilisation, destruction or sequestration elsewhere in the body (Aster, 1972). Thrombocytopenia can thus arise if production fails or if platelet loss exceeds the capacity of the bone marrow to regenerate them. A classification of thrombocytopenia is given in Table 7.2.

The haemorrhagic skin lesions of thrombocytopenic purpura may be tiny (petechiae) or extensive (ecchymoses) and are commonly more marked over the lower limbs and areas of loose skin. Mucosal haemorrhages such as

Table 7.2   Some causes of thrombocytopenia

Decreased production	Marrow aplasia
	Marrow infiltration
Shortened survival	Idiopathic thrombocytopenic purpura
	Drug induced purpura
Increased consumption	Disseminated intravascular coagulation
	Haemangiomas
Sequestration	Hypersplenism
Dilution	Massive bank blood transfusion

menorrhagia, haematuria, epistaxis, gingival, buccal and gastrointestinal bleeding are also common. Intracranial, retinal or retroperitoneal bleeding are rare but dangerous consequences of thrombocytopenia. With moderately reduced platelet counts, a tendency to easy bruising may be the only symptom; dangerous or spontaneous bleeding rarely occurs with platelet counts above 20 000/μl.

The surgeon usually encounters thrombocytopenic patients at splenectomy (which removes the main site of platelet destruction in idiopathic thrombocytopenic purpura and hypersplenism) or at incidental surgery performed in individuals with thrombocytopenic purpura of any aetiology.

In *idiopathic thrombocytopenic purpura* (ITP) platelet destruction is caused by immune mechanisms. The platelet count is low, but normal or increased numbers of megakaryocytes are present in the bone marrow. In children it often follows an infection, such as measles, rubella or mumps, and commonly runs a benign and self-limited course. In adults it is more clearly an autoimmune disease and the onset is often insidious. Sometimes the syndrome of ITP may be part of the presentation of systemic lupus erythematosus. In some adults it is a protracted, benign disease and no treatment is required.

Those with severe purpura or bleeding are treated with prednisone; the platelet count commonly increases to normal or near normal levels. A small proportion of patients does not respond to corticosteroids, and some of those who respond require unacceptably high doses to keep free of bleeding. In such patients splenectomy is the treatment of choice, as satisfactory clinical remission is obtained in the majority of those below the age of 50 (Pitney 1972).

Preoperative management is important to minimise the risk of bleeding. If steroids were administered before operation, they should be continued or resumed in increased dosage during the operative period. Surgical haemostatic care should be meticulous; it is useful to know that widespread capillary oozing (due to the defective primary haemostasis of thrombocytopenia) is effectively staunched by sustained pressure. Patients with very low platelet counts may be given platelet concentrates during surgery, preferably immediately after clamping the splenic blood vessels to avoid loss of transfused platelets into the spleen. After splenectomy platelets begin to rise steeply within two to three days, or sometimes more gradually over one to two weeks.

Table 7.3 Some congenital abnormalities of platelets

Familial thrombocytopenias	Wiskott–Aldrich syndrome
	Fanconi's anaemia
	May–Heggelin anomaly
Hereditary platelet dysfunction	Thrombasthenia
	Platelet storage pool disease
	Bernard–Soulier syndrome

Anticoagulant therapy (warfarin or low-dose subcutaneous heparin) during the peak thrombocytosis is advisable in the elderly and obese.

Many *drugs* can cause thrombocytopenia, either by a direct toxic effect on platelets or megakaryocytes, or by immune mechanisms. In most cases the platelet count returns to normal within a few days of withdrawing the drug, although with some such as gold, recovery may take many months (Pitney, 1972; Aster, 1972). Platelet transfusions are of little benefit as donor platelets may be destroyed by the same mechanism as the patient's platelets. Nevertheless, they are distinctly beneficial if surgery must be carried out.

Patients suffering from thrombocytopenia due to *bone marrow depression* or *infiltration* are likely to bleed severely at surgery, which is best avoided. Essential procedures must be covered with platelet transfusions.

Splenectomy may also be carried out if thrombocytopenia is due to *splenic sequestration*, as commonly found in portal hypertension, Felty's syndrome, various haematological diseases such as lymphoma, haemoglobinopathies, myelofibrosis, and in Gaucher's disease and other storage disorders.

Functional platelet defects

Surgery is occationally required in patients with congenital abnormalities of platelets (Table 7.3).

Patients with *familial thrombocytopenia* are usually children, sometimes with other congenital abnormalities (Chessels and Hardisty, 1974). In *hereditary platelet dysfunction* the platelet count is normal, but the platelets cannot sustain a normal haemostatic plug. These patients suffer from a lifelong bleeding tendency, severe in thrombasthenia and Bernard–Soulier syndrome, and usually mild in platelet storage pool disease (Weiss, 1975). Operations require platelet cover in the severely affected patients.

Abnormalities of platelet function may arise as a result of treatment with antiplatelet drugs; they are also often found in uraemia, myeloproliferative disorders and paraproteinaemias.

Aspirin, all non-steroid anti-inflammatory drugs, dipyridamole, anti-depressants, antihistamines and many other drugs interfere with platelet function and may cause brisk intra- and postoperative bleeding. Such drugs, particularly aspirin, should be avoided preoperatively whenever possible. The antiplatelet effects of aspirin wear off in 5 to 11 days, whereas the effect of other drugs does not last beyond 48 h (Weiss, 1972).

In *chronic renal failure* platelet dysfunction is probably caused by the presence of metabolites of urea in plasma (Rabiner, 1972). Intractable bleeding from mucous membranes and after renal biopsy is not uncommon. Platelet transfusions are of little use as normal platelets lose their function when exposed to the patient's plasma; bleeding is usually best corrected by haemodialysis.

In *myeloproliferative diseases* functionally abnormal platelets are produced by the bone marrow, and a bleeding tendency is often found in patients with normal or even greatly increased platelet counts (Lewis, Szur and Hoffbrand, 1972). Platelet transfusions are needed to cover unavoidable surgery.

The haemostatic defect in *paraproteinaemia* is complex; the abnormal protein sometimes coats platelets and interferes with their normal function (Lackner, 1973).

Platelet transfusion

Platelet replacement can be given as fresh whole blood, platelet rich plasma and platelet concentrates (Cash, 1972). Platelets lose their viability very quickly and are of little use in preparations more than 48 h old. ABO compatible and, whenever possible, Rh compatible platelets should be given as all platelet preparations contain some red cells and may cause immunisation of the recipient. If the patient is a child with a congenital platelet abnormality likely to require repeated transfusions, it is advisable to use single donor platelets obtained by plasmapheresis in order to reduce the risk of immunisation; unfortunately, this is rarely feasible.

Platelet rich plasma and platelet concentrates are prepared from fresh blood centrifuged to removed red cells; for platelet concentrates further centrifugation reduces the volume of plasma containing platelets. Platelets obtained from one donation of fresh blood are 1 unit of platelets and can be expected to raise the platelet count by about $10000/\mu l$ in an adult recipient. Platelet concentrates are pools of 5 units, and 10 units are usually sufficient for an adult at the time of surgery if clinically indicated. Larger doses may be needed in the presence of bleeding or infection, or if the patient had been transfused previously. It is necessary to repeat platelet transfusions after surgery if the count remains low (below $20000/\mu l$) and the patient is bleeding.

Coagulation Disorders

Patients may require surgical treatment who also have plasma coagulation defects. These may be inborn or acquired, and their accurate recognition is a prerequisite for successful operative management.

Congenital defects

Inborn abnormalities of coagulation are rare diseases. The commonest are haemophilia A (classical haemophilia) and von Willebrand's disease, in both of which there is a factor VIII defect, and haemophilia B (Christmas disease) in which factor IX is defective. Genetic coagulation defects generally involve a single factor, and are characterised by life-long easy bruising, painful, often spontaneous bleeding into joints and muscles, prolonged bleeding after minor injuries and operations, and a tendency to epistaxis, menorrhagia, haematuria and gastrointestinal haemorrhage.

Haemophilia A and Christmas disease are clinically indistinguishable, and are both inherited as a sex-linked recessive disorder. In Britain the estimated prevalence of haemophilia is one in about 10000 males, with Christmas disease patients numbering one-tenth of the total. The hetero-zygous female carrier typically has intermediate levels of clotting factor; some are sufficiently low to have a mild bleeding tendency. This may be disregarded until its true nature is unmasked dangerously at surgical operation. It is essential to distinguish between haemophilia A and B as modern replace-ment therapy employs different plasma materials for each, which are in-effective when used for the other.

CLASSICAL HAEMOPHILIA

Haemophiliacs possess normal amounts of factor VIII-related protein detectable immunochemically, but this protein does not have the normal clotting activity. The reduced plasma factor VIII activity in patients is between 0.0 and 0.4 international units per millilitre, i.e. between 0 and 40 per cent of average normal.[1] The clinical severity is largely determined by the plasma level of factor VIII which tends to be the same among affected members of one family. A patient who has less than 0.01 i.u./ml of factor VIII (1 per cent) has inherited severe haemophilia with frequent spontaneous

---

[1] One international unit of factor VIII is based on the activity of 1 ml of average fresh normal plasma (also described as having 100 per cent activity).

bleeding into joints, muscles and other sites, and progressive crippling if not treated. Those whose clotting activity is 2 to 5 per cent of normal are only moderately affected, and with 6 to 25 per cent of factor VIII activity a patient has mild haemophilia and bleeds excessively only if injured. Subjects with levels of 26 to 40 per cent are in practice 'masked', but like those with mild haemophilia they may bleed dangerously—even fatally—after surgical operations or major trauma unless recognised and adequately protected.

Bleeding usually starts at the end of the first year when the child becomes more active and affects knees, ankles, elbows and shoulders, often in the absence of obvious injury. The haemarthroses are painful and if left untreated lead to permanent joint disability. Buccal bleeding is common at this time. Haemorrhage into muscles and soft tissues may cause damage to nerves and arteries, with ensuing weakness, ischaemia and contracture of muscles. Gastrointestinal bleeding and painless haematuria are common. Clot formation in the renal pelvis may obstruct urinary flow and cause attacks of ureteric colic. Untreated haemophilic bleeding after surgery or trauma may persist relentlessly for many days or weeks. The bleeding starts several hours after the injury and cannot be controlled by local measures. Superficial cuts, nicks or needle punctures do not bleed excessively, since platelet–capillary function ensures a normal bleeding time.

The diagnosis is confirmed by the laboratory finding of a low plasma factor VIII activity. The traditional whole blood clotting time is prolonged only in those severely affected, but an abnormally long PTT is found in all but very mildly affected patients. While knowledge of affected male relatives on the mother's side supports the diagnosis, 40 per cent of patients have a negative family history.

The surgeon encounters haemophilia in several circumstances: (a) haemophilic bleeding may masquerade as an *acute surgical emergency*, commonly abdominal, for which the treatment is intensive factor VIII replacement and symptomatic relief of pain, dehydration and ileus. An important instance is retroperitoneal haemorrhage into the iliacus or psoas muscles presenting with pain, hypovolaemic shock, hip flexion, an iliac fossa mass and femoral nerve deficit. Intramural bowel bleeding causes vomiting, cramps, peritonism, fever and leukocytosis, and (in a known haemophiliac) evaluation of adequate replacement therapy for several hours—preferably a day—is indicated before embarking on laparotomy. The occasional occurrence of massive gastrointestinal bleeding requires similar management unless radiographic or endoscopic evidence of peptic ulcer (or other operable lesion) dictates surgical intervention under experienced haematological guidance. (b) *Coincidental* conditions may require surgery in haemophiliacs (dental extractions, traffic injury, neoplasm, etc.) and (c) operative treatment may be indicated for lesions attributable to the *bleeding state* (obstructed airway requiring tracheostomy, intussusception complicating a bowel haematoma, subdural bleeding after minor head injury). (d) Increasingly, *orthopaedic surgery* is enabling correction of disabling deformities resulting from repeated haemarthroses, wasting or contractures. (e) Paradoxically *mildly affected* haemophiliacs run the greatest surgical risk since they are as likely to bleed disastrously after major trauma or surgery, but may not say—or even know—that they are haemostatically abnormal.

Replacement therapy. The treatment of bleeding in haemophilia consists in replacing factor VIII by infusion of human plasma or factor VIII concentrates. The half-life of administered factor VIII is only about 12 h, and repeated infusions are necessary to maintain the desired factor VIII level. Factor VIII is very labile on storage, requiring prompt processing of donated blood; non-freeze-dried preparations such as plasma or cryoprecipitate must be stored at $-20°C$ or less.

Materials used. Factor VIII can be given as fresh frozen plasma, cryoprecipitate or, more recently, reconstituted freeze-dried concentrate. *Fresh frozen plasma* is prepared from individual donations and because of volume limitation cannot ordinarily be infused beyond a rise of 0.2 i.u./ml in plasma factor VIII. This may be sufficient to arrest minor spontaneous bleeding but is difficult to sustain long enough for healing of even minor surgical operations.

Cryoprecipitate is also prepared from individual fresh plasma donations. When rapidly frozen plasma is thawed at 4°C, a thick sludge (cryoprecipitate) remains till last. It contains fibrinogen, cold-insoluble globulins and about one half of the total factor VIII present in the original plasma. The supernatant plasma is removed and the few remaining millilitres of cryoprecipitate stored at $-30°C$. For use it is thawed, reconstituted in saline, and the contents of several different bags pooled. As a dose for an adult may require 30 to 40 bags, this procedure is time consuming and may involve considerable loss of factor VIII activity. The average factor VIII activity in a bag of cryoprecipitate, when a large number is pooled, is about 70 i.u. (Rizza, 1975).

Lyophilised concentrates of human factor VIII are prepared by plasma fractionation and freeze-drying. These materials come in vials containing about 250 units of factor VIII, and are stable for many months at 4°C. For use they are dissolved in 10 to 20 ml of sterile water, enabling effective haemostatic doses to be injected in a small volume of minimal osmotic load. Some concentrates derived from large plasma pools have hitherto carried an appreciable risk of transmitting serum hepatitis.

Animal factor VIII concentrates from cattle or swine have played a notable part in haemophilic surgery, but are now only used in some patients with factor VIII inhibitors, or if adequate human material is unobtainable in an emergency.

The dose of factor VIII administered and its frequency are determined by the type of bleeding, the patient's size, and by the in vivo recovery and survival of the material used. After injection the half-life of factor VIII is about 12 h.

An early, 'spontaneous' haemarthrosis or soft tissue bleed responds rapidly to a factor VIII level of 0.10 to 0.20 i.u/ml (10–20 per cent of normal) in the patient's plasma. A severe haemorrhage affecting joints, muscles or internal organ requires the plasma factor VIII to be raised to 30 to 40 per cent and maintained by repeated injection at least at half that level for three to five days. Not only does adequate replacement therapy bring about relief of pain, impaired function and pressure effects, it also helps to decide whether an acute abdomen is due solely to a haemophilic episode, or requires surgical intervention for an added complication such as intussusception or coincidental pathology.

Major surgical operations, emergency or elective, and serious injuries can be successfully managed if enough factor VIII is administered until healing is firmly established. An initial plasma level above 0.8 i.u./ml (80 per cent of normal) is aimed at. Thereafter levels exceeding 40 per cent activity are maintained for 7 to 10 days by repeated 12-hourly injections, and levels of 20 to 30 per cent for another 7 to 10 days. For abdominal surgery a total of 10 to 14 days is usually sufficient, whereas operations on bone or muscle, which heal more slowly, require factor VIII replacement for about three weeks; further intermittent administration is advisable until weight-bearing or full activity is restored.

The importance of conserving veins both for injection and blood sampling is paramount in haemophilic surgery. No infusion should stay in situ longer than 24 h, and when feasible indwelling needles should be replaced by intermittent venepuncture at alternating sites.

Dental extractions can commonly be carried out with a single large dose of factor VIII to raise plasma levels to above 0.5 i.u./ml; if the synthetic antifibrinolytic agent, EACA, is administered simultaneously and the surgical procedure is not too extensive, no further factor VIII may be needed. EACA is given in a dose of 100 mg/kg body weight every 6 h for 7 to 10 days; alternatively tranexamic acid (Forbes et al, 1972) 15 mg/kg thrice daily, which does not cause nausea, may be given.

Calculation of dosage. Various formulae have been devised based on the patient's estimated plasma volume and the desired rise in factor VIII concentration. In a surgical setting it is important to assay the initial factor VIII levels to confirm the adequacy of the calculated dose, and periodically thereafter. Rizza (1972) uses a formula based directly on the percentage plasma factor VIII rise for each unit per kilogram of administered factor VIII. This R (for recovery) value is 1.5 per cent using cryoprecipitate and 2 per cent when lyophilised human factor VIII is injected (Rizza, 1975). One can thus determine the dose of factor VIII required to attain a particular increment in plasma activity which, expressed as a percentage, will be 1.5 to 2.0 times the number of units administered per kilogram (Table 7.4).

The main *complications of replacement therapy* are serum *hepatitis*, and the development of an *inhibitor* against factor VIII. Such an IgG antibody, occurring in about 6 per cent of haemophiliacs (Rizza, 1972), usually with severe deficiency, neutralises infused factor VIII and greatly impedes replacement therapy. Its presence is suspected when injections of factor VIII raise the plasma level only slightly and transiently, or not at all. Even small surgical procedures may bleed intractably and threaten life if an inhibitor is overlooked preoperatively, or develops early in treatment. Large neutralising doses of factor VIII may stop a dangerous spontaneous bleed, but at the cost of a secondary antibody rise. The rise is not predictably averted by simultaneous immunosuppressive treatment. Haemostasis has also been promoted by concentrates of the vitamin K-dependent factors (Kurczynski and Penner, 1974). Repeated continuous-flow plasmapheresis to remove high-titre factor VIII antibody facilitates neutralisation of the remaining inhibitor (Edson et al, 1973; Mibashan et al, 1975); only with such facilities can surgery be contemplated, and even then it is best avoided.

Table 7.4 Therapeutic levels of factor VIII related to lesion treated and dose infused

Bleeding lesion	Initial factor VIII level desired (% normal)	Factor VIII dose (i.u./kg)[a]
Early, spontaneous	10–20	10–15
Severe joint, soft tissue; dental extraction	30–40	20–30
Major surgery or trauma	80–100	50–80

[a] The amount varies with the material injected and individual circumstances

Patients with haemophilia should not be given aspirin or any drugs that affect platelets as they may aggravate the bleeding tendency; they should not be given intramuscular injections except when 'covered' for operation.

The best care for haemophiliacs is provided by haemophilia centres where experienced staff is always available to give prompt treatment and appropriate advice.

VON WILLEBRAND'S DISEASE

In this congenital defect the patients have a prolonged bleeding time and low level of factor VIII clotting activity. The inheritance is autosomal dominant and affects both sexes to a variable degree in any one family. Many patients with von Willebrand's disease are only mildly affected; they have repeated nose bleeds, menorrhagia or bruising. Rarely, severely affected patients with very low factor VIII levels bleed into joints and muscles and are clinically indistinguishable from haemophilia A.

The *diagnosis* is established on the basis of low factor VIII levels, prolonged bleeding time, and family history when it is available. In addition these patients have diminished plasma levels of factor VIII-related antigen and defective platelet aggregation by ristocetin. This is an antibiotic that aggregates the platelets of all normal individuals but not those of patients suffering from von Willebrand's disease (Howard, Sawers and Firkin, 1973).

Treatment of von Willebrand's disease is similar to that of haemophilia but is generally much easier. Identical materials are used, but fortunately the levels of factor VIII show a prolonged rise for up to 72 h after the infusion and are therefore easier to maintain. The prolonged bleeding time may be corrected for a shorter time following infusion, and such platelet–capillary oozing responds, when accessible, to local compression until haemostasis is consolidated by fibrin.

CHRISTMAS DISEASE

This is factor IX deficiency or haemophilia B and is clinically indistinguishable from haemophilia A. In the United Kingdom about one in ten patients with haemophilia has haemophilia B. The diagnosis is established by demonstrating a low plasma factor IX level.

As for haemophilia A, replacement treatment is the mainstay of management. Factor IX is more stable on storage than factor VIII and also has a longer in vivo plasma half-life of 18 to 24 h. Against these advantages, the recovery of infused factor IX in the patient's blood is poor compared with the response to factor VIII infusion. A relatively larger dose must be given initially, and about half repeated daily, to maintain haemostatic levels.

Two types of material are available—plasma and lyophilised concentrates. *Plasma*, 15 to 20 ml/kg body weight, is ordinarily suitable to arrest only spontaneous bleeding, although in an emergency much more can be infused with the help of diuretics and partial plasma exchange. To achieve the higher haemostatic levels needed for surgery or accidental injury, *lyophilised concentrates* derived from human plasma fractionation must be used. These also contain prothrombin and factor X, and in some cases factor VII (Dike, Bidwell and Rizza, 1972). The aim is to maintain factor IX levels above 30 per cent of normal until the wounds have healed. This requires an initial dose of 80 u/kg of body weight (1 u is equivalent to 1 ml of average fresh normal plasma), and 40 to 50 u/kg once daily thereafter, or more frequently if indicated by assays (Rizza, 1974).

Other coagulation deficiencies are exceptionally rare, and their clinical manifestations are generally similar to those of mild haemophilia. Their identity is established by laboratory tests. Deficiencies of prothrombin, factor X and factor VII are corrected by infusion of concentrates used for Christmas disease. Fresh frozen plasma is needed in factor V, factor XI and factor XIII deficiency. Patients with factor XII deficiency rarely if ever bleed and do not require treatment. In congenital afibrinogenaemia human fibrinogen or cryoprecipitate is administered.

Acquired defects of coagulation

LIVER DISEASE

The liver is of major importance in maintaining haemostasis: it is the site of production of fibrinogen, vitamin K-dependent factors (prothrombin, factors VII, IX and X), factor V, and probably factors XI, XII and XIII, as well as of the plasma inhibitors (antithrombin III, α_2-macroglobulin and α_1-antitrypsin). The liver normally also removes active coagulation factors (Deykin, 1966) from the circulation and helps maintain a normal haemostatic balance. Liver disease can thus cause a variety of haemostatic abnormalities (Roberts and Cederbaum, 1972).

In *biliary obstruction* vitamin K, a fat-soluble vitamin, is not absorbed from the gut and the synthesis of the vitamin K-dependent factors is blocked. The low plasma levels of these factors cause a marked prolongation of the prothrombin time and moderate prolongation of the partial thromboplastin time. The defect is easily corrected by parenterally administered vitamin K, of which the naturally occurring form (vitamin K_1 or phytomenadione) is the most effective.

In *severe liver disease,* when its synthetic function fails, the plasma levels of both vitamin K-dependent factors and factor V are reduced, and vitamin K does not correct the abnormality. Fibrinogen levels are rarely affected except in advanced hepatic insufficiency. In patients with fulminant hepatitis or acute hepatic necrosis, the liver fails to clear active clotting factors from the blood and overt DIC may occur. Low fibrinogen levels, high serum FDP and reduced concentration of all coagulation factors ensue. The platelet count is commonly reduced by splenic sequestration, and in alcoholic cirrhosis by the direct toxic effect of alcohol on the bone marrow. DIC causes further thrombocytopenia, and the FDP formed may impair platelet function. In this setting bleeding, once begun, may prove intractable.

Patients with liver disease undergoing surgery are a serious haemostatic risk. If vitamin K_1 does not correct the defect, fresh blood, fresh frozen plasma, platelet concentrates and exchange transfusions can be used in an attempt to correct the defect preoperatively or to arrest bleeding. The results are often poor. Prothrombin complex concentrates should not be used as they may precipitate fatal DIC (Ménaché, 1975).

OTHER CAUSES OF VITAMIN K DEFICIENCY

Some severely ill or malnourished patients, as well as those on parenteral fluid therapy, may develop significant vitamin K deficiency. This can occur very quickly as body stores of this vitamin are negligible. Bleeding from the operative site or gastrointestinal tract may occur due to the low plasma levels of vitamin K-dependent factors. Prolonged prothrombin and partial thromboplastin time are found on laboratory investigation. The defect is rapidly corrected by vitamin K_1 administration, and in an emergency by fresh frozen plasma.

164   RECENT ADVANCES IN SURGERY

COAGULATION ABNORMALITIES IN RENAL DISEASE

In acute and chronic renal failure there is a tendency to both bleeding and thrombosis. The bleeding in uraemic patients is usually associated with platelet abnormalities (see page 157) and is best corrected by haemodialysis. In addition, very low plasma levels of factors VII, IX or X (Hardisty and Ingram, 1965), sometimes corrected by vitamin K administration, may be found in some patients. Low factor XIII (Losowsky and Walls, 1969) and raised serum FDP (Nilsson, 1974) are common findings; overt DIC is associated with some cases of acute renal failure. Correction of metabolic abnormalities and if necessary platelet transfusion are required to avoid pre- and postoperative bleeding in uraemic patients. The thrombotic tendency found in some patients is probably related to reduced plasma fibrinolytic activity (Wardle and Taylor, 1968; Larsson, Hedner and Nilsson, 1971).

CIRCULATING ANTICOAGULANTS

An autoantibody against factor VIII sometimes develops in patients with rheumatoid arthritis, drug allergy, connective tissue disorders, in women postpartum and rarely in individuals without any underlying disease. Such patients suffer from a severe bleeding disorder clinically indistinguishable from haemophilia. Steroids, immunosuppressants and large doses of factor VIII are used in the treatment (Rizza and Biggs, 1973). Occasionally the autoantibody disappears spontaneously. Surgery presents a major hazard best avoided; if inescapable, it should be dealt with in a haemophilia centre of ample resources. In patients with disseminated lupus erythematosus an autoantibody directed against prothrombin, tissue factor, or the prothrombin-activating complex of Xa–V–phospholipid, is sometimes found (Feinstein and Rapaport, 1972). Marked prolongation of prothrombin time and partial thromboplastin time is found, but there is little or no bleeding unless thrombo-cytopenia is also present.

Preoperative Evaluation

Haemostatic competence should be assessed preoperatively in every surgical patient. Recognition of this need is half its fulfilment, since the best single test of haemostatic function—other than surgery itself—is a pertinent *clinical history*. Physical examination and laboratory studies are helpful, but the latter especially complements the patient's history and do not substitute for it.

Patients with *known bleeding disorders*, whether life-long or acquired, are prepared for surgery (including needle biopsy and invasive diagnostic procedures) by laboratory confirmation of their defect, measurement of its severity, testing for clotting antibodies in haemophilia, and planning of adequate replacement or other protective measures.

In *other patients* the surgeon should determine whether any abnormal bleeding has complicated a previous haemostatic challenge, particularly tooth extraction, tonsillectomy, circumcision or accidental injury. Epistaxis, untoward bruising and menorrhagia may signify a platelet, vascular or coagulation defect justifying further study. The presence of coincidental disease, or the taking of drugs known to affect haemostasis must be ascertained preoperatively, and the extent of their influence determined and controlled.

A family history of bleeding disorder, though informative when present, is least likely to be helpful in those patients with undiagnosed mild deficiencies. It is precisely these patients, with few or no bleeding complaints and possibly no previous trauma, who merit closest questioning and a basic spectrum of laboratory tests preoperatively (p. 157). If a known deficiency exists in such a person's family, the specific assay should be performed even if the 'screening' tests are within normal limits and he (or she) is symptom-free. Previous trouble-free procedures render a serious inborn defect unlikely.

ACUTE HAEMOSTATIC FAILURE IN SURGERY

Occasionally a patient without any previous history of bleeding develops an acute generalised bleeding state at operation, immediately afterwards, or during the postoperative period. In a severe case there is intractable bleeding from the operative and drainage sites, oozing from venepunctures and catheters, extensive tracking haematomas and purpura. In less severe cases continuous bleeding from the wound may be the only manifestation, requiring rapid laboratory exclusion of a systemic defect before local re-exploration.

One of the causes of such bleeding is disseminated intravascular coagulation, but it may also be caused by massive transfusion with stored blood, liver failure (p. 143), ineffective neutralisation of heparin (after cardiopulmonary by-pass or vascular surgery) and undiagnosed preoperative haemostatic defects (p. 153) including treatment with oral anticoagulant drugs.

There is usually little time for complicated laboratory tests. Enough information for diagnosis and treatment is obtained from platelet count, one-stage prothrombin time, partial thromboplastin time and calcium thrombin time, determination of fibrinogen, and fibrin degradation products. The typical patterns of laboratory results in different conditions that may cause acute haemostatic failure are shown in Table 7.5.

Disseminated Intravascular Coagulation
(Defibrination Syndrome)

Disseminated intravascular coagulation (DIC) is due to widespread activation of coagulation in the blood. This results in consumption of coagulation factors and platelets, fibrin formation and secondary fibrinolysis (Deykin, 1970; Merskey, 1972; Rapaport, 1972). DIC is always secondary to other diseases (Table 7.6). It may occur as an acute, fulminant bleeding disorder or as a more chronic condition with both haemorrhagic and thrombotic manifestations; some patients with laboratory evidence of DIC are clinically silent.

In acute DIC there may be a sudden onset of purpura, bleeding from the gastrointestinal, urinary or genital tract, and excessive oozing from operative

Table 7.5 Laboratory tests in acute haemostatic failure

	Platelet count	Prothrombin time	Activated PTT	Calcium thrombin time	Fibrinogen	FDP
Disseminated intravascular coagulation	Low	Long	Long	Long	Usually low	Usually high
Massive transfusion	Low	Long	Long	N	N	N
Hepatocellular disease	N or low	Very long	Long	N or long	N or low	N or high
Oral anticoagulants or vitamin K deficiency	N	Very long	Long	N	N	N
Heparin	N	Long or N	Long	Long	N	N
Undiagnosed inborn defect (usually mild haemophilia)	N	N	Long or N	N	N	N

PTT = partial thromboplastin time; FDP = fibrin(ogen) degradation products; N = normal

Table 7.6 Conditions sometimes associated with DIC

Acute

Shock	Major surgery, especially thoracic
Septicaemia	Burns
Acute intravascular haemolysis (incompatible transfusion)	Placental abruption, amniotic fluid embolism, septic abortion
Acute pulmonary embolism	Heat stroke
Cardiac arrest and resuscitation	Bites of some poisonous snakes
Acute liver failure	

Chronic

Disseminated malignancy	Retained dead fetus
Pancreatic or ovarian carcinoma	Aortic aneurysm
Promyelocytic leukaemia	Giant haemangioma or haemangioblastoma

wounds. Blood loss, hypovolaemic shock and fibrin deposition in the renal microcirculation may lead to renal cortical necrosis and acute renal failure. Sometimes extensive haemorrhage and ischaemic necrosis of the skin occurs (purpura fulminans) and even limb gangrene may result. In patients with chronic DIC, especially in malignancy, thrombotic manifestations such as recurrent deep venous thrombosis or embolisation from large non-bacterial vegetations on heart valves may predominate. A proportion of patients with fibrin partially obstructing the microcirculation develop jaundice due to fragmentation of erythrocytes, so-called microangiopathic haemolytic anaemia.

Pathogenesis

DIC can be triggered directly by clot-promoting substances entering the circulation (tissue trauma, amniotic fluid embolism, snake venom), or indirectly by endotoxin or antigen–antibody complexes damaging red cells, leucocytes, platelets or vessel walls and thereby releasing procoagulant material. Factors that predispose to DIC are hypovolaemic shock, liver

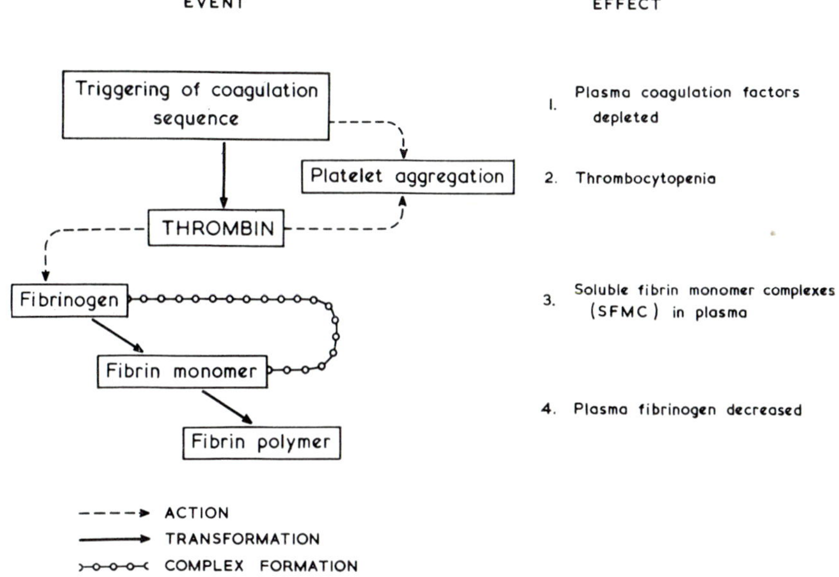

Figure 7.5   Coagulation sequence in DIC

disease, pregnancy, reduced fibrinolytic activity, and impairment of the mononuclear phagocytic system responsible for clearing procoagulants from the circulation (Evensen and Hjort, 1970).

The haemostatic abnormalities occurring in DIC are shown schematically in Figures 7.5 and 7.6.

The release of clot-promoting substances into the circulation results in the *generation of thrombin*. Thrombin splits fibrinopeptides A and B from fibrinogen, converting it to circulating fibrin monomer. This polymerises rapidly to fibrin, with concomitant lowering of plasma fibrinogen (Fig. 7.5). The deposition of fibrin in the microcirculation provokes brisk *secondary fibrinolysis*, leading to an increased concentration of *fibrin–fibrinogen degradation products* (FDP) (Fig. 7.6). Fibrin monomers released by thrombin may form soluble complexes with plasma fibrinogen; FDP produced by plasmin also form soluble fibrin monomer complexes (SFMC), which impede normal polymerisation.

Thrombin and plasmin combine in DIC to deplete the plasma of several clotting factors and fibrinogen by effecting coagulation and fibrinolysis. Platelets are aggregated and trapped in the microcirculation when widespread thrombin generation and fibrin deposition occur; they may also be involved early as a part of the triggering mechanism. The bleeding in DIC is thus the

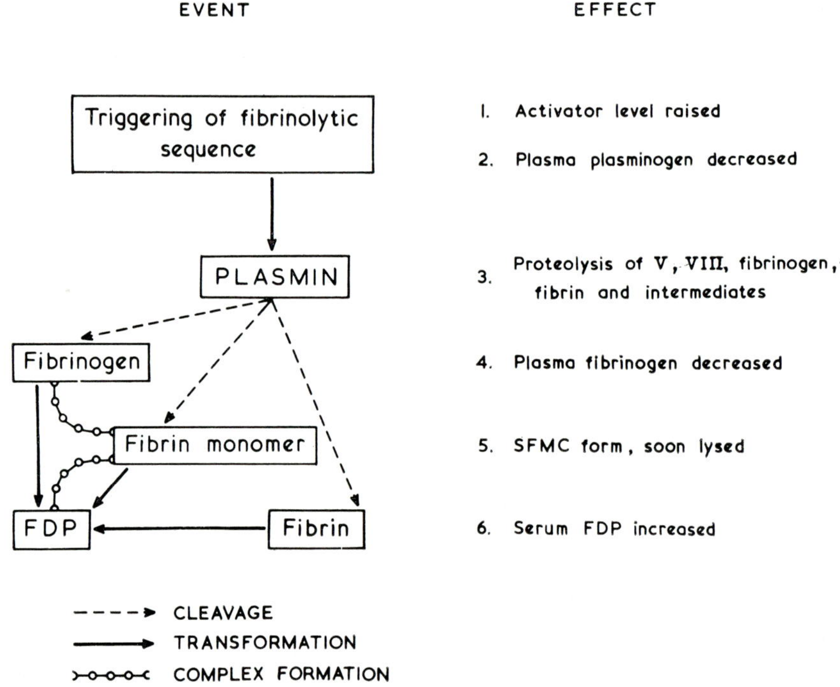

Figure 7.6 Fibrinolytic sequence in DIC, following the action of thrombin

result of multiple coagulation factor deficiencies, thrombocytopenia and the anticoagulant effect of FDP, in addition to any vessel wall damage which may coexist.

Red cells may be fragmented while passing through the fibrin mesh laid down in the microcirculation. In some cases they are damaged so severely that a haemolytic anaemia occurs, but this is not a constant feature of all DIC.

Diagnosis

In a suggestive clinical setting the prothrombin, partial thromboplastin and calcium thrombin times are prolonged and the platelet count reduced.

Thereafter fibrin monomer complexes are looked for and fibrinogen and FDP concentration measured.

The diagnosis of chronic DIC can be difficult as the results of initial tests may be normal or nearly so; recognition of the disorder is important pre-operatively to forestall or deal promptly with its escalation to an acute bleeding crisis. The condition is suspected in the presence of a persistently high FDP concentration, positive fibrin monomer test and, typically, a reduced platelet count.

Management of bleeding in acute DIC

Treatment of the causal disorder (hypovolaemic shock, septicaemia, retained dead fetus) removes the triggering mechanism (Rapaport, 1972; Flute, 1974). DIC itself does not always require active intervention. Treatment is required to stop persistent bleeding and to prevent anoxic tissue damage. Whole blood, preferably fresh, is used to replace the blood lost and to combat shock. The use of plasma expanders like dextran is undesirable during active haemorrhage as it causes haemodilution without contributing to haemostasis; indeed both platelet function and coagulation may be impaired by it. Clotting factors may be replaced with fresh frozen plasma; if cryoprecipitate or fibrinogen are given, deposition of fibrin from the infused material may lead to further tissue damage. By the same token platelet concentrates are given cautiously in the acute phase as they may form aggregates that block the microcirculation. Fibrinogen level and platelet count are monitored carefully during treatment, and fibrinogen and platelet concentrates infused if low levels persist, with bleeding, after the triggering mechanism is removed.

The decision whether to give heparin to arrest intravascular coagulation is difficult, since it may provoke further bleeding especially in major surgery or trauma. It is commonly used in patients with evidence of renal damage, in some with malignancy, e.g. promyelocytic leukaemia, or if thrombotic manifestations coexist, and in haemangiomata and purpura fulminans. It is difficult to evaluate the results of treatment. If heparin is given, low doses (maximum 10 i.u./kg body weight/h) should be administered by constant intravenous infusion under careful clinical and laboratory supervision. In patients already bleeding the aim of treatment is not to prolong the clotting time further, but to correct thrombocytopenia, fibrinogen depletion and raised FDP.

Primary Fibrinogenolysis

Primary fibrinogenolysis (Nilsson, 1974) is an extremely rare condition associated with liver disease or some carcinomas, usually of the prostate. There is systemic fibrinolysis without activation of coagulation. It should be suspected in such a patient whose laboratory signs resemble DIC except for a normal platelet count, negative fibrin monomer complex tests and extremely short euglobulin or dilute whole blood clot lysis times. Because of its rarity and uncertainty as the sole cause of systemic defibrination, the use of anti-fibrinolytic agents alone is dangerous.

Local fibrinolysis is thought to be one of the causes of bleeding after prostatectomy or bladder operations, and one of the contributory causes of menorrhagia (Nilsson, 1974).

Management

Synthetic antifibrinolytic agents (epsilon-amino caproic acid and tranexamic acid) have been used to suppress local fibrinolysis when this is considered a possibility. Both drugs are rapidly absorbed from the gastrointestinal tract and excreted in urine, where their concentration is 80 to 100 times that in plasma. Usual adult doses are 24 g of EACA or 3 g of tranexamic acid in six or three divided doses per day by mouth. The main danger is of formation of un-lysable clots in the urinary tract, as well as deep vein thrombosis and pul-monary embolism.

Bleeding Due to Massive Transfusion with Stored Blood

Bank blood contains no platelets, and little factor V or VIII, as they are lost on storage. The levels of fibrinogen and vitamin K-dependent factors are normal or only slightly reduced. Plasma protein fraction, increasingly used as a volume expander, is devoid of fibrinogen, factor V or VIII and also most of the vitamin K-dependent factors. Patients transfused with 10 units or more of stored blood or plasma protein fraction are gradually depleted of coagulation factors and platelets. The platelet count is sometimes sufficiently reduced to contribute to bleeding, which is usually provoked by low levels of factor V and VIII. Prolonged prothrombin and partial thromboplastin times in the presence of a normal calcium thrombin time point to the right diagnosis. Fresh blood, or 1 to 2 units of fresh frozen plasma should be given. Platelet concentrates may also be required in the absence of fresh blood. The platelet count becomes normal in three to five days and it is not uncommon to find a count of $1\,000\,000/\mu$l (10^{12}/litre) or more, 7 to 10 days after such an episode.

Haemorrhagic Manifestations of Extracorporeal Circulation

Cardiopulmonary by-pass affects many haemostatic parameters and haemorrhage may be a serious complication. Pathogenesis of the haemostatic defect is complex, and usually results from inadequate neutralisation of heparin, fibrinolysis, thrombocytopenia, and deficiency of clotting factors, usually II, V and VIII (Porter and Silver, 1968; Signori, Penner and Kahn, 1969; Gralnick and Fischer, 1971). Abnormalities of platelet function have also been reported (De Leval et al, 1972). The use of newer oxygenators and improved materials has reduced some of these complications, but critical bleeding is still encountered in some patients.

In open heart surgery, diverse schemes for heparin dosage are in use. It is often given as an initial dose of 300 i.u./kg body weight, and 4000 i.u. for each litre of blood in the machine. This achieves a blood level of about 4 i.u./ml with a half-life of about 2 h (Nyman, Thurnherr and Duckert, 1974); therefore half of the initial dose is added every 2 h. Neutralisation after surgery is achieved by giving protamine sulphate or chloride, and is checked by the calcium thrombin time immediately and after 2 h. The correct amount of protamine to reverse heparin anticoagulation is controversial, as the calculations may be based on the initial dose of heparin only, the initial plus supplemental doses, or on the total amount of heparin administered to the patient and to prime the pump. There are other factors that may also affect the heparin level at the time of neutralisation, such as heparin half-life in circulation (which is affected by body temperature and the duration of bypass), heparin flush for arterial and venous lines, and addition of heparinised blood. Thus, various authorities recommend from no protamine to 4 mg of protamine per each 100 i.u. of the original dose of heparin (Castenada, 1966; Osborne, 1967; Adkins and Hardy, 1967; Nyman et al, 1974; Ellison et al, 1975).

Heparin rebound

Bleeding can occur if heparin is not fully neutralised, or may result later from the 'rebound' phenomenon. Rebound is a term used to describe the reappearance of free heparin in the circulation up to 18 h after initial satisfactory neutralisation. Several mechanisms for such rebound are suggested: the splitting of heparin–protamine complexes in the body with release of free heparin; non-neutralisation by the initial protamine dose of heparin in the microcirculation and in extravascular spaces, and its systemic reappearance when normal circulation is re-established, with consequent bleeding. Rebound is more commonly found with protamine sulphate, which is more rapidly metabolised, than with protamine chloride, which is slowly eliminated (Frick and Brogli, 1966). In a recent study, Ellison et al (1975) have demonstrated that the dose of protamine required to neutralise exactly the in vitro heparin activity was consistently less than the dose required to prevent heparin rebound. As a moderate excess of protamine has not been shown to produce appreciable anticoagulant effects (Ellison, Ominsky and Wollman, 1971), it appears prudent to give enough protamine to prevent heparin rebound. The authors suggest that a safe dose for oxygenators with small prime volumes is 1 mg of protamine for each 100 i.u. of heparin given to the patient and used to prime the pump, whereas for oxygenators with large prime volumes, 0.5 mg protamine for each 100 i.u. of heparin should be sufficient.

Neutralisation of excess heparin with a calculated dose of protamine corrects the bleeding.

Overt DIC is not often found after extracorporeal circulation, probably because of the use of heparin during the by-pass. However, it has been described 2 to 10 days after surgery in patients with severe depression of cardiac output (Boyd et al, 1972). Replacement with fresh blood and the correction, if possible, of haemodynamic abnormalities may arrest the bleeding.

A fall in platelet count invariably accompanies extracorporeal circulation (Berger and Salzman, 1974), due to adherence of platelets to the surface of the extracorporeal circuit, and the sequestration of platelets in the liver and spleen. The thrombocytopenia lasts for several days and may sometimes need correction with platelet transfusions.

Abnormal Bleeding without Detectable Abnormalities

Profuse bleeding from the operative site alone may arise as a result of local abnormalities in the wound (for example, local fibrinolysis in the prostatic bed) or defective surgical haemostasis. It can also occur in the very old, ill and malnourished, when it is presumably due to the poor quality of the vessel wall which fails to contract and is highly permeable. Exploration of the wound, application of pressure when possible and adequate replacement of blood are of help.

Prevention of Acute Haemostatic Failure

Some patients and certain types of operation are particularly prone to acute haemostatic failure. They include patients with malignant disease, haematological abnormalities (leukaemia, mycloproliferative states, lymphoma, paraproteinaemias, megaloblastic anaemias or haemoglobinopathies), patients with collagen diseases or with chronic infection. The very old, very young and pregnant women are particularly at risk, as are those taking anticoagulant drugs and agents impairing platelet function.

Major operations, especially thoracotomy and in particular re-exploration, and extensive trauma or burns represent additional important groups at risk.

Prevention includes preoperative awareness of special hazards, and anticipatory measures. Pre-existing haemostatic defects due to disease or therapy must be evaluated and either corrected, or the operation deferred, or supportive measures ensured in unavoidable situations. Suitable blood replacement at and after operation, prevention of shock, treatment of infection and control of metabolic disturbance will reduce the problems of bleeding due to bank blood overtransfusion or fulminant DIC.

DRUGS USED IN THE PREVENTION AND TREATMENT OF VENOUS THROMBOEMBOLISM

Venous thromboembolism is a frequent complication of many operations and injuries. The magnitude of the problem has become apparent in the last few years with the development of sensitive and objective methods such as the radioactive fibrinogen test and phlebography for detecting and studying thrombosis (Flanc, Kakkar and Clarke, 1968; Negus et al, 1968; Kakkar et al, 1969; Nicolaides et al, 1971; Browse and Lea Thomas, 1974; Nicolaides

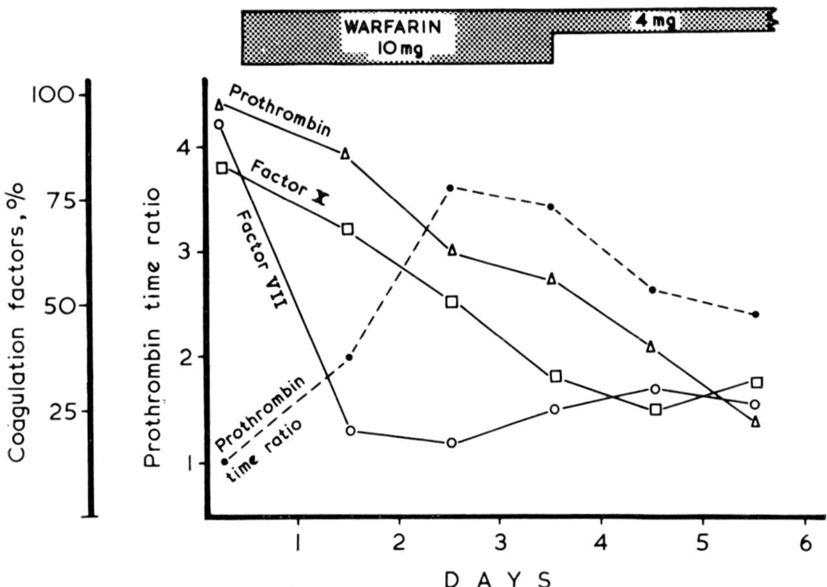

Figure 7.7 Effect of warfarin (non-loading dose) on vitamin K-dependent factors and prothrombin time ratio in a patient anticoagulated after myocardial infraction and calf vein thrombosis

and O'Connell, 1975). Many attempts have been made to prevent postoperative thrombosis, and this chapter gives a brief account of the drugs used for this purpose. It also includes the drugs used in the treatment of venous thrombosis and pulmonary embolism. All of these preparations interfere with haemostasis and may cause a severe haemorrhagic state.

Anticoagulant Drugs

Oral anticoagulants

Mechanism of action and metabolism. Oral anticoagulants are vitamin K antagonists and are chemically either coumarin or indanedione derivatives. Their site of action is the microsomes of liver cells where they interfere with a late stage of completion of vitamin K-dependent coagulation factors (prothrombin, factors VII, IX and X) and so reduce their concentration in blood. These factors, synthesised in the absence of vitamin K, cannot bind calcium and are therefore incapable of participating in the coagulation of blood (Stenflo, 1974). As shown in Figure 7.7, the rate of disappearance of the clotting factors after warfarin is given depends on their plasma half-life, factor VII falling to half its initial value after 4 h and prothrombin only after three days.

The patient is anticoagulated only when the levels of all vitamin K-dependent factors are reduced. For 72 h after the first dose of warfarin the patient is not protected from thrombosis, and this period should be covered with heparin or ancrod.

Smooth control of anticoagulation is more easily achieved with the more slowly metabolised drugs (Table 7.7). Warfarin is the most commonly used agent of this group and will form the main substance of this account.

Table 7.7   Oral anticoagulants

Pharmacological name	Proprietary name	Gastrointestinal absorption	Plasma $T_{\frac{1}{2}}$ (h)
Warfarin sodium	Marevan Coumadin	Rapid, complete	36
Phenindione	Dindevan	Rapid, complete	5
Nicoumalone	Sinthrome	Rapid, complete	8

Warfarin is almost completely absorbed from the gut and about 97 per cent of the plasma content is bound to albumin. Only the free circulating molecule is effective at the hepatic receptor sites. Warfarin is metabolised by the liver where it is hydroxylated, conjugated, and excreted in the bile. Partial reabsorption occurs and metabolic products of warfarin are excreted in the urine (Deykin, 1970).

Administration of warfarin. The *treatment* should be started with 10 mg warfarin once daily for three days (O'Reilly and Aggeler, 1968; Deykin, 1970). The customary loading dose of 30 to 40 mg is avoided as it may cause dangerous bleeding due to a rapid fall in factor VII without protecting the patient from thrombosis. Very small initial doses (2–5 mg daily) are sufficient for adequate anticoagulation in the very old, those on parenteral feeding or recovering from cardiac surgery. The maintenance dose of warfarin varies between 1 and 20 mg daily and is usually between 3 and 8 mg. It is determined by laboratory tests. Warfarin is usually given for six weeks after calf vein thrombosis and for three to six months after iliofemoral thrombosis or pulmonary embolism. Previous thromboembolic illness dictates continued treatment for a year or longer. When it is decided to cease anticoagulant treatment warfarin can be stopped without any need to tail it off gradually.

For *prophylaxis* of venous thrombosis, warfarin can be given 10 mg the night before operation, 5 mg the night of operation and then sufficient to maintain a prothrombin time ratio (see page 151) of 1.5 to 2.0 with British Comparative Thromboplastin, or about 15 per cent with Thrombotest (Harris et al, 1974; Brozović, 1975).

Changes in responsiveness to warfarin. Many drugs interact with warfarin (O'Reilly, 1974). Some that *potentiate* its anticoagulant effects like phenylbutazone, aspirin, indomethacin, acidic sulphonamides and anabolic steroids, act by *displacing warfarin from its albumin binding*. Mineral oils in laxatives, cholestyramine and broad spectrum antibiotics *reduce the availability of vitamin K* in the gastrointestinal tract, and chloramphenicol, alcohol and nortryptiline *suppress the liver enzymes that metabolise warfarin*. Phenytoin and salicylates directly *suppress the synthesis of vitamin K-dependent factors* and thus increase patients' sensitivity to warfarin. Increased responsiveness to oral anticoagulants is also found in infection, liver disease, hyperthyroidism and congestive cardiac failure, as well as in diarrhoea and in patients on parenteral nutrition, who develop vitamin K lack quite quickly in view of its negligible body stores.

Barbiturates, spironolactone and glutethimide *induce liver enzymes and cause rapid metabolism of warfarin*. This results in *decreased responsiveness*. Thiazide diuretics and oral contraceptives also make patients resistant to warfarin. Decreased responsiveness is found in pregnancy and in lactating women. Hereditary resistance to oral anticoagulant has been described in two large families (O'Reilly, 1974).

Contraindications to anticoagulant treatment. Patients who have a haemorrhagic tendency, have undergone recent surgery involving the central nervous system or eyeball, have a diastolic blood pressure over 110 mmHg, have gastrointestinal lesions liable to bleed such as peptic ulcer or oesophageal varices, or have liver disease are not suitable for anticoagulant treatment (Douglas, 1969).

Relative contraindications are inability or unwillingness to cooperate, moderate hypertension, a previous history of peptic ulcer, and renal disease. These contraindications are by no means complete, and each patient must be assessed individually.

Laboratory control of oral anticoagulants. The purpose of laboratory control is to maintain stable blood concentrations of factors II, VII, IX and X at levels which prevent thrombosis while minimising the risk from bleeding. The test most widely used in control is the prothrombin time. The therapeutic range depends largely on the method and thromboplastin used. The results are usually expressed as a *prothrombin time ratio*—the ratio of the patient's clotting time to a control. Many different thromboplastins, each giving a different 'therapeutic ratio', are available. In the United Kingdom, an excellent standardised human brain thromboplastin is available from the National Reference Laboratory for Anticoagulant Control Reagents in

Manchester (Poller, 1970). The prothrombin time ratio obtained using this British Comparative Thromboplastin is the British Ratio and its suggested therapeutic range is between 2.0 and 3.0. This range is not absolute as some patients may require a higher ratio to prevent recurrent attacks of venous thrombosis, whereas others may bleed when the ratio is no greater than 2.0.

Another commonly used reagent for measuring reduced prothrombin complex activity is Thrombotest, a commercial preparation containing bovine brain thromboplastin, absorbed bovine plasma, cephalin and calcium. As it already contains fibrinogen and factor V it is not affected by changes in these factors. Clotting time is recorded as *percentage activity* read off a graph supplied by the manufacturers. The therapeutic range is between 5 and 10 per cent, although patients with relative contraindications should be maintained at about 10 to 15 per cent. Thrombotest is of no use diagnostically to recognise slight deficiency of vitamin K-dependent factors in clinical practice.

Minor surgical interventions and dental extractions can be carried out in patients whose prothrombin time ratio is below 2.0 or whose thrombotest value is above 15 per cent.

The anticoagulant clinic. When the patient is in hospital the prothrombin time measured three times weekly during the induction period is sufficient to establish the desired therapeutic range. When the patient leaves hospital, control is best achieved through regular attendance at an anticoagulant clinic where the dose of warfarin is adjusted according to the results of the test. Patients should carry a card which includes details of the patient, his doctors and treatment record.

Complications of warfarin treatment. The commonest complications are bleeding, including haematuria, epistaxis, bruising and conjunctival haemorrhage. It is not uncommon for a patient to have repeated minor bleeds while his tests are well within the therapeutic range. The dose of warfarin in these patients must be adjusted to reduce the incidence of troublesome bleeding. Massive gastrointestinal bleeding—often due to unsuspected peptic ulcer— retroperitoneal and cerebrospinal haemorrhage are the most dangerous complications of oral anticoagulant treatment.

Apart from occasional skin rashes and diarrhoea, other complications (such as haemorrhagic skin necrosis or 'purple toe' syndrome) are extremely rare with warfarin. Agranulocytosis, renal and liver damage and exfoliative dermatitis have been reported with phenindione, and its use should therefore be avoided (Douglas, 1969).

Excessively raised prothrombin ratio. This may be due to an overdose of warfarin, administration of drugs that potentiate the effects of warfarin, intercurrent infection especially if treated by antibiotics, liver disease, renal disease, congestive cardiac failure, severe dietary restriction or conditions requiring intravenous feeding. A careful clinical history and examination is required to determine how many of these factors are responsible.

If a patient has a high prothrombin ratio without any haemorrhage it is usually enough to stop warfarin for 24 to 72 h and resume a smaller dose. If the patient is bleeding, or if the prothrombin time ratio is over 6.0 even in the absence of bleeding, warfarin should be stopped and 1 to 2 units of plasma, fresh frozen or 'cryosupernatant', administered. Four hours after the infusion of plasma the prothrombin time is repeated, and if the ratio is still in excess of 6.0 another 1 to 2 units of plasma are given. Vitamin K should not be given to patients in whom anticoagulants are to be continued, as not only does vitamin K (even if given intravenously) take about 6 h to act, but it renders the patient resistant to anticoagulant treatment for some weeks. The indications for vitamin K (in the form of the naturally occurring vitamin K_1, 20–30 mg i.v.) in addition to plasma are a suicidal overdose of warfarin, suspected cerebral bleeding, and bleeding in a patient who does not require further anticoagulation. Some patients in cardiac failure cannot tolerate infusion of plasma, and small doses (10 mg) of vitamin K_1 can be given i.v. or orally, or an intravenous dose of lyophilised prothrombin complex factors may be administered.

When drugs known to interact with warfarin need to be given, the prothrombin time should be determined every day or two during the following 7 to 10 days. The warfarin dose is then reduced or increased according to the altered prothrombin time ratio. Similarly when the interacting drug is discontinued regular prothrombin times must also be carried out during the ensuing week. Unawareness of this precaution may endanger life.

Surgical operations. A patient on oral anticoagulants undergoing major surgery should be changed to subcutaneous heparin. Warfarin is stopped 42 h before operation, and subcutaneous heparin started 48 h before operation in a dose of 5000 i.u. eight-hourly. This ensures adequate protection for most patients. Warfarin should be reintroduced five to seven days after operation. A three day overlap of heparin and warfarin is necessary.

For emergency operations, patients who are fully anticoagulated should be given 2 to 3 units of fresh frozen plasma before and during the operation. The prothrombin time ratio is checked during the operation and every 4 h during the first postoperative day; it should be less than 2.0 at all times. Warfarin can be restarted in the preoperative maintenance dose three days after the operation, or when the prothrombin time ratio falls below 1.5.

Heparin

Heparin is a naturally occuring acidic mucopolysaccharide produced by the microsomal fraction of mast cells and basophils in all tissues. Commercially it is obtained from bovine or porcine lung or intestines. As the sodium or calcium salt it is a white powder containing molecules varying in length between 6000 and 30000 daltons (Ehrlich and Stivala, 1973). Batches of heparin may vary in their specific activity from about 110 to 150 i.u./mg. Because of this variation the dose of heparin is always calculated in units and not in milligrams.

Mode of action and metabolism. When administered subcutaneously or intravenously heparin has multiple effects due to its binding and complexing with many different positively charged proteins and cations. Heparin forms a complex with a plasma protein variously called antithrombin III, anti-Xa or heparin cofactor (Rosenberg, 1975). Although this protein can neutralise thrombin in the absence of heparin, the effect is slow and incomplete. In the presence of very small amounts of heparin this protein shows a marked *anti-Xa effect*, i.e. neutralisation of activated factor X, while in the presence of higher heparin concentrations the *antithrombin effect* is immediate, thus neutralising thrombin before it can split fibrinopeptides A and B from fibrinogen. Blood is thus rendered incoagulable.

Heparin is split and inactivated in the gastrointestinal tract and hence must be administered parenterally. It acts immediately when given intravenously and has a plasma half-life of about $1\frac{1}{2}$ h (Estes, 1971), being rapidly disulphated in the liver. Smooth anticoagulation with heparin is achieved by continuous infusion, preferably with a constant-infusion pump. Intermittent dosage involves excessive initial impairment of haemostasis with inadequate anticoagulation 3 to 4 h after injection. Heparin is released slowly after subcutaneous injection and a systemic effect can be maintained for 8 to 12 h (Pitney, 1972).

Administration of heparin. For *prophylaxis* of venous thrombosis, heparin is given subcutaneously in a dose of 5000 i.u. (contained in 0.2–1.0 ml) every 8 to 12 h. The first injection is given 2 h before operation, or on admission to hospital in certain high risk patients, and the treatment continued for 7 to 21 days or until the patient is fully mobile (Kakkar et al, 1972; An International Multicentre Trial, 1975).

For *treatment* of thrombosis, much higher plasma levels of heparin must be maintained. The treatment is usually started with an intravenous injection of 5000 to 10 000 i.u., and then continued with 25 i.u./kg body weight per hour (usually 30–40 000 i.u. daily for most adults). Similar plasma levels may be achieved with subcutaneous injections of 12 500 to 20 000 i.u. twice daily, but erratic absorption and local haematomas may occur. Warfarin is started in the three final days of heparin therapy, avoiding the large loading dose. In calf vein thrombosis where heparin is given for only three days, the first dose of warfarin is given at the start of heparin treatment. The duration of heparin treatment for iliofemoral thrombosis and pulmonary embolism varies from one to three weeks (Pitney, 1972).

Contraindications to heparin treatment are similar to those for warfarin. Conventional therapeutic doses are likely to cause bleeding if given within 48 h of major surgery or within 24 h of childbirth. The elderly and those with impaired renal function or thrombocytopenia may be unduly sensitive to heparin (Douglas, 1969; Pitney, 1972).

Laboratory control of heparin treatment. Some six tests are commonly used for control of heparin levels. These are the whole blood clotting time, whole blood activated recalcification time (BART), activated partial thromboplastin time of plasma, calcium thrombin time, anti-Xa assay and protamine neutralisation test. The acceptable therapeutic range for each of these tests is given in Table 7.8; at least one should be chosen for daily use. The whole blood clotting time is used most commonly but the last two tests are probably the most sensitive. All tests are unreliable in patients with renal impairment or those being treated for disseminated intravascular clotting, where bleeding may occur even when heparin levels are well within the therapeutic range (Pitney, Pettit and Armstrong, 1970).

The control of subcutaneously administered heparin depends on the dose used. If larger doses are given the same tests as for intravenously administered heparin can be used. Laboratory control of low-dose heparin (5000 i.u. b.d. or t.d.s.) for prophylaxis of venous thrombosis is rarely needed, except in

Table 7.8   Tests used in the control of heparin treatment

Test	Acceptable therapeutic range
Whole blood clotting time	15–25 min (Pitney, 1972)
Blood activated recalcification time (BART)	2–3 min, or 2–3 × control (Reno et al, 1974)
Activated partial thromboplastin time	60–100 s, or 2–3 × control (Spector and Corn, 1967)
Calcium thrombin time	25–100 s, or 2–6 × control (O'Shea et al, 1971)
Protamine titration of heparin	0.5–1.5 i.u./ml (Pitney, 1972)
Anti-Xa assay of heparin	0.5–1.5 i.u./ml (Brozović, 1975)

patients with a low platelet count or an impaired haemostatic mechanism. The best test for measuring such low levels of heparin (0.02–0.3 i.u./ml) is the anti-Xa assay (Denson and Bonnar, 1975), but modifications of the PTT can also be used.

Complications of heparin treatment. Haemorrhage occurs in about 10 to 20 per cent of those with normal haemostasis, and in half the patients with low platelets or with uraemia (Pitney et al, 1970; Salzman et al, 1975). Other complications of heparin treatment are uncommon. They are thrombocytopenia, alopecia (4–12 weeks after heparin administration), local hypersensitivity (skin necrosis at the site of injection in patients on subcutaneous heparin), general hypersensitivity reactions, and osteoporosis in patients on high doses for long periods of time (Pitney, 1972).

Treatment of heparin overdosage and bleeding. Because of its short plasma half-life, cessation of heparin ordinarily suffices. If considered necessary protamine sulphate, a highly cationic peptide obtained from salmon or herring sperm, is an effective antidote. One milligram of protamine usually neutralises 100 i.u. of heparin, the neutralising dose being calculated from a protamine neutralisation test on the patient's plasma. Protamine is given slowly intravenously, as it can cause flushing and a fall in blood pressure. A large excess of protamine in the blood may itself be anticoagulant.

Ancrod (*Arvin*)

Ancrod is sometimes used as an alternative to heparin. It is a proteolytic enzyme obtained from the venom of the Malayan pit viper (*Angkistrodon rhodostoma*) which splits off fibrinopeptide A from the Aα chain of fibrinogen. This liberates 'pseudo'-fibrin monomers which polymerise to an unstable fibrin-like gel. Ancrod given as a slow infusion over 4 to 6 h defibrinates the patient, but the microclots formed are readily lysed by the patient's own fibrinolytic system, and high concentrations of FDP are found in the circulation. The anticoagulant effect is mediated by hypofibrinogenaemia and the presence of FDP (Kwaan and Grumet, 1975).

Administration. Two units of ancrod per kilogram of body weight are given initially as an intravenous infusion over 4 to 6 h, followed by maintenance therapy of 1 to 2 u/kg body weight every 12 h for 7 to 14 days. Three days before the end of treatment warfarin should be started in the usual dosage (Pitney, 1972).

In most patients the response of plasma fibrinogen to ancrod is remarkably predictable, and the levels of fibrinogen fall to between 20 and 50 mg/100 ml. The plasma fibrinogen may take up to three weeks to return to normal after the treatment is stopped. Fibrinogen levels may be followed once or twice weekly in case of rare resistance developing to ancrod; ordinary observation of the 'mini-clot' forming when whole blood clots in glass is sufficient guide to control.

Bleeding, bruising and oozing from venepuncture sites are the commonest complications in ancrod therapy. A small proportion of patients (apparently if given ancrod intramuscularly) develop resistance due to antibody formation, and it may be impossible to give a second course of treatment. In experimental animals ancrod impairs wound healing, so it should be used with caution after surgery (Pitney, 1972).

If rapid reversal of ancrod effect is required, a specific antivenom together with intravenous fibrinogen or plasma can be injected.

Thrombolytic Drugs

Streptokinase

Mode of action and metabolism. Streptokinase is a peptide isolated from the filtrate of cultures of certain haemolytic streptococci. It readily forms complexes with human plasminogen and plasmin and these complexes act as activators of free plasminogen. Plasmin so generated digests fibrin in thrombi and to a lesser extent fibrinogen in the circulation. The effect of streptokinase is immediate, provided all the antibodies to streptokinase in plasma have been neutralised by the initial dose (Prentice and McNicol, 1973). There is an immediate fall in plasminogen and fibrinogen concentration, with transient

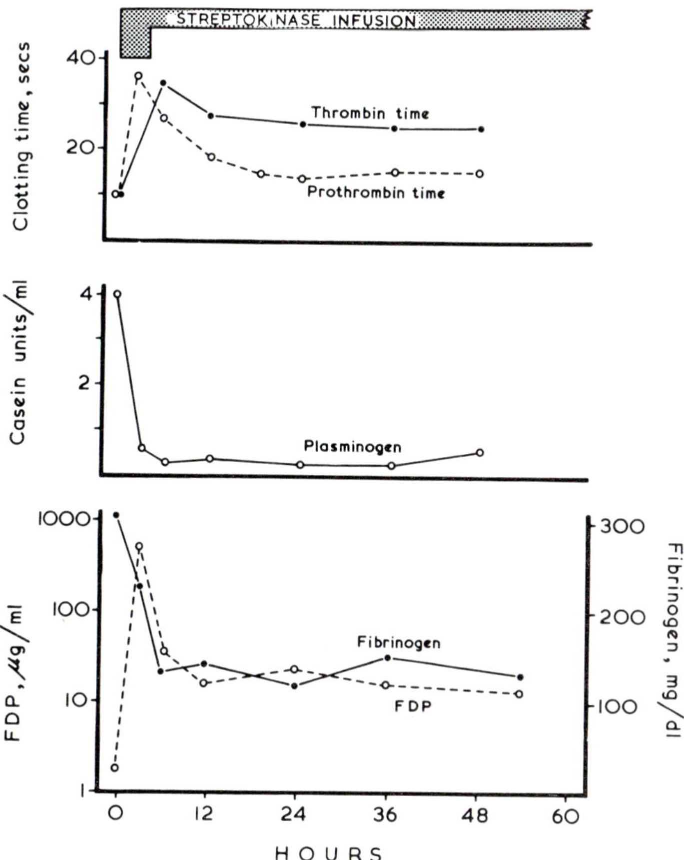

Figure 7.8   Effect of streptokinase infusion on different coagulation tests in a patient with massive iliofemoral venous thrombosis

marked shortening of euglobulin lysis time and a rise in the concentration of FDP. Slightly elevated FDP are found throughout the course of treatment. Much of the remaining plasma fibrinogen is also partially degraded by plasmin (Gaffney, Chesterman and Allington, 1974). The thrombin time is prolonged and a transient fall in factors V and VIII accompanies the induction. The changes are shown schematically in Figure 7.8.

Administration of streptokinase. Streptokinase is used in the treatment of

7

acute arterial occlusion, deep venous thrombosis and acute massive pulmonary embolism, and to lyse clots in arteriovenous shunts. Streptokinase is administered as an intravenous infusion, or in cases of pulmonary embolism through a catheter directly into the pulmonary artery. The initial dose is given to neutralise the antistreptococcal antibodies in the blood. This is either determined by a streptokinase-antibody neutralisation test, or an arbitrary dose sufficient to neutralise the antibodies in most people (usually 250 000 i.u.) is administered over 30 min. As streptokinase may cause hypersensitivity reactions, the initial dose must be covered with 100 mg hydrocortisone and 10 mg chlorpheniramine (Piriton) intravenously, repeated if necessary every 6 to 12 h. The maintenance dose is 100 to 150 000 i.u. hourly intravenously for 72 h. Longer administration is associated with an increase of bleeding complications. When the calcium thrombin time is twice the control time, usually 4 h after stopping streptokinase, intravenous heparin should be started, followed by oral anticoagulants for three to six months (Pitney, 1972), and sometimes longer according to individual indications.

Kakkar, Sagar and Lewis (1975) have reported excellent results in deep vein thrombosis with 600 000 i.u. of streptokinase administered over 15 min immediately after the infusion of 90 to 120 mg of human plasminogen. The combination of plasminogen and streptokinase was repeated once daily for five days.

Contraindications. Streptokinase should not be used within five days of major surgery or 72 h after childbirth. In patients who have received previous streptokinase treatment it is of little effect and may cause severe hypersensitivity reactions. Other contraindications are similar to those for warfarin and heparin treatment.

Laboratory control. Treatment is adequate when the thrombin clotting time is between 20 and 40 s (control 10–12 s) (Pitney, 1972). The test is first performed 4 h after the initial dose and then daily for the duration of treatment. A very long thrombin time indicates hyperplasminaemia, and the dose of streptokinase might be increased to enable more plasminogen to complex with streptokinase and avoid generation of plasmin. This is a difficult decision especially if a patient is bleeding, and many physicians prefer to stop infusing streptokinase temporarily. A short thrombin time indicates that there is no plasmin available in the circulation due to all the plasminogen having complexed with streptokinase, leaving none to be activated and generate plasmin. The dose of streptokinase should be reduced to 50 000 or 75 000 i.u. hourly. The thrombin time is repeated 4 h after modification of the dose. Other laboratory tests to monitor streptokinase treatment are time-consuming and used only if a full assessment of the fibrinolytic state is required. These tests are euglobulin clot lysis time, fibrin plate assay for activator, and plasminogen, fibrinogen and FDP assays. Many reports suggest that it is probably justifiable to omit control when using a standard dosage scheme (Pitney, 1972; Robertson and Nilsson, 1974).

Complications of streptokinase therapy. The main risk is bleeding including oozing from needle punctures, indwelling catheter sites and operative wounds, as well as menorrhagia in women. If bleeding is severe cessation of treatment and blood transfusion are preferred to the administration of anti-fibrinolytic agents such as epsilon-aminocaproic acid and tranexamic acid, which are kept for special situations such as a decision to proceed to embolectomy. EACA (100 mg/kg body weight), or tranexamic acid (10 mg/kg body weight) are given as a slow intravenous infusion. These agents are inhibitors of plasminogen activator and all clots and thrombi formed in their presence will be resistant to lysis.

Urokinase

Urokinase is the naturally occurring plasminogen activator isolated from urine. It is an enzyme which readily cleaves plasminogen into plasmin. It is not antigenic and has a greater affinity for plasminogen absorbed on to clots than for circulating plasminogen (Prentice and McNicol, 1973). The great disadvantage of urokinase is the cost of its production and the limited supply available.

Drugs that Enhance Fibrinolysis

Many substances cause the release of plasminogen activator from venous and capillary endothelium. A continuous increase in plasminogen activator may maintain the patency of the microcirculation, but most of the substances tested have only transient effects and after some weeks of administration no increase in plasminogen activator occurs. The exceptions are the combination of phenformin (a biguanide) 100 mg daily with ethyloestranol (an anabolic steroid) 8 mg daily (Fearnley, Chakrabarti and Evans, 1969), and the anabolic steroid Stanozolol alone, 10 mg daily (Davidson, McDonald and McNicol, 1971). These drugs cause a persistent increase in plasminogen activator with subsequent fall in plasma fibrinogen levels, raised FDP with reduction of platelet retention by glass beads, and lowering of serum cholesterol. They are not entirely free of side effects (occasional nausea, vomiting or fluid retention) and up to three weeks may pass before the increase in fibrinolytic activity, which limits their value in the prevention of deep vein thrombosis. Some encouraging results have been reported in patients with recurrent deep venous thrombosis (Nilsson and Isaacson, 1973) as well as in patients with ischaemic heart disease (Chakrabarti and Fearnley, 1972).

Antiplatelet Drugs

Antiplatelet drugs are agents which have been shown to inhibit various aspects of platelet function in vitro and to alter in vivo responses in which platelets play a major role (Weiss, 1972; Vermylen, De Gaetano and Verstraete, 1973). Since the formation of a platelet aggregate appears to be an early event in the formation of thrombi such drugs are of potential use as antithrombotic agents.

Many compounds show inhibitory effects on platelets; the most extensively studied drug is aspirin which has been used in prophylaxis of postoperative venous thrombosis (Salzman, Harris and DeSanctis, 1971; Report of the Steering Committee, 1972; Harris et al, 1974). The results were conflicting and aspirin probably deserves further trials. The dose recommended is 600 mg once or twice daily. Other drugs in use include dipyridamole and sulphinpyrazone. They have been used to prevent thrombosis on prosthetic devices, and in several clinical conditions such as transient cerebral ischaemic attacks, renal allograft rejection and microangiopathic disorders. In some cases encouraging results have been reported (Didisheim, Kazmier and Fuster, 1974).

Low Molecular Weight Dextran

Low molecular weight dextran (Dextran 40) is derived from a polyglucose produced by a special strain of *Leuconostoc mesenteroides*. Dextran 40 decreases blood viscosity and improves flow by disaggregating the red cells (Engeset, Stalker and Matheson, 1967) and expanding the plasma volume (Ahnefeld, Halmagyi and Uberla, 1965). It also interferes with platelet aggregation, probably through coating of the platelet surface (Cronberg, Robertson and Nilsson, 1966).

The renal molecular weight threshold for dextran is 50000, and 60 per cent of the molecules under 50000 are excreted within 6 h of infusion. The remaining larger molecules are slowly metabolised by enzymatic degradation. A small proportion is excreted into the gastrointestinal tract.

Dextran 40 is available as a 10 per cent solution in either saline or dextrose. Dextran in dextrose should never be given through the same apparatus as blood, as protein precipitation and red cell agglutination may occur.

Many different regimes are described for using Dextran 40 in the prophylaxis of deep venous thrombosis. One of these is to give a 500 to 1000 ml infusion daily for three days starting on the day of operation, and then on alternate days until discharge.

Contraindications to the use of dextran are a bleeding tendency, congestive cardiac failure and renal failure. The side effects include rare anaphylactoid reactions and occasional capillary oozing from wound surfaces.

The efficiency of Dextran 40 in preventing deep venous thrombosis needs to be proved by a large, well-controlled trial, but encouraging results have been reported from many centres (Bygdeman, Svensjö and Tollerz, 1970; Evarts and Feil, 1971; Bonnar and Walsh, 1972; Harris et al, 1974).

REFERENCES

Adkins, J. R. & Hardy, J. D. (1967) Sodium heparin neutralisation and the anticoagulant effects of protamine sulphate. *Archives of Surgery*, **94**, 175–177.

Ahnefeld, F. W., Halmagyi, M. & Uberla, K. (1965) Investigation of the assessment of colloidal volume substitution solutions. *Anaesthetist*, **14**, 137–143.

Ambrus, C. M. & Markus, G. (1960) Plasmin–antiplasmin complex as a reservoir of fibrinolytic enzyme. *American Journal of Physiology*, **199**, 491–494.

An International Multicentre Trial (1975) Prevention of fatal post-operative pulmonary embolism by low doses of heparin. *Lancet*, **2**, 45–51.

Aster, R. H. (1972) Distribution, life span and fate of platelets. In *Hematology*, ed. Williams, W. J., Erslev, A. J. & Rundles, W. R., pp. 1046–1050. New York: McGraw-Hill.

Aster, R. H. (1972) Thrombocytopenia due to enhanced platelet destruction. In *Hematology*, ed. Williams, W. J., Erslev, A. J. & Rundles, W. R., pp. 1131–1159. New York: McGraw-Hill.

Berger, S., & Salzman, E. W. (1974). Thromboembolic complications of prosthetic devices. In *Progress in Hemostasis and Thrombosis*, ed. Spaet, T. H., pp. 273–311. New York: Grune & Stratton.

Blombäck, B. & Blombäck, M. (1972) The molecular structure of fibrinogen. *Annals of New York Academy of Science*, **202**, 77–97.

Bonnar, J. & Walsh, J. (1972) Prevention of thrombosis after pelvic surgery by British Dextran 70. *Lancet*, **1**, 614–616.

Boyd, A. D., Engleman, R. M., Beaudet, R. L. & Lackner, H. (1972) Disseminated intravascular coagulation following extracorporeal circulation. *Journal of Thoracic and Cardiovascular Surgery*, **64**, 685–693.

Browse, N. L. & Lea Thomas, M. (1974) Source of non-lethal pulmonary emboli. *Lancet*, **1**, 258–259.

Brozović, M. (1975) Personal observation.

Bygdeman, S., Svensjö, E. & Tollerz, G. (1970) Prevention of venous thrombosis. *Lancet*, **2**, 419–420.

Cash, J. D. (1972) Platelet transfusion therapy. *Clinics in Haematology*, **1**, 395–412. London: W. B. Saunders Co.

Castaneda, A. R. (1966) Must heparin be neutralised following open heart operations? *Journal of Thoracic and Cardiovascular Surgery*, **52**, 716–723.

Chakrabarti, R., Bielawiec, M., Evans, J. F. & Fearnley, G. R. (1968) Methodological study and recommended technique for determining the euglobulin lysis time. *Journal of Clinical Pathology*, **21**, 698–701.

Chakrabarti, R. & Fearnley, G. R. (1972) Phenformin plus ethyloestrenol in survivors of myocardial infarction. *Lancet*, **2**, 556–559.

Chessels, J. M. & Hardisty, R. M. (1974) Bleeding problems in the newborn infant. In *Progress in Haemostasis and Thrombosis*, ed. Spaet, T. H., Vol. 2, pp. 333–365. New York: Grune & Stratton.

Cronberg, S., Robertson, B. & Nilsson, I. M. (1966) Suppressive effect of dextran on platelet adhesiveness. *Thrombosis et Diathesis haemorrhagica*, **16**, 384–387.

Dacie, J. V. & Lewis, S. M. (1975) *Practical Haematology*, 5th edn, pp. 314–403. London: Churchill Livingstone.

Davidson, J., McDonald, G. A. & McNicol, G. P. (1971) Fibrinolytic enhancement by Stanozolol. *Abstracts of the 2nd Congress of the International Society on Thrombosis and Haemostasis*, Oslo, p. 116.

De Leval, M., Hill, J. D., Mielke, C. H. & Gerbode, F. (1972) Blood platelets and coagulation mechanisms during extracorporeal circulation. *Circulation*, **45**, Suppl. II, 3.

Denson, K. W. E. (1972) In *Human Blood Coagulation, Haemostasis and Thrombosis*, ed. Biggs, R., pp. 652–661. Oxford: Blackwell Scientific Publications.

Denson, K. W. E. & Bonnar, J. (1973) The measurement of heparin. *Thrombosis et Diathesis haemorrhagica*, **30**, 471–479.

Denson, K. W. E. & Bonnar, J. (1975) Measurement of heparin in patients receiving subcutaneous heparin therapy. *British Journal of Haematology*, **30**, 139–144.

Deykin, D. (1966) The role of liver in serum induced hypercoagulability. *Journal of Clinical Investigation*, **45**, 256–263.

Deykin, D. (1970) Warfarin therapy. *New England Journal of Medicine*, **283**, 691–694, 801–803.

Deykin, D. (1970) The clinical challenge of disseminated intravascular coagulation. *New England Journal of Medicine*, **283**, 636–644.

Didisheim, P., Kazmier, F. J. & Fuster, V. (1974) Platelet inhibition in the management of thrombosis. *Thrombosis et Diathesis haemorrhagica*, **32**, 21–34.

Dike, G. W. R., Bidwell, E. & Rizza, C. R. (1972) The preparation and clinical use of a new concentrate containing factor IX, prothrombin, and factor X and of a separate concentrate containing factor VII. *British Journal of Haematology*, **22**, 469–490.

Douglas, A. S. (1969) Current status of anticoagulant treatment. In *Recent Advances in Blood Coagulation*, ed. Poller, L., pp. 107–136. London: Churchill.

Edson, J. R., McArthur, J. R., Branda, R. F., McCullogh, J. J. & Chou, S. N. (1973) Successful management of a subdural haematoma in a haemophiliac with an anti-factor VIII antibody. *Blood*, **41**, 113–122.

Ehrlich, J. & Stivala, S. S. (1973) Chemistry and pharmacology of heparin. *Journal of Pharmacological Science*, **62**, 517–544.

Ellison, N., Beatty, P., Blake, D. R., Wurzel, H. A. & Macvaugh, H. (1975) Heparin rebound. *Journal of Thoracic and Cardiovascular Surgery*, **67**, 723–729.

Ellison, N., Ominsky, A. J. & Wollman, H. (1971) Is protamine a clinically important anticoagulant? A negative answer. *Anesthesiology*, **35**, 621–629.

Engeset, J., Stalker, A. L. & Matheson, N. (1967) Turbidometric measurement of red cell aggregation and effects of Dextran 40. *Proceedings of British Microcirculation Society*, July.

Estes, J. W. (1971) The kinetics of heparin. *Annals of New York Academy of Science*, **179**, 187–204.

Evarts, C. M. & Feil, E. J. (1971) Prevention of thromboembolic disease after elective surgery of the hip. *Journal of Bone and Joint Surgery*, **53A**, 1271–1280.

Evensen, S. A. & Hjort, P. F. (1970) Pathogenesis of disseminated intravascular clotting. In *Plenary Sessions, Scientific Contributions, XIII International Congress of Haematology*, Münich, pp. 109–120.

Fearnley, G. R., Chakrabarti, R. & Evans, J. F. (1969) Fibrinolytic and defibrinating effect of phenformin plus ethyloestrenol in vivo. *Lancet*, **1**, 910–914.

Fearnley, G. R., Revill, R. & Tweed, J. M. (1952) Observations on the inactivation of fibrinolytic activity in shed blood. *Clinical Science*, **11**, 309–314.

Feinstein, D. I. & Rapaport, S. I. (1972) Acquired inhibitors of blood coagulation. In *Progress in Hemostasis and Thrombosis*, ed. Spaet, T. H. pp. 75–96. New York: Grune & Stratton.

Flanc, C., Kakkar, V. V. & Clarke, M. B. (1968) The detection of venous thrombosis in the legs using I^{125}-labelled fibrinogen. *British Journal of Surgery*, **55**, 742–747.

Flute, P. T. (1974) Acquired disorders of haemostasis. In *Blood and its Disorders*, ed. Hardisty, R. M. & Weatherall, D. J., pp. 1076–1109. Oxford: Blackwell Scientific Publications.

Forbes, C. D., Barr, R. D., Reid, G., Thomson, C., Prentice, C. R. M. & McNicol, G. P. (1972) Tranexamic acid in control of haemorrhage after dental extraction in haemophilia and Christmas disease. *British Medical Journal*, **1**, 311–313.

Frick, P. G. & Brogli, H. (1966) The mechanism of heparin rebound after extracorporeal circulation for open cardiac surgery. *Surgery*, **59**, 721–726.

Gaffney, P. J., Chesterman, C. N. & Allington, M. J. (1974) Plasma fibrinogen and its fragments during streptokinase treatment. *British Journal of Haematology*, **26**, 285–294.

Godal, C. & Abildgaard, U. (1966) Gelation of soluble fibrin in plasma by ethanol. *Scandinavian Journal of Haematology*, **3**, 342–350.

Gralnick, H. R. & Fischer, R. D. (1971) The hemostatic response to open heart operations. *Journal of Thoracic and Cardiovascular Surgery*, **61**, 909–915.

Hardisty, R. M. (1968) Treatment of nonthrombocytopenic purpuras. In *Treatment of Haemorrhagic Disorders*, ed. Ratnoff, O. D., pp. 217–235. New York: Harper & Row.

Hardisty, R. M. & Ingram, G. I. C. (1965) In *Bleeding Disorders*, p. 196. Oxford: Blackwell Scientific Publications.

Harris, W. H., Salzman, E. W., Athanasoulis, C., Waltman, A. C., Baum, S. & DeSanctis, R. W. (1974) Comparison of warfarin, low molecular weight dextran, aspirin and subcutaneous heparin in prevention of venous thromboembolism following total hip replacement. *Journal of Bone and Joint Surgery*, **56A**, 1552–1562.

Holmsen, H., Day, H. J. & Stormorken, H. (1969) The blood platelet release reaction. *Scandinavian Journal of Haematology*, Suppl. 8.

Howard, M. A., Sawers, R. J. & Firkin, B. G. (1973) Ristocetin: a means of differentiating von Willebrand's disease into two groups. *Blood*, **41**, 687–690.

Kakkar, V. V., Corrigan, T., Spindler, J., Fossard, D. P., Flute, P. T., Crellin, R. Q., Wessler, S. & Yin, T. E. (1972) Efficacy of low doses of heparin in prevention of deep vein thrombosis after major surgery. *Lancet*, **2**, 101–106.

Kakkar, V. V., Field, E. S., Nicolaides, A. N., Flute, P. T., Wessler, S. & Yin, E. T. (1971) Low doses of heparin in prevention of deep vein thrombosis. *Lancet*, **2**, 669–671.

Kakkar, V. V., Howe, C. T., Flanc, C. & Clarke, M. B. (1969) Natural history of deep vein thrombosis. *Lancet*, **2**, 230–232.

Kakkar, V. V., Sagar, S. & Lewis, M. (1975) Treatment of deep-vein thrombosis with intermittent streptokinase and plasminogen infusion. *Lancet*, **2**, 674–675.

Kurczynski, E. M. & Penner, J. A. (1974) Activated prothrombin concentrate for patients with factor VIII inhibitors. *New England Journal of Medicine*, **291**, 164–167.

Kwaan, H. C. & Grumet, G. M. (1975) The place of thrombolytic and defibrinating agents in the treatment of venous thromboembolism. In *Thromboembolism*, ed. Nicolaides, A. N., pp. 251–268. Lancaster: Medical and Technical Publishing Company.

Lackner, H. (1973) Hemostatic abnormalities associated with dysproteinemias. *Seminars in Hematology*, **10**, 125–133.

Larsson, S. O., Hedner, U. & Nilsson, I. M. (1971) On coagulation and fibrinolysis in uraemia. *Scandinavian Journal of Urology and Nephrology*, **5**, 234–242.

Lewis, S. M., Szur, L. & Hoffbrand, A. V. (1972) Thrombocythaemia. *Clinics in Haematology*, **1**, 339–358.

Lorand, L. (1972) Fibrinoligase: the fibrin-stabilising factor system of blood plasma. *New York Academy of Science*, **202**, 6–30.

Losowsky, M. S. & Walls, W. D. (1969) Abnormal fibrin stabilisation in renal failure. *Thrombosis et Diathesis haemorrhagica*, **22**, 216–222.

Macfarlane, R. G. (1964) An enzyme cascade in the blood clotting mechanism and its function as a biological amplifier. *Nature (London)*, **202**, 498–499.

Macfarlane, R. G. (1972) Introduction and theory. In *Human Blood Coagulation, Haemostasis and Thrombosis*, ed. Biggs, R., pp. 1–31. Oxford: Blackwell Scientific Publications.

Marder, V. J. (1971) Fibrinogen and fibrin degradation products. Physicochemical and physiological considerations. *Thrombosis et Diathesis haemorrhagica*, Suppl. 47, 85–93.

Ménaché, D. (1975) Clinical use of factor IX concentrates. *Thrombosis et Diathesis haemorrhagica*, **33**, 597–599.

Merskey, C. (1972) Defibrination syndrome. In *Human Blood Coagulation, Haemostasis and Thrombosis*, ed. Biggs, R., pp. 444–475. Oxford: Blackwell Scientific Publications.

Mibashan, R. S., Kernoff, L., Lowenthal, R., Whyte, G. & Thumpston, J. (1975) In preparation.

Negus, D., Pinto, D. J., LeQuesne, L. P., Brown, N. & Chapman, N. (1968) ^{125}I-labelled fibrinogen in the diagnosis of deep vein thrombosis and its correlation with phlebography. *British Journal of Surgery*, **55**, 835–839.

Nicolaides, A. N., Kakkar, V. V., Field, E. S. & Renney, J. T. G. (1971) The origin of deep vein thrombosis: a venographic study. *British Journal of Radiology*, **44**, 653–663.

Nicolaides, A. N. & O'Connell, T. D. (1975) Origin and distribution of thrombi in patients presenting with clinical deep venous thrombosis. In *Thromboembolism*, ed. Nicolaides, A. N., pp. 167–180. Lancaster: Medical and Technical Publishing Company.

Nilsson, I. M. (1974) Fibrinolysis, thrombolysis and defibrination. In *Haemorrhagic and Thrombotic Diseases*, pp. 111–121. London: John Wiley & Sons.

Nilsson, I. M. & Isaacson, S. (1973) New aspects of the pathogenesis of thromboembolism. *Progress in Surgery*, **11**, 46–68.

Nyman, D., Thurnherr, N. & Duckert, F. (1974) Heparin dosage in extracorporeal circulation and its neutralisation. *Thrombosis et Diathesis Haemorrhagica*, **33**, 102–104.

O'Reilly, R. A. & Aggeler, P. M. (1968) Studies on coumarin anticoagulant drugs. Initiation of warfarin therapy without a loading dose. *Circulation*, **38**, 169–177.

O'Reilly, R. A. (1974) The pharmacodynamics of the oral anticoagulant drugs. In *Progress in Hemostasis and Thrombosis*, ed. Spaet, T. H., pp. 175–213. New York: Grune & Stratton.

Osborne, J. J. (1967) Perfusion techniques of cardiopulmonary by-pass. In *Cardiac Surgery*, ed. Norman, J. C., pp. 91–98, New York: Meredith Publishing Company.

O'Shea, M. J., Flute, P. T. & Pannell, G. M. (1971) Laboratory control of heparin therapy. *Journal of Clinical Pathology*, **24**, 542–546.

Owen, C. A. Jr, Bowie, E. J. W. & Thompson, J. H. Jr (1975) *The Diagnosis of Bleeding Disorders.* Boston: Little, Brown & Co.

Pitney, W. R. (1972) *Clinical Aspects of Thromboembolism.* Edinburgh: Churchill Livingstone.

Pitney, W. R. (1972) Disorders of platelets. In *Tutorials in Postgraduate Medicine, Haematology*, ed. Hoffbrand, A. V. & Lewis, S. M., pp. 594–612. London: William Heinemann Medical Books Ltd.

Pitney, W. R., Pettit, J. E. & Armstrong, L. (1970) Control of heparin therapy. *British Medical Journal*, **3,** 139–141.

Poller, L. (1970) The British Comparative Thromboplastin. *Association of Clinical Pathologists Broadsheet*, 71.

Porter, J. M. & Silver, D. (1968) Alterations in fibrinolysis and coagulation associated with cardiopulmonary by-pass. *Journal of Thoracic and Cardiovascular Surgery*, **56,** 869–878.

Prentice, C. R. M. & McNicol, G. P. (1973) Fibrinolytic therapy. In *Recent Advances in Thrombosis*, ed. Poller, L., pp. 157–180. Edinburgh: Churchill Livingstone.

Rabiner, F. S. (1972) Uremic bleeding. In *Progress in Hemostasis and Thrombosis*, ed. Spaet, T. H., pp. 233–250. New York: Grune & Stratton.

Rapaport, S. I. (1972) Defibrination syndromes. In *Hematology*, ed. Williams, W. J., Erslev, A. J. & Rundles, W. R., pp. 1234–1255. New York: McGraw-Hill.

Reno, W. J., Rotman, M., Grumbine, F. C., Dennis, L. H. & Mohler, E. R. (1974) Evaluation of the BART (a modification of the whole blood activated recalcification time test) as a means of monitoring heparin therapy. *American Journal of Clinical Pathology*, **61,** 78–84.

Report of the Steering Committee of a Trial Sponsored by the Medical Research Council (1972) Effect of aspirin on postoperative venous thrombosis. *Lancet*, **2,** 441–445.

Rizza, C. R. (1972) The Clinical features of clotting factor deficiencies. In *Human Blood Coagulation, Haemostasis and Thrombosis*, ed. Biggs, R., pp. 210–224. Oxford: Blackwell Scientific Publications.

Rizza, C. R. (1974) Haemophilia and related disorders. *British Medical Journal*, **4,** 36–38.

Rizza, C. R. (1975) Unpublished observations.

Rizza, C. R. & Biggs, R. (1973) The treatment of patients who have factor VIII antibodies. *British Journal of Haematology*, **24,** 65–82.

Roberts, H. R. & Cederbaum, A. I. (1972) The liver and blood coagulation. *Gastroenterology*, **63,** 297–390.

Robertson, B. R. & Nilsson, I. M. (1974) Treatment with thrombolytics. In *Haemorrhagic and Thrombotic Diseases*, ed. Nilsson, I. M., pp. 189–200. London: John Wiley & Sons.

Rosenberg, R. D. (1975) Actions and interactions of antithrombin and heparin. *New England Journal of Medicine*, **292,** 146–151.

Salzman, E. W., Deykin, D., Shapiro, R. M. & Rosenberg, R. (1975) Management of heparin therapy. *New England Journal of Medicine*, **292,** 1046–1050.

Salzman, E. W., Harris, W. H. & DeSanctis, R. W. (1977) Reduction in venous thrombosis by agents affecting platelet function. *New England Journal of Medicine*, **284,** 1287–1292.

Sherry, S., Fletcher, A. P. & Alkjaersig, N. (1959) Fibrinolysis and fibrinolytic activity in man. *Physiological Reviews*, **39,** 343–382.

Signori, E. E., Penner, J. A. & Kahn, D. R. (1969) Coagulation defects and bleeding in open heart surgery. *Annals of Thoracic Surgery*, **8,** 521–529.

Spector, I. & Corn, M. (1967) Control of heparin therapy with activated partial thromboplastin time. *Journal of American Medical Association*, **201,** 157–159.

Stemerman, M. B. (1974) Vascular intimal components: precursors of thrombosis. In *Progress in Hemostasis and Thrombosis*, ed. Spaet, T. H., Vol. 2, pp. 1–49. New York: Grune & Stratton.

Stenflo, J. (1974) Structural comparison of normal and dicoumarol induced prothrombin. In *Prothrombin and Related Coagulation Factors*, ed. Hemker, H. C. & Veltkamp, J. J., pp. 152–158. Leiden: Leiden University Press.

Vermylen, J., De Gaetano, G. & Verstraete, M. (1973) Platelets and thrombosis. In *Recent Advances in Thrombosis*, ed. Poller, L., pp. 113–150. Edinburgh: Churchill Livingstone.

Walsh, P. N. (1972) The role of platelets in the contact phase of blood coagulation. *British Journal of Haematology*, **22,** 237–254.

Walsh, P. N. & Biggs, R. (1972) The role of platelets in intrinsic factor Xa formation. *British Journal of Haematology*, **22,** 743–760.

Wardle, E. N. & Taylor, G. (1968) Fibrin breakdown products and fibrinolysis in renal disease. *Journal of Clinical Pathology*, **21**, 140–146.
Weiss, H. J. (1972) The pharmacology of platelet inhibition. In *Progress in Hemostasis and Thrombosis*, ed. Spaet, T. H., Vol. 1, pp. 199–232. New York: Grune & Stratton.
Weiss, H. J. (1975) Platelet physiology and abnormalities of platelet function. *New England Journal of Medicine*, **293**, 531–541 and 580–588.
White, J. G. (1974) Electron microscopic studies on platelet secretion. In *Progress in Hemostasis and Thrombosis*, ed. Spaet, T. H., Vol. 2, pp. 49–99. New York: Grune & Stratton.
Zimmerman, T. F., Ratnoff, O. D. & Powell, A. E. (1971) Immunologic dfferentiation of classic hemophilia (factor 8 deficiency) and von Willebrand's disease, with observations on combined deficiencies of antihemophilic factor and proaccelerin (factor 5) and on an acquired circulating anticoagulant against antihemophilic factor. *Journal of Clinical Investigation*, **50**, 244–254.

8
MICROSURGERY

W. J. Rich

A magnified view of the surgical field is firmly established as essential in some areas of surgical endeavour. The operating microscope offers great potential not only for the improvement of accepted operative techniques but also for the realisation of entirely new developments in surgery. Those surgeons who are regularly using the operating microscope know that there must be many fields of surgical endeavour where the potential offered by the microscope is as yet untouched.

The otolaryngologists can rightly claim the credit for the introduction of the microscope to surgery. Nylén (1921) and Holmgren (1922) used the microscope to operate on the labyrinth in otosclerosis. Apart from Hinselmann, who in 1925 used the binocular microscope for colposcopy, the otolaryngologists were alone in developing and exploiting microsurgical techniques for the next three decades; Cawthorne in 1941 was using a dissecting microscope for operations on the facial nerve. In 1950 Perritt of Chicago used a binocular dissecting microscope for ophthalmic surgery. Zeiss in 1953 produced their Op. Mi. I surgical microscope and differing surgical specialities began to realise that the operating microscope had potential in their fields (Table 8.1). Ophthalmology with Barraquer in 1956, vascular surgery with Jacobson and Suarez in 1960, neurosurgery with Kurze in Los Angeles and plastic surgery

Table 8.1 Progress to surgical applications of the microscope

1590–1621	Janssen Drebbel Van Leenwenhoek Robert Hook	Compound microscope	
1702	Zahn	Binocular microscope	Botanical studies
1886	Zehender	Binocular head-mounted magnifying spectacles	Ophthalmology
1921	Nylén	Monocular operating microscope	Middle ear surgery
1922	Holmgren	Binocular operating microscope	Middle ear surgery
1925	Hinselmann	Binocular microscope	Colposcopy
1950	Perritt	Binocular microscope	Ophthalmic surgery
1953	Zeiss	Operating microscope I	Widespread adoption and development in surgery

with Burke in 1962 in California were specialties which then began to use the microscope.

It is interesting that, as in so many fields of medicine, widespread acceptance lags far behind discovery and development. It is now 200 years since the invention of the compound microscope and 50 years since the first use of an optically satisfactory operating microscope. The reasons for this delayed appreciation seem to lie in the lack of flexibility of the microscope itself, the microscope and instrument manufacturers and the surgeons themselves. It is only now that the appreciation of the potential of microsurgery on the one hand and special requirements and constraints on the other is bringing about the realisation that here is a really valuable asset to modern surgery in many fields.

HISTORICAL

History of the Use of Magnification in Surgery

The principle of magnification must have been known in very ancient times; what is thought to be a magnifying lens was found in the excavations of Nineveh (770 B.C.). Spectacles were in use about A.D. 1300 and can be seen in a painting by Thomas Von Madena in 1352. The compound microscope is attributed to different individuals between 1590 and 1631, among them Janssen of Holland, Galileo in 1610 and Drebbel of Holland in 1621. Certainly much initial work was carried out at that time with basic observations on botanical and biological specimens. Magnifying spectacles were introduced by the ophthalmologist Zehender (1887), but they suffered the disadvantage, which persists today, of discomfort and lack of stability of the field.

ADVANTAGES OF MICROSURGERY

Some of the advantages which a magnified view of the operating field gives to the surgeon are obvious. Tissues can be examined with clarity and in detail; dissection, mobilisation and suturing can be performed with greater accuracy and less trauma than is possible with unaided vision.

Other advantages are perhaps less obvious but lie in the evolution of completely new techniques, in new instruments and new equipment—some of which is proving to be of benefit in non-microsurgical applications—and in the ready facility the microscope provides for teaching and recording of surgical procedures.

MODERN OPERATING MICROSCOPES

The range of operating microscopes available today is wide and still evolving to suit different applications. At the simplest, telescopic spectacles (Fig. 8.1) can be worn by the surgeon; the value is severely restricted by the fact that the surgeon must keep his head at the exact focal distance from the operating field and any movement of his head produces apparent movement of the field. A normal field of vision is retained around the miniature telescopes which may be cemented on to the surgeon's own spectacles. Their use is limited to applications requiring low-power magnification intermittently during the course of the operation.

A simple operating microscope, for example the Zeiss Op. Mi. I (Fig. 8.2), is suitable for many applications, although many specialties have found it necessary to add to its complexity in order to satisfy their special needs. The binocular eyepieces can be straight or inclined in relation to the microscope

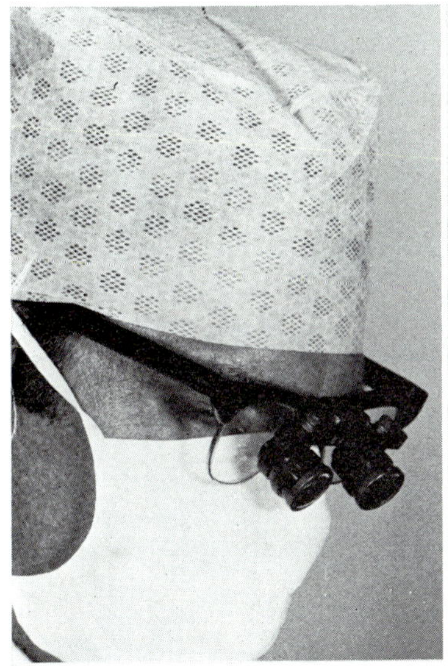

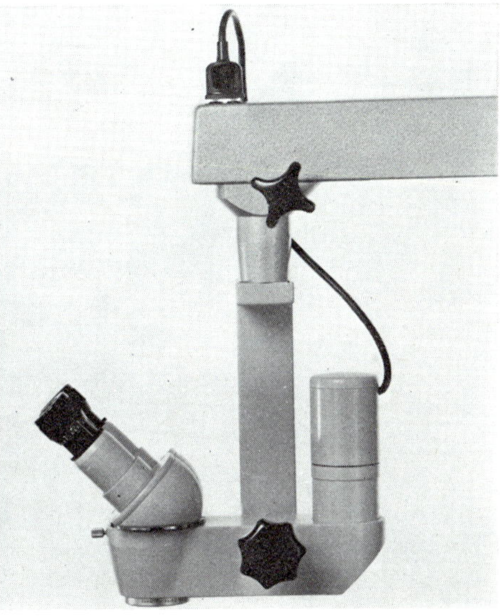

Figure 8.1   Telescopic spectacles (Keelers, London)

Figure 8.2   Simple operating microscope (Zeiss Op. Mi. 9)

body, and are adjustable for the refractive error and interpupillary distance of the surgeon. The body of the microscope contains an optical system which allows magnification to be changed between approximately $\times 6$ and $\times 40$, the exact value depends upon the power of the eyepieces and objectives used. The focal length of the single objective lens is chosen according to the operating distance which is required. Thus in neurosurgery and ear, nose and throat surgery, where the field is often in a deep cavity, the most useful objective lenses are those with long focal lengths (300–400 mm), whereas in surface applications such as ophthalmic or plastic surgery 175 or 200 mm focal length lenses are more suitable. A powerful coaxial light is incorporated in the body of the microscope. The mounting of the simple microscope must combine ready adjustability with rigidity, and may be from a heavy floor-based stand with several interlinking arms and counterbalanced vertical movement which may be locked in position.

Many refinements which add to the performance of the microscope, and to its complexity, have been introduced and are necessary in certain applications. An examination of some of the parameters which affect microsurgery will indicate the advantages and disadvantages of such refinements.

Stereoscopic vision

This is of fundamental importance to the surgeon; without it he would be quite unable to judge the depth of the tissues, where to suture and where to

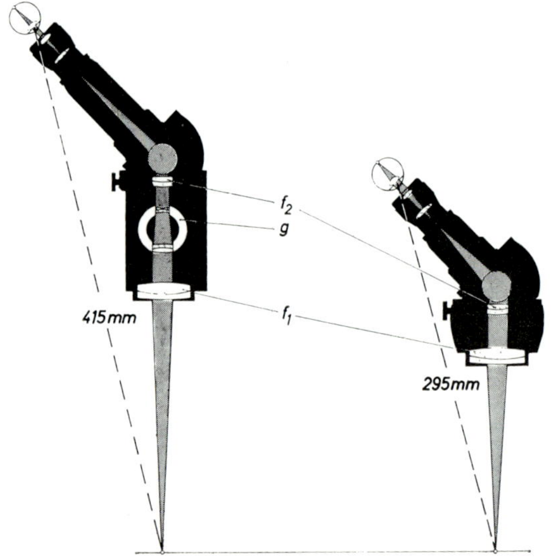

Figure 8.3   Angled eyepieces

cut or manipulate. A great advantage of the microscope is that stereoscopic appreciation of depth can be retained even though the surgeon may be working through an extremely small surgical approach. The unaided surgeon cannot retain stereoscopic vision through a narrow opening because the interpupillary distance of his own eyes is too great. The binocular surgical microscope enables the independent light pathway to be retained for each eye at very small angular separation. Thus, even through an opening as small as 5 mm diameter, the surgeon retains good stereoscopic separation.

Field of vision

This is governed by the magnification employed; at ×6 magnification the diameter of the field is 3 cm, at ×40 magnification it is 5 mm. The effective field which the surgeon covers, however, is greatly increased by mobility of the microscope. The extent to which the microscope interferes with the surgeon's wider view of the non-magnified field depends on the bulk of the microscope body and is greatly reduced by employing angled eyepieces (Fig. 8.3).

Magnification

The range of magnification found useful in present applications is between ×6 and ×40. For many uses a fixed magnification is perfectly satisfactory, but variation during surgery by steps or a continuously variable zoom lens is essential for some procedures. Two important corollaries accompany

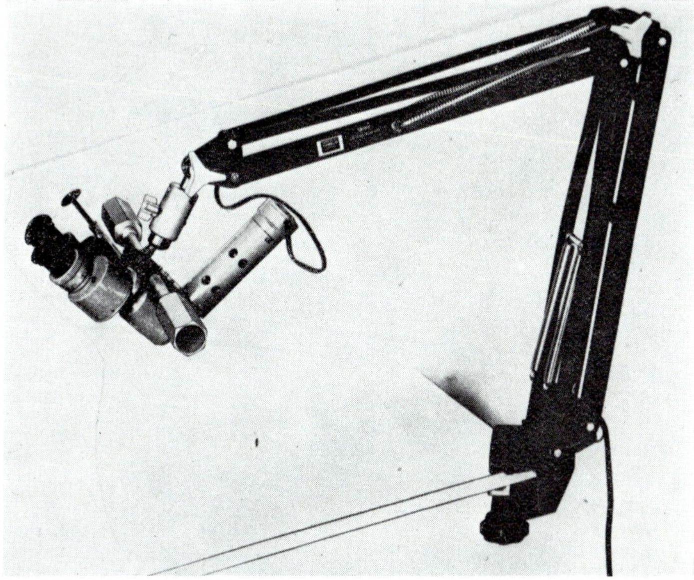

Figure 8.4   Lightweight portable microscope, which may be clamped to the operating table (Mentor, Hamblin, London)

increased magnification. One is reduction of the depth of focus so that at high magnification extremely accurate focusing is necessary and may require frequent adjustment; the other is the need for greatly increased illumination as magnification increases.

Focal distance

The comfort of the surgeon requires a distance of 150 to 200 mm between the eyepieces of his microscope and his hands; in superficial operations a 175 or 200 mm objective lens will give this comfortable distance and adequate clearance for instruments between the operating field and the microscope; in deeper operations a longer focus lens is necessary to enable this clearance to be maintained and to give access for long instruments. The objective lens can be changed with ease on most microscopes.

Mounting and adjustment of the microscope

Some of the constraints imposed by the microscope can be overcome or minimised by attention to mounting and controls. It is desirable both that the microscope is held rigidly at the desired position to give a focused view of the surgical field, and that the surgeon is able to alter the angle or area of field under observation and change focus or magnification with the minimum of distraction from his surgical task. Mounting of the microscope from an arm

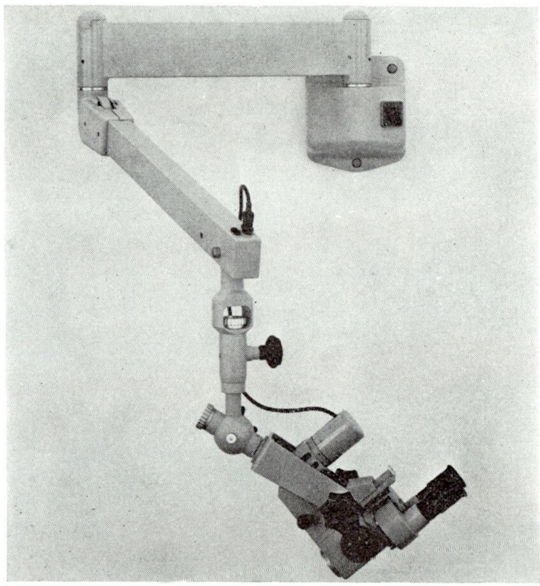

Figure 8.5 Wall-mounted simple microscope suitable for casualty or paediatric use (Zeiss)

clamped to the operating table (Fig. 8.4) has the advantage of simplicity but may restrict mobility and is not rigid enough for the more bulky microscope and its ancilliary equipment. This method, or a wall mounting (Fig. 8.5), are very suitable for casualty department or paediatric applications. A floor stand has the advantage of mobility within the theatre area, but the disadvantage of bulk and cables on the theatre floor, and the possibility of capsize. Ceiling mounting of the microscope (Fig. 8.6) is perhaps the ideal, since not only is the theatre floor clear of cables and bulky equipment, but the microscope can be raised out of the way when not in use. Adjustment of focus, magnification and position of the microscope can be performed manually by controls on the microscope, but foot controls, either on a separate panel (Fig. 8.7) or incorporated into the surgeon's chair (Fig. 8.8), avoid the necessity for the surgeon to move his instruments from the field. A foot controlled servomotor can be fitted to move the microscope or the theatre table itself in an X–Y horizontal axis. The surgeon's operating chair can also be used as a stable base on which to mount the microscope; this again reduces the demand for floor space in the theatre but does limit the movement of the surgeon to some degree. An interesting and promising simplification which allows greatly increased mobility for the surgeon is that recently introduced by Pierse (Fig. 8.9) of fixing the microscope by rigid arm to the surgeon's chair and making it possible for the surgeon to adjust the focus by the simple effort of leaning forwards or backwards on the hydraulically clamped seat.

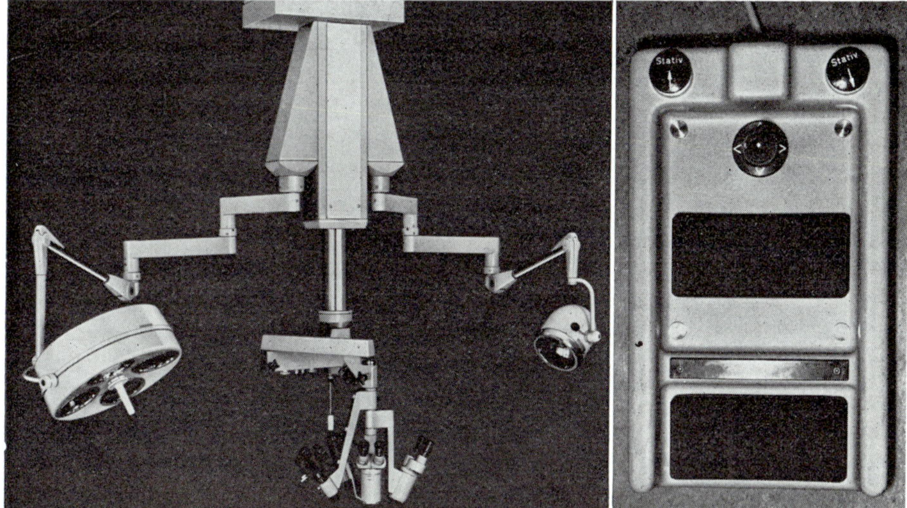

Figure 8.6   Ceiling-mounted microscope (Zeiss)

Figure 8.7   Foot control panel. Pedals for focus and magnification and miniature joy-stick for X–Y movement (Zeiss)

Horizontal movement may readily be accomplished by the surgeon rolling his chair sideways or backwards and forwards.

STERILISATION

The operating microscope is a potential source of surgical infection. The surgeon's hands or instruments may be inadvertently contaminated by touching non-sterilised apparatus, or dust from it may fall directly into his surgical field. In some situations it is reasonable for the surgeon to handle the microscope by sterilised caps which fit on to the essential controls, and the objective of the microscope can be similarly protected by a sterilised guard. Some surgeons feel able to handle the microscope after it has been isolated in a plastic bag containing formalin tablets for 24 h prior to use. Cold formalin has been shown, however, to be an inadequate method of producing sterility, and this technique cannot be recommended. A satisfactory method for most applications is to cover the entire microscope head with a transparent plastic drape (Fig. 8.10)—the surgeon can see and manipulate the controls, a cut-out is made around the eyepieces and the objective and the drape held around them with sterilised plastic bands. This is effective for even very bulky apparatus,

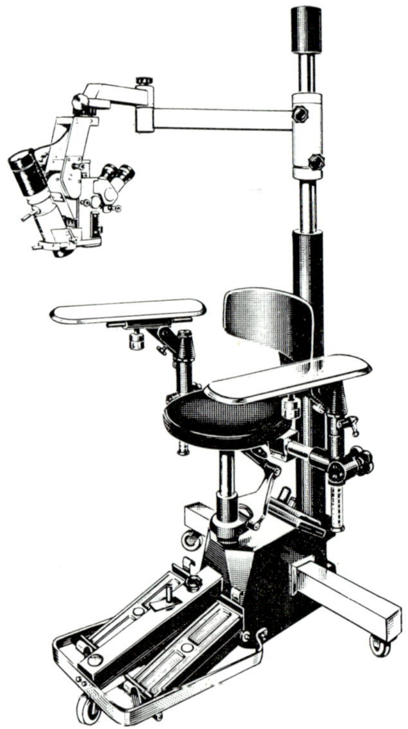

Figure 8.8   Chair mounting. A stable base also incorporating foot controls and arm rests for the surgeon (Möller–Wedel)

though attention must be given to adequate air space around the light source in order to allow convection of heat.

LIGHTING

High intensity illumination is required, and even more so if light is required for photography or a second observer which will introduce a beam splitter in the optical system. In many applications limited access to the surgical field makes coaxial illumination essential, and indeed this type of illumination is satisfactory for most purposes. In some applications, particularly when working on tissue planes at a relatively superficial level, oblique illumination can be helpful because it accentuates the judgement of depth. Ophthalmologists sometimes use oblique light reduced to a narrow slit in width so that an 'optical section' can be seen in transparent tissues such as cornea, and this gives very accurate depth judgement. Fibreoptic cables are bringing very considerable improvements in lighting conditions so that a powerful light source can be remotely placed from the surgical field. By this means a cool, powerful light is brought by thin fibre cable right to the surgical field, where

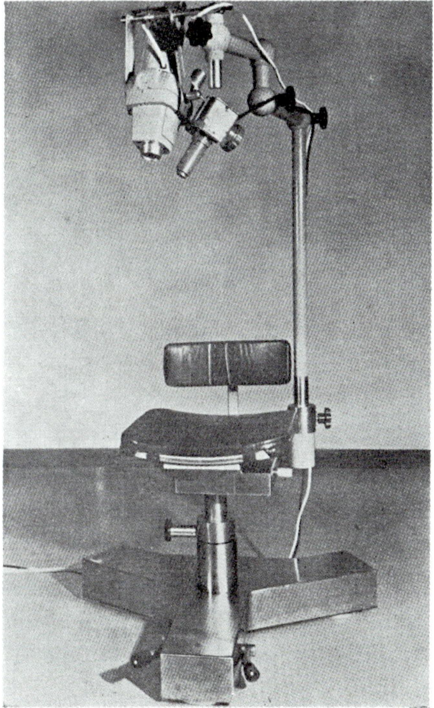

Figure 8.9 Chair microscope (Pierse)

it can be guided by an assistant. Indeed the optical fibre may be incorporated in the instrument itself to bring the light to the very tip (Fig. 8.11). Fibreoptics furthermore allow the possibility of oblique or retro-illumination, even at a great depth in a surgical wound, and this is a very valuable asset to microsurgery.

INSTRUMENTS

The magnified view brings to the surgeon realisation of the trauma produced by surgical instruments, and from this the questioning as to whether the instruments used are really the most efficient for their task. Very considerable advances have already been made and some of these are producing a feed-back into the non-microsurgical techniques. The traditional tissue-holding forceps which have sharp interdigitating teeth can be seen to inflict considerable damage, while ridge or beak-tipped forceps (Fig. 8.12), which hold the tissue just as firmly, inflict minimal tissue trauma. Needle holders which can hold a microneedle rigidly and allow easy manipulation within a small area have been developed in various fields of application, for example the needle-holder shown in Fig. 8.13 is designed so that easy rotation between finger and thumb will allow the curve of the needle to follow its natural arc through the tissues

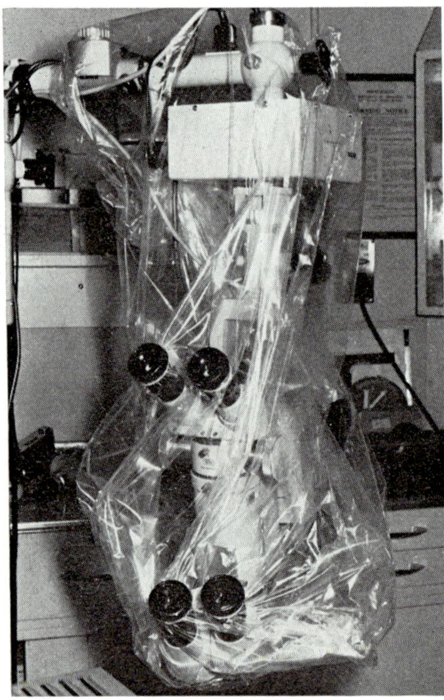

Figure 8.10   Sterile drape around the entire microscope allows manipulation of all controls

rather than being involved in traumatic pushing and pulling. Each field has developed its own special instruments. Particularly valuable in vascular micro-surgery is a two-pronged fork (Yasargil) which can be placed against the blood vessel wall to give counter pressure against the passage of the needle. Tissue-cutting instruments have been greatly improved and miniaturised with the development of microscissors (Fig. 8.14) and the use of razor blade fragments and even a diamond-tipped knife.

The technical advances in needles and sutures have been responsible for many microsurgical advances; atraumatic needles are universally employed in microsurgery with tips and cross-sections appropriate to their use. Thus for vascular surgery a round-bodied needle, and for corneal surgery a cutting

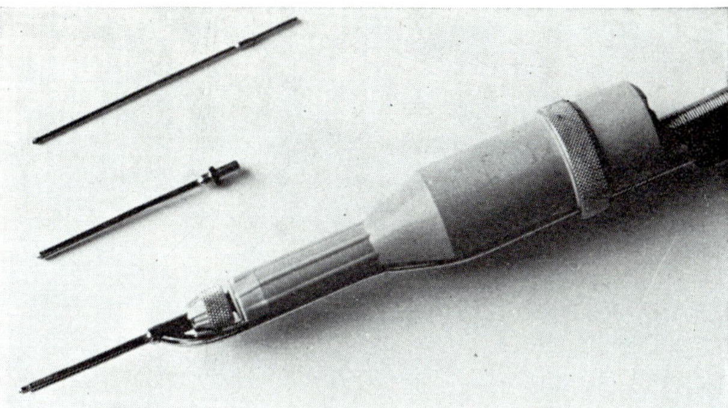

Figure 8.11 Suction cutter for vitreous surgery, incorporating fibreoptic illumination at the cutting tip (Storz)

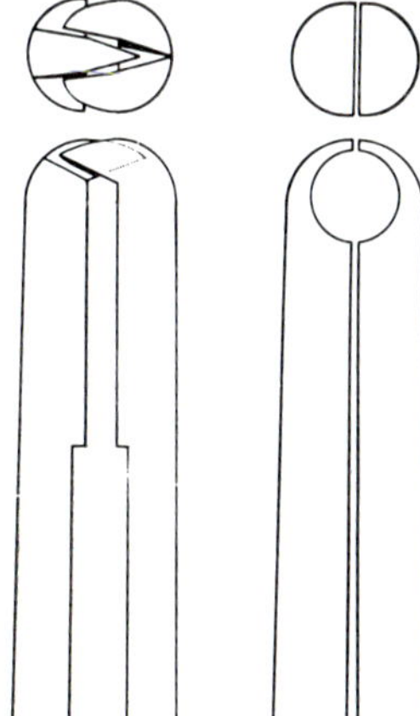

Figure 8.12 Forceps tip. Beak or ridge tip is less traumatic than traditional toothed forceps

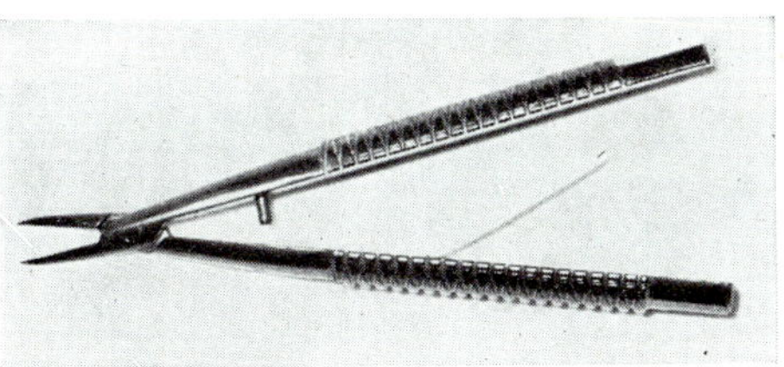

Figure 8.13 Titanium microsurgical needle-holder (MICRA, Ethicon)

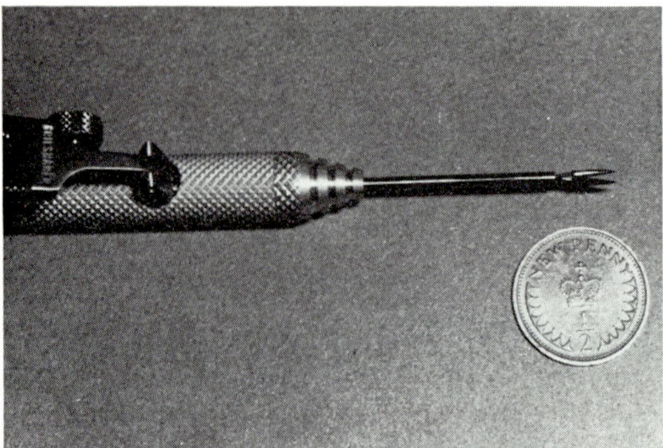

Figure 8.14   Microscissors (Greishaber)

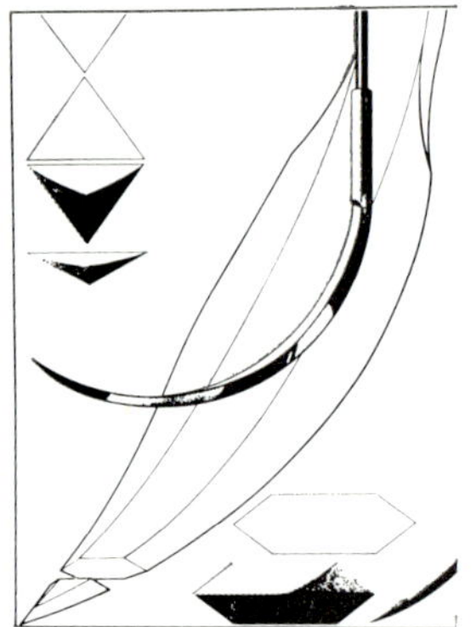

Figure 8.15   Engineering requirements of microsurgical needles. Cross-section of a needle designed to enter tissues with ease but to maintain a long tract without cutting out

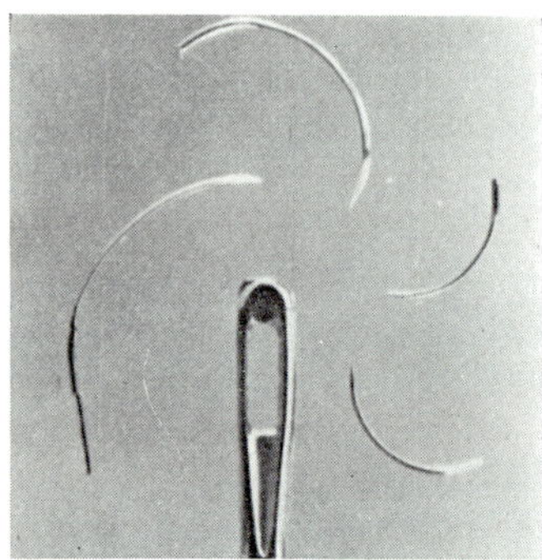

Figure 8.16   Microsurgical needles: 4 and 5 mm round and cutting needles compared with the 'eye' of a 55 mm needle (Ethicon)

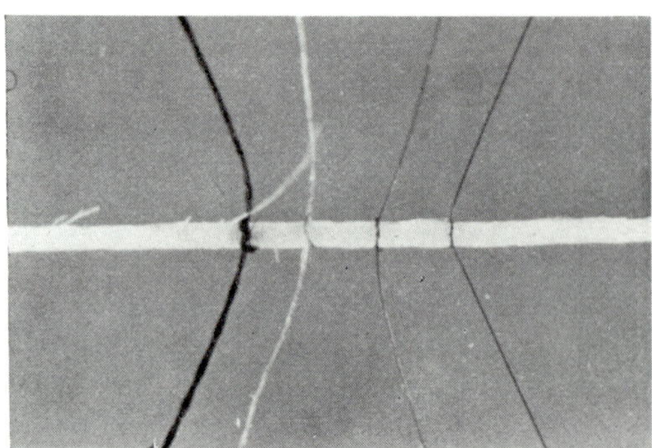

Figure 8.17   Suture materials: 2/0 linen with 7/0 silk, 8/0 silk, 9/0 nylon and 10/0 nylon (Ethicon)

tip with flat tissue-cleaving surfaces (Fig. 8.15) is used, while the needle itself may be as short as 3 mm in length and only 0.10 mm in diameter for some of the microvascular applications. The ability of the industry to provide these needles (Fig. 8.16), reliable, sharp and in presterilised packaged form is indeed a major advance.

Suture materials themselves have been the subject of wide experimentation and, while stainless steel is proving suitable for some applications, nylon as fine as 10/0 or 24 μm in diameter (Fig. 8.17) is not only strong and well tolerated, but also has useful properties of elasticity. Attention has to be paid to suture-tying techniques when using new types of suture materials, and nylon in particular requires three half-hitches on the first knot if a tendency to slip is to be avoided with certainty. A mini sucker can be very useful in certain applications. Bipolar cautery allows pinpoint coagulation across the smaller vessel walls, and this is very much more useful in a microsurgical field than is unipolar cautery or diathermy, which has a far more extensive field of tissue damage. It is possible for the microsurgeon to pick up a small blood vessel between the teeth of a very fine forceps and to apply the current to produce very selective coagulation. Skilled modern engineering advice has been brought into the design of microsurgical instruments with the result that new materials are being introduced, such as titanium which offers the advantages of great hardness, together with resistance to corrosion and lightness.

The care of microsurgical instruments is of particular importance since their tips are finely engineered and naturally easily damaged. With proper attention and protection, there is no reason why they should not last well. It is useful to have an ultrasonic cleaning bath rather than to use traumatic brushing techniques to clean blood and tissue away from the tips of instruments. It is also very useful to store the instruments in racks so that the tips cannot possibly be dislodged or damaged.

THE MICROSCOPE AS A TEACHING AID

The microscope offers enormous scope for teaching and recording. A beam splitting prism in the microscope can take in exactly the surgeon's view of the operating field to a variety of teaching and recording systems and thus reach a wider audience than the surgeon and his assistants. An observer's viewing arm from the beam splitter allows superb viewing for teaching only one or two observers. A compact colour television camera (Fig. 8.18) can be mounted on the beam splitter without intrusion and the operation can be watched on a monitor in the theatre or elsewhere. Quite an amazing increase in efficiency and interest accompanies such a sharing of the operation scene with the whole surgical team. Videotape recording of the operation is not a fanciful encumberance but a most valuable teaching aid; examination of technique, replayed immediately after the operation with analysis of particular problems and points, adds to surgical experience more effectively than opportunities to repeat such operative procedures on occasions separated by considerable time. Videotapes may be kept for recording or teaching, but most often are replayed and then reused for the next operating session. A 35 mm camera for transparencies or a cine camera can record the operation, being attached by the beam splitter to the microscope body. Such recording does not interfere with the surgery in any way, and the microscope lighting itself is sufficient for good photography.

In a very real way the use of the microscope in an operating theatre does contribute to the learning processes and interest of all involved.

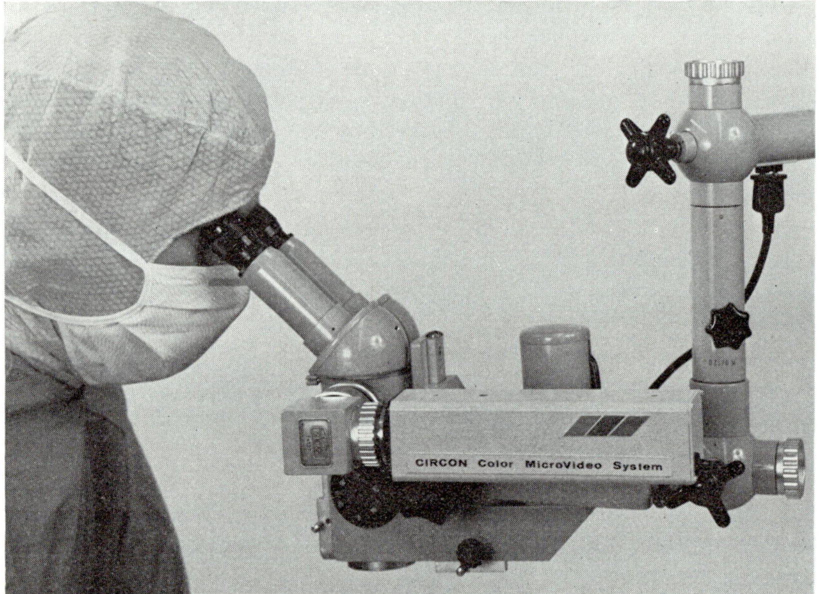

Figure 8.18   Colour television camera mounted on a beam splitter on the microscope (Circon)

THE ASSISTANT

In some microsurgical situations an assistant can be of little practical value to the surgeon, for example in a deep cavity as in many neurosurgical applications where there is really only room for the surgeon's own activities. In other situations an assistant is not only helpful but absolutely essential, for example in controlling suction during vitreous surgery or cutting sutures in cataract surgery. In order to act efficiently the assistant must be able to see the surgical field, and if he has to manoeuvre he must have a stereoscopic view—so either a stereoscopic beam splitter or a separate microscope becomes necessary for the assistant. A uniocular view of the surgeon's field can easily be obtained

by an assistant or other observers through an eyepice from a beam splitter
in the optical system, and is of great value for teaching.

CURRENT MICROSURGICAL APPLICATIONS

Otolaryngology

The stereoscopic view down a very narrow approach and excellent coaxial
lighting provided by the operating microscope make its use invaluable in this
field. Middle-ear surgery, fenestration, stapes operations, tympanoplasties,
and the approach to an acoustic neuroma via the external auditory canal are all
fields in which its use is routine. Similarly, the very narrow and deep access
to the pituitary fossa would not be possible without the stereopsis of the
microscope. Surgery of the larynx is aided by a long focus objective lens.

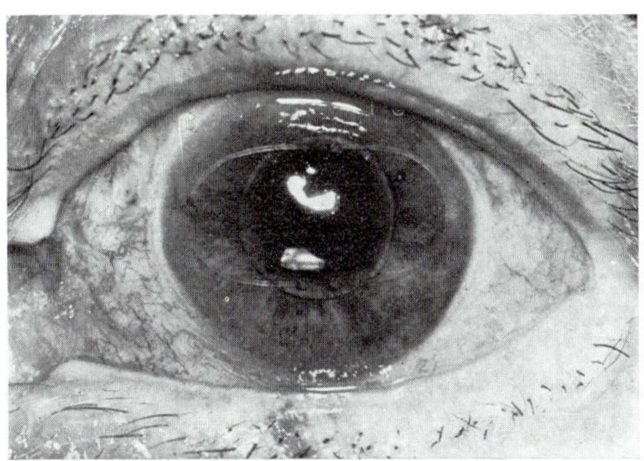

Figure 8.19   Intraocular acrylic lens sutured to the iris with 10/0 nylon

Ophthalmology

The accuracy of suturing techniques made possible with microsurgical
equipment has not only produced radical improvement in visual and structural
results following cataract surgery and keratoplasty, but has also led to the great
advance of very early mobilisation and discharge from hospital of the predominantly elderly type of patient. Entirely new operations such as implantation of an acrylic intraocular lens sutured to the iris (Fig. 8.19), trabecu-
lectomy drainage operation for glaucoma, operations direct on the canal of
Schlemm, or vitrectomy have become possible simply because the surgeon
can see minute detail.

Neurosurgery

Especially in applications where the field can be kept relatively free from
blood, the microscope is becoming widely accepted. Intracranial aneurysms
can be more accurately ligated, and danger points and threatened bleeding

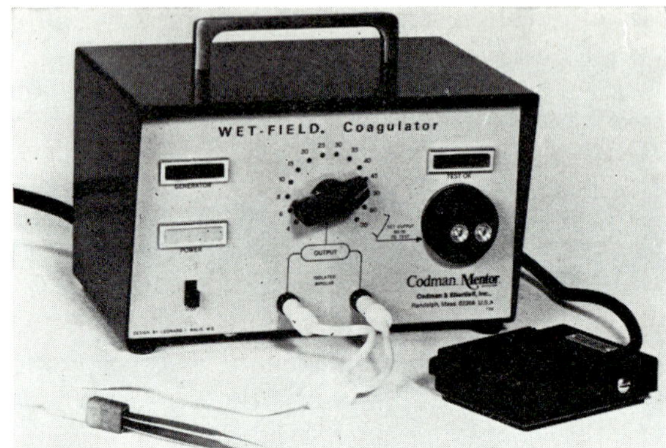

Figure 8.20   Bipolar cautery (Codman–Mentor, Hamblin)

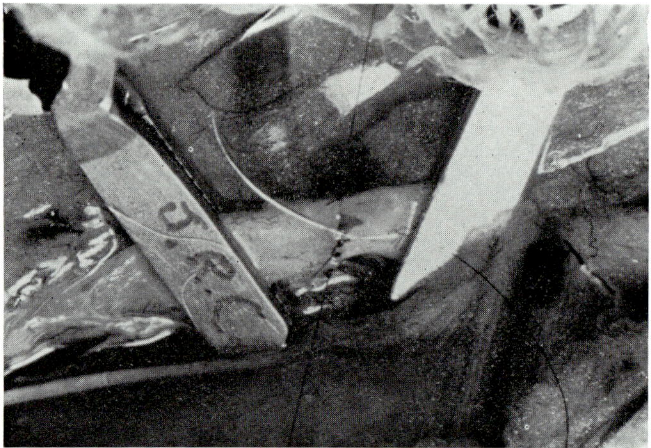

Figure 8.21   Small vessel anastomosis in hand surgery (by courtesy of J. R. Cobbett, East Grinstead)

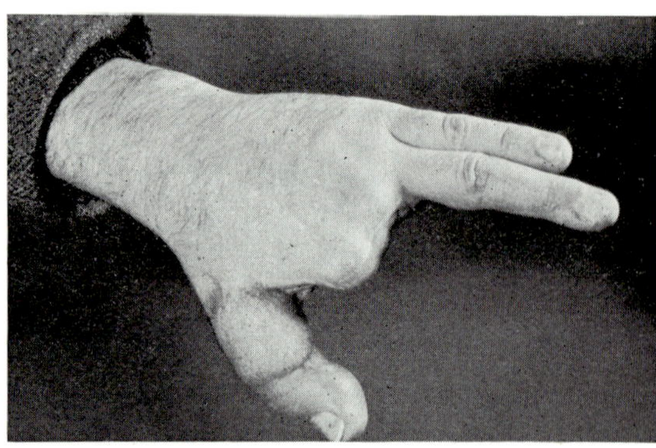

Figure 8.22   Great toe to thumb transplant (by courtesy of J. R. Cobbett, East Grinstead)

better anticipated. Neurosurgeons find the bipolar cautery with microtip particularly helpful in this field (Fig. 8.20). Thrombectomies, embolectomies and by-pass anastomoses have been performed. Surgery on tumours, particularly of the spinal cord, can be very confidently helped by the aid which the microscope provides to dissection of tissue planes and the avoidance of bleeding, because the surgeon can see vessels before he is in danger of cutting them.

Plastic surgery

Work pioneered by J. R. Cobbett uses microsurgical techniques for limb surgery, with anastomosis of small vessels (Fig. 8.21) and nerves and even transplantation of a great toe for use as a thumb (Fig. 8.22).

Vascular surgery

An increasing number of vascular surgeons are coming to realise the value of the microscope in their field. Thus some are using it for renal anastomoses, carotid surgery and small vessel surgery. It is technically possible to anastomose vessels as small as 1 mm in diameter, and this means that vessels in many parts of the body hitherto hardly considered operable may indeed be suitable for vascular surgery.

Gynaecology

Colposcopy is perhaps not a surgical operation, although it was one of the earliest uses of the microscope in this field. Perhaps the most exciting is the careful dissection and anastomosis of the ovarian tube which now is being performed by microsurgical techniques.

Urology

Ureteric anastomosis and sphincter surgery have felt the benefit of microsurgical technique. Anastomosis of the vas deferens might be treated with advantage in the same way.

Other applications

Casualty—operations for removal of foreign bodies and repair surgery.

Paediatrics—for cauterisation of minute vessels and surgery on very small babies.

Dermatology—for diagnosis and treatment of lesions.

These three are all specialties in which appreciation of the microscope is beginning to develop and in which its use will expand rapidly as the advantages become apparent.

THE FUTURE

Microsurgical developments are certain to play an important part in surgical advances. The possibility of vascular anastomosis and replacement of really small blood vessels brings the possibility of important advances in almost every field of surgery. Simplification of the microscope may come through such developments as the bifocal microscope, or a non-optical system of magnification using a stereo television camera, compact and remote from the field of surgery. This requires little illumination to provide a stereo image for the surgeon in any position and at any magnification he requires, and is simply controlled by electronic means. Micromanipulators are receiving attention, and fibreoptic illumination is certain to bring increasing benefits.

These are exciting prospects.

REFERENCES

Cawthorne, T., quoted by Sahmbaugh, G. E. (1967) *Surgery of the Ear*, 2nd edn, p. 179. Philadelphia: Saunders.
Holmgren, G. (1923) *Acta otolaryngology, Stockholm*, **5,** 460.
Nylén, C. D. (1954) *Acta otolaryngology, Stockholm*, Suppl. 116, 226.
Perritt, R. A. (1950) American Academy of Ophthalmology and Otolaryngology, Course No. 288.

9
SURGERY AND THE HYPERBARIC ENVIRONMENT

D. N. Walder

A few years ago the publication of articles by Boerema et al (1956), Boerema (1961) and Illingworth et al (1961) resulted in a renewed interest in the possible advantages of treating some surgical conditions, and even operating, in a hyperbaric environment. Treating patients by raising the ambient pressure had been originally suggested by Henshaw as early as 1662, probably on the general assumption that if air was essential to life then an increase in its concentration might be effective in the treatment of disease.

No great interest had been shown in the idea until the middle of the nineteenth century when Pravaz (1840) built a large pressure chamber in which to treat patients at Lyons in France. The fashion spread and before long there were 50 or more pressure chambers throughout Europe (Gowdey, 1966) including one in London at the Brompton Hospital (Williams, 1885). The excess pressure in these early chambers was usually quite small, typically $\frac{1}{4}$ to $\frac{1}{3}$ bar, though at least one chamber (Junod, 1834) could be taken to an ambient pressure of 3 or even 4 bar. The chambers were mainly used for the treatment of respiratory conditions although pressure was also considered beneficial in deafness, cholera, metrorrhagia and rickets amongst other conditions.

The first reports claiming the beneficial effects of using oxygen as opposed to air in pressure chambers began to appear in 1887 when Valenzuela described the results of treating patients with pneumonia. This was followed by Haldane who reported in 1895 the dramatic effect of hyperbaric oxygen in protecting experimental animals against carbon monoxide poisoning. Unfortunately oxygen was not available in sufficient quantities to be generally used for therapeutic purposes until the 1920s.

As might be imagined, a good deal of over optimism about the therapeutic value of raised atmospheric pressure therapy was generated at first. Fortunately, in the background, Paul Bert was investigating the matter scientifically and in 1878 his very important book *La Pression Barometrique* was published. The significance of this work may be gauged from the fact that an English translation of the original text appeared in 1941, over 60 years later. Paul Bert's work did not however prevent Cunningham in 1927 bringing hyperbaric therapy into disrepute by making such grandiose claims for its value that he was publicly attacked by the American Medical Association Bureau of

Investigation in a report published in 1928. Undaunted, Cunningham went on to built a 72-room, six-storey, spherical pressure chamber in Cleveland, Ohio, USA, for the treatment of patients.

Hyperbaric surgery

The first hyperbaric operating room was used by a French surgeon called Pean and was described by Fontaine in 1879. This mobile chamber could accommodate 10 to 12 people (Fig. 9.1) and amongst its advantages was mentioned the fact that patients recovered from their anaesthetic more quickly and cyanosis and asphyxia were absent. Postanaesthetic excitement and vomiting were also markedly decreased. It was said to facilitate the reduction of hernias and was recommended for use when operating on patients with asthma, emphysema, chronic bronchitis and anaemia.

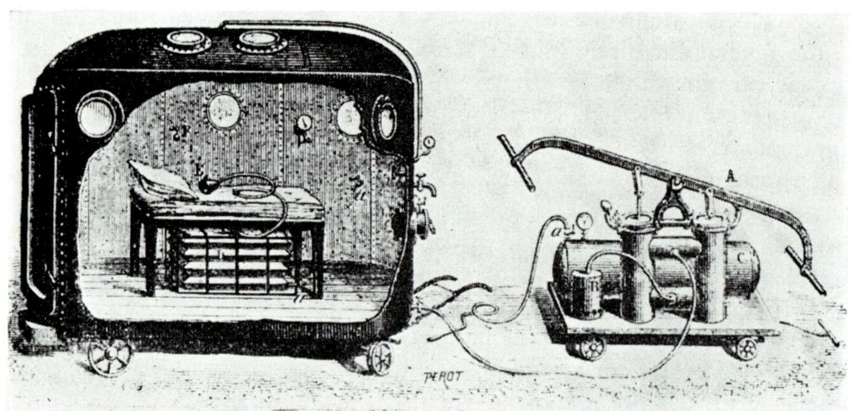

Figure 9.1   Mobile hyperbaric operating room (1879). Note the manual compressor and the anaesthetic gas container and mask

Boerema's object in establishing a chamber in Amsterdam in the 1950s (Fig. 9.2) was to make use of the oxygen storage effect expected in patients breathing 100 per cent oxygen at pressure. He hoped that it would enable the surgeon to submit his patient to longer periods of cardiac arrest than would otherwise be possible, whilst operating on the heart. Other applications of hyperbaric oxygen therapy both surgical and medical were quickly suggested and are mentioned later.

It is usual to limit the working pressure of this type of hyperbaric chamber to an absolute pressure of 3 bar (i.e. 2 bar above atmospheric pressure) because above this prolonged breathing of undiluted oxygen becomes dangerous. It is of course only the patient who breathes pure oxygen, as the surgeon, anaesthetist, assistants and other personnel in the chamber are exposed only to air at pressure. The risks to them are similar to those of compressed air workers.

Occupational hyperbaric exposure

Whilst the therapeutic value of a hyperbaric environment was first being explored, a civil engineer named Triger introduced at Chalon (France) in the late 1830s the novel idea of using air under pressure to facilitate the construction of shafts, tunnels and caissons for bridge foundations through water-bearing ground (Triger, 1841). As a consequence the labourers engaged in the construction also had to be exposed to the raised pressure. They have therefore come to be called compressed air workers. Almost at once illness

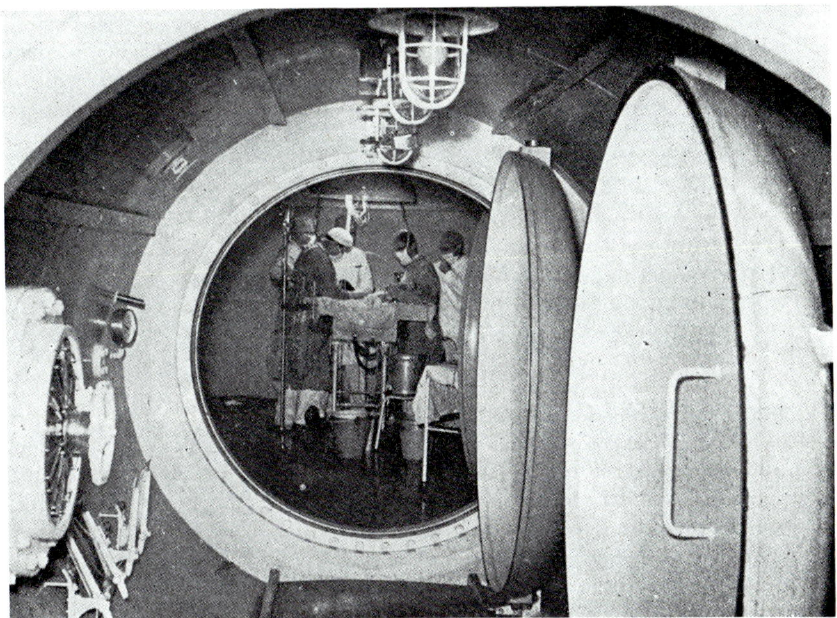

Figure 9.2 Boerema's pressurised operating theatre (1956) (reproduced, with permission, from Boerema, Brummelkamp and Meijne, 1964, *Clinical Application of Hyperbaric Oxygen.* Amsterdam: ASP Biological and Medical Press)

was noticed amongst the men engaged in this work and the first record of acute symptoms affecting men, as a result of working at pressure, was published in a report by Trouessart in 1845). In 1854 Pol and Wattelle recorded that it was 'the return to atmospheric pressure (i.e. the decompression) which had to be dreaded', though even before this Bouhy (1847) had realised that compressed air workers who became ill could be relieved by putting them back to pressure in the working place.

It is now recognised that in addition to the immediate dangers of acute decompression sickness, which may come on during decompression or within a few hours of its completion, there is also the risk that men who work under increased pressure may eventually (i.e. after a few months) also suffer from an aseptic necrosis of bone which has come to be known as caisson disease of bone. Although a few sporadic papers about caisson disease of bone were published from 1911 (Bornstein and Plate) onwards it was not until 1966 that the full extent of the problem began to become apparent (Decompression Sickness Panel, 1966). Some years later the position in Great Britain was reviewed by Walder (1970).

Perhaps more topical because of its relevance to the recovery of oil from the North Sea is the fact that divers can also suffer from decompression sickness and bone necrosis. This latter condition was not reported in divers until 1941 (Grutzmacher) and has only recently started to receive the detailed attention which it deserves (Harrison, 1971; Walder, 1974).

Another condition which may affect divers and which sometimes requires operative treatment is persistent vertigo following injury to the inner ear.

A new problem which will involve surgery and the hyperbaric environment and which is currently attracting a good deal of attention stems from the fact that the work of the diver in the North Sea is changing from that concerned with prospecting and drilling to that concerned with heavy construction work. In the latter the risk of injuries to the diver is obviously higher.

More than 1000 divers are involved, and many of them work at depths in excess of 200 m (>20 bar). Such diving requires decompression times of the order of two to three days for quite short 'bottom times'.

As a consequence there has been a change from the so-called 'excursion diving', in which the diver goes down for an hour or so and then immediately starts his decompression and ascent to the surface to what is known as 'saturation diving'. In this the diver lives at pressure in a dry compression chamber situated at the surface on the oil rig platform or deck of a ship or barge for many days. From time to time as required he is lowered in a 'diving bell' (submersible decompression chamber, personnel transfer capsule, submersible work chamber) at the same pressure to the place of work. He then goes out into the sea to do his task and returns again to the 'diving bell'. He can then be transported vertically back to the deck compression chamber into which he transfers without any change in pressure. Here he waits until next required. After a spell lasting 10 days or more of such on-call diving duty at constant pressure his tissues are essentially saturated at the ambient pressure, hence the term 'saturation diving'. Since at the end of a long, deep 'excursion dive' the decompression required would only be slightly shorter than that at the end of a saturation dive to the same depth, the system saves both time and therefore money. However, the two factors, heavy construction work and long periods at high pressure with the necessity of several days decompression before the diver can be safely brought out into free air, result in a potential problem. That is, how to manage a serious injury or an acute surgical emergency when it occurs during a saturation dive (Society for Underwater Technology Report, 1976). This will be discussed later.

HYPERBARIC PHYSIOLOGY

Although there may be some therapeutic advantages in exposing a patient to a moderately raised ambient pressure there are also many dangers. If doctors and others are to attend the patient whilst at pressure they must also accept the dangers.

The professional compressed air worker and diver often have to submit themselves to pressures much greater than those used for the treatment of patients. The risks they run are therefore greater and consequently their remuneration is high.

At atmospheric pressure when breathing air the tissues of the body are normally in equilibrium with the gases of the air. Both oxygen and nitrogen dissolve in the tissues of the body to an extent which depends upon (a) the partial pressures of the gas, and (b) its solubility in the tissues. This dissolved gas is present in addition to the oxygen carried by chemical combination with the haemoglobin of the blood.

The degree to which the haemoglobin is saturated depends on the partial pressure of oxygen in the breathing gas. Since man's haemoglobin is already 98 per cent saturated when he is breathing air at atmospheric pressure, little additional carriage of oxygen by the haemoglobin results from either increasing the pressure at which air is breathed or indeed increasing the proportion of oxygen in the breathing mixture. When the ambient pressure is raised the amount of oxygen in solution in the blood (normally about 0.28 ml/100 ml blood) increases in proportion to the partial pressure of oxygen in the breathing gas (Henry's law). This then passes into solution in the tissues until a new equilibrium is reached.

Similarly if breathing air the amount of nitrogen in solution in the blood (normally about 0.98 ml/100 ml blood) increases and will also pass into solution in the tissues until equilibrium is reached. Any rise in oxygen or nitrogen pressure in the breathing gas will be reflected by a rise in the amounts dissolved in the blood and tissues.

The possibility of having more oxygen at a higher partial pressure than normal in the blood and hence in the tissues is the basis for the interest in hyperbaric therapy. There are however some complicating factors which must be taken into consideration.

Oxygen poisoning

If the partial pressure of inspired oxygen is too high a condition known as oxygen toxicity may result. There are two types. First there is the effect on the brain which results in convulsions. This is thought to be due to interference with the enzyme systems of the brain cells (Wood, Radomski and Watson, 1971). Men differ widely in their sensitivity to this condition, and they can also change their susceptibility from day to day. Second, there is an effect on the lungs, which leads to alveolar collapse. This is thought to

8

be due to interference with the production of surfactant (Gilder and McSherry, 1974). Both these effects are related to the duration of exposure to, as well as to the partial pressure of, oxygen.

In recent years the acceptable safe limits of partial pressure of oxygen in the breathing gas have been gradually reduced as more experience has been gained. For patients undergoing hyperbaric oxygen therapy breathing pure oxygen Kindwall (1970) recommends sessions of 2 h duration at an absolute pressure of 2 bar and 90 min duration at an absolute pressure of 3 bar. These exposures seem excessively long when compared to the duration of exposure to pure oxygen allowed by the US Navy for the treatment of decompression sickness when 30 min is all that is allowed at an absolute pressure of 3 bar. For saturation diving it is usual to control the proportion of oxyegn in the breathing gas so that its partial pressure never exceeds an absolute value of 0.6 bar, even though the total absolute pressure may be as high as 100 bar.

Nitrogen narcosis

When the partial pressure of nitrogen in the breathing gas exceeds that present in air at an absolute pressure of 6 bar it begins to have a narcotic effect which progresses as the pressure increases until eventually unconsciousness supervenes. As in oxygen poisoning there is considerable individual variation: some men are seriously affected by air at an absolute pressure of only 4 bar whereas a few are not affected until the air absolute pressure reaches 8 bar.

This is not a serious problem in the hyperbaric oxygen therapy chamber in which the absolute pressure does not usually exceed 3 bar, nor for compressed air workers where the maximum gauge pressure is limited by law (Statutory Instrument No. 61, 1958) to 50 lb/in^2 (approximately an absolute pressure of 4.4 bar) although the effect may be present to a small degree and could affect decision making when at pressure (Walder, 1966b).

However, for divers wishing to go deeper than 50 m (an absolute pressure of 6 bar) the nitrogen in the breathing mixture must be replaced by some other inert gas (Statutory Instrument No. 1229, Offshore Installations Regulations, 1974). In fact helium is most commonly used and deep diving is carried out almost exclusively with helium–oxygen mixtures. Interestingly enough not only does nitrogen narcosis become a problem at 50 m but it is also at about this pressure that the resistance of breathing apparatus to the flow of gases rises so much that the work of breathing starts to become an important factor. By changing to helium–oxygen mixtures instead of air this effect is also avoided.

Unfortunately the use of helium brings with it some disadvantages. One is that it has a high thermal conductivity so that at great depths the body can lose more heat via the respiratory tract that it can generate by maximum activity. This problem is too large to be overcome by the use of heated diving suits alone. Only by heating the inspired gases as well can the heat loss be compensated and the man prevented from becoming hypothermic. A second disadvantage of using helium in the breathing gas is that it affects speech which becomes like that of Donald Duck. So bad is this effect at great depths that communication becomes a severe problem. Fortunately there are electronic devices which are capable of unscrambling the speech and reconstructing it so that it becomes almost identical with normal speech. An excellent helium speech unscrambler designed and manufactured in Great Britain is available commercially.

Decompression sickness

As has already been explained, at greater than normal pressures more oxygen and nitrogen go into solution in the body tissues than normal until such time as the partial pressures of the gases in solution in the tissues come into equilibrium with the partial pressures of the gases being breathed. At this point the man is said to be saturated for that particular pressure. Because saturation of the various tissues takes place in an exponential manner but at different rates it is conventional to describe the tissue response by means of tissue half times.

If he goes to a higher pressure (or deeper in the sea) he will take into solution yet more gas and if he goes to a lower pressure (less deep in the sea) or returns to atmospheric pressure his tissues will be temporarily supersaturated with respect to the ambient pressure, and will remain in this state until the body has had time to clear the excess gas from the tissues via the circulation and lungs. Supersaturation of the tissues with oxyegn is not usually of great importance since oxygen is being continually used by the body and so can be readily disposed of. Nitrogen on the other hand is not involved in the body metabolism. If the supersaturation of the tissues with nitrogen exceeds some critical value (usually expressed as a ratio of tissue pressure to ambient pressure) there is the possibility that bubbles will arise either in the tissues or in the circulation or in both, and give rise to the signs and symptoms of decompression sickness. At least that is the classical story that we are told!

For years the direct evidence that such bubbles occur in man during too fast a decompression came mainly from postmortem dissections. Unfortunately when bubbles were seen in such circumstances it was never clear whether they had been introduced into the body through cut surfaces or not. Scepticism of the bubble explanation became so great that research workers began to seek for other mechanisms to account for the decompression sickness. Then in the later 1960s several centres reported the use of ultrasonic devices to detect bubbles in the intact man (Evans, 1975). Using such devices it seemed that not only do bubbles arise during a decompression which results in decompression sickness but they are also often present during a decompression which appears to be uneventful and is therefore thought to be safe (Evans, Barnard and Walder, 1972).

The symptoms of acute decompression sickness become evident either during a decompression or within an hour or two of its completion. For convenience we have come to think of decompression sickness as consisting of two types.

In type I, usually called 'the bends' the man suffers from pain in a limb usually in the region of a major joint. The pain may be so severe that the sufferer urgently seeks treatment, or it may be mild (the 'niggles'), when he may be tempted to 'ride it out'. This latter practice should be discouraged. In type I decompression sickness there is no constitutional upset. The man looks and feels perfectly well—it is just that he has an unpleasant pain. Treatment is by recompression.

Type II decompression sickness on the other hand must be taken much more seriously. This condition may involve (1) the central nervous system, producing paraesthesia and paraplegia, and visual scotomata may also occur; (2) the respiratory system, when the man looks blue, may have an irritating cough and has respiratory embarrassment (sometimes known as 'the chokes'), and (3) the cardiovascular system when the man may have all the signs and symptoms of an acute coronary artery occlusion. In type II decompression sickness there is nearly always a constitutional upset. The man looks and feels ill. He may be permanently disabled or even die unless treated quickly and correctly by recompression.

As type II attacks have been reported following exposure to absolute pressures as low as 1.4 bar (4 m water) this is clearly a potential hazard for those who work in hyperbaric operating chambers.

Acclimatisation

A man's susceptibility to decompression sickness is greatest when he starts subjecting himself to pressure. If he dives or exposes himself to pressure regularly, that is daily or every other day for a period of time, his susceptibility to decompression sickness gradually falls until it reaches a minimum. If he then stops this type of work for a while his susceptibility will increase again so that when he restarts he will again have to acclimatise (Walder, 1966a). Acclimatisation to work at one pressure does not necessarily acclimatise a man to work at another pressure.

High pressure nervous syndrome

It has been found that when descending to depths beyond 50 m on helium–oxygen mixtures it is at first possible to descend at a rate of 30 m/min but as the depth increases such a rate of descent results in what is known as the high pressure nervous syndrome or HPNS (Fructus et al, 1969). In this the subject develops tremors of the limbs which can become so gross that function and particularly fine manipulative activities are seriously interfered with. To avoid the onset of this condition it is necessary to descend slowly so that several hours may be required to reach a depth of 200 m in a fit state to start work on arrival. HPNS must clearly be considered when planning surgery at greatly increased pressures (see later).

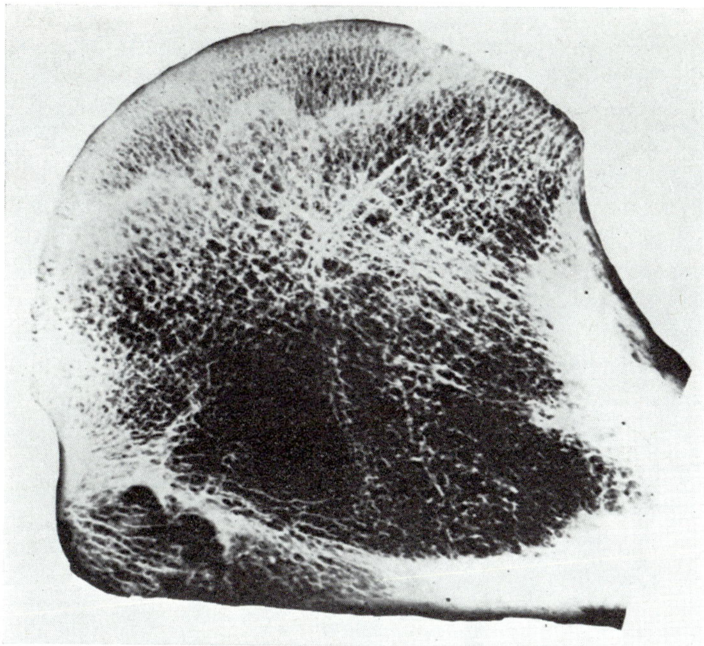

Figure 9.3A   A slab radiograph of a humeral head. The contour of the head is well preserved but a dense line can be seen crossing the head. This is an A_3 lesion

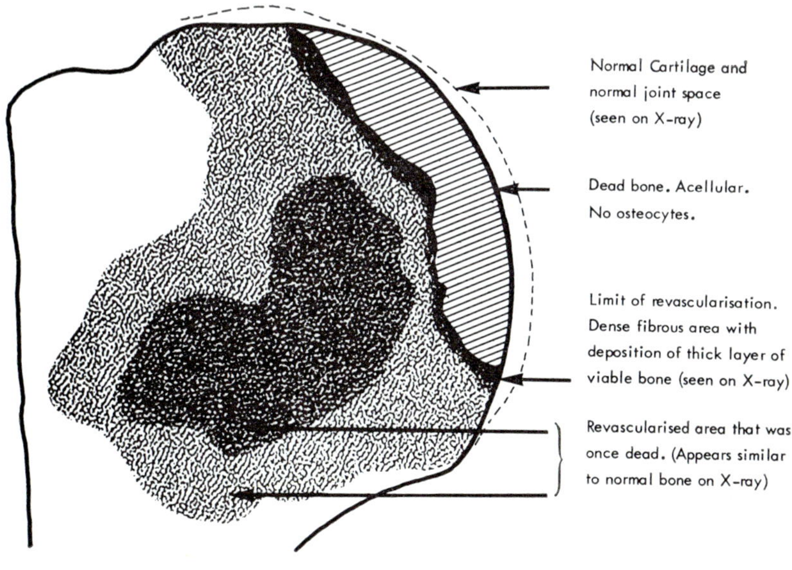

Figure 9.3B   A diagram illustrating the full extent of the lesion as revealed by histology (adapted from McCallum and Walder, 1966, *Journal of Bone and Joint Surgery*, **48B**, 207–235)

Aseptic bone necrosis

An insidious and potentially serious chronic complication of exposure to pressure is aseptic necrosis of bone (also known as caisson disease of bone and dysbaric osteonecrosis). Although this condition can be detected on radiographic examination it is not until at least four to five months after the causal incident that the signs begin to appear. The reason for the delay is that a considerable structural change has to take place in bone before anything abnormal can be seen on a radiograph. It is now thought that the changes which are seen represent the end result of the attempts by the body to repair the area of bone which was infarcted and therefore only indicate the tip of an iceberg (Fig. 9.3). It is suggested that the infarcting agent is a gas bubble, though other suggestions have been made, for example that it is a fat globule (Jones and Sakovich, 1966) or some denatured blood constituent (Philp,

Table 9.1   Radiological classification of bone necrosis in divers and compressed air workers

(A)   Juxta-articular lesions
1.   Dense areas, with intact articular cortex
2.   Spherical segmental opacities
3.   Linear opacity
4.   Structural failures
(i) Translucent subcortical band
(ii) Collapse of articular cortex
(iii) Sequestration of cortex
5.   Osteoarthritis
(B)   Head, neck and shaft lesions
1.   Dense areas
2.   Irregular calcified areas
3.   Translucent areas

Inwood and Warren, 1972). Another mechanism suggested for the aetiology of bone lesions in hyperbaric workers is that osmotically induced fluid shifts (Hills, 1972) occurring during the compression/decompression cycles result in the precipitation of bone salts in the Haversian canals, to narrow blood vessel passages and cause ischaemia.

The sites mainly affected by aseptic bone necrosis as a result of hyperbaric exposure are the shafts of the femur, tibia and humerus and the juxta-articular regions of the head of the humerus and the head of the femur.

A piece of dead bone in the centre of a shaft of a long bone may be of little significance, but if there is an area of dead bone beneath an articular surface the day-to-day trauma and forces that have to be withstood by the joint may result in collapse of the articular surface and the development of pain, limitation of movement and secondary osteoarthritis. A classification of the bone lesions which can occur is given in Table 9.1.

There is in Newcastle upon Tyne an MRC Decompression Sickness Central Registry where the radiological records of compressed air workers and divers are kept for study in connection with a research programme into the cause and prevention of this condition. An attempt is being made to keep a constant watch on North Sea divers by annual radiological checks in order to identify those with damaged bones as early as possible. Once a lesion has been identified it is difficult to know what is the best management. In those cases where the juxta-articular lesion has led to the collapse of the humeral or femoral head (there have been no such cases in North Sea divers so far but there have been many such cases in compressed air workers) little has been successful other than total joint replacement. Understandably there has been reluctance to adopt this line of treament in men who are usually only in their mid-twenties or thirties.

Much effort is at present being exerted to develop a technique of early diagnosis of these lesions—earlier that is than radiography will allow—in the hope that it may be possible to bring about full repair if the treatment of the condition is started early enough. Although radioisotope scanning could be helpful it has limitations as a screening procedure (Cox and Walder, in press). Studies of the urinary excretion of hydroxyproline as an early indicator of bone damage are at present underway.

Fortunately aseptic necrosis of bone does not seem to have occurred in hyperbaric oxygen therapy chamber personnel (Ledingham and Davidson, 1969) probably due to the limited duration of exposures allowed and the strict control of the decompression procedures.

CLINICAL APPLICATION OF HYPERBARIC OXYGEN

The treatment of decompression sickness must be primarily by recompression. The fact that such therapy almost invariably brings about relief of the symptoms is strong evidence that bubbles are involved in its aetiology since what else would be so pressure sensitive. Until recent years the recommended regimen was to return the subject to working pressure or even a little higher and then to commence a long slow so-called therapeutic decompression which, hopefully, would allow the excess gases in the body to be dispelled without further bubble formation or growth. With increasingly deep dives, going back to the working pressure and then starting a slow decompression could result in significantly more gas being taken into solution by the diver and an even slower decompression being required. Following the suggestion of Behnke and Shaw (1937) the use of oxygen at pressure in the treatment of decompression sickness became established. Using pure oxygen for the breathing gas results in the creation of the maximum possible pressure differential between the excess inert gas (nitrogen or helium) in the patient's tissues and the alveolae, so that the inert gas will diffuse out as fast as possible. Oxygen treatments are limited in depth and time of breathing oxygen and are shorter than the conventional type of decompression (RN Diving Manual,

1972). To treat a patient who does not respond to oxygen therapy requires the expertise of a specialist in underwater medicine.

For some years now Cockett has been drawing attention to the haemoconcentration which occurs in decompression sickness and advocating the use of plasma expanders as well as recompression in its treatment. He also advocates the use of heparin and has even been so bold as to suggest that decompression sickness can be successfully treated without recompression by the use of heparin alone in selected cases (Cockett et al, 1971). Although admitting that there is good evidence that such measures are excellent and in some cases essential, in the author's opinion it is not yet justifiable to withhold pressure as a component of the treatment if a chamber is available.

Only a very few of the clinical applications suggested for hyperbaric oxygen therapy have withstood critical appraisal of the objective investigator. In spite of this it is still used in situations where the evidence for its value is unproven.

Boerema's original purpose in establishing a hyperbaric chamber in Amsterdam to increase the time for elective cardiac arrest turned out to be a disappointment because the extra time was insignificant even when hyperbaric oxygen therapy was combined with hypothermia. Bernhard et al (1966) in Boston, also put this idea into effect and reported favourably on its value when operating on children with cyanotic congenital heart disease. It was later established however that many other factors had been at work and in any case there were no control subjects for this study.

From the surgical point of view the most important application is in the treatment of anaerobic bacterial infections. On theoretical grounds it is clear that every anaerobic infection should be inhibited in an environment of high oxygen tension. This is true only if the oxygen can gain access to the bacteria or its toxin, and organisms located deep in avascular tissue are not affected by changes in the tension of oxygen in the ambient atmosphere.

In practice it is claimed that *Clostridium welchii* infections respond dramatically to hyperbaric oxygen therapy (Boerema and Groeneveld, 1970). There are possibly three reasons for this. First, the toxin is very sensitive to oxygen and is rapidly destroyed in its presence; second, high tissue oxygen tensions inhibit the rate of growth of the organism although they do not kill it, and third, the raised ambient pressure reduces the muscle fascia stripping effects so that spread of the infection is reduced. Unfortunately even in the case of gas gangrene infections most of the evidence is anecdotal albeit well documented. There can be no doubt however that a combination of surgical intervention, the use of antibiotics and oxygen therapy is a successful combination for the treatment of gas gangrene.

The treatment of the other major anaerobic infection, tetanus, by the addition of hyperbaric oxygen to the treatment regimen has not met with such success.

As far as aerobic infections are concerned it would appear that no generalisations can be made because whilst at one partial pressure of oxygen the in vivo rate of growth of one organism might be inhibited, at another it might be enhanced.

Micro air embolism

A condition indistinguishable from type II decompression sickness can also occur in man as a result of accidental gas trapping in the lungs (Fig. 9.4) during a reduction in ambient pressure (Walder, 1964). The trapped gas expands to create shearing forces in the lung which lead to rupture and passage of air from the lung into the circulation. Hyperbaric therapy is essen-

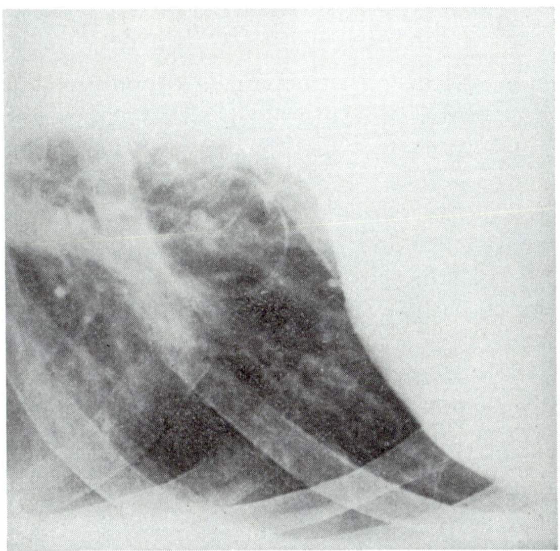

Figure 9.4   Postdecompression radiography of a man who suffered from symptoms indistinguishable from type II decompression sickness after only a brief exposure to pressure. A lung cyst due to air trapping can be seen

tial and should not be withheld on the grounds that the patient has not been exposed to a 'significant' pressure or has not been at pressure for a 'significant' length of time. Serious cases have resulted from a few moments exposure to an absolute pressure of less than 2 bar.

There is also a place for hyperbaric therapy in the treatment of accidental air embolus. As with decompression sickness, a dramatic improvement can be achieved in a patient with an air embolism by exposing him to raised pressure and giving oxygen to breathe. Satisfactory oxygen treatment regimes are those advocated by the British Navy for the management of decompression sickness.

It has often been suggested that hyperbaric oxygen therapy has a part to play in the treatment of shock. Cowley et al (1965) claimed a better survival rate in dogs with haemorrhagic shock and in rats with traumatic shock treated by hyperbaric oxygen, but they found that bacteraemic shock in dogs was not influenced by hyperbaric oxygen therapy. There are few if any clinical reports of the use of hyperbaric oxygen therapy in shock.

Much effort has gone into investigating the role of hyperbaric oxygen in wound healing. It appears doubtful whether it makes any difference to the rate of healing, but there is good evidence that it enhances the speed of epidermal regeneration (Winter and Perrins, 1970). It also prolongs the survival of split skin grafts (Perrins, 1970) but there is considerable doubt as to its effect on blue skin flaps. It seems to have a small effect on the rate of healing of burns though the evidence is tenuous (Grossman and Yanda, 1973).

At one time it appeared that hyperbaric oxygen therapy might be of value in reducing cerebral oedema but it subsequently transpired that the effect was secondary to the cerebral vasoconstriction which it brought about (Miller and Ledingham, 1970) so that the apparent benefit was secondary to an undesirable effect.

Beneficial effects on the ischaemic lesion of peripheral vascular disease have been claimed (Schraibman and Ledingham, 1970) but objective evidence is hard to come by. Much has also been claimed for hyperbaric oxygen therapy in the treatment of chronic osteomyelitis but here again the results are difficult to evaluate (Bingham et al, 1973).

Many more purely medical applications for hyperbaric therapy have also been advocated at various times but these too are of doubtful value. For example, its effect in acute myocardial infarction still remains equivocal in spite of trials in which attempts were made to include controls (Thurston and Greenwood, 1973).

Another major area in which the value of hyperbaric oxygen therapy has been claimed to be of value is that of radiation therapy for cancer. In fact one of the pioneers of this form of therapy was Churchill-Davidson in London, whose first papers on the subject were published in 1955 and 1957, well before the surgical interest created by Boerema and Illingworth. Unfortunately, again, the evidence has never been sufficient to silence the sceptics.

Ear problems

It is well known to hyperbaric chamber personnel, caisson workers and divers that inability or failure to open the Eustachian tubes when the ambient pressure is changing will prevent the middle ear from equalising its pressure with the ambient pressure and result in pain in the ear. If the increase in the ambient pressure is allow to continue, the drum will be forced inwards and will eventually burst. Similarly, failure to vent the middle ear during a reduction in ambient pressure may also result in a burst drum.

Other sites where pain is generated if pressure differentials are allowed to develop are in the sinuses and behind faulty tooth fillings.

It is not so well recognised that inner ear disturbances can also occur in association with the middle ear damage (Edmonds, 1973). This may be followed by partial or even total sensorineural hearing loss. Not only is the cochlea involved but also the vestibular apparatus since a few cases present with rotational vertigo and most cases show vestibular dysfunction when tested by electronystagmography. It is now recognised that both cochlear and vestibular disturbances are basically the result of the development of a fistula of the round window. The importance of appreciating this is that the condition is treatable and not only can further deterioration be prevented but sometimes improvement brought about. The treatment consists of sealing the fistula.

The postulated mechanism is as follows. Most of the cases occur during the compression phase with the subject having difficulty in equalising the middle ear pressures through the Eustachian tube (Freeman and Edmonds, 1972). The middle ear space contracts in accordance with Boyle's law and the movable membranes bulge into the middle ear. There are associated mucosal haemorrhages and congestion. Under these conditions, the subject may perform an over-zealous Valsalva manoeuvre in an attempt to inflate the middle ear and relieve the pain associated with the 'ear squeeze'. The Valsalva manoeuvre involves a considerable rise in intrathoracic and CSF pressure. The latter is transmitted to the perilymph of the ear via a patent cochlear aqueduct or the internal auditory meatus (Goodhill, 1971). The rise in the perilymph pressure is transmitted through the compartmented membranous labyrinth and to the oval and round windows. The round window is unsupported, microscopically thin and already stretched into the middle ear. It receives an added pressure wave transmitted via the CSF from the Valsalva manoeuvre and ruptures.

Postdecompression precautions

Since the risk of decompression sickness is maximal at the end of decompression and takes some hours to subside it is normal to advise subjects who have recently been exposed to hyperbaric conditions to remain near a recompression chamber for a period which is related to the severity (i.e. pressure and duration) of their hyperbaric exposure. It is also inadvisable to fly in aircraft or indeed rapidly ascend mountains, as by cable car, soon after an exposure to pressure as this can provoke an attack of decompression sickness.

Fire precaution in pressure chambers

Wherever an oxygen-enriched atmosphere is used and that includes a chamber pressurised with air, the strictest precautions are essential to avoid fire. Ignition sources must be eliminated and as far as possible inflammable materials excluded from the chamber. Although an automatic fire fighting system may be fitted, fires develop so rapidly under hyperbaric conditions that such systems cannot be totally relied upon. Prevention is the key.

THE MANAGEMENT OF SERIOUS INJURIES AND ACUTE SURGICAL EMERGENCIES IN DIVERS

Little is known about the effect of damaged tissue on decompression time but almost certainly an ill or injured diver in the middle of a 10 day saturation dive at 200 m from an oil rig in the North Sea will require even longer than normal before he can be brought safely out of the pressure chamber. As has been explained this could mean a delay of several days. Careful consideration must therefore be given to the way in which an ill or injured diver should be managed. Hopefully it may be possible after careful assessment to treat the diver conservatively and delay operative measures. Before accepting this line of action however it will almost certainly require that a doctor or surgeon enters into the pressure chamber to make a detailed assessment of the patient's condition. If treatment is to include intravenous fluid replacement and naso-gastric suction, for example, the doctor will probably have to stay with the patient to supervise this therapy during the subsequent decompression.

In the case of a severe avulsion injury when prompt operative measures may be unavoidable there would be two possibilities.

The first would be to arrange to operate in the deck compression chamber on the oil rig. The disadvantages are obvious—space would be very limited, there would be a long distance from the base hospital, sterility would be difficult to establish and maintain, light would be poor and finally but most important from the economic point of view, all work on the rig might have to stop until the deck compression chamber could be freed again to allow the normal diving programme to go ahead. The second would be to transfer the patient under pressure from the deck chamber in a portable pressure chamber capable of carrying both the patient and a doctor or other medical attendant by ship or helicopter to a land-based large hyperbaric operating theatre situated near a major hospital. There the patient would again be transferred under pressure, this time from the portable chamber to a pressurised operating theatre chamber. The emergency surgery could then be carried out under first-rate conditions. Finally after the operation the necessary decompression could be carried out and the patient eventually transferred to an ordinary ward for convalescence at lesiure. Such a system would be expensive both to set up and to maintain but the economic advantages of such a scheme in allowing the decompression chamber complex on the oil rig to resume its normal function would easily compensate for this.

To be of universal use the portable pressure chamber with all its ancillary life support system would have to be designed so that it could connect on to all known deck compression chambers operating in the North Sea as well as to one or more 'mother' operating chambers ashore. Such equipment would be heavy (up to 10000 kg) and the distances to be transported great—perhaps 500 km round trip. Special rescue ships or helicopters would have to be provided and made available 24 h a day.

Whatever method is adopted to manage these problems, doctors and surgeons who are willing and physically fit to go into the pressure environment to assess and deal with the ill and injured divers must be available. A form of medical examination for fitness to dive in the North Sea has been established and a rigorous standard is set. The medical personnel will have to meet these requirements for fitness. As has already been mentioned, acclimatisation is an important factor in ensuring rapid and safe excursions to pressure so that those intending to do this sort of work will have to arrange to keep in training by carrying out regular practice exposures to pressure. This in itself will be very time consuming, added to which each emergency could entail an unscheduled absence away from normal work for several days at a time. Travelling time apart, to get to 200 m pressure equivalent could take several hours—transfer under pressure from oil rig to mother chamber could take another 6 h. This would then be followed by the operating period, and finally decompression of the patient, doctors and assistants which might take another three to four days.

It all seems rather futuristic but although such a scheme will probably only be called into action once in many months the alternative is so bleak (that is to abandon the diver to conservative treatment) that in the author's opinion the services suggested will have to be provided on humanitarian grounds, if on no other.

REFERENCES

American Medical Association Bureau of Investigation (1928) The Cunningham 'tank treatment'. The alleged value of compressed air in the treatment of diabetes mellitus, pernicious anaemia and carcinoma. *Journal of American Medical Association*, **90**, 1494–1496.

Behnke, A. R. & Shaw, L. A. (1937) The use of oxygen in the treatment of compressed air illness. *U.S. Navy Medical Bulletin*, **35**, 61–73.

Bernhard, W. F., Norman, J. C., Ishizuka, R. & Carr, J. G. (1966) Evaluation of hyperbaric surgery in infarcts with congenital cardiac defects. In *Proceedings of the 3rd International Congress on Hyperbaric Medicine*, ed Brown, I. W. & Cox, B. G., pp. 345–351. Washington: National Academy of Sciences.

Bert, P. (1878) *La Pression Barometrique*. Paris: Masson.

Bingham, E. L., Mullen, J. E., Winans, R. C. & Hart, G. B. (1973) The treatment of refractory osteomyelitis with hyperbaric oxygen: a progress report. In *Proceedings of the 5th International Hyperbaric Congress*, ed. Trapp, W. G., Banister, E. W., Davison, A. J. & Trapp, P. A., pp. 264–269. Burnaby: Simon Fraser University.

Boerema, I., Knoll, J. A., Meyne, N. G., Lokin, E., Kroon, E. & Huiskes, J. W. (1956) High atmospheric pressure as an aid to cardiac surgery. *Archivum chirurgicum Neerlandicum*, *Arnhem*, **8**, 193–211.

Boerema, I. (1961) An operating room with high atmospheric pressure. *Surgery*, **49**, 291–298.

Boerema, I. & Groeneveld, P. H. A. (1970) Gas gangrene treated with hyperbaric oxygenation. In *Proceedings of the 4th International Congress on Hyperbaric Medicine*, ed. Wada, J. & Iwa, T., pp. 255–262. London: Baillière, Tindall & Cassell.

Bornstein, A. & Plate, E. (1911) Uber chronische gelenkveranderungen, entstanden durch presslufterkrankung. *Fortschritte auf dem gebiete der Röntgenstrahlen*, **18**, 197–206.

Bouhy, M. (1847) Rapport sur l'explosion d'un cylindre à air comprimé sur l'avaleresse No. 7, située dans la concession de Douchy (Nord). *Annales des mines*, Fourth series, **2**, 121–148.

Churchill-Davidson, I., Sanger, C. & Thomlinson, R. H. (1955) High pressure oxygen and radiotherapy. *Lancet*, **1**, 1091–1095.

Churchill-Davidson, I., Sanger, C. & Thomlinson, R. H. (1957) Oxygenation in radiotherapy. II. Clinical applications. *British Journal of Radiology*, **30**, 406–422.

Cockett, A. T. K., Pauley, S. M., Saunders, J. C. & Hirose, F. M. (1971) Coexistence of lipid and gas emboli in experimental decompression sickness. In *Proceedings of the 4th Symposium on Underwater Physiology*, ed. Lambertson, C. J., pp. 245–250. New York: Academic Press.

Cowley, R. A., Attar, S., Blair, E., Esmond, W. G., Michaelis, M. & Ollodart, R. (1965) Prevention and treatment of shock by hyperbaric oxygenation. In *Hyperbaric Oxygenation*, ed. Whipple, H. E., pp. 673–683. New York: Academy of Sciences.

Cox, P. T. & Walder, D. N. (1976) Strontium scanning in caisson disease of bone. In *Proceedings of the 5th Symposium on Underwater Physiology and Medicine*, ed. Lambertson, C. Bethesda, Maryland.

Cunningham, O. J. (1927) Oxygen therapy by means of compressed air. *Anesthesia and Analgesia*, **6**, 64–66.

Decompression Sickness Panel (Medical Research Council) (1966) Bone lesions in compressed air workers. *Journal of Bone and Joint Surgery*, **48B**, 207–235.

Edmonds, C. (1973) Inner ear barotrauma. In *Proceedings of the 5th International Hyperbaric Congress*, ed. Trapp, W. G., Banister, E. W., Davison, A. J. & Trapp, P. A., pp. 874–882. Burnaby: Simon Fraser University.

Evans, A., Barnard, E. E. P. & Walder, D. N. (1972) Detection of gas bubbles in man at decompression. *Aerospace Medicine*, **43**, 1095–1096.

Evans, A. (1975) Ultrasonic surveillance of decompression. In *The Physiology and Medicine of Divers and Compressed Air Workers*, ed. Bennett, P. B. & Elliott, D. H., Ch. 22. London: Baillière & Tindall.

Fontaine, J. A. (1879) Emploi chirurgical de l'air comprimé. *L'Union Médicale* **28** (3), 445–448.

Freeman, P. & Edmonds, C. (1972) Inner ear barotrauma. *Archives of Otolaryngology*, **95**, 556–563.

Fructus, X., Naquet, R., Gosset, A., Fructus, P. & Brauer, R. W. (1969) Le syndrome nerveux des haut pressions. *Marseille Medicine*, **106**, 509–512.

Gilder, H. & McSherry, C. K. (1974) Pulmonary surfactant synthesis, the effect of high oxygen tensions. In *Proceedings of the 5th International Hyperbaric Congress*, ed. Trapp, W. G., Banister, E. W., Davison, A. J. & Trapp, P. A., pp. 73–83. Burnaby: Simon Fraser University.

Goodhill, V. (1971) Sudden deafness and round window rupture. *Laryngoscope*, **81**, 1462–1474.

Gowdey, C. W. (1966) A second look at hyperbaric oxygenation. *Modern Medicine*, **11**, 949–973.

Grossman, A. R. & Yanda, R. L. (1973) The hyperbaric oxygen treatment of burns. In *Proceedings of the 5th International Hyperbaric Congress*, ed. Trapp, W. G., Banister, E. W., Davison, A. J. & Trapp, P. A., pp. 300–303. Burnaby: Simon Fraser University.

Grutzmacher, K. T. (1941) Veranderungen am schultergelenk als folge von druckluftcrkrankung. *Röntgen-Praxis*, **13**, 216–218.

Haldane, J. S. (1895) The relation of the action of carbonic oxide to oxygen tension. *Journal of Physiology*, **18**, 201–217.

Harrison, J. A. B. (1971) Aseptic bone necrosis in Naval clearance divers. Radiographic findings. *Proceedings of the Royal Society of Medicine*, **64**, 1276–1278.

Henshaw. (1857) In *Compressed Air as a Therapeutic Agent in the Treatment of Consumption, Asthma, Chronic Bronchitis and Other Diseases*, ed. Simpson, A. Edinburgh: Sutherland & Knox.

Hills, B. A. (1972) Clinical implications of gas induced osmosis. *Archives of Internal Medicine*, **129**, 356–362.

Illingworth, C. F. W., Smith, G., Lawson, D. D., Ledingham, I. McA., Sharp, G. R. & Griffiths, J. C. (1961) Surgical and physiological observations in an experimental pressure chamber. *British Journal of Surgery*, **49**, 222–227.

Jones, J. P. & Sakovich, L. (1966) Fat embolism of bone. *Journal of Bone and Joint Surgery*, **48A**, 149–164.

Junod, V. T. (1834) Recherches physiologiques et thérapeutiques sur les effects de la compression et de la raréfaction de l'air, tant sur le corps et sur les membres isolés. *Review Medicale France Etrange*, **3,** 350–368.

Kindwall, E. P. (1970) *Hyperbaric Medicine Procedures.* Milwaukee: St Luke's Hospital.

Ledingham, I. McA. & Davidson, J. D. (1969) Hazards in hyperbaric medicine. *British Medical Journal*, **2,** 324–327.

Miller, J. D. & Ledingham, I. McA. (1970) The effect of hyperbaric oxygen on intracranial pressure in experimental cerebral oedema. In *Proceedings of the 4th International Congress on Hyperbaric Medicine*, ed. Wada, J. & Iwa, T., pp. 453–455. London: Baillière, Tindall & Cassell.

Perrins, D. J. D. (1970) The influnece of hyperbaric oxygen on the survival of split skin grafts. *Proceedings of the 4th International Congress on Hyperbaric Medicine*, ed. Wada, J. & Iwa, T., pp. 369–376. London: Baillière, Tindall & Cassell.

Philp, R. B., Inwood, M. J. & Warren, B. A. (1972) Interactions between gas bubbles and components of the blood: implications in decompression sickness. *Aerospace Medicine*, **43,** 946–953.

Pol, B. & Wattelle, T. J. J. (1854) Mémoire sur les effects de la compression de l'air appliquée au creusement des puits à houille. *Annales d'hygiène publique et de médecine légale (industrille et sociale)*, **1** (2), 241–279.

Pravaz, M. (1840) Mémoire dur l'emploi du bain de l'air comprimé associé à la gymnastique dans le traitment du rachitisme, des affections strumeuses et des surdités catarrhales. *L'expérience*, **5,** 177–192.

R.N. Diving Manual (1972) BR2806. London: HMSO.

Schraibman, I. G. & Ledingham, I. McA. (1970) Blood flow and oxygen consumption in the ischaemic foot. The effect of hyperbaric oxygen and regional intravenous vasodilator infusion. In *Proceedings of the 4th International Congress on Hyperbaric Medicine*, ed. Wada, J. & Iwa, T., pp. 457–459. London: Baillière, Tindall & Cassell.

Society for Underwater Technology (1976) Hyperbaric rescue in the North Sea. *Journal of the Society for Underwater Technology*, 12–17.

Statutory Instrument No. 61 (1958) *Factories. The Work in Compressed Air*, Special Regulation 1958. London: HMSO.

Statutory Instrument No. 1229 (1974) *Offshore Installations*. The Offshore Installations (Diving Operations) Regulations 1974. London: HMSO.

Thurston, J. G. B. & Greenwood, T. W. (1973) Results of a controlled trial of hyperbaric oxygen in acute myocardial infarction. In *Proceedings of the 5th International Hyperbaric Congress*, ed. Trapp, W. G., Banister, E. W., Davison, A. J. & Trapp, P. A., pp. 726–733. Burnaby: Simon Fraser University.

Triger, E. (1841) Mémoire sur un appareil à air comprimé pour le percement des puits de mines et autres travaux, sous les eaux et dans les sables submergés. *Comptes rendus aux Hébdominaire Séance du Academie de Science, Paris*, **13,** 884–896.

Trouessart, M. (1845) Rapport sur les puits à air comprimé de M. Triger. *Bulletin de la Societe industrial d'Angers et du déport de Maine-et-Loire.*

Valenzuela (1887) quoted by Gowdey, C. W. (1966) A second look at hyperbaric oxygenation. *Modern Medicine*, **11,** 949–973.

Walder, D. N. (1964) Some dangers of a hyperbaric environment. In *Proceedings of the 2nd International Congress on Hyperbaric Oxygenation*, ed. Ledingham, I. McA., pp. 5–9. London: Livingstone.

Walder, D. N. (1966a) Adaptation to decompression sickness in caisson work. In *Proceedings of the 3rd International Biometeorological Congress*, ed. Tromp, S. W. & Weihe, W. H., pp. 350–359. London: Pergamon.

Walder, D. N. (1966b) Some problems of working in an hyperbaric environment. *Annals of the Royal College of Surgeons of England*, **38,** 288–307.

Walder, D. N. (1970) Caisson disease of bone in Great Britain. In *Proceedings of the 4th International Congress on Hyperbaric Medicine*, ed. Wada, J. & Iwa, T., pp. 83–87. London: Baillière, Tindall & Cassell.

Walder, D. N. (1974) Management and treatment of osteonecrosis in divers and caisson workers. In *Proceedings of the Symposium on Dysbarism-related Osteonecrosis*, ed. Beckman, E. L. & Elliott, D. H., pp. 195–199. Washington, DC: US Government Printing Office.

Williams, C. T. (1885) The compressed air bath and its uses in the treatment of disease. *British Medical Journal*, **1**, 769–772, 824–828, 936–939.

Winter, G. D. & Perrins, D. J. D. (1970) Effects of hyperbaric oxygen treatment on epidermal regeneration. In *Proceedings of the 4th International Congress on Hyperbaric Medicine*, ed. Wada, J. & Iwa, T., pp. 363–368. London: Baillière, Tindall & Cassell.

Wood, J. D., Radomski, M. W. & Watson, W. J. (1971) A study of possible biochemical mechanisms involved in hyperbaric oxygen-induced changes in cerebral amino-butyric acid levels and accompanying seizures. *Canadian Journal of Biochemistry*, **49**, 543–547.

10
REGIONAL RENAL HYPOTHERMIA

J. E. A. Wickham

When any operative procedure on the kidney requires incision of the renal substance, the prudent surgeon has usually attempted to control the renal circulation by means of a vascular clamp placed across the whole renal pedicle.

Whole pedicle clamping is however unsatisfactory for two reasons. Firstly, the kidney remains congested with the entrapped blood which tends to ooze from the cut parenchyma and subsequently obscure the operative field, whilst secondly, and more importantly, should the vascular occlusion be prolonged, deterioration of renal cellular function quite rapidly follows. The degree of deterioration is progressive with time, and Table 10.1—constructed from an accumulation of the effect of vascular arrest on renal function in many species—gives some idea of the limitations of such prolonged occlusion.

It is obvious that short periods of vascular arrest of around 15 min are permissible and cause little ultimate functional damage to the kidney, but prolonged occlusion is dangerous. It should be noted that the studies reported above were all performed on normal kidneys, whilst in the clinical situation the organ to be treated is frequently damaged with an already diminished starting function.

For minor procedures involving parenchymal incision, therefore, it may well be satisfactory to stop the circulation for a short period of time without harm. If, however, it is intended to work on the organ for prolonged periods in a dry vascular field, then these short periods of ischaemia are quite inadequate to permit the slower and more meticulous operative technique that is required in much of present day renal surgery.

Table 10.1 Deterioration after vascular occlusion

Ischaemia time (min)	Degree of initial depression of function (%)	Time for recovery
10	Just measurable	One hour
20	40–50	One week
30	60–70	Ten days
60	70–80	Some kidneys will permanently lose function and never fully recover
120	Complete	Nearly 100% kidneys rendered functionless

To extend this permissible ischaemic period therefore some form of protection is required and of the various methods explored in the last 20 years, undoubtedly that of simple renal cooling has been the most successful.

In 1962 when I was first attracted to the idea of using some form of regional renal cooling with controlled pedicle clamping to produce a dry operative field, the optimum temperature to which to cool the kidney was not known. Regional cooling has been used clinically by several workers and had usually been achieved by packing the kidney in crushed sterile ice or surrounding it

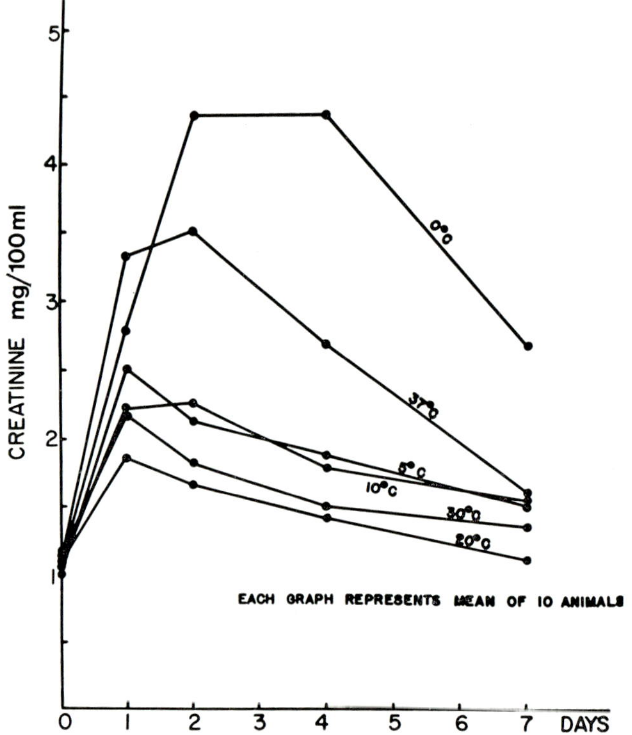

Figure 10.1   Protective effect of temperature on renal function. Serial serum creatinine measured in rabbits subjected to 45 min renal artery clamping

with plastic bags of sterile cooled saline. Both of these methods appeared somewhat crude with questionable control of renal temperature and there appeared to be two problems worthy of investigation.

1. To determine the optimum temperature to which to cool the kidney to obtain maximum protection of function.
2. To develop a simple method of achieving controlled hypothermia to the required temperature.

To answer the first question a series of experiments were therefore carried out using the rabbit kidney. In these the remaining kidney of unilaterally nephrectomised animals was subjected to a standard period of ischaemia whilst at the same time being cooled to a controlled temperature level. Groups of 10 animals each were cooled to 30, 20, 10, 5 or 0°C with a fixed ischaemia time of 45 min. Renal function was subsequently estimated by serum creatinine levels.

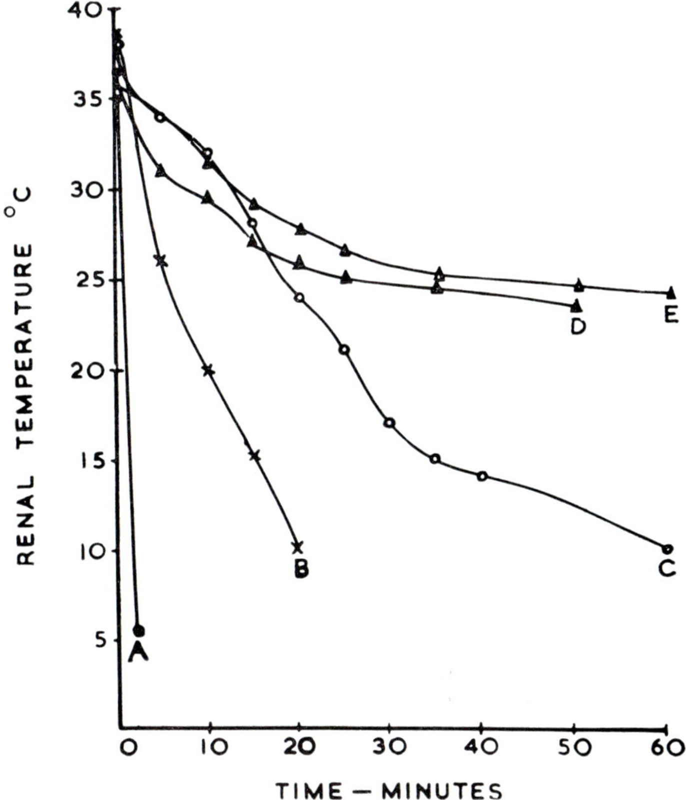

Figure 10.2 Rates of cooling—human kidney. A, cold intravascular perfusion; B, external parenchymal cooling (Markland and Parsons, 1963)

From these experiments the optimum temperature for preservation appeared to be around the 10 to 20°C level (Fig. 10.1), little further improvement in protection being obtained by using the lower temperature ranges (Wickham, Hanley and Joekes, 1967). More recent and sophisticated experiments in the dog by Ward (1975) have also confirmed a level of 15°C as being the optimum in this respect.

With cooling to the 15 to 20°C level, preservation of undisturbed renal function could be achieved for periods of up to 3 h, a time certainly sufficient for most operative procedures.

The need to achieve only a modest lowering of temperature to obtain protection was important for it allowed the use of an external parenchymal cooling method rather than any need for intra-arterial perfusion of the organ. Also Markland and Parsons (1963) had already shown that the human kidney could be externally cooled to 20°C in approximately 10 min and this appeared to be a realistic time span to use in the clinical situation (Fig. 10.2). Previous methods of ice packing, although effective, provided only poor control of temperature and were necessarily somewhat messy to use at operation.

I therefore attempted to develop a simple form of external cooling device that would be safe, cheap, simple to sterilise and easy to apply and remove from the kidney surface as well as providing good and rapid control of renal

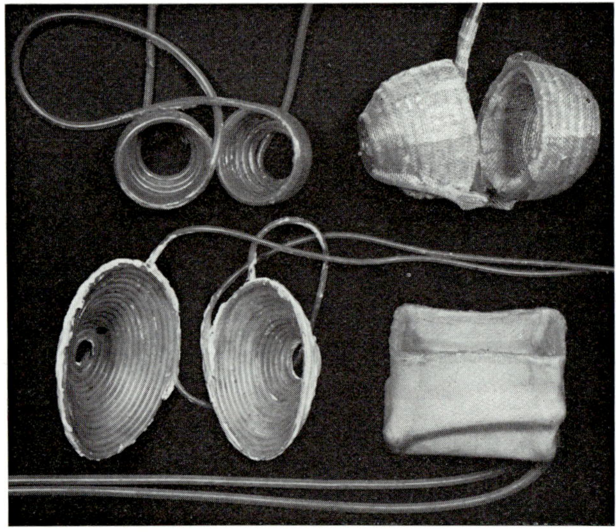

Figure 10.3   Prototype heat exchanger coils

core temperature at the desired level. Over a period of a year or so an apparatus was produced which consisted of three main parts.

1. Paired plastic heat exchange coils designed to surround the kidney so that a cooled liquid could be conveyed to and from
2. an external coolant source with circulatory pump.
3. A telethermometer probe for recording renal core temperature.

The heat exchange coils

Many configurations were tried (Fig. 10.3) culminating in the development of a pair of saucer shaped pads made from a continuous length of small bore rubber tubing (Fig. 10.4). This shape was found to fit easily into the wound to envelop the kidney satisfactorily and worked well with an ethyl alcohol/

dry ice cooling mixture. Latterly the coolant fluid was changed to water circulating in a large volume at high speed and the coil configuration was altered to achieve a better wide bore flow pattern (Fig. 10.5). This final version consists of two saucer shaped PVC cups covered on their inner surfaces with a soft plastic membrane. Coolant is led to the centre of these coils, flows over the membrane, and returns to the external source. The coils fit snugly round the kidney which sinks into the soft membrane thus maintaining a very close contact with the circulating coolant. The coils are initially prepared by gamma ray sterilisation, but may be reutilised after exposure to ethylene oxide or by soaking in Hibitane solution.

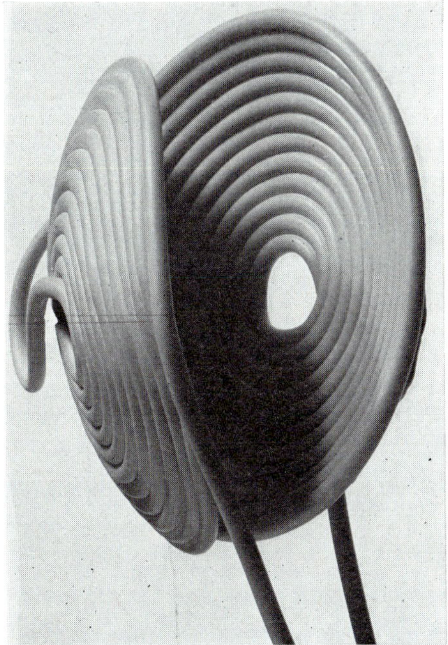

Figure 10.4   First coils used for human hypothermia

The coolant source and pump

This was initially a simple plastic container into which a dry ice/ethyl alcohol mixture was placed (Fig. 10.6). The temperature of this reservoir was very low at $-40°C$ and the coolant was circulated at slow speed by a simple Watson–Marlow roller pump. Line temperature was monitored and the pump speed regulated electronically to produce a coil surface temperature of about 2°C.

Later it was decided to use iced water instead of alcohol to offset the possible risk of super cooling both the coils and the kidney surface to below zero temperatures. Two machines were produced, one with an electrical refrigerator to cool the water and finally, in the production machine (Fig. 10.7), a return was made to a simple reservoir into which water and ice cubes or dry ice could be placed to produce a reservoir temperature of 1 to 2°C. From this reservoir water is circulated by a high speed electrical pump to the plastic coils at a volume of about 1500 ml/min to give a surface temperature at the coil of about 2 to 4°C.

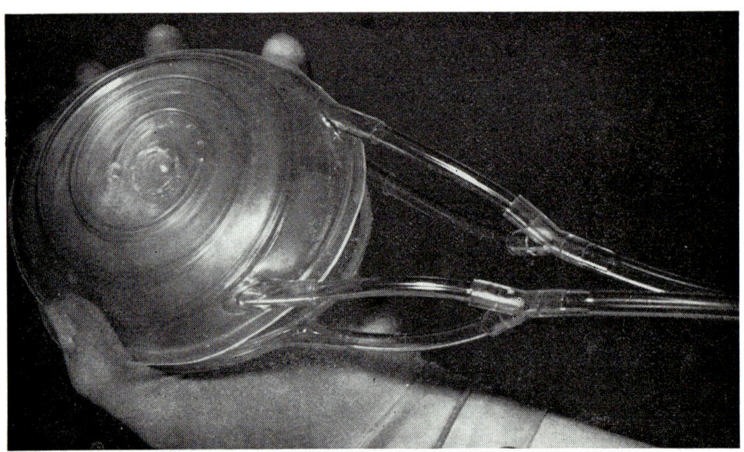

Figure 10.5   Production heat exchanger coils (Peter Steer Ltd)

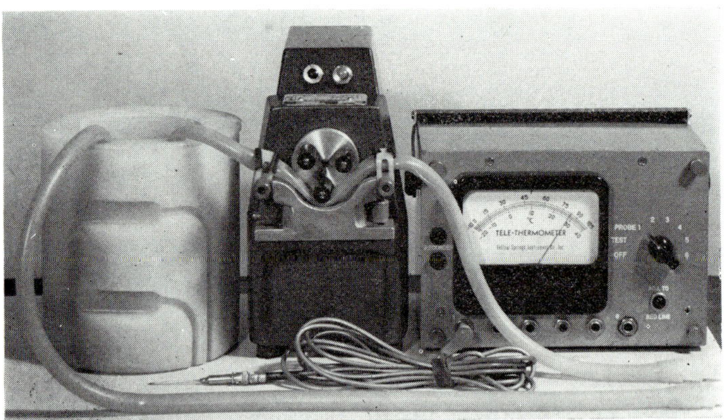

Figure 10.6   Prototype coolant system

Telethermometer

This has been a simple hypodermic needle type of thermometer with only the needle tip registering the temperature in degrees Celsius of the area of kidney into which it is inserted. In the final production model of the cooling apparatus, the telethermometer is able to record both kidney temperature and water bath temperature.

Having achieved a satisfactory and simple apparatus which worked well on the canine kidney, I first applied the technique to the clinical situation in 1965. Since that time, with the various modifications indicated, the method has been used continuously and, at the time of writing, some 300 kidneys have been operated on.

The Method and Use of the Apparatus in the Clinical Situation

When any operation on the kidney requires a period of prolonged ischaemia,

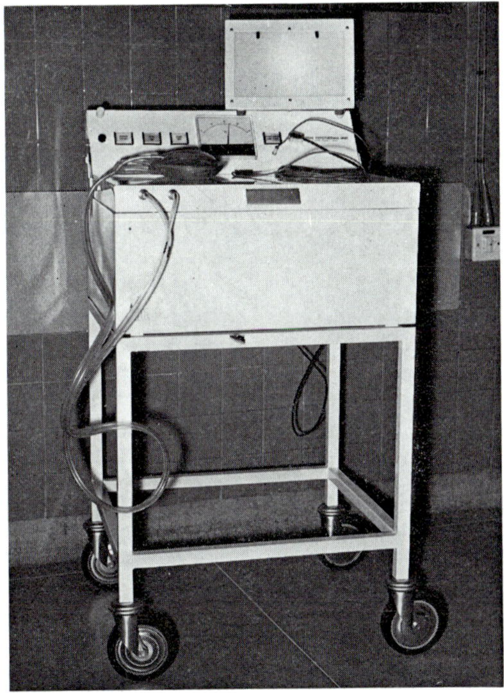

Figure 10.7   Production model regional hypothermia machine (Manor Dynamics Ltd)

such as a complicated nephrolithotomy or the local excision of a renal tumour, the procedure used is extremely simple.

The kidney is exposed through the conventional oblique loin incision or through a posterior lumbotomy. The wound margins are usefully held open by the author's self-retaining contoured ring retractor which enables both the operator's and the assistant's hands to remain free for manipulation of the kidney itself (Fig. 10.8).

The kidney is fully mobilised and the renal pedicle dissected to expose the renal artery clearly and any ancillary arterial vessels supplying the kidney. It is most important for the achievement of successful hypothermic protection that all vascular inflow to the organ is arrested before cooling commences. If even a small polar artery to the organ is left uncontrolled, the trivial amount of warm blood conveyed to the kidney may be sufficient to preclude the achievement of an adequately lowered core temperature. Failure to appreciate this point is perhaps the major reason why some workers have found difficulty with the technique and have not obtained satisfactory renal cooling.

At this stage in the procedure we have found it convenient to enclose the kidney in a small elastic net sling (Fig. 10.8). This is available commercially as 'Net-E-Last' size B (Roussell). The Net-E-Last is secured to the kidney by a purse string tape around its lower margin and when in place allows the

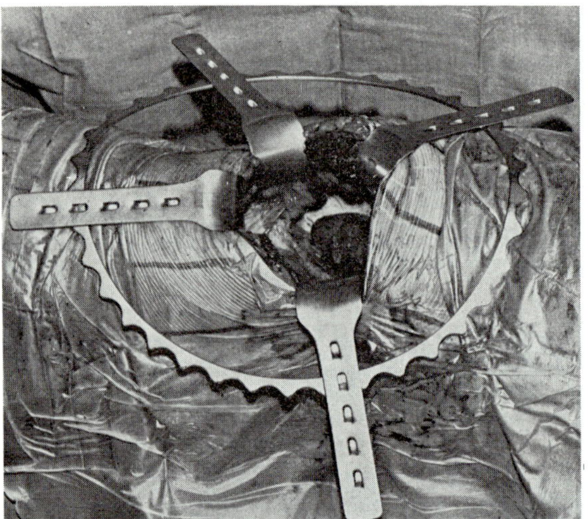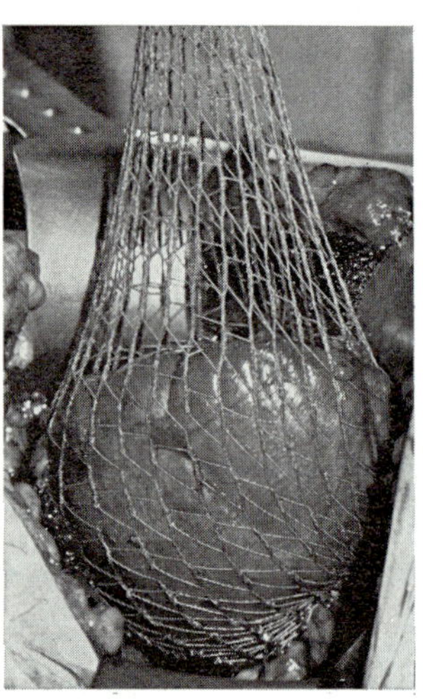

Figure 10.8   Ring retractor and Net-E-Last sling

assistant to stabilise the organ so that the operator can work with both hands unencumbered.

The renal artery or arteries only are then occluded with small bulldog clamps and the two halves of the heat exchanger coils placed on either side of the organ and gently compressed together so that the kidney sinks into the plastic membrane on the inner side of the coils (Fig. 10.9). Circulation of the ice water coolant is then started and the telethermometer probe inserted into a suitable medullary area of the kidney. Cooling is continued until the core temperature of the organ has reached the 15 to 20°C level which in the normal sized kidney takes an average of about 8 to 10 min. Large solitary kidneys with a very thick parenchyma and hydro- and pyonephrotic kidneys containing considerable amounts of calculous material may require a slightly more prolonged period of cooling.

When the desired temperature has been achieved, circulation of the coolant is stopped and the coils and thermometer are removed. The kidney should now be blanched, cold to the touch, and is normally diminished in size due to extrusion of contained blood from the intrarenal vasculature.

The kidney is now immediately ready and unencumbered for the performance of any operative procedure that is required.

Rewarming occurs to about 30°C over a period of 25 to 30 min when it is advisable to replace the coils for a further period of cooling. Recooling to 15°C is then much more rapid and usually takes 4 to 5 min. A further re-application of the coils is extremely simple in contradistinction to the difficulty and messiness of achieving recooling with the ice slush method.

At the conclusion of the operative procedure, and after any necessary reconstruction of the renal parenchyma has been completed, the arterial

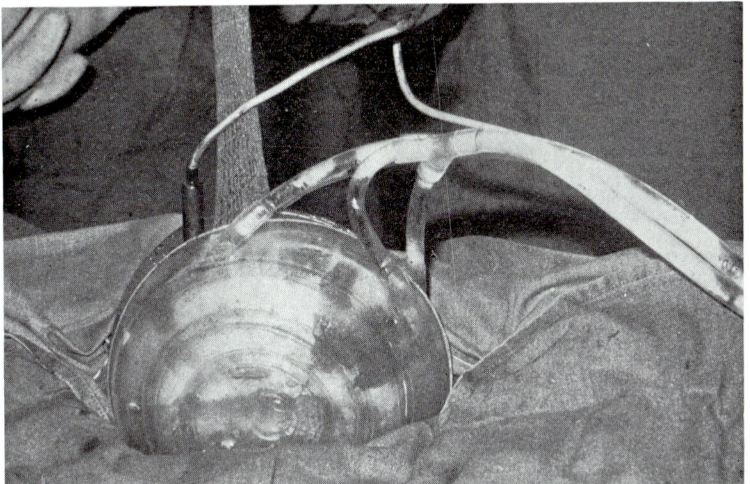

Figure 10.9   Coils in situ around the kidney

clamps are removed. The kidney normally reperfuses with arterial blood very rapidly and a normal core temperature of around 36 to 37°C is achieved within about 2 to 3 min.

Indications for the Use of Regional Renal Hypothermia

With increasing experience over the last eight years the indications for the use of this technique have become more clearly defined. There is little doubt that with the availability of this method it is now possible to perform a detailed and careful exploration of the interior of the kidney and to move into the much more rewarding area of 'intrarenal conservative' rather than purely ablative surgery.

In descending order of frequency we have used the method for

1. Removal of cast and multiple calculi from the peripheral renal collecting system.
2. Excision of renal cell carcinoma from solitary and bilaterally involved kidneys.
3. Excision of intrarenal arteriovenous malformations and aneurysms.
4. Occasionally for the correction of renal artery stenosis.

All these procedures have required prolonged renal circulatory arrest with deep incision of the renal substance. There is obviously no point in using the

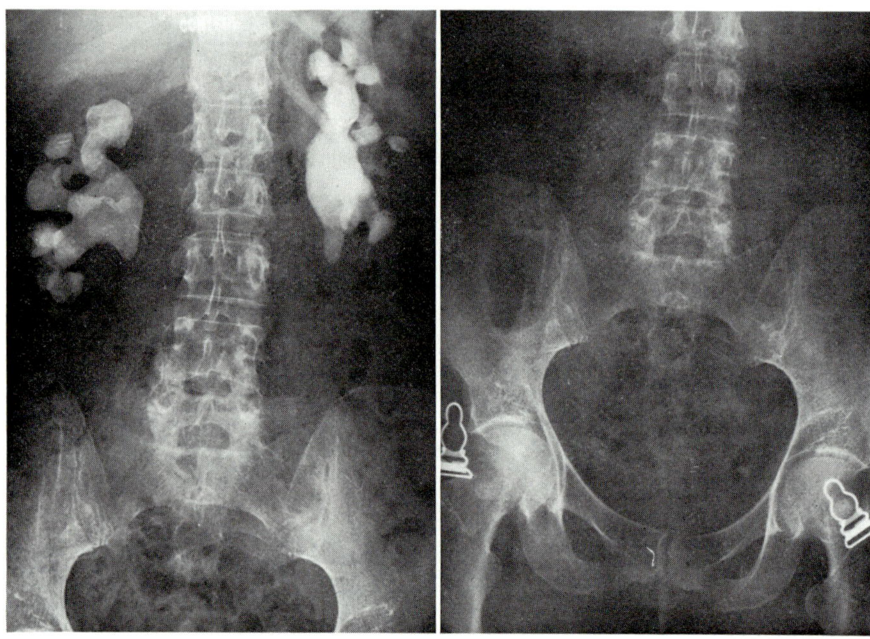

Figure 10.10   Plain x-ray of bilateral staghorn calculi of 20 years duration

Figure 10.11   Postoperative plain x-ray of patient shown in Fig. 10.10

technique when the renal substance does not need to be disturbed, for instance when a calculus needs removal from the renal pelvis or from a grossly hydronephrotic calyx. Here the conventional sinus approach is completely adequate.

Removal of cast and multiple calculi

This has been the most frequent indication for using renal cooling and we have at the time of writing experience of somewhat over 200 cases treated in this manner. The first 100 cases treated have been studied in some detail (Wickham, Coe and Ward, 1974) and a brief description of the method and the results achieved may give some indication of the usefulness of the technique.

Most of these initial 100 patients suffered from cast or multiple stones in the kidney such that complete clearance of these required incision of the parenchyma to clear the peripheral collecting system (Fig. 10.10). Many of these patients had been symptomatic for years and suffered from recurrent loin pain, fever, frequency and haematuria. The average age of the patients treated was 40 years, with a range of 16 to 67 years, whilst 15 patients had bilateral stones and bilateral operations.

Regional hyopthermia was achieved as described above and due to the clean dry field available for surgery, it was possible to achieve removal of all macroscopic fragments of calculus in 91 per cent of cases (Fig. 10.11). There were no deaths in this series and evaluation of pre- and postoperative renal function by 24 h creatinine clearance tests showed a statistically significant

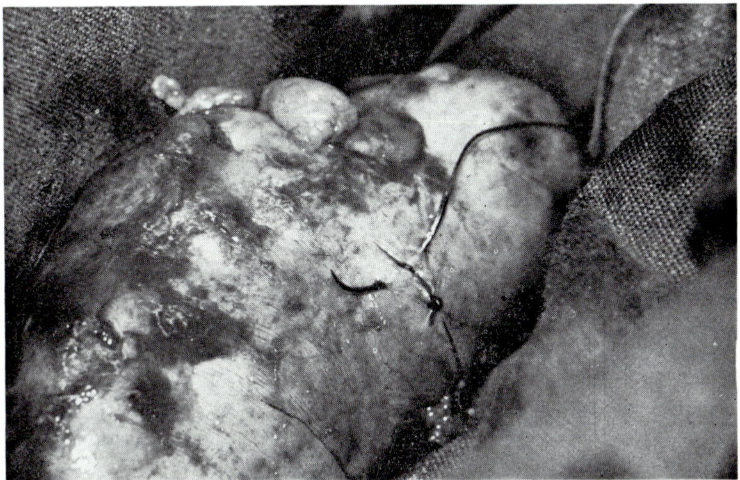

Figure 10.12   Capsular closure of nephrotomy with no need for haemostatic suturing

long-term increase in renal function over the whole series. In this 100 cases no kidney was lost. In the subsequent 100 cases, one kidney failed to function postoperatively and one was removed for secondary haemorrhage and again there was no mortality.

The sustained and even improved renal function in this series was very gratifying. In part we are sure this has been due to the ability to avoid inflicting further parenchymal damage to the kidney during the procedure. All incisions to remove peripheral calculi have been made radially in the renal substance and parallel to the natural line of the intralobar arteries; most nephrotomies being only 2 to 3 cm long. A few minutes examination of any selective renal angiogram provides convincing evidence that this is the most logical way to avoid damage to the intrarenal vessels. Due to the clear dry field it is possible to visualise directly the main intrarenal vasculature and to place the paren- chymal incision so that transection of intralobar vessels can be minimised and nephron function maximally preserved. Due, we feel to this more planned approach, there has been quite a dramatic lack of haemorrhage on declamping the renal artery despite the fact that the parenchyma after incision has been routinely closed with a fine 4 'O' chromic stitch applied to the capsule only (Fig. 10.12). There has been no indication whatever to use the grossly

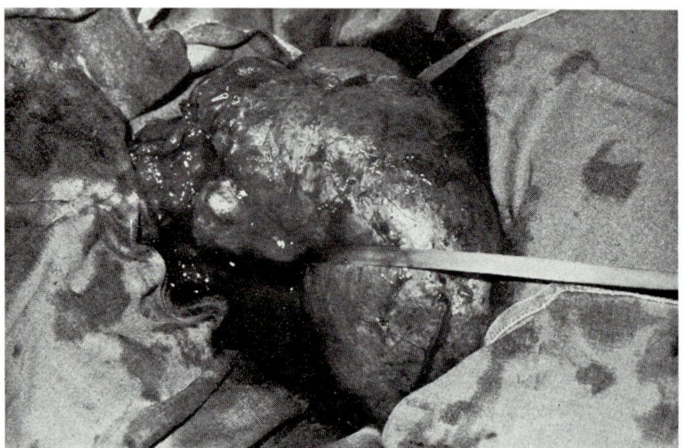

Figure 10.13   Tumour mass in solitary kidney

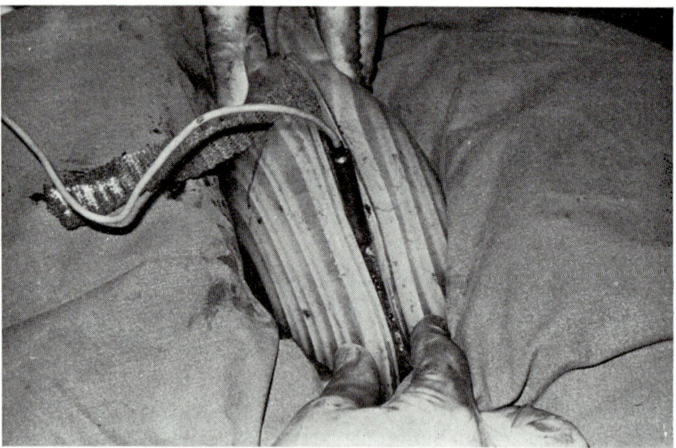

Figure 10.14   Cooling coils applied to kidney

traumatic transparenchymal mattress stitches that were previously required to achieve renal haemostasis after such crude manoeuvres as renal bivalving for stone extraction.

With careful postoperative follow-up and appropriate antibiotic treatment, practically all of these patients have been rendered free of urinary tract infection and, more importantly, have been rendered free of persistent pain and discomfort. In some cases there has been dramatic improvement in creatinine clearance from as little as 10 ml/min up to 65 ml/min.

It is true to say that this sort of result could not have been achieved without a technique permitting a meticulous intrarenal toilet of all macroscopic fragments of calculus. I have published evidence elsewhere of the importance

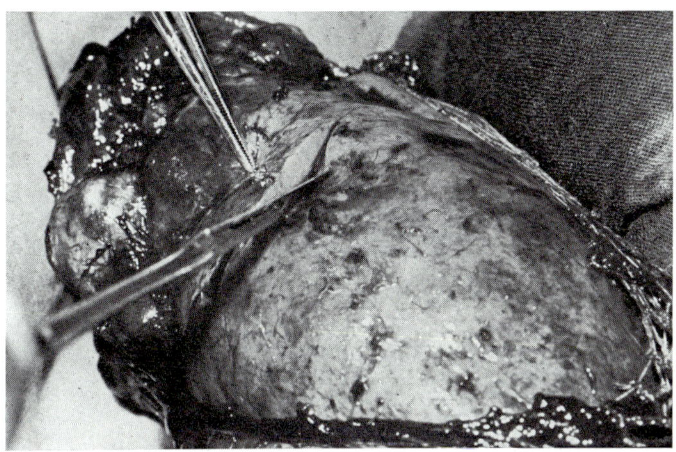

Figure 10.15   Commencement of tumour excision

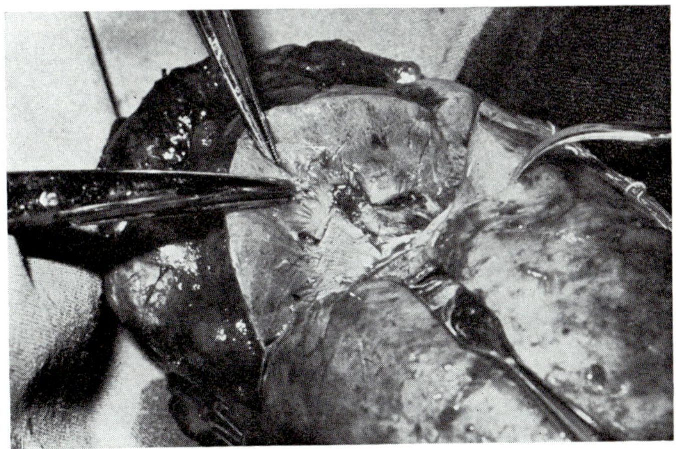

Figure 10.16   Further excision of tumour mass with clear rim of normal kidney. Note dry field

of the removal of all fragments (Wickham and Mathur, 1971) of stone for the prevention of calculus recurrence, particularly when the aetiology of the stone has almost certainly been due to pre-existing urinary tract infection.

Excision of renal cell carcinoma and transitional cell tumours
When a patient presents with a tumour in a solitary kidney or even bilateral

renal tumours, it has in the past been regarded as a situation which is not amenable to surgical correction.

With the assistance of the hypothermic technique, however, it is now possible to deal with this situation and to excise the tumour-containing area of the kidney whilst conserving maximum function in the remaining tissue.

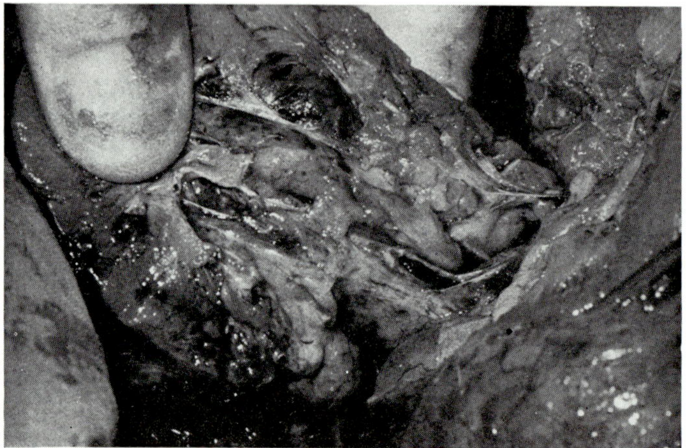

Figure 10.17   Tumour mass almost mobilised. Note blood clot in collecting system

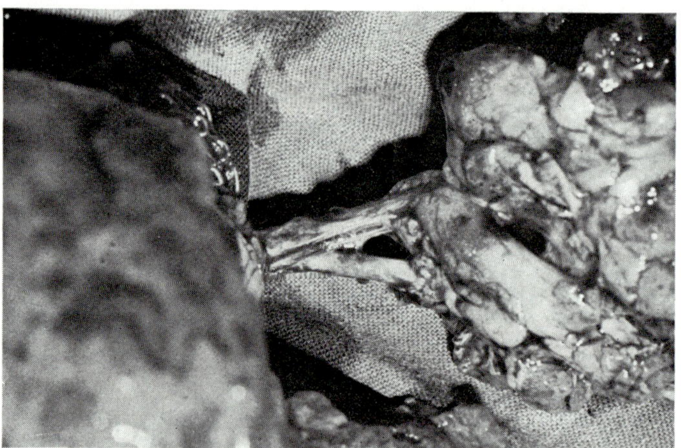

Figure 10.18   Tumour separated from major feeding vessels. Again note dry field

There is now evidence that a more aggressive attitude to the treatment of such patients can result in the salvage of those hitherto regarded as inoperable (Wickham, 1975).

I have dealt with a number of these patients using regional hypothermia in the mobilised organ as already described above. Conventional segmental partial nephrectomy is seldom possible in these patients as tumour tissue frequently extends across the vascular territories of several branches of the renal artery. In order to conserve a maximum amount of normal functioning renal tissue it has been found necessary to excise the tumour mass or masses by a very careful sharp dissection leaving a minimal rim of normal tissue around the tumour (Figs. 10.13 to 10.19). This manoeuvre is best undertaken with some form of visual aid such as magnifying operating spectacles to ensure a complete excision of tumour. Clearly such a procedure would be impossible to perform without some means of vascular arrest and hypothermic protection. One case operated upon illustrates this point, five tumours being excised from the parenchyma of a solitary kidney with a total ischaemia time of 2 h 15 min. At the end of the procedure a complete reconstruction of the intrarenal collecting system was necessary but the patient is alive and well with good renal function two years later.

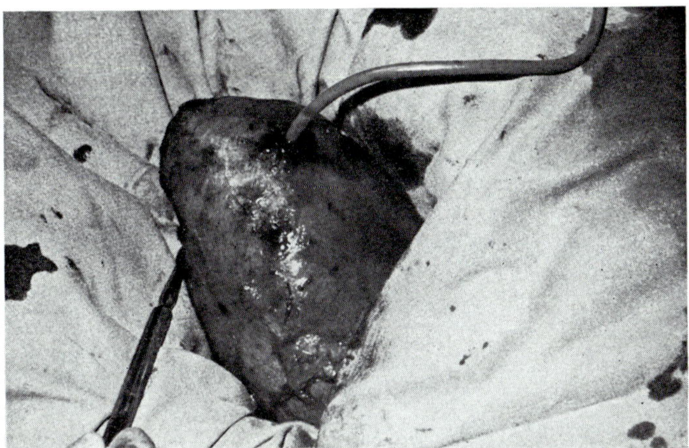

Figure 10.19   Kidney reconstructed with nephrotomy tube. Note absence of haemorrhage on declamping

It is worth noting with regard to operations such as this that where medullary areas of the kidney are incised it is impossible not to transect major tributaries of the intrarenal venous drainage system. This may lead to profuse venous bleeding due to reflux from the renal vein or its major branches, and it is wise at the time of induction of cooling deliberately to occlude the main venous drainage of one or more veins with small bulldog clips. After the arteries have been clamped, the transected ends of such veins may be easily visualised following the resection of the tumour and specifically ligated before declamping and haemostasis of the parenchyma achieved by oversewing with fine 4 'O' chromic cat gut.

Transitional cell tumours in solitary kidneys may likewise be dealt with by excision of the tumour-bearing segment of the kidney. The well-known characteristic of such tumours to appear in other areas of the collecting system of the renal tract might perhaps encourage a more conservative approach

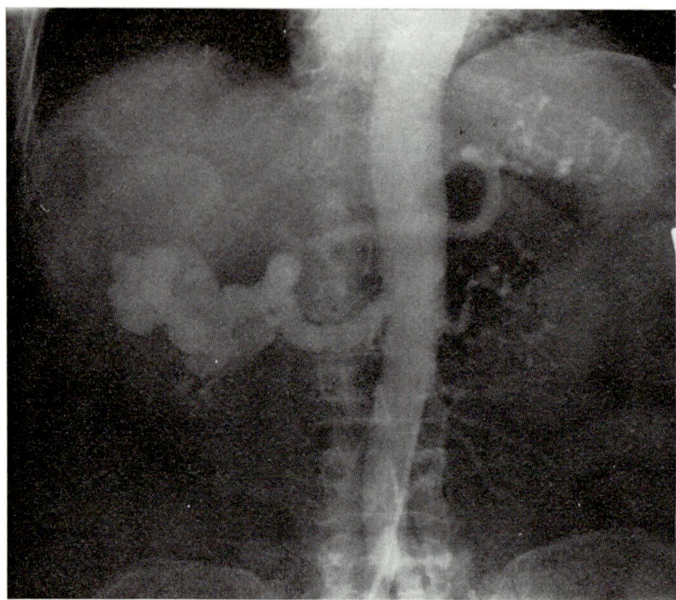

Figure 10.20   Renal angiogram, arterial phase, to show A/V malformation right kidney

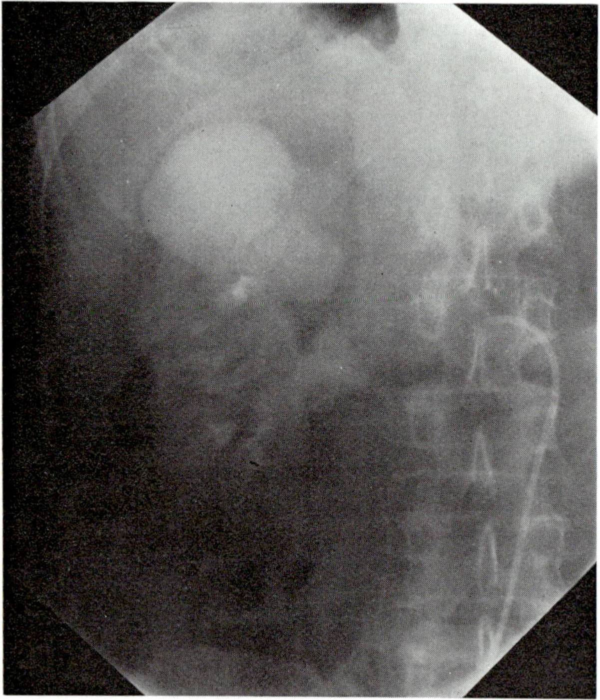

Figure 10.21   As in Figure 10.20—venous phase of angiogram

to their management if they could be shown to be localised to a particular area of the collecting system of a kidney even when the contralateral organ is apparently normal. The conventional management of such tumours by complete nephroureterectomy seems perhaps a little radical when a tumour focus is localised to a single calyx. Petkovic (1972) has advocated local excision of such lesions pointing out the frequency with which further tumours can occur in the contralateral organ. I have performed local resection of such lesions under hypothermic control, conserving the major functioning part of the involved kidney in case subsequent tumour emergence requires removal of further renal tissue.

Clearly this sort of surgery cannot be undertaken without renal ischaemia coupled with hypothermic protection.

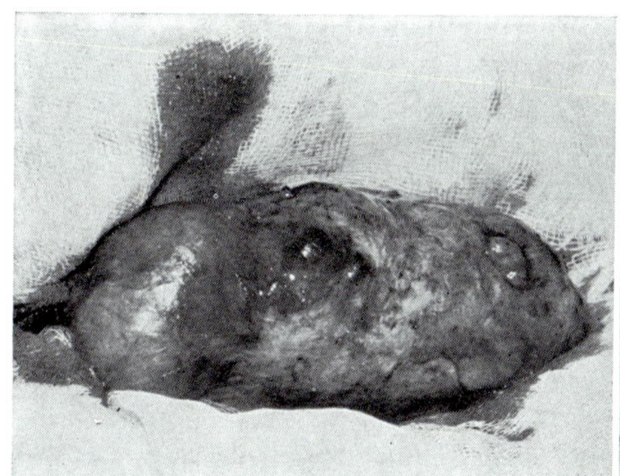

<table>
<tr><td>Figure 10.22   Kidney exposed to show large A/V malformation at upper pole</td><td>Figure 10.23   Feeding vessels to malformation exposed</td></tr>
</table>

Vascular malformations

On several occasions excision of congenital arteriovenous fistulae has been undertaken utilising regional hypothermia rather than resorting to total nephrectomy (Figs. 10.20 to 10.25).

The kidney is cooled as described above, both arterial and venous inflows to the malformation being controlled. The branches of the vessels supplying the malformation are then dissected under direct vision and exposed by incision and retraction of the overlying parenchyma. When fully displayed the feeding vessels are ligated under magnification if necessary, the malformation excised and the parenchyma reconstructed. One or two of the malformations dealt with by this manoeuvre have been of considerable size with measured blood flows of up to 1.0 litre/min and clearly not amenable to surgery except with vascular control and an unhurried operative approach.

Recently with the advent of magnification renal angiography, I have been able to deal with several patients who have presented with persistent upper tract bleeding from one kidney, a situation quite frequently dealt with by

9

ablative nephrectomy. Careful angiography has demonstrated the presence of a small haemangioma or minute branch artery aneurysm which has apparently ruptured through the epithelial lining of a minor calyx. In these cases, due to the ability of hypothermia to provide protection during a careful dissection and exploration of these small branch arteries, I have been able to identify the lesion after incision of the parenchyma, ligate the affected vessel and remove the local lesion. Subsequently the parenchyma has been reconstructed with negligible loss of renal tissue and no detectable effect upon renal function. This seems to be a far preferable technique to either total or partial nephrectomy with sacrifice of much normal renal tissue. Again the ability to be able to approach such a problem unhurriedly is provided by the hypothermic technique.

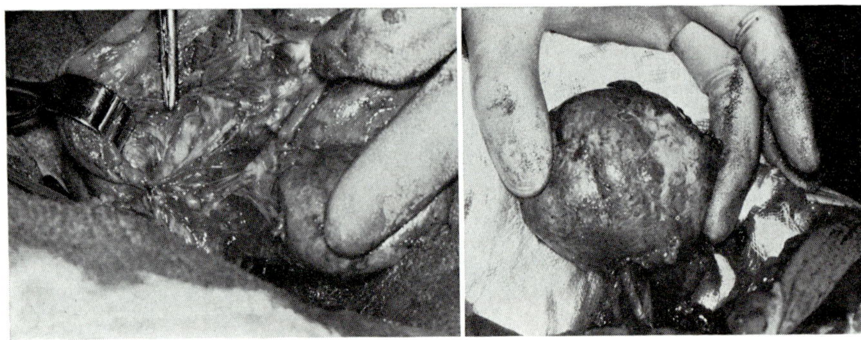

Figure 10.24   Malformation almost completely excised. Note absence of bleeding

Figure 10.25   Kidney reconstructed and declamped showing absence of haemorrhage

Renal artery stenosis

Occasionally if reconstruction of a renal artery stenosis has entailed some particular problem requiring circulatory arrest to the kidney for a period longer than about 15 min, the hypothermic technique has been utilised to provide protection whilst the arterial reconstruction is undertaken. The method has also been used when a renal artery has been involved at the upper end of an abdominal aortic aneurysm. Here the renal artery has been detached from the aneurysmal mass, the kidney cooled and the renal vessels later reimplanted directly into the graft or into adjacent iliac vessels.

Bench Surgery

The concept of removing the kidney, placing the organ on a small operating table, correcting a pathological lesion and then reimplanting the organ in the iliac fossa as in conventional renal transplantation, appears a superficially attractive manoeuvre.

The operative technique is certainly feasible and very adequate protection to function of the ex-vivo organ can be afforded by simple hypothermia such as described above, or by perfusion with hypothermic perfusates of intra-cellular ionic composition such as that described by Collins or Sacks. Alternatively, the kidney may be constantly perfused extracorporeally by a Belzer or Gambro type of renal perfusion machine. Consideration, however, of the number of situations where such a technique would be really useful are found to be somewhat limited.

There are few calculi and few renal tumours that cannot be very satisfactorily removed in situ as described above. The prolongation of the operative procedure necessitated by the bench surgery technique is considerable, often stretching to 5 or 6 h compared with the 2 to 3 h for the in situ operation. Further a generous extension of the primary incision or the necessity to make a second major incision can contribute considerably to the overall morbidity of the technique.

To my mind the indications for bench surgery would appear to be:

1. Where there is for any reason a considerable defect in the ureter, especially in the upper or middle thirds. In such a situation the kidney can be 'moved down' to the pelvis from its normal lumbar position and the shortened length of ureter can be implanted directly into the bladder. Thus the need for an ileal loop interposition with its resultant problems of infection can be avoided.
2. For the correction of renal arterial defects close to the aorta or upon the intrarenal vessel within the kidney such that extensive magnification and reconstruction is required and an in situ operative correction may be impossible.

In most clinical situations an *in situ* operative technique is fully adequate to deal with most forms of intrarenal pathology.

Conclusion

The development of regional renal hypothermia from an experimental to a fully practical clinical technique has enabled an entirely different approach to be made to various problems of renal surgery in the last few years.

It has stimulated a much more conservative approach to the preservation of renal tissue and has enabled the surgeon to operate in a clear dry field without hurry or anxiety about deteriorating renal function in an ischaemic situation. It has permitted a meticulous rather than purely ablative approach to the renal parenchyma and opened up an exciting new field of 'intrarenal' surgery.

REFERENCES

Markland, C. & Parsons, F. M. (1963) Preservation of kidneys for homotransplantation. *British Journal of Urology*, **35**, 457.

Petkovic, S. D. (1972) Conservation of the kidney in operations for tumours of the renal pelvis and calyces. A report of 26 cases. *British Journal of Urology*, **44**, 1–8.

Ward, J. P. (1975) Determination of the optimum temperature for regional hypothermia. *British Journal of Urology*, **47**, 17.

Wickham, J. E. A. (1968) A simple method for regional renal hypothermia. *Journal of Urology*, **99**, 246.

Wickham, J. E. A. (1975) Conservative renal surgery for adenocarcinoma. The place of bench surgery. *British Journal of Urology*, **47**, 25.

Wickham, J. E. A., Coe, N. & Ward, J. P. (1974) One hundred cases of nephrolithotomy under hypothermia. *Journal of Urology*, **112**, 702.

Wickham, J. E. A., Hanley, H. G. & Joekes, A. M. (1967) Regional renal hypothermia. *British Journal of Urology*, **39**, 727.

Wickham, J. E. A. & Mathur, V. K. (1971) Hypothermia in the conservative surgery of renal disease. *British Journal of Urology*, **43**, 648.

11
TESTICULAR TUMOURS

J. P. Blandy

Because testicular tumours are so rare, few surgeons have the opportunity to see more than a very small number, and may be unaware of the remarkable improvement which has taken place in their prognosis over the last few years. Because this improvement is limited to men whose disease is detected early, before distant metastases have appeared, it is of crucial importance that we should be aware of the presentation of these tumours, and of the essential steps in their management. Serious delays in treatment still occur, and tragic errors are still made in early management: tumours are still being removed through a scrotal incision, or, worse, biopsied via the scrotum, and we are still asked whether any further treatment is necessary in the case of a teratoma after orchidectomy.

AETIOLOGY

The well-documented rarity of testicular tumours among Negroes in Africa and in America is confirmed in recent studies both in adults and in children (Li and Fraumeni, 1972; Sherman, Ciaverra and Cohen, 1973; Berg et al, 1973). Clearly an important genetic influence affects the incidence of these tumours, and this is echoed in the occasional familial example (Gulley, Kowalski and Neuhoff, 1974; Silber, Cittan and Friedlander, 1972). Similarly, the long recognised association between the undescended testis and malignancy suggested even to Pott that there was some constitutional defect common to both disorders. Recently Whitaker (1970) has attempted to quantify the risk of malignancy in the undescended testis. His first attempt led to the conclusion that a man with an undescended testis ran a 1:1000 chance of subsequent malignancy, but more recently he has revised this estimate, taking into account the cumulative nature of the hazard from year to year. Indeed, it seems possible that the risk during a man's lifetime may be as high as 1:30 (Whitaker, 1975). Even in this context, the influence of the genetic defect is considerably modified by the unusual environment in which the undescended testis finds itself, and Whitaker's review of the evidence suggests that orchidopexy, especially when done before puberty, may somewhat mitigate the risk of subsequent malignant change.

Of all environmental influences perhaps the one subject for most debate is that of trauma, because as many as one in ten patients report a severe injury to the testis at some time prior to noticing their tumour. Of course nobody can put this question to the test of experiment, and the debate remains more for the armchair or the courtroom than the surgical ward (Thomas, 1972). Other influences in the environment may go unrecognised: Clemmesen (1968) noted in Denmark a doubling of the death rate from tumour of the testis in the city of Copenhagen, but not in the rural areas. We could not find any evidence of such an increase in Britain (Blandy, Hope-Stone and Dayan, 1970) and Lipworth and Dayan (1969) found that, if anything, country areas were more prone to the disease than towns in the United Kingdom. Nevertheless environmental pollution could be an important influence: cadmium has been the subject of considerable concern among ecologists of recent years, and it was with cadmium that Roe (1964) induced testicular tumours in the rat. We should also pay attention to the possible hazards of treatment of oligospermia with hormones, since testicular tumours have been discovered in men given clomiphene (Reyes and Faiman, 1973) as well as gonadotrophins (Rubin, 1973). Levick and Levick (1971) questioned whether these tumours were perhaps unusually common among addicts of LSD, but as with the occasional discovery of a tumour in an infertile patient, it is difficult to know whether the association is merely one of chance. In infertile men testicular tumours have been found sufficiently often to make one wonder: we have had two such patients at the London Hospital and others were reported by Bunge and Bradbury (1965) as well as by Shakkebaek (1972) as accidental findings in a testicular biopsy done in the routine investigation of infertility.

Classification

In recent years there has been some resolution of the conflict between the different systems of classification operating on either side of the Atlantic, now that each system has been revised, and is republished, or is about to be. The standard North American system, that of Dixon and Moore (1952) promulgated by the US Armed Forces Institute of Pathology in Washington, has been revised and brought up to date by Mostofi and Price (1973) in a new version of the USAFIP fascicle. Meanwhile the British system, first published by Collins and Pugh (1964) on behalf of the Testicular Tumour Panel and Registry, has been revised and has been published by Pugh (1976).

In theory at least, both systems now agree as to what they understand by seminoma, and although they differ in points of detail and terminology, there is general agreement about the rarer non-germinal cell tumours. Differences persist in the classification of the non-seminomatous germinal cell tumours or, broadly speaking, the teratomas. In both schemes, recognition is given to the 1 or 2 per cent of extremely well-differentiated tumours which have all the characteristics of benign dermoids, and the exceedingly malignant tumours which have the features of trophoblast and syncytiotrophoblast—again a very small group amounting to only 2 or 3 per cent.

In the USAFIP system the majority of teratomas are divided into two main categories, teratocarcinoma and embryonal carcinoma. In the revised British system, they are divided into malignant teratoma, intermediate and undifferentiated (this latter category incorporating the old subgroups MTIB and MTA). For practical purposes one would expect considerable agreement in these two classifications, and indeed that is what was found in the course of a recent study (Blandy et al, 1976) (Table 11.1).

It is however not so simple: while it is all very well to lay down rules for the classification of testicular tumours, it is quite another thing to interpret and apply them, and considerable room for error and variation arises in the application of any system of classification. In the context of tumours of the testicle there is a particular area where error may arise, and it concerns those tumours in which sheets of undifferentiated cells occur without identifying features. One pathologist may well assign such a section to the category

Table 11.1   Comparison between American and British schemes for classification of teratoma testis

American system (Mostofi and Price, 1973)	Teratoma differentiated (TD)	Malignant teratoma intermediate (MTI)	Malignant teratoma undifferentiated (MTU)	Teratoma trophoblastic
Teratoma mature	2	1	0	0
Teratocarcinoma with embryonal carcinoma	0	49	0	0
Embryonal carcinoma	0	0	49	0
Teratoma immature	0	4	0	0

The header spans: British system (Pugh, 1976) covering the TD, MTI, MTU columns.

seminoma: another will classify it as an undifferentiated or embryonal carcinoma. For this reason it is well to look closely at the overall proportion of cases in a given series which have been put down as seminoma. One sees astonishing variations: but on the whole one finds 35 to 40 per cent of tumours in the seminoma category in most North American series; whereas in most Scandinavian and British series the proportion is nearer 60 per cent (Table 11.2) (Miller and Seljelid, 1971). Of course, there may be valid local variations due to differences in genetic make-up of the population, or in age structure, or, as in the case of the British Testicular Tumour Panel and Registry, in case selection: but it is much more likely that there is a variation in the subjective opinions of pathologists working in isolation from each other on either side of the Atlantic. The author is bound to admit that observer variation seems to him the most likely explanation: and if this is so, then it follows that there is a proportion of disputable cases labelled seminoma by some and embryonal carcinoma by others. We shall return to this issue later, for it is of some importance when trying to decide what is the best form of treatment for a given teratoma.

One group of seminomas are however not in dispute, and they have been given increasing recognition recently, since they carry a more favourable prognosis. These are the spermatocytic seminomas. They are uncommon, and occur in the older age group—usually in men over 65—and are sometimes bilateral (Scobie, 1970).

Table 11.2 Variation in the percentage of germinal cell tumours designated as seminoma in different reported series from the literature

%	
87	Navarro & Martinez (1964) *XIIIe Congrès Soc. Int. Urol.*, **1,** 96
84	Correa & Tallman (1965) *XIIIe Congrès Soc. Int. Urol.*, **2,** 96
74	Easson & Russell (1968) *Brit. med. J.*, **1,** 1704
70	van Welkenhuyzen & Henry (1965) *XIIIe Congrès. Soc. Int. Urol.*, **2,** 44
68	Cox (1954) *Brit. J. Urol.*, **26,** 350
60	Notter & Ranudd (1964) *Acta Radiol.*, **2,** 273
59	Danish Cancer Registry (1969) Clemmesen, *Acta Path. Microbiol Scand.*, Suppl. 209, xxi
58	Ekman et al (1965) *Urol. Int.*, **20,** 129
58	Nedelec et al (1964) *XIIIe Congrès. Soc. Int. Urol.*, **1,** 58
57	London Hospital (1976) Blandy et al, *Current Controversies in Surgery* (in press)
57	Fantoni & Martinazzi (1964) *Arch. De Vecchi.*, **43,** 467
55	Jomain et al (1964) *J. Urol. néphrol. (Paris)*, **70,** 304
54	Mackay & Sellers (1966) *Canad. Med. Ass. J.*, **94** (ii), 889
52	Reddy & Ranganayakamma (1966) *Indian J. Cancer*, **3,** 255
50	Boctor et al (1969) *Cancer (Phila)*, **24,** 870
50	Benbanaste (1965) *Acta Urol. Belg.*, **33,** 317
48	Robson et al (1965) *J. Urol.*, **32,** 291
45	Vechinski et al (1965) *Amer. J. Roentgenol.*, **95,** 494
40	Pugh (1976) *Pathology of the Testes*, Blackwell Scientific Publications.
38	Mostofi & Price (1973) *Tumors of the Male Genital System*, p. 78. U.S. Armed Forces Institute of Pathology
36	Maier et al (1969) *J. Urol.*, **101,** 356

Testicular Tumours in Boys

In most large collected series, as in that from our own hospital (Fig. 11.1), the age incidence of germinal tumours follows a familiar pattern, with two peaks—for seminoma and teratoma. But this obscures a very important, if rare, subgroup of testicular tumours in boys, which has lately been the subject of an important and comprehensive review by Brosman and Gondos (1975) based on a study of 414 tumours of the testis in children. They point out that only two-thirds of these tumours arise in germinal cells, in which group seminomas do not occur; about one-third are virtually benign teratomas; and the remainder—amounting to perhaps about half of the entire group—are a particular kind of embryonal carcinoma which, from its resemblance to the yolk sac tumour of the mouse, is called a yolk sac carcinoma. This specially designated tumour occurs in the first two to three years of life, and it metastasizes much as does a malignant embryonal carcinoma in the adult. On the basis of a review of the outcome of therapy in 199 cases, Brosman and Gondos recommend retroperitoneal node dissection when there is evidence of spread. There is some dispute as to whether these yolk sac tumours occur in adults though Talerman (1974) has reported three cases, associated with seminoma.

The other important group of testicular tumours encountered in childhood are those arising from other than germinal cells: thus Sertoli cell tumours occurred in 22 of their 414 cases, Leydig cell tumours in 48, and the remainder had paratesticular tumours such as leiomyosarcoma and rhabdomyosarcoma arising from coverings of the testis and spermatic cord.

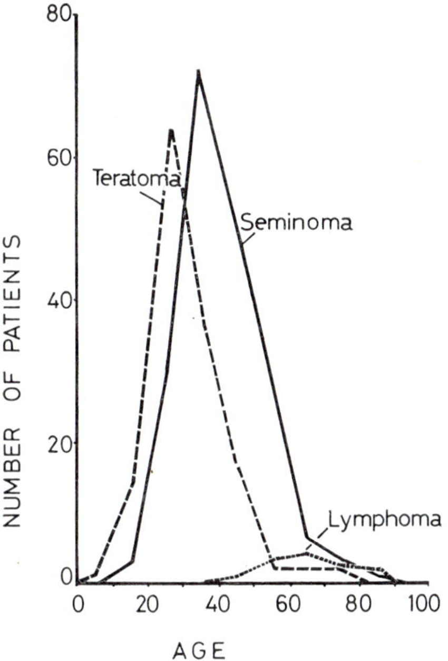

Figure 11.1   Age incidence of testis tumours: the London Hospital 1952 to 1972 (combined tumours included in teratomas)

Leydig and Sertoli cell tumours

In the past, one of the questions which gave rise to controversy was whether Leydig or Sertoli cell tumours were truly benign. The problem is not confined to the testis, for in other endocrine organs it is often difficult to know whether a given tumour is essentially hyperplastic, neoplastic, or hypertrophic, particularly when, as in the Leydig cell tumour, extragonadal rests of Leydig cells are normal, and hyperplasia is a common finding in association with undescended testis and adrenal hyperplasia (Bahuleyan and Harlal, 1969; Earll, Newman and DiRaimondo, 1969). Nevertheless undoubted metastases can occur with either of these unusual testicular tumours, though the event is a very rare one. Livesay, Branch and Eaton (1972) record what they believe is the twelfth case with metastases of a Leydig cell tumour, and Koppikar and Sirsat (1973) the ninth example in a Sertoli cell tumour.

Paratesticular tumours

A true seminoma may occur in what clinically seems to be the epididymis, but the epididymis may also give rise to true adenoma and carcinoma from its own tubules (Broth, Bullock and Morrow, 1968; Price, 1971). Since it is also the site for some vestigial Müllerian structures it can give rise to the so-called adenomatoid tumour, which is thought to arise in Müllerian duct structures (Miller and Lieberman, 1968). Most of the adult paratesticular tumours arise in the coverings of the cord: our cases at the London Hospital were reviewed by Grant Williams and Banerjee (1969): unlike the boyhood rhabdomyo-sarcoma, when the adult ones were malignant they tended to be leiomyo-sarcomas or fibrosarcomas. None of them is common, and none of them can be trusted to be benign.

Extragonadal origin of testicular tumours

The long argument about the cause for those abdominal metastases which prove to be teratoma or seminoma, in the patient who seems to have both testes which are normal, has taken a new turn. A few years ago, thanks to the studies of Azzopardi et al (1961, 1965) we were taught that most of these metastases began in a small primary tumour in the testis, which then healed, to leave only an inconspicuous scar. More recently Utz and Buscemi (1971) and Johnson et al (1973) reviewing some 37 of these unusual cases, including 3 in the pineal and 19 in the mediastinum, have argued convincingly for the view that some at least of them are due to rests of testicular blastema remaining in the site of the primitive gonadal ridge.

The phenomenon of scarring does raise another interesting consideration, for the writer has recently seen two patients in whom the first symptom was not a swelling of the testis, but a shrinking of it: the specimen removed in each case showed scarring and fibrous replacement of a considerable part of the seminoma which was present. The moral is clear—any symptom, however bizarre or unexpected, when it affects the testis, must be taken seriously, and must raise a doubt in the mind of the examining surgeon that perhaps there is an underlying tumour.

DIAGNOSIS

The tragedy of so many tumours of the testis is not so much that there was anything new or unusual about them but simply that the possibility of malignancy had not been entertained seriously by the surgeon. Three errors deserve particular notice.

Tumour mistaken for inflammation

Between 4 and 16 per cent of all large series of cases form a group in whom the signs and symptoms were misinterpreted as inflammation. In my experience it has been quite impossible to distinguish some of these inflammatory tumours from a severe epididymo-orchitis of several days standing, or a neglected torsion. So long as the diagnosis is unsure, and so long as the inflammation is not obviously limited to the epididymis, then it is clear that the rule must be to explore the testis unless it is certain that there is urinary infection, or some other gross and obvious cause for inflammation. Occasionally tuberculous epididymo-orchitis is encountered, or one of the rare granulomas of the testis, but in every case, orchidectomy is the right treatment when the testis is involved. In the only case where I have made the correct pre-operative diagnosis of a sperm granuloma, and attempted to conserve the testis, pain and continuing local features made orchidectomy necessary within 10 days.

Neglected injury of the testis

Another curious blind spot in surgical education has been the subject of the injured testis. Every article on the subject of the proper management of the injured testis since the classical observations of Atwell and Ellis (1961) has only reiterated the message, namely, that the best way to preserve the injured testis is to explore it at once, evacuate the haematocele, repair the laceration in the visceral tunica vaginalis and retain as many testicular tubules as can be kept inside it. There is no justification, unless the patient is in extremis, for treating a haematocele 'expectantly'. The only expectation the patient can look forward to is atrophy of the injured testis and loss of its function. A policy of prompt exploration would not only preserve otherwise healthy testes, but would bring to light the occasional tumour whose presenting feature has been a swelling which followed a recent injury. The most unwise and unhelpful thing is to attempt to aspirate the haematocele: not only does the swelling not go down, but if there is tumour present it will be disseminated into the tissues of the scrotum.

Scrotal aspiration or excision

Alas, this is still the most common of the three tragic errors in dealing with tumours of the testis which is still encountered even today. Again, through some odd quirk of ignorance, quite a number of surgeons have never been convinced that it is both wrong and dangerous to perform a scrotal orchidectomy, and worse still to perform a trans-scrotal biopsy. This is not a new message, and the impassioned plea of Stephen in 1958 certainly deserved widespread attention. Not only does meddling with a tumour of the testis through a scrotal incision invite local recurrence in the scrotal skin, but it opens up the lymphatic catchment area of the scrotum to the tumour cells, and condemns the patient to an extra burden of therapy. In cases when a tumour is being treated by radiation, this will involve no more than the discomfort of radiation dermatitis of the groin and scrotum, and the unnecessary sterilisation of the contralateral testis which might otherwise have been protected. But in centres where radical node dissection is believed to be correct, the surgical blunder of a scrotal incision makes it necessary for the unfortunate patient to undergo a radical groin node dissection. The disadvantages of scrotal incisions are not merely theoretical. On looking through our records at the London Hospital I found that of 38 men (referred from other centres for radiotherapy) in whom the testis had been removed through a scrotal rather than an inguinal incision, no less than 12 had developed recurrent tumour in the inguinal nodes or the scrotum. Of the 252 others with an inguinal orchidectomy only one developed a recurrence, at the medial end of a rather low incision. Herr, Silber and Martin (1973) and Fraley (1976) have also commented on this sorry error.

It is pointless to dwell on the catalogue of signs and symptoms which may be the unusual presenting features of a tumour of the testis: most of them have been described previously (Blandy et al, 1970). To that list one might add the occasional case with what seems to be a spontaneous rupture of the testicular tumour (Watkins, 1970; Cutajar, 1972) which may cause a haemoperitoneum if the testis is abdominal. The sensible rule to have every testis sectioned when it is removed in the course of herniorrhaphy, or because it is undescended, will bring to light an occasional tumour. One other clinical sign, not previously noted, is the cutaneous manifestation of malignancy—acanthosis nigricans—described in the context of the testis for the first time by Braun and Schlang (1970).

Much of the delay in obtaining the right treatment for the patient rests neither with the patient himself, nor with his general practitioner, but with the first surgeon he sees. Utley and his colleagues in Christchurch, New Zealand, have shown that a firm policy of early diagnosis of swellings in the testis can pay off handsomely not only in testes saved from loss by torsion, but in an 85 per cent clinical stage 1 diagnosis rate for testicular tumours (Utley et al, 1972, 1974).

Chevassu's Manoeuvre

In his plea for early diagnosis and radical surgery, Chevassu recognised that it was not always easy to be sure whether there was a lump in the testis or not, and that the only way to be sure was to explore it. If this policy is followed, as I believe it ought to be, rigorously and ruthlessly, even the most experienced surgeon will from time to time find himself holding a testis in his hand which is not obviously a tumour, and which he does not therefore feel confident enough about to remove. If the wound is then carefully isolated with towels, the testis may be sliced open along its anterior border. This may reveal a tell-tale sphere of seminoma lying entirely surrounded by testis, when one is present. A pathologist colleague in the operating room to give moral support is of more value at this juncture than a frozen section (which may give rise to error). If nothing is found wrong, the testis may be carefully closed with a continuous running catgut suture along the tunica vaginalis. As Chevassu showed in his dogs, and as I can now confirm in three patients, the testis does not subsequently atrophy. Let me add, however, that the need for this manoeuvre arises very very seldom.

Clinical Staging

Once the suspected tumour has been removed and histological confirmation obtained, the next task is to attempt to determine how far the tumour has spread, i.e. assess its clinical stage. The system formerly in use in most British centres has been fully described previously (Blandy et al, 1970), and was based on that used by Boden and Gibb (1951). However, recent developments in lymphangiography have confused the former simplicity of this system of staging, and it is important when setting out to compare one form of treatment with another to be sure exactly what criteria are being used in determining the clinical stage.

A good many studies have been carried out now where the lymphangiographic changes have subsequently been checked against the findings at retroperitoneal node dissection: the range of error is wide. Cosgrove and Metzger (1975) reported a false positive rate of up to 50 per cent: Jonsson, Ingemansson and Ling (1973) had three mistakes in 22 examples: Fein and Taber (1969) reported 33 per cent of false negatives: Maier and Schamber (1972) had 9 errors in 69. In other centres, where lymphographic staging is widely used, no check is made on the accuracy of the lymphographic interpretation by node dissection, though we are frequently and solemnly informed that with sufficient skill and experience mistakes do not occur.

One of the more sensible objections to the use of pedal lymphography in evaluating the stage of spread of a testicular tumour is that the foot lymphatics are different from those of the testis. Direct injection of the lymphatics of the spermatic cord is perfectly feasible (Chiappa et al, 1966), but until recently has been prohibitively time consuming. Now a simplified and more rapid version has been developed by Kuisk et al (1970) which is said to take only 30 minutes to complete.

There certainly is a need to be able to detect and perhaps to quantify retroperitoneal node metastases. Palpation at operation even under anaesthesia is notoriously unreliable. Separation of the ureters and kidneys will be shown in the urogram, but will only detect quite bulky tumour. The use of alpha-feto-protein as a diagnostic aid has been very disappointing (Merrin et al, 1973). Something on the lines of the uptake by invaded lymph nodes of a radioactive isotope such as the gallium[67] used in a pilot study by Bailey et al

(1973) would be a great advantage, especially if it worked consistently, and could pick out lymph nodes with small deposits in them.

As it is, we have in current use, three systems of staging of tumour. The standard clinical stage; the stage which accepts lymphangiographic findings as being true; and the 'surgical' staging which provides histological evidence of tumour in the retroperitoneal tissue (Fig. 11.2). It is obvious that these three systems each have their own errors, each overlap to a greater or lesser extent, and are all very fallible. Even the accuracy of surgical staging must to some extent reflect the zeal and industry of the pathologist assigned to the

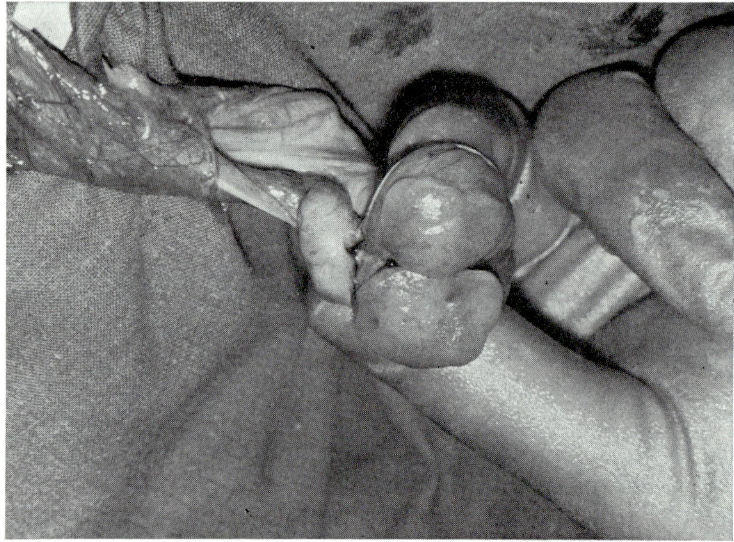

Figure 11.2   Chevassu's manouvre: with a clamp on the cord, the testicle is delivered through an inguinal incision. When there is still doubt as to the presence of a tumour within the testis, it is then sliced open and inspected. A seminoma may be completely surrounded by healthy testicular tissue (as here). Frozen section is hardly ever necessary

boring task of trying to find small metastases in a jumble of retroperitoneal fibrofatty tissue. There are very few centres where this particular chore is accorded a high priority in the pathological institute, and none (as far as I know) where every specimen is subjected to step sectioning (Wilkinson and Hause, 1974).

TREATMENT

The Controversy Over Treatment of Retroperitoneal Nodes

It ought to surprise a detached observer that surgeons on either side of the Atlantic can hold such diverse opinions with such vehemence, on the question of how retroperitoneal metastases ought to be treated, when their methods of detecting them are so extremely unreliable and slipshod. Yet this is exactly the position today. The young man who comes to my department with an embryonal carcinoma will receive radiotherapy after his simple orchidectomy: if he goes to many North American centres he will undergo radical node dissection, supplemented (if the nodes show evidence of tumour) by radiotherapy in most centres. And yet the surgeons are not unusually unintelligent; they do not lack for goodwill, and each believes that he is doing the best for his patient. This Looking-Glass situation needs to be explained.

No argument about seminoma—or is there?

The first ray of hope for men with testicular tumours was seen in the 1930s when radiotherapy began to be given as a routine to retroperitoneal nodes in clinical stage 1. At first the improvement was limited to seminomas, and before long the cure rate obtained by radiotherapy in seminoma became so manifestly excellent, that radical node dissection was entirely abandoned for these tumours. Today, even in the diehard centres of radical node dissection, if a tumour is categorised as a pure seminoma (without bits of teratoma in it) then the patient is treated by radiotherapy alone, and is excused laparotomy. As we have pointed out above this begs the whole question of the observer error inherent in the diagnosis of a seminoma, and there is strong reason to suppose that many a tumour called seminoma in one centre would be regarded as embryonal cell carcinoma in another.

Teratomas are radioresistant—or are they?

One very interesting phenomenon in modern surgery is the extent to which dogma can be accepted despite want of evidence. One such dogma asserts that non-seminomas are radioresistant. This took its origin in the early days of radiotherapy, and the authority cited is always Friedman (1950) though nowhere is the experimental or clinical data given upon which this statement was based. However, once the pejorative term *radioresistant* has been coupled with *teratoma* it needs more than mere evidence to break the association. As we have pointed out earlier, about half the non-seminomas with which we have to deal are the relatively more differentiated (at least in certain areas) malignant teratoma intermediate group or teratocarcinomas in North American usage. Even granting the enormous errors inherent in the idea of 'clinical stage 1' the results of simple orchidectomy and radiotherapy obtainable in most modern English centres approaches 90 per cent crude survival rate (Fig. 11.3, Table 11.3). In some centres which make extensive use of, and trust, staging by lymphangiography, the stage 1 results are even better, and those in stage 2 are also encouraging. If evidence were needed, here is surely clear rebuttal of the dogma that all teratomas are radioresistant.

Of course, the fact remains that the results are not very good for the bad teratomas—the embryonal carcinomas and malignant teratoma undifferentiated group (Fig. 11.4, Table 11.4). At first glance, they are not as good as

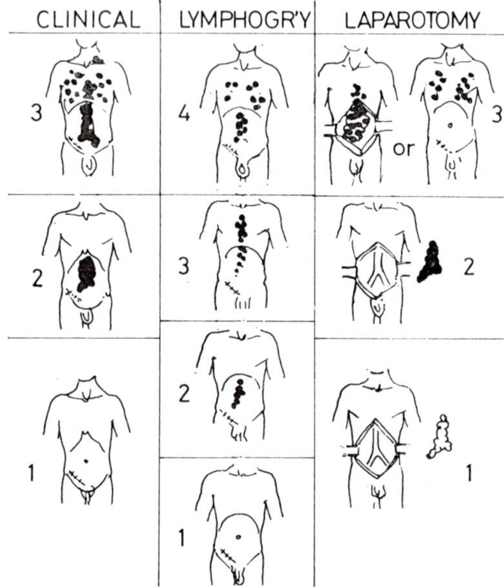

Figure 11.3 The 'staging' of testicular tumours depends upon the method used to detect retroperitoneal metastases: many impalpable lymph node metastases are missed in clinical staging, which relies upon abdominal palpation and excretion urography: lymphography will detect some of these—but not as many as histological examination of the nodes removed at operation. The claims for some of the results of treatment by node dissection (compared with radiotherapy) may well be the result of differences in the methods of staging used in different series

Table 11.3 Survival of malignant teratoma intermediate tumours

	Years					
	< 1	1	2	3	4	5
Clinical stage 1						
Survived	49	45	43	41	39	38
Number at risk	49	47	47	46	44	43
Crude survival (%)	100	95	92	89	89	89
Clinical stage 2						
Survived	10	5	3	3	3	2
Number at risk	10	10	7	7	7	6
Crude survival (%)	100	50	43	43	43	33
Clinical stage 3						
Survived	8	1	0	0	0	0
Number at risk	8	8	7	7	7	7
Crude survival (%)	100	13	0	0	0	0
All stages						
Survived	67	51	46	44	42	40
Number at risk	67	65	61	60	58	55
Crude survival (%)	100	78	75	73	72	72

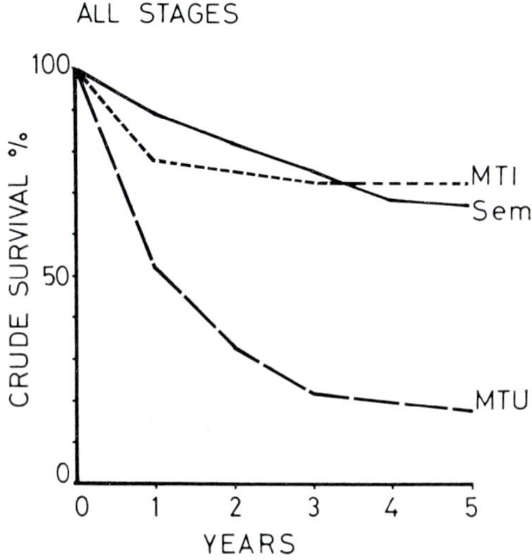

Figure 11.4   Crude survival rates for malignant teratoma intermediate, malignant teratoma undifferentiated, and seminoma in all clinical stages, treated by inguinal orchidectomy and radiotherapy

Table 11.4   Survival of malignant teratoma undifferentiated tumours

	Years					
	<1	1	2	3	4	5
Clinical stage 1						
Survived	28	21	13	8	6	5
Number at risk	28	28	27	23	21	20
Crude survival (%)	100	75	48	35	29	25
Clinical stage 2						
Survival	10	7	4	2	2	2
Number at risk	10	10	6	5	5	5
Crude survival (%)	100	70	67	40	40	40
Clinical stage 2						
Survived	18	1	0	0	0	0
Number at risk	18	18	18	17	14	13
Crude survival (%)	100	5	0	0	0	0
All stages						
Survived	56	29	17	10	8	7
Number at risk	56	56	51	45	40	38
Crude survival (%)	100	52	33	22	20	19

those of radical node dissection for surgical stage 1 cases (Staubitz et al, 1974). There may be a place for radical retroperitoneal node dissection in these tumours: let us look at it further.

Radical retroperitoneal node dissection—its claims

As has been known for 65 years, the lymphatic drainage of the testis is to the para-aortic nodes on either side of the aorta, and to the internal iliac nodes on the side of the tumour by way of the lymphatics of the vas. One of the difficulties which arises in understanding the claims of radical node dissection is that many of its most vehement protagonists, notably the pupils of the late much-loved and well-respected Wyland Leadbetter, have practised a unilateral node dissection (Walsh et al, 1971; Skinner and Leadbetter, 1971; Fraley, 1975). Even when the more logical transabdominal approach of Patton, Seitzman and Zone (1960) was used, it could do not more than remove two-thirds of the potentially involved nodes (Tavel et al, 1963) and indeed the proposition that a surgeon can remove all the lymphatics and lymph nodes by any 'radical en bloc' operation is one which is being more and more open to doubt not only in relation to the testis, but also to the breast, neck and cervix.

Of course no theoretical argument would signify if the results of surgical node dissection were better than those of radiotherapy for the same kind of tumour in the same stage of spread. But here we run up against the impossibility of comparing results, when the proponents of node dissection work in North America and those of radiotherapy in Europe. As we have discussed, even the application of the same histological system in different centres does not overcome the difficulty of the disputed group of cases here called seminoma and there embryonal carcinoma. The fact that the results of radiotherapy have to be put in terms of clinical staging, or at best, of lymphographic staging, whereas the results of surgery are expressed according to whether or not the nodes are invaded by tumour, means that it is quite impossible to compare similar stages of tumour spread.

As we have seen, because radiotherapy rules out the possibility of being sure about the state of involvement of the retroperitoneal nodes, one can only guess at the presence of lymph node metastases: hence in clinical stage 1 there will be a good many with histologically positive nodes, and others in whom the nodes are not only histologically positive but actually fixed and inoperable.

Where node dissection is the favoured method of treatment for teratoma, at laparotomy as many as 25 per cent of patients prove to be inoperable because the nodes are fixed, or extend above the diaphragm. Such cases are excluded from consideration of the results of operation, and are placed in the surgical category stage 3. Of the patients in whom nodes are removed, perhaps half are found to have histological evidence of tumour, and about half are negative on routine sectioning of the surgical specimen. Again, the results will be expressed according to the surgical staging: stage 1 will be those with negative nodes, stage 2 with positive nodes: but all of these plus a proportion in stage 3 will have been included in the clinical (radiotherapy) category stage 1.

Since, in general, the practice has been for cases with histological nodes to receive radiotherapy after node dissection (with the notable exception of Staubitz's cases) the comparison of forms of treatment is clouded even further.

How then do results of treatment compare? We have recently attempted

CLINICAL STAGE 1

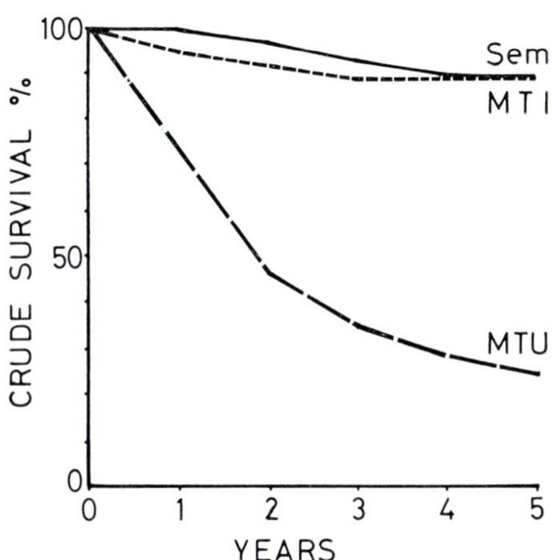

Figure 11.5   Crude survival rates for malignant teratoma intermediate, malignant teratoma undifferentiated, and seminoma presenting without 'clinical' evidence of metastases and treated by inguinal orchidectomy and radiotherapy

Table 11.5   Survival of seminoma after orchidectomy and radiotherapy

	Years					
	<1	1	2	3	4	5
Clinical stage 1						
Survived	106	105	98	91	83	80
Number at risk	106	105	101	98	93	90
Crude survival (%)	100	100	97	93	89	89
Clinical stage 2						
Survived	38	29	25	21	15	15
Number at risk	38	35	35	35	35	35
Crude survival (%)	100	83	72	60	43	43
Clinical stage 3						
Survived	18	6	2	1	1	1
Number at risk	18	17	16	16	16	16
Crude survival (%)	100	35	7	7	7	7
All stages						
Survived	162	140	125	113	99	96
Number at risk	162	157	153	149	144	141
Crude survival (%)	100	89	82	76	69	68

to make this comparison (Blandy et al, 1976) in a study in which our results have been presented on the basis of clinical staging, in terms of crude survival rates. These figures presented here would be much improved if we excluded those patients who had emigrated, gone to jail, or who had died of other unrelated causes. As shown in Table 11.5 the five-year survivals for the more differentiated tumours compare well with those for seminoma (where nobody disputes that radiotherapy is the treatment of choice). For the undifferentiated tumours the results are much worse. It is my belief that the results are worse because of inaccurate staging: and that if these patients had been explored, about a tenth of them would have been found to be inoperable, and positive nodes would have been present in half of the remainder. By juggling the figures on this basis we can arrive at an estimated five year survival of four out of six which is comparable with what can be achieved by surgical excision of the nodes in the best hands. Such a comparison would be as misleading as it would be futile. But it is important to note the results obtained at the Royal Marsden Hospital, expressed on the basis of lymphographic staging, which suggest that if there are no positive lymph nodes in the retroperitoneal tissue, even the anaplastic teratomas have an excellent response to radio-therapy (Peckham, 1975). Any differences in the results obtained in our hands, and those obtained elsewhere with surgical node dissection could easily be explained on the basis of the remarkable variations in methods used to stage the tumours and differences in the interpretation of the systems used to classify them histologically.

One fact which suggests that this may be the true explanation of the apparently poor results in current methods of treating embryonal carcinoma with radiation, is that the patients who die, die with widespread blood-borne metastases; they do not come up with an abdominal mass at some time between their first course of treatment and the onset of haematogenous secondaries. Our clinical impression over the last 15 years study of these patients has always been that the bad tumours spread early and through the blood stream.

In recent years our policy of treatment has been to offer radical node dissection to those patients in the anaplastic MTU/embryonal carcinoma group if their abdominal mass fails to go away with radiotherapy, or if such a mass appears in a patient in whom no lung metastases can be found. Such patients are very rare. The contrary course of events has been much more common—where a man originally thought to have a stage 1 tumour, develops a crop of pulmonary metastases even before he has finished his course of radiotherapy. One cannot imagine that radical node dissection would have improved such a man's chances.

One interesting feature is brought to light by this policy of delayed node dissection. Histological study of the tissue which is removed several months after the original course of treatment will often show a considerable change in its histological appearance: instead of being made up of wildly malignant tissue, the retroperitoneal mass may appear to be no more sinister than a dermoid cyst. Such differentiation has been reported before both after radiation and after chemotherapy in embryonal carcinoma (Dees, 1973; Willis and Hajdu, 1973).

Until an agreed multicentre trial can be started in which to compare the results of radiotherapy versus node dissection for the embryonal carcinoma/

MTU cases, it does not seem possible to decide which is the right treatment to use. Fortunately Maier and his colleagues at the Walter Reed Army Hospital have just such a randomised prospective trial in progress.

Chemotherapy

One cannot emphasise too strongly that the extraordinary improvement which has taken place in the results of treatment of seminoma and intermediate teratocarcinoma applies only to patients seen early, before there is widespread involvement with tumour. For patients who come up too late, or in whom needless delay has occurred in making the diagnosis, the outlook is still grim. Here death is the result of unchecked blood-borne spread, and the only hope for the patient is to find a method of therapy which can act on blood-borne metastases.

The possibility of discovering some agent, or combination of agents, which will be effective against testicular tumours, has been the target of intense study in several centres, and the results are by no means all hopeless. Very anaplastic seminoma and embryonal carcinoma may occasionally show prolonged remission for periods beyond two years (Foley et al, 1972). Of the many chemotherapeutic agents which have been tried, the combination of vincristine, actinomycin D, and methotrexate seems to be the most promising at the time of writing, though the number of possible combinations of different drugs which can be tried suggests that a better permutation may yet remain to be found (Smithers, 1972; Whitmore, 1973). As cancer chemotherapy gradually develops (and as we are today mercifully spared the presentation of three month results expressed in terms of subjective improvement) so we begin to see a definite pattern of benefit emerging for our patients. Cancer chemotherapy is not now made insupportable for the patient: such therapy no longer means offering treatment that is worse than the natural history of the disease, and we begin to see remissions of such duration that it is possible to think, with a measure of confidence, that perhaps the patient may be cured. Alone in this most promising field, the chemotherapy of chorioncarcinoma of the testis stands out as a signal disappointment in contrast to the brilliant results in trophoblastic tumours of women (Goldstein and Piro, 1972).

Immunotherapy

Disillusionment with the applications to cancer therapy of the results of immunological studies in animals should not blind us to the possibility that one day these studies may prove to be valuable in solid tumours. A few disconnected gleams of hope can be observed even in the unrewarding field of testicular tumours. First, spontaneous remissions can occur (Birkhead and Scott, 1973) though they are remarkably uncommon: second, cases are on record where a previously undetectable testicular tumour, after transplantation, will flourish and spread in the immunosuppressed recipient (Leb and Howell, 1971). Thirdly, we have evidence that marked lymphocyte infiltration in a seminoma carries with it a significant improvement in prognosis (Blandy et al, 1970). We may be a long way off the vaccine for teratoma which we would like to possess, but there is at least some evidence that in these tumours we may one day be able to apply those principles of immunology which are so promising in the laboratory, to our patients in the ward.

Conclusion

For the present the most important single thing we can offer the patient with a testicular tumour is early diagnosis, prompt and correct orchidectomy, with radical radiotherapy to the retroperitoneal nodes, supplemented by chemotherapy for those tumours which have already reached the bloodstream. Perhaps, in certain highly selected types of anaplastic teratoma, we should add retroperitoneal node dissection, though this must remain for the time being a matter for debate until current clinical trials are finished.

ACKNOWLEDGEMENTS

It is a pleasure to thank my colleagues Drs Hope-Stone, Shanks, Mantell and Tresidder for permission to refer to cases under their care, and to cite work done in collaboration with Drs E. A. Molland and D. Pollock.

The illustrations are all reproduced, with permission, from Fraley (1976) *Current Controversies in Urology*, Chapter 21, published by W. B. Saunders Company, Philadelphia.

REFERENCES

Atwell, J. D. & Ellis, H. (1961) Rupture of the testis. *Brit. J. Surg.*, **49**, 345–346.

Azzopardi, J. G., Mostofi, F. K. & Theiss, E. A. (1961) Lesions of testes observed in certain patients with widespread chorioncarcinoma and related tumours. *Amer. J. clin. Path.*, **38**, 207–225.

Azzopardi, J. G. & Hoffbrand, A. V. (1965) Retrogression in testicular seminoma with viable metastases. *J. clin. Path.*, **18**, 135–141.

Bahuleyan, K. & Harlal, K. R. (1969) Bilateral interstitial cell tumour of testes. Report of a case with brief review of literature. *Indian J. Surg.*, **31**, 187–190.

Bailey, T. B., Pinsky, S. M., Mittemeyer, B. T., Borski, A. A. & Johnson, M. (1973) A new adjuvant in testis tumor staging: gallium-67 citrate. *J. Urol.*, **110**, 307–310.

Berg, J. W., Godwin, J. D., McKay, F. W. & Percy, C. L. (1973) Testis cancer in negroes. *Lancet*, **1**, 782–783.

Blandy, J. P., Hope-Stone, H. F. & Dayan, A. D. (1970) *Tumours of the Testicle*. London: William Heinemann Medical Books.

Blandy, J. P., Chapman, R. H., Pollock, D. & Molland, E. (1976) The management of tumors of the testis. In *Current Controversies in Surgery* (in press).

Birkhead, B. M. & Scott, R. M. (1973) Spontaneous regression of metastatic testicular cancer. *Cancer*, **32**, 125–129.

Boden, G. & Gibb, R. (1951) Radiotherapy and testicular neoplasms. *Lancet*, **2**, 1195–1197.

Braun, E. M. & Schlang, H. A. (1970) Acanthosis nigricans associated with testicular carcinoma. *J. Amer. med. Ass.*, **211**, 660–661.

Brosman, S. & Gondos, B. (1975) Testicular tumors in children. *Reviews in Paediatric Urology*, ed. Johnston, J. H. & Goodwin, W. E., pp. 131–171. Amsterdam: Excerpta Medica; New York: American Elsevir Publishing Co.

Broth, G., Bullock, W. K. & Morrow, J. (1968) Epididymal tumors. 1. Report of 15 new cases including review of literature. 2. Histochemical study of the so-called adenomatoid tumor. *J. Urol.*, **100**, 530–536.

Bunge, R. G. & Bradbury, J. T. (1965) An early human seminoma. *J. Amer. med. Ass.*, **193**, 960–962.

Chevassu, M. (1906) *Tumeurs du testicule*, Thèse de Paris, No. 193. Steinheil.

Chiappa, S., Uslenghi, C., Galli, G., Ravasi, G. & Bonadonna, G. (1966) Lymphangiography and endolymphatic radiotherapy in testicular tumours. *Brit. J. Radiol.*, **39**, 498–572.

Clemmesen, J. (1968) A doubling in mortality from testis carcinoma in Copenhagen 1943–1962. *Acta path. microbiol. scand.*, **72**, 348–349.

Collins, D. H. & Pugh, R. C. B. (1964) Classification and frequency of testicular tumours *Brit. J. Urol.*, **36**, Suppl.

Cosgrove, M. D. & Metzger, C. K. (1975) Lymphangiography in genitourinary cancer. *J. Urol.*, **113**, 93–95.

Cutajar, C. L. (1972) Spontaneous rupture of testicular teratoma. *Brit. med. J.*, **1**, 154–155.

Dees, J. E. (1973) Metastatic embryonal cell carcinoma of testis: an apparent 8-year cure. *J. Urol.*, **110**, 90–92.

Dixon, F. J. & Moore, R. A. (1952) Tumours of the male sex organs. *Atlas of Tumor Pathology*, **VIII**, 31B, 32. Washington, DC: Armed Forces Institute of Pathology.

Earll, J. M., Newman, S. G. & DiRaimondo, V. C. (1969) Bilateral testicular tumors in untreated congenital adrenocortical hyperplasia. *J. Amer. med. Ass.*, **209**, 937–939.

Fein, R. L. & Taber, D. O. (1969) Foot lymphography in the testis tumor patient: a review of 50 cases. *Cancer*, **24**, 248–255.

Foley, J. F., Lemon, H. M., Miller, D. M. & Kessinger, A. (1972) The treatment of metastatic testicular tumors. *J. Urol.*, **108**, 439–442.

Fraley, E. (1976) The management of tumors of the testis. *Current Controversies in Urology*, Chapter 21. Philadelphia: Saunders.

Friedman, M. (1950) Tumors of testis: relation of histogenic classification to radiosensitivity and prognosis. *Proc. New York Path. Soc.*, 27th April 1950, pp. 33–41.

Goldstein, D. P. & Piro, J. (1972) Combination chemotherapy in the treatment of germ cell tumors containing choriocarcinoma in males and females. *Surg. Gynec. Obstet*, **134**, 61–66.

Gulley, R. M., Kowalski, R. & Neuhoff, C. F. (1974) Familial occurrence of testicular neoplasms: a case report. *J. Urol.*, **112**, 620–622.

Herr, H. W., Silber, I. & Martin, D. C. (1973) Management of inguinal lymph nodes in patients with testicular tumors following orchiopexy, inguinal or scrotal operations. *J. Urol.*, **110**, 223–224.

Johnson, D. E., Laneri, J. P., Mountain, C. F. & Luna, M. (1973) Extragonadal germ cell tumors. *Surgery*, **73**, 85–90.

Jonsson, K., Ingemansson, S. & Ling, L. (1973) Lymphography in patients with testicular tumours. *Brit. J. Urol.*, **45**, 548–554.

Koppikar, D. D. & Sirsat, M. V. (1973) A malignant Sertoli cell tumour of the testis. *Brit. J. Urol.*, **45**, 213–217.

Kuisk, H., Blackard, C. E., Schenk, D. C. & Panning, W. P. (1970) A method of funicular (testicular) lymphography by eliminating indicator dye. *Radiology*, **96**, 198–201.

Leb, D. E. & Howell, R. S. (1971) Carcinoma of the testis in a renal transplant recipient. *Amer. J. med. Sci.*, **262**, 171–174.

Levick L. J. & Levick S. N. (1971) Testicular choriocarcinoma in L.S.D. users: coincidence or cause? *J. Amer. med. Ass.* **217**, 475–476.

Li, F. P. & Fraumeni, J. F. (1972) Testicular cancers in children: epidemiological characteristics. *J. Nat. Cancer Inst.*, **48**, 1575–1581.

Lipworth, L. & Dayan, A. D. (1969) Rural preponderance of seminoma in England and Wales. *Cancer*, **23**, 1119–1121.

Livesay, J. E., Branch, H. E. & Eaton, W. L. (1972) Interstitial cell carcinoma of the testis: a case report. *Amer. J. Roentgenol.*, **115**, 728–731.

Maier, J. G. & Schamber, D. T. (1972) The role of lymphangiography in the diagnosis and treatment of malignant testicular tumors. *Amer. J. Roentgenol.*, **114**, 482–491.

Merrin, C., Sarcione, E., Bohne, M. & Albert, D. J. (1973) Alpha-fetoprotein in testicular tumors. *J. Surg. Res.*, **15**, 309–312.

Miller, F. & Lieberman, M. K. (1968) Local invasion in adenomatoid tumors. *Cancer*, **21**, 933–939.

Miller, A. & Seljelid, R. (1971) Histological classification and natural history of malignant testis tumors in Norway 1959–1963. *Cancer*, **28**, 1054–1062.

Mostofi, F. K. & Price, E. B. (1973) Tumors of the male genital system. *Atlas of Tumor Pathology*, 2nd Series, Fascicle 8. Washington, DC: United States Armed Forces Institute of Pathology.

Nicholson, T. C., Walsh, P. C. & Rotner, M. B. (1974) Lymphadenectomy combined with preoperative and postoperative cobalt 60 teletherapy in the management of embryonal carcinoma and teratocarcinoma of the testis. *J. Urol.*, **112**, 109–110.

Patton, J. F., Seitzman, D. N. & Zone, R. A. (1960) Diagnosis and treatment of testicular tumors. *Amer. J. Surg.*, **99**, 525–532.

Peckham, M. (1975) Personal communication.

Pott, P. (1779) *The Chirurgical Works of Percivall Pott*. London: Lowndes et al.

Price, E. B. (1971) Papillary cystadenoma of the epididymis: a clinico-pathologic analysis of 20 cases. *Arch. Path.*, **91**, 456–470.

Pugh, R. C. B. (1976) *Pathology of the Testis*. Oxford: Blackwell Scientific.

Reyes, F. I. & Faiman, C. (1973) Development of a testicular tumor during cis-clomiphene therapy. *Canad. med. Ass. J.*, **109**, 502.

Roe, F. J. C. (1964) Cadmium neoplasia: testicular atrophy and Leydig cell hyperplasia and neoplasia in rats and mice following the subcutaneous injection of cadmium salts. *Brit. J. Cancer*, **18**, 674–681.

Rubin, S. O. (1973) Malignant teratoma of testis in a subfertile man treated with HCG and HMG. *Scand. J. Urol. Nephrol.*, **7**, 81–84.

Scobie, W. G. (1970) Orchioblastoma: a report of 6 cases. *Brit. J. Urol.*, **42**, 332–335.

Shakkebaek, N. E. (1972) Possible carcinoma-in-situ of the testis. *Lancet*, **2**, 516–517.

Sherman, F. P., Ciaverra, V. A. & Cohen, M. J. (1973) Testis tumors in Negroes. *Urology*, **2**, 318–320.

Silber, S. J., Cittan, S. & Friedlander, G. (1972) Testicular neoplasm in father and son. *J. Urol.*, **108**, 889.

Skinner, D. G. & Leadbetter, W. F. (1971) Surgical management of testis tumors. *J. Urol.*, **106**, 84–93.

Smithers, D. W. (1972) Chemotherapy for metastatic teratomas of the testis. *Brit. J. Urol.*, **44**, 217–228.

Staubitz, W. J., Early, K. S., Magoss, I. V. & Murphy, G. P. (1974) Surgical management of testis tumor. *J. Urol.*, **111**, 205–207.

Stephen, R. A. (1958) Malignant testicular tumours. *Ann. Roy. Coll. Surg. Engl.*, **23**, 71–88.

Talerman, A. (1974) Yolk sac tumor associated with seminoma of the testis in adults. *Cancer*, **33**, 1468–1473.

Tavel, F. R., Osius, T. G., Parker, J. W., Goodfriend, R. B., McGonigle, D. J., Jassie, M. P., Simmons, E. L., Tobenkin, M. I. & Schulte, J. W. (1963) Retroperitoneal node dissection. *J. Urol.*, **89**, 241–245.

Thomas, H. (1972) Testicular tumours. *Brit. J. Urol.*, **44**, 124.

Utley, W. F. & Goldstein, A. M. (1972) An unselected series of patients with testicular tumours—results of treatment of 100 cases. *Brit. J. Urol.*, **44**, 124.

Utley, W. F. & Donohue, P. (1974) *Torsion of the Testis* (in press).

Utz, D. C. & Buscemi, M. F. (1971) Extragonadal testicular tumors. *J. Urol.*, **105**, 271–274.

Walsh, P., Kaufman, J. J., Coulson, W. F. & Goodwin, W. E. (1971) Retroperitoneal lymphadenectomy for testicular tumors. *J. Amer. med. Ass.*, **217**, 1953–1966.

Watkins, G. L. (1970) Massive haemoperitoneum resulting from rupture of a seminoma in an undescended testis. *J. Urol.*, **103**, 447–448.

Whitaker, R. H. (1970) The management of the undescended testicle. *Brit. J. Hosp. Med.*, **4**, 25–37.

Whitaker, R. H. (1975) Cryptorchidism and testicular cancer. Presented at Association of Surgeons, Annual Meeting. Cardiff.

Whitmore, W. F. (1973) La chimiothérapie dans les tumeurs du testicule. *XVIe Congrès de la Société Internationale d'Urologie*, Tome 2 (2), p. 485.

Wilkinson, E. J. & Hause, L. (1974) Probability in lymph node sectioning. *Cancer*, **33**, 1269–1274.

Williams, G. B. & Banerjee, R. (1969) Paratesticular tumours. *Brit. J. Urol.*, **41**, 332–339.

Willis, G. W. & Hajdu, S. I. (1973) Histologically benign teratoid metastasis of testicular embryonal carcinoma. *Amer. J. Clin. Path.*, **59**, 338–343.

12
NEW DEVELOPMENTS IN IMMUNOPATHOLOGY

J. L. Turk J. E. Castro

The 'specific adaptive immune response' is a reaction found in vertebrates for the recognition and rejection of foreign macromolecules. Whether this has been developed in phylogeny primarily as an adaptation for the more efficient elimination of infecting microorganisms, or whether it occurs as a reaction to invasive metastasising tumours has not yet been determined. However, much of the response as seen in man can be found in fishes as primitive as the lamprey, and these are amongst the more primitive creatures that have been found to develop tumours. Although invertebrates can distinguish between 'self' and 'not self', the type of recognition involved may be quite distinct from that in higher vertebrates. In certain invertebrates lethal factors are present all the time and these creatures protect themselves by a process of 'self recognition' involving the neutralisation of these lethal factors (Acton, 1974). There is also a suggestion that non-specific mediators such as the complement system and lymphokines may have evolved quite early in evolution. A primitive form of cell-mediated immunity as evidenced by specific allograft rejection has now been demonstrated in at least two types of advanced invertebrates, annelids and echinoderms (Uhlenbruck, 1974). However, immunological memory and classical immunoglobulin (IgM) production appear to be a particular characteristic first found in primitive fishes. Lymphocytes responding to phytohaemagglutinin in the same way as mammalian T-lymphocytes are found in protochordates (Cooper and du Pasquier, 1974). As there has been a consistent failure to observe tumorigenesis and cancer in invertebrates, it is generally thought now that the earliest form of immune response was an antiparasitic function rather than an immunosurveillance mechanism against cancer (Uhlenbruck, 1974).

Self and not self

All immune responses involve a mechanism of specific recognition of antigen followed by its rejection, mediated through the population of cells commonly called 'lymphocytes'. However, the term lymphocyte and its particular morphological appearance gives little indication of the complex activity of this cell type. An immune response can be thought of as having three phases which are best demonstrated in graft rejection, but which are common to all immune responses whether the end result is cell-mediated immunity or the production and action of humoral antibody in the periphery. These three phases are those of (1) recognition, (2) amplification by proliferation of specifically activated lymphocytes, and (3) rejection. The means by which a lymphocyte recognises a foreign antigen as being 'not self' as opposed to 'self' is poorly understood. There is, however, no doubt that the difference between 'self' and 'not self' may depend on very small differences in the chemical nature of a molecule. It has long been recognised that the covalent linkage of a simple chemical group or hapten to a 'self' molecule is enough to allow it to be recognised as 'not self'. These molecules need be no larger than the dinitrophenyl group. However, even the binding of simple metals such as nickel or mercury may be all that is needed. It has been suggested in the past that at least one lymphocyte capable of recognising each possible foreign grouping is present in the body and it is the switching on and stimulation of proliferation of such lymphocytes, when they recognise the foreign antigen, that constitutes the fundamental basis of an immune response. However, such a unidirectional hypothesis can no longer be accepted as the only view.

JARGON BOX

Noun	*Adjective*	*Meaning*
Autograft	autochthonous	Graft from individual to himself
Syngeneic homograft	syngeneic	Graft within genetically identical inbred strains of animals or identical twins
Allogeneic homograft or allograft	allogeneic	Graft within same species, however between genetically different individuals
Xenograft	xenogeneic	Graft between animals of different species

As will be discussed later, the demonstration of positive suppression by 'suppressor' lymphocytes indicates that an immune response might be stimulated as much by the *switching off* of suppressor cell activity as by the switching on of a specific population of effector cells. Such a concept would be more in keeping with the more primitive forms of immune response described above. The recognition of 'self' need not be the result of 'tolerance' due to the elimination of a potentially destructive clone of cells, but to the generation of a population of specific suppressor cells during embryonic development. The concept of a balance between effector and suppressor elements as a means of homeostasis in the immune response may be vital in the protection of self antigens from immune rejection. However, whether the specific proliferation of lymphocytes in an immune response is the result of switching off of a positive suppression or the result of the direct stimulation of the cells to pro-liferation, the effect must be triggered by a chemical reaction involving the recognition of the antigen as 'self' or 'not self'. This must involve a specific recognition molecule. Although the chemical nature of the specific recognition site and the frequency of its presence in a random population of lymphocytes has not yet been determined, a considerable amount of knowledge is accumulating about the genetic control of its appearance. Much of this information in man has been derived from a study of lymphocyte activating determinants in the mixed lymphocyte reaction and a comparison of its inheritance with that of histocompatibility antigens. Over the last few years it has been possible to map some of the genes controlling the major histocompatibility systems in both the mouse and in man (Festenstein and Demant, 1974). It has been found that the lymphocyte activating determinants in man or immune response (Ir) genes in mice are frequently linked to those genes that result in the antigenic expression of histocompatibility.

So far we have considered immunological mechanisms within the context of their protective function. However, a major aspect of immunological action is related to tissue damage that occurs during or as a result of the immune response. Terms such as hypersensitivity reaction and allergy are used to describe these phenomena. One might define an allergic or hypersensitivity phenomenon as 'local tissue damage occurring in tissues at the site of rejection or attempted rejection of that which is *not self*, due to the release of non-specific pharmacological agents'. An example of this is the delayed hypersensitivity reaction to mycobacterial protein that occurs during rejection of tubercle bacilli in the immune individual which is caused by the local release of non-specific 'lymphokines' into the tissues. These agents are primarily released in the activation of macrophages to eliminate invading mycobacteria. However, their release into the surrounding tissues produces a strong local inflammation. A similar phenomenon occurs in hypersensitivity to pollens where IgE reaginic antibody reacting with the pollen antigen results in degranulation of mast cells and the local release of histamine and similar vasoactive agents into the surrounding tissues. The local anaphylaxis that develops will manifest itself in the upper respiratory tract as hay fever and bronchial asthma.

THE CONTROL OF SPECIFIC IMMUNE RESPONSE

In syngeneic animals the ability to recognise antigens as immunogens is governed by the product of individual dominant genes termed immune response (Ir) genes. Mouse strains (McDevitt and Chinitz, 1969) possessing the relevant Ir genes always produce cellular and humoral responses against the determinants of the appropriate antigens. The most useful antigens for identification of Ir genes in mice are (1) synthetic polypeptides of restricted structural heterogeneity, (2) alloantigens with only slight differences from their appropriate autologous antigens, and (3) low doses of multideterminant antigens that only express more immunogenic determinants at the low dose.

Ir genes are in close relationship to genes controlling major histocompatibility specificities and mixed lymphocyte reactivity (MLR) (McDevitt and Benacerraf, 1969; Benacerraf and McDevitt, 1972). In mice (McDevitt et al, 1972) the major histocompatibility locus has been subdivided into four regions—K, I, S and D. The I region is located between I and D and by analysis with recombinants it has been subdivided into three subregions Ir-IA, Ir-IB and IC (Shreffler and David, 1975). Originally by genetic engineering experiments and more recently by antisera to Ia, many Ir genes have been shown to be located in Ir-IA or Ir-IB but other Ir genes cannot be distinguished from the K region. It has also been suggested that regions exist for MLR-r (mixed lymphocyte reaction responder), MLR-S (stimulator) which may be IA itself, ECS (effector cell stimulator) which may be IC and LADS (lymphocyte activity determinants) which may be situated between S and D regions. These observations in mice apply to other species studies, particularly rhesus monkeys (Balner et al, 1973) where Ir genes have been shown to control the response to the linear copolymer of glutamyl alanine or dinitrophenyl conjugate of glutamyl lysine (Dorf et al, 1974). Such data are interesting because of the phylogenetic relationship to man.

There is little doubt that Ir gene products are expressed on some T cells (McDevitt and Benacerraf, 1969) for Ir genes are necessary for development of cellular immunity to specified antigens and it has been shown that they are also concerned with the recognition and response to the carrier portion of hapten:carrier conjugates. Furthermore, animals that are unable to mount a response to a particular antigen because they lack the appropriate Ir gene may still form antibodies against determinants on that antigen when immunised with the antigen bound to an immunogenic carrier (Kapp, Pierce and Benacerraf, 1973) to which its helper T cells are able to respond and tetra-parental mice from responders and non-responders behave as responders. Although non-responder mice are unable to stimulate cell-mediated and helper cell responses to a particular antigen, they can stimulate specific T suppressor cells (Gershon, Maurer and Merryman, 1973). Whether this is a generalised phenomenon is not clear; if so it has considerable implications for how Ir genes work and could influence immunological responses in the direction of either immunogenicity or tolerance. Because of this, Ir gene products may play a significant role in the pathogenesis of conditions which involve immune responses. Already Ir genes have been shown to influence the response to tumour specific antigens (Lilly and Pincus, 1973; Sato et al, 1973) and to influence development of autoimmune thyroiditis in mice (Vladiatiu and Rose, 1974). They also influence the manifestations of experimental allergic encephalitis in rats (Williams and Moore, 1973), lymphocytic choriomeningitis in mice (Oldstone, Mitchell and McDevitt, 1973) and allergies to ragweed antigen (Levine, Sternber and Fotino, 1972). In humans preliminary evidence suggests that multiple sclerosis (Jersild et al, 1973) and ragweed pollenosis (Blumenthal et al, 1974) may be influenced by Ir.

The expression of Ir gene products on B cells is a matter for debate (Shearer, Mozes and Sela, 1972) but it has been suggested that the Ia is on B cells but not T cells, on foetal but not adult livers, on epidermis and sperms but not erythrocytes or platelets. It has been clearly shown that Ir products are not expressed on macrophages. It is possible that one or more of the multiple I region specificities might be concerned with cell interactions between T cells, B cells and macrophages.

Recently presumed Ia antibodies have been prepared in rats and their effects on allograft survival studied (Dawes, 1974). Administration of such antibodies, in this species, caused indefinite survival of auxillary heart allografts instead of the 8 to 12 days in untreated control rats. In humans similar sera prolonged skin graft survival in HLA identical, MLR different combinations.

SPECIFIC HOMEOSTASIS OF THE IMMUNE RESPONSE—NEW IDEAS ON IMMUNOLOGICAL TOLERANCE

The concept of a series of specific checks and balances in the immune response has been crystallising over the last few years as a result of the accumulation of information from a number of different sources. However, much of our recent knowledge has developed from a reassessment of the mechanism of immunological unresponsiveness, as a result of increasing dissatisfaction with currently held hypotheses. Clarification of the status of certain immunological phenomena that did not conform to current dogma has added to a new reassessment of the immune response. This approach has been simplified by the identification of different populations of lymphocytes capable of interaction at varying levels in the immune response.

The division of the immune response into two distinct mechanisms, those mediated by humoral antibody and the cell-mediated immune response, is fundamental to any understanding of immunological mechanisms. An awareness that certain immunological mechanisms were not mediated by antibody was slow in developing. Although this concept was inherent in the work of Römer and Joseph (1910) on immunisation in tuberculosis, it was not until 1925 that Zinsser and Mueller separated the 'bacterial allergies' from 'anaphylactic reactions', suggesting that the former were mediated by some mechanism other than serum antibody. The passive transfer of contact sensitivity and later the tuberculin reaction by mononuclear cell suspensions (Landsteiner and Chase, 1942; Chase, 1945), indicated the possible function of the lymphocyte as the specific mediator of these reactions, playing a role equivalent to the immunoglobulin molecule in antibody-mediated reactions. The implication of a similar mechanism in skin allograft rejection (Billingham, Brent and Medawar, 1954) showed the unforeseen importance of cell-mediated immunity equal to that of humoral antibody. This was confirmed by the demonstration of a similar process underlying allogeneic tumour graft rejection (Mitchison, 1953).

Throughout these early studies immunity, whether cell-mediated or due to antibody, was always considered as a positive unidirectional force in which the effector mechanism showed a narrow specificity for the antigen determining site. The only difference in specificity that could be detected between the two types of immune reaction was an indication that the lymphocyte receptor might react with a broader determining group on the antigen than the antigen recognition site of the immunoglobulin molecule. In certain states this would include part of the carrier molecule as well as the smaller surface chemical group or hapten. This produced a situation referred to as 'carrier specificity'.

Immunological tolerance and enhancement

An interest in the negative aspect of the immune response was stimulated by the experiments of Billingham, Brent and Medawar (1953) when they demonstrated that injection of allogeneic cells into neonatal mice would induce a state of 'immunological tolerance' to a skin graft from a donor of the same strain. A similar state of unresponsiveness had been induced earlier in adult guinea-pigs to 2,4-dinitrochlorobenzene by giving the sensitiser by mouth (Chase, 1946). At that time there was much interest in the clonal hypothesis of the immune response and it was accepted that immunological tolerance occurred as a result of elimination of reactive clones by the high dose of antigen administered. The greater complexity of immunological tolerance was recognised when it was found that unresponsiveness might also be induced in an animal by doses of antigen lower than the optimum for immunisation as well as doses above the optimum. This led to the concept of 'low dose tolerance' as well as that of 'high dose tolerance' (Mitchison, 1964). In all these studies immunological unresponsiveness was considered as a negative phenomenon in which there was an elimination of potentially reactive cells.

The concept of immunological 'unresponsiveness' as a positive force, as positive as immunological 'responsiveness', developed in the field of tumour immunology as a result of a study of the phenomenon known as 'immunological enhancement'. In this, the term 'enhancement' refers to 'enhancement of tumour growth' as a result of diminution of the effectiveness of the immune response in controlling tumour growth. The initial observation was that syngeneic tumour grafts that had been in contact with specific antisera showed enhanced growth and were protected from the host's immunological response directed against them. Enhancement could also be induced by injection of the antiserum directly into the host or by active immunisation of the host with a tumour extract before tumour transplantation. The antibody was considered to modify the graft in such a way that it was no longer susceptible to the homograft reaction (Kaliss, 1958). It was later suggested that the effect of antibody might also be to inhibit the immune response directed against the tumour and to lower the proportion of lymphocytes that could have an inhibitory effect on the tumour (Snell, 1963). Hellström, Hellström and Allison (1971) considered the possibility that a mechanism similar to immunological enhancement might be involved in mice made

tolerant to skin allografts following neonatal injection of allogeneic lymphocytes. They demonstrated that such mice had lymphocytes which were
specifically cytotoxic in vitro to target cells of the strain to which they were
tolerant and that these were specifically inhibited by serum from the same
animals. This indicated the possibility that tolerance in these animals was
maintained by the presence of either an enhancing antibody or immune
complexes in the circulation that might specifically block cell-mediated
allograft rejection. The concept that immunological enhancement was due
to a block of cell-mediated immunity by circulating immune complexes
formed between antibody and soluble antigen derived from the graft, was
introduced by Sjögren et al (1971) who demonstrated that the blocking
activity of serum was due to immune complexes rather than just antibody
alone, and Baldwin, Price and Robbins (1972) who demonstrated the
lymphocyte blocking activity of immune complexes formed at equivalence in
vitro.

These studies were the first to indicate a modulating effect of one form of
the immune response on another. In this case there was a modulating effect
of aspects of the humoral antibody response on aspects of the cell-mediated
immune response.

B and T-lymphocytes

Further progress in this field depended on the definition of different
populations of lymphocytes and an analysis of their role in the different
immunological responses. The first steps in this direction was the demonstration of the role of the thymus in the control of skin graft rejection in mice
(Miller, 1961) and the role of the bursa of Fabricius in controlling antibody
production in the chicken (Glick, Chang and Jaap, 1956). Subsequently it
became increasingly obvious that lymphocytes were divided into two main
classes, T-lymphocytes which were thymus dependent and gave rise to the
effector cells in cell-mediated immunity, and B-lymphocytes which were
dependent on the integrity of the bursa in the chicken and were precursors
of plasma cells in mammals as well as the chicken (Roitt et al, 1969). T-
lymphocytes can be distinguished from B-lymphocytes by the receptors
on their cell membranes. Thus T-lymphocytes in mice have a specific antigen,
the θ-antigen, on their surface and form spontaneous rosettes with sheep
erythrocytes; B-lymphocytes carry easily detectable immunoglobulin on the
cell membrane and have receptors for the Fc fragment of the immunoglobulin
molecule as well as for complement. T-lymphocytes and B-lymphocytes
are found in distinct areas of lymphoid tissue. T-lymphocytes are specifically
depleted from their specific areas in neonatally thymectomised animals and
those treated with antilymphocyte serum. Both these procedures have little
effect on the B-lymphocyte population.

In addition to T-cells being the effector cells in cell-mediated immunity,
cooperation between T-lymphocytes and B-lymphocytes is necessary for full

expression of B-lymphocyte function. Maximum antibody production towards certain antigens is only obtained if there is a parallel T-lymphocyte response to the same antigen or in the case of a hapten–protein complex to the carrier protein. The exact mechanism of T-cell/B-cell cooperation is poorly understood but involves the release of a specific humoral factor resembling an immunoglobulin molecule and the cooperation of an intermediate cell, probably a macrophage. Evidence is accumulating to suggest that the T-lymphocytes which cooperate with B-lymphocytes are a different population from those that form the effector cells of cell-mediated immunity.

The cooperative effect of T-cell function on B-cell antibody production contrasts with the suppressive effect of B-cell derived antibody on T-cell function as shown in the phenomenon of immunological enhancement. These may both be considered as examples of the specific regulatory effect of the one lymphocyte subpopulation on the other. However, there is increasing evidence that immunological unresponsiveness can occur as a result of T-cell action as well as B-cell action. The presence of suppressor T-cells have now been demonstrated in a number of experimental systems in which they have been shown to have a regulatory function on effector T-cell as well as B-cell function. The systems in which suppressor T-cells were studied first, include the depression of antibody response in normal mice to sheep erythrocytes (Gershon and Kondo, 1971) and prolonged allotypic suppression (Jacobson et al, 1972). Recently suppressor T-cells have been studied extensively as mediators of immunological tolerance in chemical contact sensitivity in the mouse (Asherson, Zembala and Barnes, 1971; Zembala and Asherson, 1973). In this system it was demonstrated that passive transfer of lymph node cells from mice made unresponsive to picryl chloride by multiple injections of picryl sulphonic acid, could specifically suppress the ability of normal mice to be sensitised with picryl chloride. In subsequent experiments it was shown that these suppressor cells were susceptible to antiserum prepared against the θ-antigen which was specific for T-cells (Raff, 1969), indicating that these cells were T-lymphocytes. In further experiments suppressor T-lymphocytes were shown to act by interfering with the ability of the recipients' own effector T-cells to manifest a reaction in the periphery without interfering with central T-lymphocyte proliferation. Soluble factors have now been found in supernatants and extracts of suppressor T-cells that might play a role in this inhibition of immune reactivity in vivo. These have been demonstrated for allotypic suppression of tumour rejection as well as contact sensitivity. Such immunosuppressive factors are antigen specific and of low molecular weight ($\sim 50\,000$). In the contact sensitivity model in the mouse they can be absorbed on to normal peritoneal exudate cells. However, when 'armed' these cells develop a non-specific ability to block contact sensitivity to unrelated antigens (Zembala, 1974).

In addition to the suppressive effect of enhancing antibody, B-cells can have a direct modulating effect on T-cell function. It has now been discovered that during a number of situations where animals are immunised so as to develop delayed hypersensitivity, there is not only stimulation of effector T-lymphocytes, but also a parallel stimulation of B-lymphocytes which interact with the T-cells to suppress the reaction. Initially the animals may show modified reactivity. However, later on the B-cell response may be so great as to damp down the T-cell response, so that the animal may show Arthus reactivity due to reaction of antigen with antibody, but the delayed hypersensitivity reaction may be completely suppressed. Such a situation occurs in the guinea-pig immunised with ovalbumin in Freund's incomplete adjuvant (OA/FIA) (Turk and Parker, 1973). Initially one week after immunisation the animals show a modified delayed hypersensitivity reaction (Jones–Mote hypersensitivity). After two weeks this reactivity is often completely absent. In such an experimental model it has been possible to suppress B-cell function without interfering with T-cell function. This can be achieved by taking advantage of the susceptibility of dividing cells to the drug cyclophosphamide (CY). Resting B-cells have a greater turnover rate than resting T-cells and are therefore more susceptible to CY (Turk and Poulter, 1972). It is thus possible to produce a temporary relative depletion of B-cells without affecting T-cell function. These animals fail to make antibody when immunised with OA/FIA but develop increased delayed hypersensitivity which persists for two weeks instead of being lost. Moreover, they can be returned to normal reduced reactivity by the transfusion of cell suspensions containing B-cells from normally immunised donors. However, if the B-cells are removed by passage through an anti-immunoglobulin coated column, such suspensions are inactive (Katz, Parker and Turk, 1974). Suppressor cells have been shown to act at least at two points on the immunological arc. There is no doubt that in states of immunological unresponsiveness there is central suppression of specific T-cell proliferation (Turk and Stone, 1963). However, in passive transfer studies in which suppressor cells are transfused just before skin testing, it can be shown that both suppressor T-cells (Zembala and Asherson, 1973) and suppressor B-cells (Katz et al, 1974) can act in the periphery. In these situations there may be direct competition between the receptors for antigen on suppressor cells with those on effector cells, or suppressor cells acting through intermediary cells, possibly macrophages, might produce non-specific pharmacological mediators that damp down peripheral reactivity. Similar increased delayed hypersensitivity reactions can be produced if guinea-pigs are sensitised with the contact sensitising agents 2,4-dinitrofluorobenzene or oxazolone after B-cells have been temporarily reduced by CY treatment. Similarly B-cell depleted mice have also been shown to develop stronger delayed hypersensitivity to sheep red cells (Kerkhaert, 1974; Lagrange, Mackaness and Miller, 1974).

10

Unresponsiveness

In these studies, suppressor cells were eliminated by removing a specific population of cells before stimulation of suppressor cell production. However, from the clinical point of view it would be important to disturb the balance in a situation where suppressor cell action was so strong as to inhibit immune responsiveness completely. Such a situation has been studied in at least one model of immunological tolerance, that induced to a contact sensitiser by the systemic injection or oral administration of large doses of the sensitiser, before attempted contact sensitisation (Polak and Turk, 1974; Polak, Geleick and Turk, 1975). As has been mentioned above, the injection of oral administration of massive doses of hapten produces a state in which the animal becomes completely unresponsive to further contact sensitisation. There is not only an absence of peripheral responsiveness, but it can also be shown that there is a complete inhibition of specific T-cell responsiveness in the draining lymph nodes. Two possible mechanisms exist for this suppression. In the first, there could be a complete inhibition of proliferation of potentially responsive clones of lymphocytes. One might refer to this as a process of 'negative' unresponsiveness. The second possibility is that suppressor cells act centrally to suppress effector T-cell responsiveness as well as suppressing the peripheral reactions induced by effector T-cells. One might refer to this process as one of 'positive' unresponsiveness. In such a situation unresponsiveness might be reversed if one was able to inhibit the action of suppressor cells. Experiments were designed to take advantage of the observation that cyclophosphamide (300 mg/kg) in a single dose would inhibit the action of suppressor cells as a feedback mechanism in a normal state of contact sensitivity (Turk, Parker and Poulter, 1972). It was found that animals made tolerant by intravenous injection or oral feeding of the hapten, could be induced to show contact sensitivity by giving them a single injection of cyclophosphamide (250 mg/kg) three days before attempted sensitisation. However, if the gap between the injection of CY and attempted sensitisation was prolonged to two weeks, the tolerant state persisted (Polak and Turk, 1974). Once tolerance had been broken, sensitivity persisted. It was shown, moreover, that the ability to become sensitised was associated with a return of the specific proliferative capacity of T-cells within the lymph node draining the site of application of the sensitising agent. This would indicate that the action of the drug was on a population of proliferating cells that were acting in a positive manner to suppress specific T-cell proliferation in response to antigenic stimulation. One might go on to suggest that in such a state of tolerance the action of suppressor cells normally acting as part of a feedback homeostatic mechanism, had been stimulated to such an extent that they completely inhibited normal T-cell responsiveness to antigen. The action of cyclophosphamide was to remove this check and allow normal effector T-cell responsiveness.

Such a model has therefore far-reaching importance in clinical medicine.

If one supposes that the body's defence mechanism against tumours is the proposed immunosurveillance mechanism involving cell-mediated immunity, then failure of such defence could be due to the stimulation of suppressor cells by tumour-specific soluble antigens released from the tumour. If the balance between suppressor elements and effector elements is in favour of the suppressors, tumour growth is encouraged. However, if the suppressor elements can be eliminated without affecting the effector elements, as in the above models, the body's defence mechanisms might be put into a position that they could control or eliminate the proliferating growth. At the present time the use of cyclophosphamide in this way can only be considered as a model, as it has to be used in such a dose that it is toxic to a proportion of animals treated. However, it is hoped that in time a compound might be found that can inhibit suppressor cells without affecting effector elements and without the generalised toxicity of the compounds used in these experimental models.

THE MECHANISM OF IMMUNOLOGICAL TISSUE DAMAGE

The idea that the deposition of immune complexes in the tissues might underline a number of well-known clinical conditions has only recently been generally accepted in clinical medicine. However, the concept of disease mechanisms resulting from deep-seated immunological damage has been put forward by allergists since the turn of the century. It is now recognised that in many situations allergic tissue damage may result from a process developed as a mechanism for the protection of the body from invasion by pathogenic microorganisms and the uncontrolled proliferation of neoplastic cells. However, it is a particular quirk of nature that the disease process that occurs from invasion of these microorganisms is not the result of damaging substances that they release or, as in the case of viruses, from destruction of host cells during intracellular growth. In many of these situations local tissue damage may result from the activation of enzyme pathways which in the first place are able to neutralise the invading organism, but because of their inability to distinguish between their target and surrounding tissue can damage healthy tissues either in the vicinity of their release or even at some distance.

Immunological processes consist of two phases, the recognition and the rejection of that which is foreign. The first phase is specific to the foreign substance that is recognised as being 'not self' by cells of the lymphocyte series. These cells then go through a phase of proliferation and differentiation, which is a means of amplification of the response. If the response is of T-lymphocytes, specifically sensitised lymphocytes are formed capable of reacting in a cell-mediated immune process resulting in the specific rejection of the foreign invader, generally a facultative or obligate intracellular parasite, such as a mycobacterium or a virus. In the case of a B-lymphocyte response the result of the process of cellular proliferation and differentiation is the presence of a population of plasma cells secreting specifically reactive antibodies which join and augment the circulating pool of immunoglobulins. The reaction between specifically sensitised T-lymphocytes or humoral antibody with the antigen is the only specific event in the rejection phase of the immune reaction. In the case of a cell-mediated immune response, this reaction causes the release of macrophage activating and tissue damaging factors from lymphocytes that are glycoprotein in character and referred to generally as 'lymphokines' (Dumonde et al, 1969). These lymphokines act to activate macrophages to eliminate invading organisms, but their release also results in the development of inflammatory changes in the surrounding tissues which, in the skin, can be recognised typically as those of delayed hypersensitivity (Pick et al, 1969). Such reactions are typified by a heavy infiltrate with mononuclear cells, both lymphocytes and macrophages.

The equivalent pharmacological agents released during the reaction between antibody and antigen depends on the nature of the immunoglobulin involved. If the antibody is IgE, there will be release of vasoactive amines, plasma kinins and prostaglandins, all of which are capable of producing local tissue damage of the anaphylactic type. However, if reaction is with IgG or IgM there will be activation of the complement cascade. Complement consists of a series of enzymes with their activators and inhibitors. Complement can cause both the elimination of invading organisms and also a considerable amount of local tissue damage. The key component of complement is the third component referred to as C3. This powerful agent is one of those that is chemotactic to polymorphonuclear leucocytes and also promotes the phagocytosis of microorganisms. However, it can produce tissue damage by a property referred to as anaphylatoxin. C3 can be activated through the 'classical' pathway involving C1, C4 and C2. It can also be activated by microorganisms non-specifically through an 'alternate' pathway involving the serum protein properdin bypassing C1, C4 and C2. Once C3 is activated the cascade results in the release of further chemotactic agents, and can eventually cause the death of microorganisms and tissues with which there is sufficiently close contact.

The Arthus reaction

Tissue damage can be the result of immune complex formation and complement activation locally. Such a reaction in the skin is referred to as an Arthus reaction. This is a localised area of cutaneous vasculitis surrounded by an intense infiltrate of polymorphonuclear leucocytes. In such lesions immunoglobulin and C3 may be demonstrated in the lesion, especially in relation to the damaged vessels. Immune complexes may also be formed in the circulation, and if these are in antigen excess they will tend to localise preferentially on the basement membrane of blood vessels at certain sites in the body. The association of the symptom complex of vasculitis, glomerulonephritis and arthritis with the presence of circulating immune complexes as a result of injections of foreign serum in both animals and man has been known for many years. It has frequently been referred to as 'chronic serum sickness'. More recently this symptom complex has been associated with an increasing number of different aetiological agents which include infectious organisms, drugs and autoantigens such as DNA. These conditions may occur together as in systemic lupus erythematosus, or separately. Occasionally they may be associated with myocarditis, cardiac valvulitis and uveitis, and in certain rheumatic conditions.

A number of techniques have been used to demonstrate the association of these lesions with the deposition of circulating immune complexes. These may be divided into those which demonstrate the complexes deposited at the site of tissue damage. Antigen, antibody and C3 (β_{1C} globulin) have been demonstrated mainly on the basement membrane of glomerular lesions in the kidney or as deposits in other tissues such as the skin and joints by immuno-fluorescent techniques or the use of electron microscopy. However, it is likely that if such complexes are present in the circulation, they can also deposit at the site of non-specific inflammation. This might account for the preferential localisation of arthritis in some joints rather than others. In this case immune complex deposition may exaggerate a pre-existing mild inflammation. The demonstration of antigen in these lesions is frequently more difficult than the demonstration of immunoglobulin and complement. The immune complex basis of glomerulonephritis has been demonstrated conclusively in a number of conditions including systemic lupus erythematosus, streptococcal glomerulonephritis and malarial nephrosis.

The other approach to the demonstration of immune complexes as a cause of disease has been their demonstration in the circulation. Striking success using this approach has been the demonstration by Almeida and Waterson (1969) of aggregates of hepatitis B virus antigen in the circulation using electron microscopy, and the association of these in some cases with polyarteritis nodosa (Gocke et al, 1970). The use of radioimmunoassay techniques can also allow more direct demonstration of specific antigen antibody complexes. However, in a large number of systems the presence of circulating immune complexes can only be inferred by indirect means. These generally depend on the demonstration of material in the circulation that can fix complement or the presence of reduced levels of haemolytic complement and C3 in the serum. Serum containing circulating complexes is anticomplementary and can also be shown to contain material that will precipitate in gel with the C1q component of complement (Agnello, Winchester and Kunkel, 1970).

Clinical patterns of hypersensitivity

The association of arthritis or glomerulonephritis with a number of infectious conditions is well known in clinical medicine. These include the arthritis following mumps, shigella dysentery and gonococcal infection. In certain of these conditions it can be shown that immune complex disease occurs as an association with a defect in host resistance against the infectious agent. This frequently arises where resistance depends primarily on cell-mediated immune mechanisms, as in infection with certain viruses and mycobacteria.

The condition 'erythema nodosum leprosum' that occurs in patients with lepromatous leprosy has a number of features that particularly illustrate this concept. *Mycobacterium leprae* depends on cell-mediated immune processes for its elimination. As a result, there is a spectrum of clinical manifestation depending on the degree of cell-mediated immunity manifested by the patient. In the high resistance or 'tuberculoid' form of the disease the lesions in the skin and nerves are due to an intense local delayed hypersensitivity reaction caused by the same mechanism that is effecting the elimination of the infecting organism. At the other extreme of the spectrum in 'lepromatous' leprosy there is a specific failure of cell-mediated immunity to *M. leprae*. This failure of host resistance is associated with massive proliferation of the organism within macrophages. The accumulation of these macrophages stuffed with organisms causes the typical nodular lesions of this form of the disease. Despite a failure of cell-mediated immunity there are high levels of antimycobacterial antibody in the circulation. The lesions of erythema nodosum leprosum (ENL) occur only in this form of the disease, especially within six months of the onset of sulphone therapy. At this time there is considerable disintegration of infectious organisms and release of soluble mycobacterial antigen into the circulation capable of forming immune complexes. The lesions of ENL in the skin are those of an intense necrotising vasculitis surrounded by a massive polymorphonuclear leucocyte infiltrate. Immunofluorescent techniques demonstrate granular deposits containing immunoglobulin, C3 and occasionally mycobacterial antigen in the lesions with a particular perivascular distribution (Wemambu et al, 1969). In addition, some of the patients may develop arthritis, neuritis and a severe uveitis, as well as fever and proteinuria. Occasionally there may be a dissociation between the systemic and the cutaneous manifestation of the disease. This would indicate a likelihood that the cutaneous manifestations are due to local immune complex deposition as in the Arthus reaction in experimental animals, whereas the systemic manifestations could be due to the deposition of circulating immune complexes as in chronic serum sickness or systemic lupus erythematosus. Thus in a chronic infection such as leprosy, the conditions for the development of immune complex disease are dependent on there being a failure of host resistance. A similar situation may be observed in secondary syphilis, where arthritis, uveitis and other symptoms associated with immune complex disease occur during a phase of low host resistance and heightened antibody formation (Friedmann and Turk, 1975).

However, not all immune complex diseases of infectious origin occur in situations where there is a failure of host resistance of the cell-mediated immune type. In recent studies in West Africa (Whittle et al, 1973), observations were made on the incidence of arthritis (6.6 per cent), cutaneous vasculitis (1.7 per cent) and episcleritis (0.9 per cent) following meningococcal infection in 717 patients. These complications occurred within the first 12 days of the illness, with a mean time of onset of six days for arthritis, seven days for cutaneous vasculitis and nine days for episcleritis. At these times the patients were beginning to develop a humoral antibody response in a disease where host resistance is considered to be due to antibody rather than cell-mediated immunity. Further investigation of four of these patients showed a marked fall in serum C3 levels at this and deposits of immunoglobulin and C3 were also observed in the synovial tissues and a skin biopsy.

THE IMMUNOLOGICAL BASIS OF GRANULOMA FORMATION

A granuloma may be defined as a localised area of chronic inflammation containing a predominance of cells of the macrophage–histiocyte series with or without the addition of other inflammatory cells. The macrophages are derived from circulating monocytes originating from cells in the bone marrow. Granuloma formation may be induced non-specifically by foreign bodies or localised deposits of insoluble colloidal material. In other situations granuloma formation may occur as a direct result of the toxic action of substances such as silica compounds increasing the permeability of the lysosomal membrane. Whereas the injection of antigen–antibody complexes in antigen excess induces transient acute inflammatory reaction of the Arthus type, characterised by a marked polymorphonuclear leucocyte infiltrate (Cochrane and Weigle, 1958), the injection of similar immune complexes at equivalence will give rise to local granuloma formation (Spector and Heesom, 1969). The immunological basis of granuloma formation in chronic infections has been defined in a series of experiments on the development of schistosome granulomas in mice (Warren, Domingo and Cowan, 1967; Domingo and Warren, 1967). The transformation of undifferentiated macrophages into 'epithelioid cells' in these granulomata appears to be related to the development of delayed hypersensitivity and the reaction is reduced in neonatally thymectomised animals. The non-specific reaction to plastic beads, however, is the same in thymectomised as in normal mice. The immunological basis for epithelioid cell formation is further emphasised by in vitro studies on macrophage cultures. It has been shown that in these cultures macrophages will transform into cells resembling epithelioid cells in the presence of a cell-mediated immune reaction (Blanden, 1968; Godal, Rees and Lamvik, 1971). Macrophages 'activated' in this way have an increased capacity to phagocytose and eliminate ingested microorganisms including mycobacteria. Macrophage activation in cell-mediated immunity is produced by the non-specific mediators or 'lymphokines' that are secreted by sensitised T-lymphocytes reacting with antigen. The changes observed in these cells include increases in activity of enzymes of the hexose monophosphate shunt, Krebs cycle and also lysosomal enzymes (Nathan, Karnovsky and David, 1971; Nath, Poulter and Turk, 1973). Activated macrophages can show enzyme activity twice to four times that of normal cells.

Granulomas generally occur at the site of immunological reactions in which there is delayed elimination of the irritating complex. Such granulomas are associated with marked lymphocytic infiltration as well as epithelioid changes in the macrophages. Granulomas of this type are found especially in infections with mycobacteria and similar obligate or facultative intracellular parasites. They also occur round the ova of helminths such as schistosomes. In the latter situation they can lead to fibrotic changes in organs such as the liver. Granulomas due to the deposition of inorganic substances may also be immunologically derived as in the case of those caused by zirconium, which only form in people who have been previously sensitised to the metal. However, although beryllium is a powerful sensitising agent there is no evidence that granulomas formed by this substance in the lung are due to immunological mechanisms, and are probably due to a direct toxic action similar to that which occurs in silicosis.

TUMOUR IMMUNOLOGY

The relation between tumour antigens and fetal antigens

Much of the early work on tumour antigenicity was confused because of the failure to appreciate the fact that tumours, like most other tissues, exhibit transplantation antigens. Only when autografts or syngeneic tumours are studied can consideration be given to those antigens that are characteristic of tumours. In animals this was possible after introduction of inbred mouse strains and in 1953 Foley produced the first evidence for specific antigenicity of experimental tumours, findings that were soon confirmed by others (Prehn and Main, 1957; Old and Boyse, 1964).

Experiments to demonstrate tumour-specific antigens involve a demonstration that pretreatment with a syngeneic tumour will influence the growth of a subsequent challenge with the same tumour. Pretreatment may involve ligation or excision of the initial tumour after it has reached a critical size, but before dissemination (Klein et al, 1960); injection of a low dose of cells which is too low to induce an overt tumour, or injection of tumour cells that have been treated chemically or physically to prevent growth and division. If pretreatment alters the growth of an inoculation of tumour cells that would normally initiate an overt tumour in a non-treated recipient, then such pretreatment has caused an immune response to the characteristic antigens of the tumour. If pretreatment alters the growth of a tumour which is different from the one used for pretreatment, then cross reactivity between the tumours used for pretreatment and challenge is said to occur.

There are also in vitro techniques for detection of tumour antigens. Some involve the demonstration of tumour antibodies by membrane immunofluorescence (Morton et al, 1968), complement fixation (Eilber and Morton, 1970) or cytotoxicity (Bloom, 1970), whilst others demonstrate lymphocyte cytotoxicity (Hellström et al, 1971a; Currie, Lejeune and Fairley, 1971). Although antibodies to tumour antigens have been demonstrated by a variety of techniques their significance in vivo is poorly understood. Most attempts at passive transference of tumour immunity by sera have failed and in some circumstances enhancement of tumour growth occurs. There are many tests for measurement of cell-mediated immunity to tumours; the majority involve a cytotoxic assay that measures the ability of lymphocytes to lyse tumour cells or inhibit their growth but the relevance of such observations to the in vivo situation is not clear. Leukaemia cells and cultured lymphoblastic cells from patients with lymphoma, leukaemia or infective mononucleosis stimulate blastogenesis when tested against responder lymphocytes of the same donor. The blastogenic response of lymphocytes from patients with leukaemia to stimulation by leukaemia cells is of favourable clinical prognostic significance as is the presence of circulating serum factors that inhibit blastogenesis (Gutterman, Rosen and Butler, 1973). Other tests involve the action of lymphokines, which are humoral substances elaborated by specifically sensitised lymphocytes on contact with antigen (Dumonde et al, 1969). Inhibition of macrophage migration by the products of sensitised lymphocytes is one of the best studied in vitro correlates of delayed hypersensitivity (Andersen, Bjerrum and Bendixen, 1970).

The existence of tumour specific transplantation antigens against autochthonous methylcholanthrene induced sarcoma has been demonstrated by transplantation techniques (Reiner and Southam, 1967). Similar antigens have been demonstrated for tumours induced by other polycyclic hydrocarbons, other types of chemical carcinogens, irradiation and implanted cellophane (Klein, Sjögren and Klein, 1963) or millipore filters. The initial view was that these induced tumours express individually distinct neoantigens whereas the antigens on virus-induced tumours were cross-reacting. It is now known that chemically induced tumours express both individually characteristic tumour antigens and also cross-reacting antigens and there is increasing evidence that at least some of these cross-reacting antigens are phase specific or fetal antigens (Coggin, Ambrose and Anderson, 1970). The inappropriate expression of normal tissue antigens has been found in a variety of animal tumours. Examples of these phase-specific antigens are thymus-leukaemia antigen (Boyse, Old and Stockert, 1968), Gix antigen (Stockert, Old and Boyse, 1971) and fetal antigens. The TL antigen can be detected serologically on normal thymus cells from some mouse strains (TL positive) but not others (TL negative). Leukaemias developing in TL negative mice frequently carry the TL antigen and it is probable that there is a repressed structural gene coding for TL determinant which is only depressed by the malignant process. The Gix antigen is similar and occurs in the serum of rats immunised with a syngeneic virally induced tumour. It has specificity for the thymocytes of certain mouse strains.

Baldwin (Baldwin, Glaves and Pimm, 1971) have shown by immuno-fluorescence that chemically induced tumours have fetal antigens on their surface. Integral to appreciating the significance of demonstrating these fetal antigens is a demonstration that adult syngeneic animals are capable of mounting an immune response against them.

Cytotoxic tests in vitro have demonstrated that lymphocytes from tumour bearers are sensitised against fetal antigens. When fetal tissues are implanted in mice made deficient in cell-mediated immunity (Castro et al, 1974) it was observed that they grow considerably larger than in normal, immuno-logically competent adults. There is also a marked difference in the variety of histological types of tissues found in these implants; for in the normal mice identifiable tissues were limited and a lymphocyte infiltrate was found at the junction of the fetal implant with host tissue. This may be contrasted with the appearance of fetal implants in immunologically depressed mice where histological types of tissues could be identified and no infiltrate could be seen at the junction of the graft and recipient tissue. This finding, together with the observation that pretreatment with fetal tissues would modify the growth of a second fetal tissue implant, suggests that early syngeneic fetal tissues may provoke a transplantation reaction in normal mice. Parmiani and Della Porta (1973) have examined the effects of immunisation with fetal tissues in a different way. They pretreated adult mice with syngeneic adult tissues, sarcoma or fetus or with allogeneic adult tissues and observed the effects of these treatments on litter size, premature birth and viability of progeny. There was a significant reduction in the frequency of pregnancies and in the litter sizes after sarcoma or fetal tissues but not after treatments with adult tissues. It is suggested that these effects result from the induction of a specific immune cytotoxic action on embryo cells after sensitisation to fetal antigens by pretreatment with embryonic or tumour tissues.

The relationship between fetal and tumour antigens has been examined in a variety of ways (Stonehill and Benditch, 1968). In 1916, Schöne showed a relationship between immunisation with fetal tissues and growth of tumours. More recent workers, using genetically defined mice, have confirmed the relationship between fetal and tumour antigens. Most have found that pretreatment with fetal tissues protects against subsequent tumour challenge (Coggin, Ambrose and Anderson, 1971), but some have found that tumour growth is enhanced and others have found no significant effects (Buttle and Frayne, 1967). The reason for these contradictory results are not known.

It has recently been shown that embryo-immune rats are capable of limiting metastatic growth of tumours (Baldwin, unpublished). This may result because intravenous inoculation of tumour cells may facilitate direct contact with cytotoxic effect or mechanisms, or in addition, tumour cells may be unable to lodge in the lungs due to mechanisms other than those of an immunological nature.

In 1965 Gold and Freedman reported a series of studies concerned with the antigenic analysis of human adenocarcinoma of the colon. Antitumour serum was prepared in rabbits and rendered tumour specific by absorption. It was found that colon carcinomas were antigenic and a similar antigen was found in fetal gut, liver and pancreas during the first trimester. With the development of sensitive radioimmune assays similar antigens were found in the circulation of patients with colon cancers and it was hoped that this would be a useful diagnostic test. However, the test has been found to lack specificity for it is found to be positive in 73 per cent of patients with cancer of colon and rectum, 92 per cent with pancreatic cancer and 60 per cent with cancer of the liver. It is also detected in patients with non-malignant diseases, 9 per cent of patients with colonic polyps, 21 per cent with colonic inflammation, 42 per cent with cirrhosis and 53 per cent with acute pancreatitis. The most useful aspects of measurement of carcinoembryonic antigen at present is in the early detection of recurrent tumour (Laurence and Neville, 1972; MacSween et al, 1972).

There are many other fetal antigens and alpha-fetoprotein is one which is probably more tumour specific. This protein is found in 31 to 78 per cent of the sera of patients with carcinomas, 80 per cent with testicular tumours, 22 per cent with pancreatic carcinomas and 17 per cent with gastric cancers. The level does not appear to be raised in patients with inflammatory diseases (Laurence and Neville, 1972).

Viral antigens

The tumour specific transplantation antigens of tumours induced by both DNA and RNA viruses is the same for all tumours induced by a single virus, but differs in tumours induced by different viruses.

Tumours induced by DNA viruses (polyoma, SV 40, adenoviruses 3, 7, 12, 18 and 31, etc.) have similar immunological findings. These viruses induce neoplasms in vivo or in vitro which do not then produce infectious virus. Tumours induced by DNA virus have three neoantigens. Tumour specific transplantation antigens, which are cell surface antigens, T antigens which are first detected in the nucleus and persist in the malignant cell. Both these may be detected by serological methods and can be differentiated from the third group of neoantigens, the complement-fixing viral particle antigens, by physical and immunological maneouvres (Black et al, 1963; Daphendi, Ephrussi and Koprowski, 1964). Furthermore with the exception of adenovirus 12, tumours without demonstrable infective virus do not elicit the production of viral antibodies (Heubner et al, 1964).

RNA viruses (mouse leukaemia virus, chicken sarcoma virus, Bittner virus) differ considerably from DNA viruses, both in structure and manner of replication. Unlike the DNA viruses there is continued production of infectious RNA viruses in most neoplasms induced by them. It is, therefore, difficult to distinguish between tumour specific antigens and viral antigens.

Most if not all autochthonous human tumours may be demonstrated to be antigenic, for instance by the use of a variety of techniques, antibodies have been demonstrated against malignant melanoma (Lewis et al, 1969), osteosarcoma (Morton et al, 1968), Burkitt's lymphoma (Klein et al, 1963) and adenocarcinoma of the colon, lung, lip and breast amongst others (Hellström et al, 1966).

Immunosurveillance

Immunosurveillance as a mechanism for control of cancer was suggested by Green in 1954 and elaborated by Burnet (1970) thus, 'A major function of the immunological mechanism is to recognise and eliminate foreign patterns of behaviour arising in the body by somatic mutation or some other equivalent process'. This concept suggests that a mutant cell, which is potentially responsible for overt tumour development, has at least one antigen with a biochemical sequence differing from that normally found in the host. An immunological response is, therefore, mounted against this antigen and if there is sufficient of it, a clone of immunologically competent cells appears and eliminates the abnormal mutants.

There is general agreement that some form of surveillance occurs continuously but the points of debate are whether or not the surveillance mechanism requires immunological rejection rather than elimination by non-immunological mechanisms and whether it has specificity. There is evidence both for and against these contentions. For example, the effect on tumour induction and growth, of manoeuvres that suppress cell mediated immunity have been studied. Nehlsen (1971) gave a group of mice long-term rabbit antimouse antithymocyte serum (ATS). She found the incidence of tumours after this treatment was not increased but when mice given ATS were exposed to an oncogenic virus (polyoma) the incidence of tumour was very high compared with appropriate controls. There are some exceptions to the association of increased tumour incidence with immunosuppression. A decreased incidence of tumours induced by mammary tumour virus has been observed following neonatal thymectomy. In addition, the low incidence of papillomas induced by the Shope papilloma virus was not increased by immunosuppression. Balner and Dersjant (1969) have reported similar results, for mice given ATS alone developed no more tumours than the control untreated mice whereas those given ATS and a chemical carcinogen developed more tumours and at an earlier time than mice given carcinogen alone. Generally it has been difficult to facilitate the induction of tumours by chemical carcinogens after immunosuppression but this may be related to the immunosuppressive effects of the oncogenic drugs themselves.

The finding that mice deprived of cell mediated immunity and exposed to an oncogenic agent develop more tumours is evidence in favour of immuno-surveillance. However, the observation that immunosuppressed mice do not have more tumours than untreated mice is evidence against the theory.

In human patients taking immunosuppressive drugs after renal transplanta-tion there is an increased incidence of tumours. Penn (1975) reported an overall corrected incidence of 5.6 per cent compared with an incidence of 0.058 per cent for a normal age-matched population. The distribution of the histological types of these tumours is markedly different from that found in the normal population for nearly 50 per cent of the tumours were mesenchymal in origin and many of these were reticulum cell sarcomas. This abnormal distribution of tumours suggests that the mechanisms operating in immuno-suppressed patients may be different from those involved in oncogenesis in the normal population. The finding may be partially explained by the suggestion that some of the agents used for immunosuppression are them-selves oncogenic, that immunosuppressed patients are subject to opportunist viral infections (some of which may be oncogenic) or the antigen drive of allogenic transplanted organs may contribute to the development of tumours, particularly lymphomas or reticulum cell sarcomas (Hoover and Fraumeni, 1973).

The importance of host resistance to tumours has been demonstrated in other ways. Stimulation of immune reactivity by specific immunisation or non-specific immunopotentiation causes a decreased incidence of tumours (Castro, 1974a, b) and prolongation of their induction time after infection with some oncogenic viruses. However, attempts to prevent chemical carcino-genesis by immunological means have failed. Complementary evidence for the importance of host resistance comes from the relationship between congenital or acquired immunodeficiency disease and tumour development (Gatti and Good, 1970; Good and Finstead, 1969).

There is an increased incidence of both lymphoreticular and solid tumours in these diseases but particularly those like ataxia telangectasia or the Wiskott–Aldrich syndrome that affect cell mediated immunity (Fialkow, 1967). There is also an increased incidence of tumours at the extremes of life and a relative decrease of immunity has been documented in ageing animals and humans.

Circumstantial evidence for the importance of immunity against human tumours comes from the occasional cases of spontaneous regression of primary tumours that occurs and the regression of metastases that rarely occurs after excision of the primary tumour (Everson and Cole, 1966). The difference between the reported incidence of clinical tumours and the higher incidence found unexpectedly during postmortem suggests that people are developing tumours that regress. The frequent infiltration of tumours by lymphocytes (Black, Opler and Speer, 1954; Lukes, 1964) and demonstration of immuno-logical reactivity by in vitro tests is further evidence of an immunological response against human tumours.

Stimulation of tumour growth by the immune response

Recently Prehn (1972) has suggested that stimulation of the immune response may stimulate tumours to develop. Although specific immune reactivity may sometimes be adequate to control a neoplasm, lesser degrees of immune reactivity may promote growth of latent tumours. If the immunological response to tumours is biphasic in this way a similar reaction would be expected with other immunological reactions. A possible example has been reported with respect to the parasite *Plasmodium berghei* infection in mice (Sheagren and Monaco, 1969). It has been found that antilymphocyte serum decreased the number of parasites and prolonged the life of infected hosts but only in situations where there was little natural resistance. In mouse strains with more immunity antilymphocyte serum shortens life from this same infection. These data are similar to the situation with mouse mammary tumours (Prehn, 1971). C_3H mouse mammary tumour produced by milk agent is quite immunogenic when grown in C_3H mice which lack the virus but when grown in a subline which contains virus it has very little immunogenicity. Attempts at immunisation against the tumour implants in virus-containing mice sometimes lead to enhanced tumour growth and irradiation or neonatal thymectomy may decrease the growth of transplants of this tumour. In the C_3H mice, in which the tumours are more immunogenic, reduction of immune capacity by thymectomy or irradiation increased tumour growth. The results could, however, be explained by alteration in the balance between blocking factors and cellular immunity. There are other data that support the immune stimulation theory. When thymectomised, x-irradiated mice were injected with various numbers of spleen cells from specifically immunised mice but mixed with a constant number of target cells, different results were obtained dependent on the proportions of the cell populations (Rosenau and Moon, 1964). Small numbers of immune spleen cells caused acceleration of tumour growth when compared with controls of non-immune spleen cells or spleen cells from animals immunised against different non-cross-reacting tumours. Large numbers of specifically immune spleen cells, however, produced inhibition of tumour growth. Such data suggests that early in the course of disease, or in situations where the immune reaction to tumour is weak, stimulation of tumour growth may occur whereas inhibition of tumour growth occurs at other times.

The in vitro experiments of Jeejeebhoy (1974) gave similar results. At early stages of tumour development when lesions were not palpable the cellular antitumour immune responses of mice were found to be capable of specifically stimulating tumour growth in vitro. However, when the tumours enlarged and were palpable, it was found that the stimulatory pattern seen early in tumour development had changed to an inhibitory one.

Escape from surveillance

That tumours develop in animals and man and grow progressively and kill the host is an all too common observation in clinical practice. If immunological surveillance exists there must be escape mechanisms by which tumours evade the control of immune responses. There are several suggested mechanisms of escape from immunological surveillance.

It is pertinent to ask whether surveillance operates selectively against some tumours or whether it is relevant to all tumours and also to question its importance in vivo. Tumours which arise spontaneously seem to be considerably less antigenic than induced ones: tumour immunologists tend to concentrate on antigenic or biologically unsuccessful tumours whereas tumour growth under natural conditions favours less antigenic or non-antigenic tumours.

Immunosurveillance may be highly efficient in destroying antigenic tumours but may be ineffective against other tumours. Evidence for the effectiveness of surveillance in vivo is limited. However, Lappé (1968) found that when mouse skin was treated with 3-methylcholanthrene and grafted on to syngeneic mice the outcome was affected by treatment of the recipient. Irradiation decreased the latent period whereas non-specific stimulation with BCG lengthened the latent period and increased the number of spontaneous regressions of these skin papillomas.

When antigenic autochthonous tumours are exposed to immunological reactions that do not entirely eliminate them, immunoresistance may develop (Hauschka et al, 1956). This diminished sensitivity to rejection may develop in the same way that bacteria develop resistance to chemotherapeutic agents, selective pressures favouring those cells expressing less antibody binding sites on their surface. It has indeed been shown by binding tests that immunoresistant cells do, in fact, show a decrease in the number of relevant antibody binding sites for each cell rather than a complete antigenic loss. Other phenotypic changes that resemble immunoresistance may develop—for example, when faced with a persistent immunological reaction the surface of the tumour cell is altered or modulates so that it is no longer expressing a configuration which will be recognised by the sensitised lymphoid cells (Boyse and Old, 1969). This was first detected in the case of the TL antigen in mice, but it has not yet been confirmed for human tumours. Another mechanism for immunoresistance is that the target molecules on the surface of tumour cells may be continuously shed into the surrounding extracellular fluid (Currie and Basham, 1972; Thomson, Steele and Alexander, 1973). The cell surface will then be comparatively immunoresistant and the locality flooded by excess antigen. Tumours which shed antigen most rapidly are presumably those of low immunogenicity and those that metastasise most rapidly.

The concept of tumours sneaking through is based on the observations of Old et al (1962). They found that medium sized inocula of antigenic tumour cells were rejected whereas large inocula and very small numbers of cells would grow progressively. The large dose of tumour cells overwhelm the immune mechanism but a small number of cells can grow to an irreversible tumour colony before an immune reaction is mounted. This may be a very important mechanism in the natural establishment of tumours and it may be that vascularisation is the time when the nascent tumour colony becomes invulnerable to immune attack.

It has been suggested by Folkmann (1974) that tumour growth occurs in two phases; the first is an avascular one whereby nutrients and waste are exchanged by simple diffusion and during this stage growth of tumours is slow. Whilst the tumour colony is still small proliferation from the host vascular system begins and most tumours are vascularised after reaching 1 to 2 mm diameter. Tumour vascularisation occurs by an ingrowth of host vascular channels into the tumour and once vascularisation is established rapid growth of the tumour occurs. In an established tumour it is mainly the vascular endothelium that is exposed to immunological attack by the host defences, but because vascularisation results from host vascular ingrowth it is recognised as 'self'.

The successful escape of tumours from surveillance can also result from changes in the host. In animals the response to various antigens has been shown to be different in different animal populations which are then designated high or low responders: a similar response may be true for tumour antigens (Zaleski and Klein, 1975). The mechanisms which effect the altered response to antigens are not clear but evidence from studies with Marek's disease in chickens, which results from horizontal infection with a herpes virus, suggest that some factors may operate through cell-mediated immunity. The clinical manifestation of the infection may be a highly malignant disease, a benign lymphoproliferative condition or no disease at all. In susceptible animals thymectomy does not increase the high incidence of malignant disease but it does increase the incidence in normally resistant chicks.

Exogenous administration of immunosuppressants can also diminish the host-immune response and the effects of this on tumour incidence has already been discussed. However, patients with tumours show a non-specific depression of immune responses or anergy (Williams and Castro, 1975). Whilst the occurrence of both cellular and humoral immunosuppression in tumour-bearing patients has some prognostic significance the mechanisms causing this immunosuppression are not clearly understood. Tumour extracts, circulating serum factors and tumour-induced ascites will cause immunological depression in vitro and in vivo and the immunosuppression is greatest when the serum or ascites are from patients showing anergy. It has also been suggested that suppressor cells may contribute to anergy. However, the central question in immunosuppression and cancer is whether subjects that develop cancer are intrinsically immunosuppressed or whether the growing tumour itself, either directly or indirectly, induces a state of immunosuppression (Castro, 1974). There is evidence for both possibilities: the finding of depressed immunological reactivity in patients with very early and in situ cancer suggest inherent immunosuppression in patients developing cancer, whilst the correlation between the stage of the disease and frequency of anergy suggests factors association with the tumour inducing immunosuppression.

Successful adaptation of tumours may be due to systemic factors which block the usual interaction of host defences and tumour cells, therefore protecting the tumour from destruction. Several serum factors have been incriminated in this inhibitory activity, blocking antibodies (Hellström et al, 1971b), antigen–antibody complexes (Baldwin and Embleton, 1971) and excess soluble antigen (Currie and Basham, 1972) have all been invoked.

Effector mechanisms of tumour destruction

It is frequently assumed that tumour immunity is simply a variant of transplantation immunity and is mediated by the same mechanisms. The data to support this assumption for tumour specific immunity are minimal and the immunological mechanisms of tumour cell destruction are not known and there is disagreement as to the relative roles of the separate components of the immunological apparatus in this process. It has not been possible to implicate any one cytotoxic mechanism in the immune elimination of tumours and different mechanisms seem to be dominant in different situations.

The importance of T lymphocytes is clear, for specifically sensitised T-lymphocytes are able to destroy tumour cells in an in vitro assay (Grant, Evans and Alexander, 1973) and in vivo. They can transfer immunity to non-immune animals and infusion of syngeneic or allogeneic immune lymphocytes into tumour-bearing animals sometimes has therapeutic effects. T-cell cytotoxic cells recognise target cell antigens and cell killing in vitro is paralleled by protection in vivo, for sensitised T-cells can be transferred to mice made deficient of T-cells by irradiation and this transfer confers protection.

There is also considerable evidence for cytotoxic cells other than T-lymphocytes (Woodruff, Dunbar and Ghaffar, 1973). For example, neonatally thymectomised rats are able to generate cytotoxic lymphocytes against Rous sarcoma antigens in the colony inhibition assay. Experiments based on studies with differential radio resistance and kinetics of cytotoxicity suggest there are several types of effector cells.

One cytotoxic mechanism is effected by thymus independent cells, now designated K-cells, which have no direct affinity for target cell antigen but they are triggered to kill by antigen bound to the target cells (MacLennon, 1972). K-cells develop independently of the thymus, they are not actively adherent to glass and they are not phagocytic. Several types of cells may be active in the assay, B-cells, polymorphonuclear cells and null cells (Greenberg et al, 1973). The antibody involved is lymphocyte-dependent antibody (LDA) and is found only in the IgG fraction and cytotoxicity is independent of complement. Because antibodies must have an intact Fc fragment it has been suggested that the Fc fragment of an IgG molecule attaches to the target cell (Larsson and Perlmann, 1972). Even in the presence of adequate numbers of antibody producing cells, antibody production is dependent upon sufficient numbers of T-helper cells. Although transfer of antibody alone will confer protection in vivo it is not clear whether this is due to collaboration with effector cells and the significance in vivo of killing by thymus-independent lymphocytes in concert with lymphocyte-dependent cytotoxic antibody has yet to be established.

A second type of serum that promotes cytotoxicity has been termed 'unblocking' serum by Bansal and Sjögren (1957). This is thought to represent the interaction of free antibody with blocking complexes. They found that serum from patients who were disease free or 'cured' seldom contained blocking activity. When such serum samples were mixed with serum samples from patients with progressive disease, which normally had blocking activity, this blocking activity was abrogated. Unblocking activity in vitro has been correlated with tumour regression in vivo (Bansal and Sjögren, 1972). The exact mechanism of unblocking is not known but there are several possible explanations. One possibility is that cytotoxic antibody in the presence of complement causes direct lysis of tumour cells. It is more likely that un-blocking serum is antitumour antibody which saturates the available antigen sites in the soluble antigen: antibody complexes and prevents interaction with immune lymphocytes. If this is the case it suggests that blocking is not due to antibody alone. The final possibility is that unblocking activity is equivalent to antibody-dependent cellular cytotoxicity. Tumour cells can be rapidly destroyed by antibodies alone in the presence of complement in in vitro systems. Lymphoma and leukaemia cella are very sensitive to such attack whereas sarcoma cells are resistant. The role of this cytotoxic mechanism is far from clear and even in vitro the culture conditions of the test are all important. In general, tumour-specific cytotoxic antibodies cannot be detected in tumour-bearing animals but in the very immunogenic lymphomas induced by the oncorna viruses antibodies can be detected in the earlier stages of tumour growth (Currie, 1973) but in chemically induced sarcomas they can never be found whilst the tumour is in situ. In some patients with human tumours, complement-dependent cytotoxic antibodies can be found in the early phases of tumour growth but disappear with extension of the disease.

Apart from a cytotoxic effect antibodies may have functions other than cytotoxicity that may be beneficial to the host. Inhibition of tumour cell growth is one action but it is often difficult to distinguish this from a slow lytic effect and its in vivo significance is not clear. Inhibition of tumour cell motility by antibody is another phenomenon easily demonstrated in vitro and if the effects are also found in vivo they could be important in limiting the local and metastatic spread of tumours (Currie and Sime, 1973).

The role of macrophages in tumour destruction is not clear, but evidence suggests a critical role in initiating and maintaining immune reactions (Feld-man and Palmer, 1971). Resistance of animals to tumour parallels reticuloendothelial phagocytic activity and during growth of transplanted syngeneic tumours there is an increased production (Baum and Fisher, 1972) and function of macrophages (Old et al, 1961) which result from changes in cellular factors rather than opsonins (Kampschmidt and Pulliam, 1972). Although stimulation of reticuloendothelial function protects against some tumours the mechanism underlying these observations is not clear. There is morphological evidence from electron microscopic studies of macrophage–lymphocyte interactions at the onset of the immune responses (Salvin, Sell and Nishio, 1971), and it is accepted that macrophages process antigens for lymphocytes (Askonas and Rhodes, 1965) but they have other functions which may be important for control of tumours. It has been shown that macrophages recovered from suitably immunised hosts are activated by contact with the tumour cells used for immunisation and after this they kill non-specifically (Evans and Alexander, 1970). Even unrelated tumour cells are unable to grow in their presence. The relationship of in vitro macrophage cytotoxicity to the tumour protection observed in vivo is complex for the interaction of macrophages with other cell types makes it difficult to establish their importance in tumour cell destruction (Unanue and Cerottini, 1970; Levis and Robbins, 1970).

There are probably many other immunological effector mechanisms that may be important: the importance of mast cells, neutrophils, immunoblasts (Hall and Morris, 1963) and other cells still remains to be elucidated.

Immunotherapy

Because most human tumours are antigenic, the central problem of immunotherapy is to make existing immunity more effective in the control of tumour growth and to this end the goal of immunological control of tumours is the potentiation or depression of the separate arms of the immune response to different degrees and at will. This goal has yet to be achieved and several approaches to immunotherapy have been tried. It may be specific, designed to cope with a particular tumour, or non-specific when the overall immunological reactivity of the host will be changed. Such treatments may be combined. Many of the approaches for specific immunotherapy are applicable to non-specific therapy dependent on whether they are directed at a specific tumour antigen or a cross-reacting antigen found on several tumours.

Specific immunotherapy can be passive (Evans et al, 1962), adoptive (Blamey, 1968) or active. In passive therapy, antiserum specific to a particular tumour may be used. In adoptive therapy donors are sensitised and cytotoxic cells transferred. For active therapy, tumour cells, or fractions of them, may be given in order to stimulate the host to produce an exaggerated response against a particular tumour antigen.

Tumour antisera may be raised in syngeneic recipients or even allogeneic and xenogeneic recipients followed by specific absorption. When antibodies are used, selective production of cytotoxic as opposed to enhancing sera is an unsolved problem, which is important both to tumour and transplantation biologists (Fuller and Winn, 1973). Several features are important in the preferential stimulation of antibodies having a particular biological function: for example, the dose of antigen used to raise antibody, its route of administration to the animal in which antibody is being raised and the time interval between priming and harvesting. In the recipient, the dosage of antibody and its route of administration are also important in obtaining biological reaction. Attempts to physically separate cytotoxic from enhancing immunoglobulins have been unsuccessful.

Despite these difficulties specific cytotoxic or cytostatic antibodies may be useful in the treatment of tumours (Smith, 1971). Carefully timed serum samples could be taken from a patient and the cytotoxicity determined in vitro. Those samples might then be used in vivo to treat residual or recurrent tumour. Alternatively, allogeneic serum from patients with histologically similar or cross-reacting tumours could be used and even xenogeneic sera specifically absorbed might be useful.

Non-specific immunotherapy may be localised to the tumour alone or generalised in the recipient as a whole. With present knowledge four non-specific immunological manoeuvres might retard tumour growth. They are:

1. Increased or improved localisation of cytotoxic or cytostatic antibodies.
2. Suppression of blocking factors.
3. More effective macrophage activity.
4. More effective cell-mediated immunity.

Cytotoxic antibodies can be stimulated against specific tumour antigens. As discussed previously some of the antigens on virus-induced tumours are cross-reacting, showing virus specificity. Antibodies raised against this virus genome might, therefore, be useful in tumours of different histological types but induced by the same virus. They might also be useful when directed against other common antigens like fetal antigens.

When antitumour antibodies are used in vivo they seem to be more effective when tumour cells are in dissociated form. The failure of antisera to destroy or inhibit established solid tumours could be a problem of antibody distribution so that the antibody and tumour cells do not make contact. Such contact could be facilitated by combining cytotoxic antibodies with pharmaceutical agents which would improve their penetration or, alternatively, by infusion or regional perfusion of the tumour. The combination of antibody administration with other immunological manipulations might facilitate tumour inhibition or destruction.

An alternative use for antitumour antibodies is to use them as vehicles for transporting antitumour agents to the tumour surface so that a high concentration of such agents is obtained at the tumour site whilst the generalised systemic side effects of the antitumour agents are minimised (Davies, Manstone and Buckham, 1974; Davies, 1974). Preliminary results reported by those using melanoma antibody linked with chlorambucil are encouraging (Ghose et al, 1967).

There are theoretically more approaches to the removal of blocking factors than stimulation of antibody formation of a particular biological class. With removal of blocking factors the normal antitumour mechanisms may be able to eliminate tumour cells. Selective suppression of those cells which are responsible for antibody production has been claimed after the use of cyclophosphamide (Turk and Poulter, 1972) and in animals antisera have been raised against antibody producing cells (Raff, Nase and Mitchison, 1971). In practice, however, use of these antisera is disappointing. Once blocking factors are present they may be removed by use of unblocking sera (see page 294), immunoabsorption, or by plasmaphoresis. Antigen–antibody complexes, if they are important, could be dissociated with the added benefit that the liberated antibody might itself be cytotoxic.

Despite the lack of knowledge on how macrophages are involved in tumour cell destruction there is considerable evidence that agents which stimulate macrophage function have powerful antitumour effects. *Corynebacterium parvum* when given intravenously or intraperitoneally, for example, increased spleen and liver size and histological examination of these organs showed enlargement was due to increased macrophages (Castro, 1974a). Concomitant with these changes resistance to animal or human tumours may develop (Woodruff and Boak, 1966; Smith and Scott, 1972). Furthermore, the anti-tumour effects of *Corynebacterium parvum* were maintained despite adult thymectomy or treatment with antilymphocyte serum, manoeuvres which inhibit cell-mediated immunity, indeed animals treated with *Corynebacterium parvum* show depression of cell-mediated immunity. Whilst not excluding the necessity of a small limiting number of cells responsible for cell-mediated immunity, these data suggest that the increased antitumour activity of mice treated with *Corynebacterium parvum* is not related to an increase of thymus processed cells (Castro, 1974b).

Despite the demonstration of antitumour activity without increase of cell-mediated immunity there is no doubt as to the importance of cell-mediated immunity in some tumour situations (Goldstein et al, 1972; Rouse, Rölling-hoff and Warner, 1972). For example, orchidectomy of male mice increased cell-mediated immunity (Castro, 1974c) and protected against the induction of tumours by oncogenic chemicals and the growth of transplanted tumours (Castro, 1974d). Other methods for stimulation of cell-mediated immunity are possible. Adoptive transfer of allogeneic lymphocytes from subjects im-munised against tumours or subjects that have undergone spontaneous or surgical cure of tumours may be used (Curtis, 1971; Sumner and Foraker, 1960) but only with limited success because of the short life-span of transferred allogeneic lymphocytes.

Transfer factor, which is a non-dialysable, non-antigenic, non-immuno-globulin extract of circulating leucocytes of 10 000 mol. wt obviates these problems (Lawrence, 1972). Administration of transfer factor in vivo converts non-sensitive recipient circulating lymphocytes to a responsive state to specific antigens including tumour antigens (Baram and Mosko, 1962). However, suitable donor sources are not readily available, it is difficult to assay and populations of cells which respond to transfer factor may not be present in the recipient. So far, reports of the use of transfer factor for treating tumours have been limited to anecdotal case reports (Levin et al, 1972; Thompson, 1971) particularly of patients with malignant melanoma (Brandes, Galton and Wiltshaw, 1971) and although some success has been claimed the specificity of transfer factor has recently been questioned. It has been suggested that it is acting as a non-specific potentiator of immune responses.

Most immunological adjuvants act on several components of the immune system (Old et al, 1961; Jurin and Tannock, 1972) but selective stimulation of cell-mediated immunity has been claimed for lentinan, a polysaccharide extracted from the edible Japanese mushroom (*Lentinus edodes*) (Chihara et al, 1970; Dresser, 1973).

Because of these difficulties in stimulating intrinsic cell-mediated responses attempts have been made to cause stimulation by altering antigenicity of tumour cells: for example, by acetoacetylation (Prager et al, 1971), enzymatic changes in the cell surface (Bekesi, Arneault, Holland, 1971) or by gluteraldehyde treatment. Sanderson and Frost (1974) have demonstrated the use of gluteraldehyde-treated cells for the induction of immunity to a methylcholanthrene-induced syngeneic mouse tumour, and found considerable protection. The incorporation of virus into tumour cells (Lindenmann and Klein, 1967; Lindenmann, 1973) is another approach to increasing tumour immunogenicity. It has been observed that mice that recover from transplantation of tumours after viral oncolysis were immune when challenged with uninfected tumour cells. It is possible that the virus used in oncolysis might act as a carrier for haptenic determinants of tumour cells and evidence for this explanation has been provided by the observation that antiviral antibody added in excess to a virus oncolysate inhibited the antitumour response. The possibility that antigens become incorporated into the virus envelope is the most easily tested explanation for adjuvanticity of viruses but it is not the only possible mechanism, for it could result from increased immunogenicity of host cell debris. Host antigens become attached to the viral proteins and the resulting molecules could carry antigenic determinants which are characteristic of the host cell in addition to the possible carrier–hapten type. Other less specific interactions are possible: effects of neuraminidase in uncovering new antigenic sites after removal of sialic acid are well established (Simmons and Rois, 1971) and also the nucleic acids of viruses themselves have adjuvant effects. Local immunostimulation, perhaps by attraction of specialised cells to critical sites, is also possible; some bacteria have been shown to act in this way (Nathanson, 1971) and it is probably also true for most viruses.

A combination of specific and non-specific therapy has been the most common approach to immunotherapy in clinical practice (Mathé, 1973). The rationale for the treatment is that non-specific adjuvants will generally boost the immune response including any reaction to specific antigens.

Immunotherapy of human cancer

An important distinction must be made between immunotherapy of established tumours and immunoprophylaxis. These two forms of treatment merge imperceptibly when immunological treatments are used as an adjunct to conventional treatments with surgery or chemotherapy to prevent recurrent disease. True immunoprophylaxis has not been practised but Rosenthal et al (1972) reported a retrospective analysis of the incidence of death from leukaemia in a population which received BCG in infancy and compared this with the leukaemia death rate in a similar population that did not receive BCG. In a retrospective study in Chicago from 1964 to 1969 one death from leukaemia was recorded from 54 414 infants aged 0 to 6 years who were vaccinated at birth, a rate of 0.31/100 000/year. In contrast 21 deaths from leukaemia were recorded in 172 986 infants who did not receive BCG. The retrospective nature of the study with the inherent problems of selection is an area of criticism in this investigation but similar results have been reported from Canada, although other studies have found no differences in leukaemia in groups receiving BCG compared with those who were not vaccinated (Cormstock, 1971; Kinlen and Pike, 1971).

Intralesional therapy

The development of an acute inflammatory reaction within or around a tumour and induced by a delayed cutaneous hypersensitivity reaction to an exogenous sensitising agent will cause regression of the effected lesion. In this way dinitrochlorobenzene can cause complete regression of basal cell carcinomas (Klein, 1969). This concept has been widely adopted and many different agents have been applied or injected into many tumour types. BCG (Morton et al, 1970) and vaccinia virus (Milton and Lane-Brown, 1966) when injected into cutaneous nodules of malignant melanoma can frequently cause rejection of the injected lesions. In all responding patients the disease was limited to the skin and subcutaneous tissues. Sequential biopsies of tumour nodules following BCG inoculation revealed tumour regression to be associated with a granulomatous mononuclear cell infiltration. Rarely, regression of uninjected distant lesions can occur.

The mechanisms of tumour regression following intralesional immunotherapy with BCG is unclear. There is probably no direct antitumour activity and the most likely explanation is that tumour cells are killed by cytotoxic factors liberated as a result of the localised inflammatory response to BCG. There is, as yet, no evidence that intralesional BCG is of any greater value than surgery, diathermy or cryosurgery.

Systemic immunotherapy

BCG has also been used for the treatment of systemic disease, despite the fact that animal experiments have failed to show a beneficial effect on solid tumours. There have been many inadequately controlled trials of BCG in established tumours. In a randomised, controlled clinical trial for treatment of acute lymphoblastic leukaemia in childhood no therapeutic effect was shown (Heyn et al, 1973; MRC, 1971). A controlled clinical trial of BCG in Burkitt's lymphoma (Ziegler and Magrath, 1973) also showed no benefit and BCG used as an adjunct to cyclophosphamide for the treatment of metastatic breast cancer conferred no additional beneficial effect (Nemato, Rosner and Dao, 1975).

In contrast BCG combined with irradiated leukaemic blast cells prolonged survival of patients with acute myeloblastic leukaemia who were in remission (Powles et al, 1973). Similar results have been reported when BCG was given without irradiated cells (Vogler and Chan, 1974). Gutterman et al (1973) reported active immunotherapy of recurrent (stages III and IV) melanoma with intradermal BCG administered by scarification. There was a significant decrease in the relapse rate and a significant improvement in survival of patients treated with Tice BCG compared with similar patients treated by surgery alone. There was only slight improvement in patients treated with Pasteur BCG. High doses of Tice BCG induced striking improvements in patients who did not show anergy. It appears that the strain of BCG used, the number of viable organisms injected, the frequency and duration of treatment and the methods of administration all affect the results of treatment with BCG. The possibilities of enhancement of tumour growth and liver granulomas resulting from treatment with BCG must always be considered.

Active immunotherapy has recently been tested as an adjunct to surgery and radiotherapy in treatment of glioblastoma multiforme (Bloom, Peckham and Richardson, 1973). There was no evidence of benefit. The use of adoptive immunotherapy has also been disappointing. Andrews et al (1967) immunised donors with tumours and then transferred thoracic duct lymphocytes into recipients with leukaemia or malignant melanoma. No beneficial therapeutic effects were observed. Nadler and Moore (1969) cross-immunised pairs of patients with tumour cells and subsequently cross-infused peripheral blood lymphocytes but on close examination there appears to be little evidence of benefit and theoretically the alloantigens of infused lymphocytes should ensure their rapid destruction.

Many other forms of immunological treatment have been used in patients with tumour. Transfer factor, Levamisole, immune RNA (Alexander and Delorme, 1971) and neuraminidase are but a few. Reports are frequently limited to anecdotal case reports and further laboratory and clinical studies are required. Generally when multiple treatments are available for a given condition the reason is that none of them is completely or uniformly effective. This is certainly the case for immunotherapy and still surgery and other conventional therapies remain the first line of treatment for patients with cancer. However, the new ideas of immunology have called into question some of the established dogma of conventional treatment. Not the least of these is the surgical approach to regional lymph nodes. It would seem at present that in the light of present knowledge there can be no justification for not treating involved lymph nodes; similarly there is no evidence to justify the removal of uninvolved nodes. However, it is not always clear, even with sophisticated diagnostic methods, whether nodes are involved. Even in this situation it is hard to justify extensive surgery unless randomised controlled clinical trials have shown a significant prolongation of survival.

It has been suggested that irradiation and chemotherapy should not be used because of their immunosuppressive effects. In the presence of a tumour mass it is most unlikely that immune response is effective and only when the tumour bulk has been reduced will immunological reactions assume importance. It is more important to kill tumour cells than to spare the immune response and once the tumour bulk is reduced immunotherapy can be expected to be most beneficial.

REFERENCES

Acton, R. T. (1974) Primitive recognition systems. *Progress in Immunology, II*, ed. Brent, L. & Holborow, J., Vol. 2, pp. 287–291. Amsterdam: North Holland Publishing Co.

Agnello, V., Winchester, R. J. & Kunkel, H. G. (1970) Precipitin reactions of the C1q component of complement with aggregated γ-globulin and immune complexes in gel-diffusion. *Immunology*, **19**, 909–919.

Alexander, P. & Delorme, E. J. (1971) The use of irradiated immune lymphoid cells for immunotherapy of primary tumours in rats. *Israeli Journal of Medical Science*, **7**, 239–245.

Almeida, J. D. & Waterson, A. P. (1969) Immune complexes in hepatitis. *Lancet*, **2**, 983–986.

Andersen, V., Bjerrum, O., Bendixen, G., Schiødt, T. & Dissing, I. (1970) Effects of autologous mammary extracts on human leukocyte migration in vitro. *International Journal of Cancer*, **5**, 357–362.

Andrews, G. A., Congdon, C. C., Edwards, C. L., Gengozian, N., Nelson, B. & Vodopick, M. (1967) Preliminary trials of clinical immunotherapy. *Cancer Research*, **27**, 2535–2541.

Asherson, G. L., Zembala, M. & Barnes, R. M. R. (1971) The mechanism of immunological unresponsiveness to picryl chloride and the possible role of antibody mediated depression. *Clinical and Experimental Immunology*, **9**, 111–121.

Askonas, B. A. & Rhodes, J. M. (1965) Immunogenicity of antigen containing ribonucleic acid preparations from macrophages. *Nature (London)*, **205**, 470–474.

Baldwin, R. W. & Embleton, M. J. (1971) Demonstration by colony inhibition methods of cellular and humoral immune reactions to tumour specific antigens associated with aminoazo-dye-induced rat hepatomas. *International Journal of Cancer*, **7**, 17–25.

Baldwin, R. W., Glaves, D. & Pimm, M. V. (1971) Tumour associated antigens as expressions of chemically induced neoplasia and their involvement in tumour–host interaction. *Progress in Immunology*, **1**, 907–914.

Baldwin, R. W., Price, M. R. & Robbins, R. A. (1972) Blocking of lymphocyte-mediated cytotoxicity for rat hepatoma cells by tumour specific antigen–antibody complexes. *Nature New Biology*, **238**, 185–187.

Balner, H. & Dersjant, H. (1969) Increased oncogenic effect of methylcholanthrene after treatment with antilymphocyte serum. *Nature (London)*, **224**, 376–378.

Balner, H., Dorf, M. E., de Groot, L. & Benacerraf, B. (1973) The histocompatibility complex of the rhesus monkey, 3. Evidence for a major M.L.R. locus and histocompatibility linked genes. *Transplantation Proceedings*, **5**, 1555–1560.

Bansal, S. C. & Sjögren, H. O. (1972) Counteractions of the blocking of cell mediated tumour immunity by inoculation of unblocking sera and splenectomy and immunotherapeutic effects on primary polyoma tumours in rats. *International Journal of Cancer*, **9**, 490–509.

Baram, P. & Mosko, M. M. (1962) Chromatography of the human tuberculin delayed type hypersensitivity transfer factor. *Journal of Allergy*, **33**, 498–506.

Baum, M. & Fisher, B. (1972) Macrophage production by the bone marrow of tumour bearing mice. *Cancer Research*, **32**, 2813–2817.

Bekesi, G., Arneault, G. St & Holland, J. P. (1971) Increased immunogenicity of leukaemic L 1210 cells after vibriocholera neurominidase. *Proceedings of the American Association for Cancer Research*, **12**, 47.

Benacerraf, B. & McDevitt, H. O. (1972) Histocompatibility linked immune response genes. *Science*, **175**, 273–279.

Billingham, R. E., Brent, L. & Medawar, P. B. (1953) Actively acquired tolerance of foreign cells. *Nature*, **172**, 603–606.

Billingham, R. E., Brent, L. & Medawar, P. B. (1954) Quantitative studies on tissue transplantation immunity. II. The origin, strength and duration of actively and adoptively acquired immunity. *Proceedings of the Royal Society, B*, **143**, 58–80.

Black, P., Opler, S. R. & Speer, F. D. (1954) Microscopic structure of gastric carcinomas and their regional lymph nodes in relation to survival. *Surgery, Gynecology and Obstetrics*, **98**, 725–734.

Black, P., Rowe, W. P., Turner, H. C. & Heubner, R. J. (1963) A specific complement fixing antigen present in SV 40 tumour and transformed cells. *Proceedings of the National Academy of Science*, **50**, 1148–1156.

Blamey, R. W. (1968) Experiments in tumour immunology. *British Journal of Surgery*, **55**, 769–771.

Blanden, R. V. (1968) Modification of macrophage function. *Journal of the Reticuloendothelial Society*, **5**, 179–202.

Bloom, E. T. (1970) Quantitative detection of cytotoxic antibodies against tumour specific antigen of murine sarcoma induced by 3-methylcholapthrane. *Journal of the National Cancer Institute*, **45**, 443–446.

Bloom, H. J. G., Peckham, M. J. & Richardson, H. E. (1973) Glioblastoma multiforme: a controlled trial to assess the value of specific active immunotherapy in patients treated by radical surgery and radiotherapy. *British Journal of Cancer*, **27**, 253–267.

Blumenthal, M. N., Amos, D. B. & Norcen, N. (1974) Genetic mapping of Ir locus in man: linkage to second locus of HLA. *Science*, **184**, 1301–1303.

Boyse, E. A. & Old, L. J. (1969) Some aspects of normal and abnormal cell surface genetics. *Annual Review of Genetics*, **3**, 270–290.

Boyse, E. A., Old, L. J., Stockert, E. (1968) Genetic origin of tumour antigens. *Cancer Research*, **28**, 1280–1287.

Brandes, L. J., Galton, D. A. G. & Wiltshaw, E. (1971) New approach to immunotherapy of melanoma. *Lancet*, **2**, 293–295.

Burnet, F. M. (1970) *Immunological Surveillance*. Oxford, London, New York, Toronto, Sydney: Pergamon Press.

Buttle, G. A. H. & Frayne, A. (1967) Effect of a previous injection of homologous embryonic tissue on the growth of certain transplantable mouse tumours. *Nature*, **215**, 1495.

Castro, J. E. (1974) Immunosuppression and cancer. *Progress in Immunology, II*, ed. Brent, L. & Holborow, J., Vol. 5, pp. 364–370. Amsterdam: North Holland Publishing Co.

Castro, J. E. (1974a) The effect of *Corynebacterium parvum* on the structure and functions of the lymphoid system in mice. *European Journal of Cancer*, **10**, 115–120.

Castro, J. E. (1974b) Antitumour effects of *Corynebacterium parvum*. *European Journal of Cancer*, **10**, 120–128.

Castro, J. E. (1974c) Orchidectomy and the immune response. II. Response of orchidectomised mice to antigens. *Proceedings Royal Society of London B*, **185**, 437–451.

Castro, J. E. (1974d) Orchidectomy and the immune response. III. The effect of orchidectomy on tumour induction and transplantation in mice. *Proceedings of the Royal Society of London, B*, **186**, 387–398.

Castro, J. E., Hunt, R., Lance, E. M. & Medawar, P. B. (1974) Implications of the fetal antigen theory for fetal transplantation. *Cancer Research*, **34**, 2055–2060.

Chase, M. W. (1945) The cellular transfer of cutaneous hypersensitivity to tuberculin. *Proceedings of the Society for Experimental Biology and Medicine, New York,* **59,** 134–135.

Chase, M. W. (1946) Inhibition of experimental drug allergy by prior feeding of the sensitising agent. *Proceedings of the Society for Experimental Biology and Medicine, New York,* **61,** 257–259.

Chihara, G., Hamuro, J., Maeda, Y. Y., Arai, F. & Fukuoka, F. (1970) Fractionation and purification of the polysaccharides with marked antitumour activity, especially lentinan, from *Lentinus edodes. Cancer Research,* **30,** 2776–2781.

Cochrane, C. G. & Weigle, W. O. (1958) The cutaneous reaction to soluble antigen–antibody complexes. *Journal of Experimental Medicine,* **108,** 591–604.

Coggin, J. H., Ambrose, K. R. & Anderson, N. G. (1970) Fetal antigen capable of inducing transplantation immunity against S.V. 40 hamster tumour cells. *Journal of Immunology,* **105,** 524–526.

Coggin, J. H., Ambrose, K. R. & Anderson, N. G. (1971) Immunisation against tumours with fetal antigens. *Proceedings of the First Conference and Workshop on Embryonic and Fetal Antigens in Cancer,* Oak Ridge National Laboratory, Oak Ridge, Tennessee, 24th–26th May 1971, pp. 185–202 U. SAEC Teport Conference 710527.

Comstock, G. W. (1971) Leukaemia and B.C.G. *Lancet,* **2,** 1062–1063.

Cooper, E. L. & du Pasquier, L. (1974) Primitive vertebrate immunology, *Progress in Immunology, II,* ed. Brent, L. & Holborow, J., Vol. 2, pp. 297–301. Amsterdam: North Holland Publishing Co.

Currie, G. A. (1973) The role of circulating antigen as an inhibitor of tumour immunity in man. *British Journal of Cancer,* **28,** Suppl. 1, 153–161.

Currie, G. A. & Basham, C. (1972) Serum mediated inhibition of the immunological reactions of the patient to his own tumour; a possible role for circulating antigen. *British Journal of Cancer,* **26,** 427–478.

Currie, G. A., Lejeune, F. & Fairley, G. H. (1971) Immunisation with irradiated tumour cells and specific lymphocytecytotoxicity in malignant melanoma. *British Medical Journal,* **2,** 305–332.

Currie, G. A. & Sime, G. C. (1973) Syngeneic immune serum specifically inhibits the motility of tumour cells. *Nature (New Biology),* **241,** 284–285.

Curtis, J. E. (1971) Adoptive immunotherapy in the treatment of advanced malignant melanoma. *Proceedings of the American Association for Cancer Research,* **12,** 52.

Daphendi, V., Ephrussi, B. & Koprowski, H. (1964) Expression of polyoma induced cellular antigen(s) in hybrid cells. *Nature,* **203,** 495.

Davies, D. A. L. (1974) The combined effect of drugs and tumour specific antibodies in protection against a mouse lymphoma. *Cancer Research,* **34,** 3040–3043.

Davies, D. A. L. (1974) Genetic control of cell surface antigens. *Proceedings of II International Congress of Immunology,* pp. 364–367.

Davies, D. A. L., Manstone, A. J. & Buckham, S. (1974) Protection of mice against syngeneic lymphomata. I. Use of antibodies. *British Journal of Cancer,* **30,** 297–304.

Domingo, E. O. & Warren, K. S. (1967) The inhibition of granuloma formation around *Schistomsoma mansoni* eggs. II. Thymectomy. *American Journal of Pathology,* **51,** 757–767.

Dorf, M. E., Balner, H., de Groot, L. & Benacerraf, B. (1974) Histocompatibility linked immune response genes in the rhesus monkey. *Transplantation Proceedings,* **6,** 119–123.

Dresser, D. W. (1973) The target for the action of an adjuvant. In *Immunopotentiation,* ed. Julie Knight. Amsterdam: Associated Scientific Publishers.

Dumonde, D. C., Wolstencroft, R. A., Panayi, G. S., Mathew, M., Morley, J. & Howson, W. T. (1969) 'Lymphokines': non-antibody mediators of cellular immunity generated by lymphocyte activation. *Nature,* **224,** 38–42.

Eilber, F. R. & Morton, D. L. (1970) Immunologic studies of human sarcomas. *Cancer,* **26,** 588–596.

Evans, R. & Alexander, P. (1970) Co-operation of immune lymphoid cells with macrophages in tumour immunity. *Nature (London),* **228,** 620–622.

Evans, G. A., Gorman, L. R., Ito, Y. & Weiser, R. S. (1962) Antitumour immunity in the Shope papilloma carconoma complex of rabbits. I. Papilloma regression induced by homologous and autologous tissue vaccines. *Journal of the National Cancer Institute,* **29,** 277–285.

Everson, T. C. (1964) Spontaneous regression of cancer. *Annals of the New York Academy of Science*, **114**, 721–735.

Everson, T. C. & Cole, W. H. (1966) *Spontaneous Regression of Cancers*. Philadelphia: Saunders.

Feldman, M. & Palmer, J. (1971) The requirement for macrophages in the secondary immune response to antigens of small and large size in vitro. *Immunology*, **21**, 685–699.

Festenstein, H. & Demant, P. (1974) Antigenic recognition in cell-mediated immune reactions. *Progress in Immunology, II*, ed. Brent, L. & Holborow, J., Vol. 2, pp. 45–55. Amsterdam: North Holland Publishing Co.

Fialkow, P. J. (1967) Immunologic oncogenesis. *Blood*, **30**, 338–394.

Foley, E. J. (1953) Antigenic properties of methylcholanthrene induced tumours in mice of strain of origin. *Cancer Research*, **13**, 853–837.

Folkmann, J. (1974) Tumour angiogenesis. *Advances in Cancer Research*, ed. Klein, G. & Weinhause, S., **19**, 331–358.

Friedmann, P. S. & Turk, J. L. (1975) A spectrum of lymphocyte responsiveness in human syphilis. *Clinical and Experimental Immunology*, **21**, 59–64.

Fuller, T. C. & Winn, H. J. (1973) Immunochemical and biologic characterization of allo-antibody active in immunologic enhancement. *Transplantation Proceedings*, **5**, 585–588.

Gatti, R. A. & Good, R. A. (1970) Aging, immunity and malignancy. *Geriatrics*, **25**, 158–168.

Gershon, R. K. & Kondo, K. (1971) Infectious immunological tolerance. *Immunology*, **21**, 903–914.

Gershon, R. K., Maurer, P. H. & Merryman, C. F. (1973) A cellular basis for genetically controlled immunologic unresponsiveness in mice: tolerance induction in T cells. *Proceedings of the National Academy of Science*, **70**, 250–254.

Ghose, T., Cerini, M., Carter, M. & Nairn, R. C. (1967) Immunoradioactive agent against cancer. *British Medical Journal*, **1**, 90–93.

Glick, B., Chang, T. S. & Jaap, R. G. (1956) The bursa of Fibricius and antibody production. *Poultry Science*, **35**, 224.

Gocke, D. J., Hsu, K., Morgan, C., Bombardieri, S., Lockshin, M. & Christian, C. L. (1970) Association between polyarteritis and Australia antigen. *Lancet*, **2**, 1149–1153.

Godal, T., Rees, R. J. W. & Lamvik, J. O. (1971) Lymphocyte-mediated modification of blood derived macrophage function in vitro; inhibition of growth of intracellular myco-bacteria with lymphokines. *Clinical and Experimental Immunology*, **8**, 625–637.

Gold, P. & Freedman, S. O. (1965) Specific carcinoembryonic antigens of the human digestive system. *Journal of Experimental Medicine*, **122**, 467–481.

Goldstein, P., Wigzell, H., Blomgren, H. & Svedmyr, E. A. J. (1972) Cells mediating specific in vitro cytotoxicity. II. Probably autonomy of the Thyme processed lymphocytes (T-cells) for the killing of allogeneic target cells. *Journal of Experimental Medicine*, **135**, 890–906.

Good, R. A. & Finstead, F. (1969) Essential relationship between the lymphoid system of immunity and malignancy. *Journal of the National Cancer Institute*, Monograph 31, 41–58.

Grant, C. K., Evans, R. & Alexander, P. (1973) Multiple effector role of lymphocytes in allograft immunity. *Cellular Immunology*, **8**, 136–146.

Green, H. N. (1954) An immunological concept of cancer: a preliminary report. *British Medical Journal*, **2**, 1374–1380.

Greenberg, A. H., Shen, L., Hudson, L., & Roitt, I. M. (1973) Antibody dependent cell mediated cytotoxicity due to a 'null' lymphoid cell. *Nature (New Biology)*, **242**, 111–113.

Gutterman, J. U., Rosen, R. B. & Butler, W. T. (1973) Immunoglobulin on tumour cells and tumour induced blastogenesis in human acute leukaemia. *New England Journal of Medicine*, **288**, 169–175.

Gutterman, J. U., Mavligit, G., McBride, C., Frti, E., Freireich, E. J. & Hersch, E. M. (1973) Active immunotherapy with B.C.G. for recurrent malignant melanoma. *Lancet*, **1**, 1208–1212.

Hall, J. G. & Morris, B. (1963) The lymph-borne cells of the immune response. *Quarterly Journal of Experimental Physiology*, **48**, 235–247.

Hauschka, T. S., Kvedar, B. J., Grinnel, S. T. & Amos, D. B. (1956) Immunoselection of polyploids from predominantly diploid cell populations. *New York Academy of Science*, **63**, 683–705.

Hellström, I., Hellström, K. E. & Allison, A. C. (1971) Neonatally induced allograft tolerance may be mediated by serum-borne factors. *Nature*, **230**, 49–50.

Hellström, I. E., Hellström, K. E., Pierce, G. D. & Young, J. P. (1966) Cellular and humoral immunity to different types of human neoplasms. *Nature*, **220**, 1352.

Hellström, I. E., Hellström, K. E., Sjögren, H. O. & Warner, G. A. (1971a) Demonstration of cell mediated immunity to human neoplasms of various histological types. *International Journal of Cancer*, **7**, 1–16.

Hellström, I. E., Hellström, K. E., Sjögren, H. O. & Warner, G. A. (1971b) Serum factors in tumour free patients cancelling the blocking of cell mediated immunity. *International Journal of Cancer*, **8**, 185–191.

Heubner, R. J., Pereira, Allison, A. C., Hollingshead, P. & Turner, H. G. (1964) Production of type specific C antigen in virus free hamster tumour cells induced by adenovirus type 12. *Proceedings of the National Academy of Sciences, U.S.A.*, **51**, 742–750.

Heyn, R., Bergej, W., Joo, P., Koron, M., Nesbit, M., Short, N., Breslow, N. & Hammond, D. (1973) B.C.G. in the treatment of acute lymphocytic leukaemia (A.L.L.). *Proceedings of the American Association for Cancer Research*, **14**, 45.

Hoover, R. & Fraumeni, J. F. (1973) Risk of cancer in renal transplant recipients. *Lancet*, **2**, 55–57.

Jacobson, E. B., Herzenberg, L. A., Riblet, R. & Herzenberg, L. A. (1972) Active suppression of immunoglobulin allotype synthesis. II. Transfer of suppressing factor with spleen cells. *Journal of Experimental Medicine*, **135**, 1163–1176.

Jeejeebhoy, H. F. (1974) Stimulation of tumour growth by the immune response. *International Journal of Cancer*, **13**, 665–678.

Jersild, C., Fog, T., Mansen, G. S., Thomsen, M., Svejigaard, A. & Dupont, B. (1973) Histocompatibility determinants and multiple sclerosis with special reference to clinical course. *Lancet*, **2**, 1222–1224.

Jurin, J. & Tannock, I. F. (1972) Influence of vitamin A on immunological response. *Immunology*, **23**, 283–287.

Kaliss, N. (1958) Immunological enhancement of tumour homografts in mice: a review. *Cancer Research*, **18**, 992–1003.

Kampschmidt, R. F. & Pulliam, L. A. (1972) Changes in the opsonin and cellular influence on phagocytosis during the growth of transplantable tumours. *Journal of the Reticuloendothelial Society*, **2**, 1–10.

Kapp, J. A., Pierce, E. W. & Benacerraf, B. (1973) Genetic control of immune responses in vitro. II. Cellular requirements for the development of primary plaque forming cell responses to the random terpolymer 1-glutaric acid 60-1-alanine 30-1-tryosine 10 (GAT) by mouse spleen cells in vitro. *Journal of Experimental Medicine*, **138**, 1121–1132.

Katz, S. I., Parker, D. & Turk, J. L. (1974) B-cell suppression of delayed hypersensitivity reactions. *Nature*, **251**, 550–551.

Katz, S. I., Parker, D., Sommer, G. & Turk, J. L. (1974) Suppressor cells in normal immunisation as a basic homeostatic mechanism. *Nature*, **248**, 612–614.

Kerckhaert, J. A. M. (1974) Influence of cyclophosphamide on the delayed hypersensitivity in the mouse after intraperitoneal injection. *Annales d'Immunologie*, **125C**, 559–568.

Kinlen, L. J. & Pike, M. C. (1971) BCG vaccination and leukaemia. *Lancet*, **2**, 398–402.

Klein, E. (1969) Hypersensitivity reactions at tumour sites. *Cancer Research*, **27**, 2351–2362.

Klein, E., Klein, G., Nadkarni, J. S., Jadkarni, J. J., Wigzell, H. & Cliffora, P. (1968) Surface IgH-kappa specificity on a Burkitt lymphoma cell in vitro and in derived culture lines. *Cancer Research*, **28**, 1300–1310.

Klein, G., Sjögren, H. O., Klein, E. & Hellström, K. E. (1960) Demonstration of resistance against methylcholanthrene induced sarcomas in the primary autochthonous host. *Cancer Research*, **20**, 1561–1572.

Klein, G., Sjögren, H. O. & Klein, E. (1963) Demonstration of host resistance against sarcomas induced by implantation of cellophane films in isologous (syngeneic) recipients. *Cancer Research*, **23**, 84–92.

Lagrange, P. H., Mackaness, G. B. & Miller, T. E. (1974) Potentiation of T-cell mediated immunity by selective suppression of antibody formation with cyclophosphamide. *Journal of Experimental Medicine*, **139**, 1529–1539.

Lamon, E. W., Skurzak, H. M., Klein, E. & Wigzell, H. (1972) In vitro cytotoxicity by a non-thymus processed lymphocyte population with specificity for a virally determined tumour cell surface antigen. *Journal of Experimental Medicine*, **136**, 1072–1079.

Landsteiner, K. & Chase, M. W. (1942) Experiments on transfer of cutaneous sensitivity to simple compounds. *Proceedings of the Society for Experimental Biology and Medicine, New York*, **49**, 688–690.

Lappé, M. A. (1968) Evidence for the antigenicity of papillomas induced by a 3-methycholanthrene. *Journal of the National Cancer Institute*, **40**, 823–846.

Larsson, A. & Perlmann, P. (1972) Study of Fab and F(ab)₂ from rabbit IgG for capacity to induce lymphocyte mediated target cell destruction in vitro. *International Archives of Allergy and Applied Immunology*, **43**, 80–88.

Laurence, D. J. R. & Neville, A. M. (1972) Fetal antigens and their role in the diagnosis and clinical management of human neoplasms and a review. *British Journal of Cancer*, **26**, 335–355.

Lawrence, H. S. (1972) *Transfer Factor in Advances in Immunology*, ed. Dixon, F. J. & Kankel, H. G. London: Academic Press.

Levin, A. S., Spitler, L. E., Wybran, J., Fudenberg, H. H., Hellström, I. & Hellström, E. (1972) Treatment of osteogenic sarcoma with transfer factor. *Clinical Research*, **20**, 568.

Levine, B. B., Sternber, R. H. & Fotino, M. (1972) Ragweed hay fever: genetic control and linkage to HLA haplotypes. *Science*, **178**, 1201–1203.

Levis, W. R. & Robbins, J. M. (1970) Effect of glass adherent cells on the blastogenic response of 'purified' lymphocytes to phytohaemagglutinin. *Experimental Cell Research*, **61**, 153–158.

Lewis, M. G., Ikonopisov, R. L., Nairn, R. C., Phillips, T. M., Fairley, G. H., Bodenham, D. C. & Alexander, P. (1969) Tumour specific antibodies in human malignant melanoma and their relationship to the extent of the disease. *British Medical Journal*, **3**, 547–552.

Lilly, F. & Pincus, T. (1973) Genetic control of murine viral leukemogenesis. *Advances in Cancer Research*, **17**, 231–277.

Lindenmann, J. (1973) The use of viruses as immunological potentiators. In *Immunopotentiation*, ed. Julie Knight. Amsterdam: Associated Scientific Publishers.

Lindenmann, J. & Klein, P. A. (1967) *Immunological Aspects of Viral Oncogenesis*. New York: Springer.

Lukes, R. J. (1964) Hodgkin's disease. Prognosis and relationship of histologic features to clinical stage. *Journal of the American Medical Association*, **190**, 914–915.

MacLennan, I. C. M. (1972) Antibody in the induction and inhibition of lymphocyte cytotoxicity. *Transplantation Reviews*, **13**, 67–90.

MacSween, J. M., Warner, N. L., Bankhurst, A. D. & Mackay, I. R. (1972) Carcinoembryonic antigen in whole serum. *British Journal of Cancer*, **26**, 356–360.

Mathé, G. (1973) Attempts at using systemic immunity adjuvants for experimental and human therapy. In *Immunopotentiation*, ed. Julie Knight. Amsterdam: Associated Scientific Publishers.

McDevitt, H. O. & Benacerraf, B. (1969) Genetic control of specific immune response. *Advances in Immunology*, *II*, p. 31.

McDevitt, H. O. & Chintz, A. (1969) Genetic control of the antibody response relationship: between immune response and histocompatibility (H.2) type. *Science*, **163**, 1207–1208.

McDevitt, H. O., Deak, B. D., Shreffler, D. C., Klein, J., Stimfling, G. H. & Snell, G. D. (1972) Genetic control of the immune response. Mapping of the Ir–1 locus. *Journal of Experimental Medicine*, **135**, 1259–1278.

Miller, J. F. A. P. (1961) Immunological function of the thymus. *Lancet*, **2**, 748–749.

Milton, G. W. & Lane-Brown, M. N. (1966) The limited role of alternated smallpox virus in the management of advanced malignant melanoma. *Australian and New Zealand Journal of Surgery*, **35**, 286–290.

Mitchison, N. A. (1953) Passive transfer of transplantation immunity. *Nature*, **171**, 267–268.

Mitchison, N. A. (1964) Induction of immunological paralysis in two zones of dosage. *Proceedings of the Royal Society B*, **161**, 275–297.

Morton, D. L., Malmgren, R. A., Holmes, E. C. & Ketcham, A. S. (1968) Demonstration of antibodies against human malignant melanoma by immunofluorescence. *Surgery*, **64**, 233–240.

Morton, D. L., Eilber, F. R., Joseph, W. L., Wood, W. C., Trahan, E., Ketcham, A. S. (1970) Immunological factors in human sarcomas and melanomas: a rational basis for immunotherapy. *Annals of Surgery*, **172**, 740–749.

MRC (1971) Treatment of acute lymphoblastic leukaemia. *British Medical Journal*, **4**, 189–194.

Nadler, S. H. & Moore, G. E. (1969) Immunotherapy of malignant disease. *Archives of Surgery*, **99**, 376–381.

Nath, I., Poulter, L. W. & Turk, J. L. (1973) Effect of lymphocyte mediators on macrophages in vitro. A correlation of morphological and cytochemical changes. *Clinical and Experimental Immunology*, **13**, 455–466.

Nathan, C. F., Karnovsky, M. L. & David, J. R. (1971) Alteration of macrophage functions by mediators from lymphocytes. *Journal of Experimental Medicine*, **133**, 1356–1376.

Nathanson, L. (1971) Experience with BCG in malignant melanoma. *Proceedings of the American Association for Cancer Research*, **12**, 99.

Nehlsen, S. L. (1971) Prolonged administration of anti-thymocyte serum in mice. I. Observations on cellular and humoral immunity. *Clinical and Experimental Immunology*, **9**, 63–77.

Nemato, T., Rosner, D. & Dao, T. (1975) *Proceedings of the XI International Cancer Congress* (in press).

Old, L. J., Benacerraf, B., Clarke, D. A., Carswell, E. A. & Stockert, E. (1961) The role of the reticulo-endothelial system in the host reaction to neoplasia. *Cancer Research*, **21**, 1281–1300.

Old, L. J. & Boyse, E. A. (1964) Immunology of experimental tumours. *Annual Review of Medicine*, **15**, 167.

Old, L. J., Boyse, E. A., Clarke, D. A. & Carswell, E. A. (1962) Antigenic properties of chemically induced tumours. *Annals of the New York Academy of Sciences*, **101**, 80–106.

Old, L. J., Boyse, E. A., Oettgen, H. F. (1966) Precipitating antibody in human serum to an antigen present in Burkitt's lymphoma cells. *Proceedings of the National Academy of Science*, U.S.A., **56**, 1699–1704.

Oldstone, M. B. A., Mitchell, G. F. & McDevitt, H. O. (1973) H-2 linked genetic control of disease susceptibility murine lymphocytic choriomeningitis virus infection. *Federation Proceedings*, **32**, 964.

Parmiani, G. & Della Porta, G. (1973) Effects of antitumour immunity on pregnancy in the mouse. *Nature (New Biology)*, **241**, 26–28.

Penn, I. (1975) Cancer in immunosuppressed patients. *Transplantation proceedings*, **VII** (1), Suppl. 1, 553.

Pick, E., Krejci, J., Cech, K. & Turk, J. L. (1969) Interaction between sensitised lymphocytes and antigen in vitro. I. The release of a skin reactive factor. *Immunology*, **17**, 741–767.

Polak, L., Geleick, H. & Turk, J. L. (1975) Reversal of tolerance in contact sensitisation by cyclophosphamide: tolerance induced by prior feeding with DNCB. *Immunology*, **28**, 939–942.

Polak, L. & Turk, J. L. (1974) Reversal of immunological tolerance by cyclophosphamide through inhibition of suppressor cell activity. *Nature*, **249**, 654–656.

Powles, R. L., Crowther, D., Bateman, C. J. T., Beard, M. E. J., McElwain, T. J., Russel, J., Lister, T. A., Whitehouse, J. M. A., Wrigley, P. F. M., Pike, M., Alexander, P. & Hamilton-Fairley, G. (1973) Immunotherapy for acute myelogenous leukaemia. *British Journal of Cancer*, **28**, 365–376.

Prager, M. D., Derr, I., Swann, A. & Cotropia, J. (1971) Immunisation with chemically modified cancer cells. *Proceedings of the American Association of Cancer Research*, **12**, 2.

Prehn, R. T. (1971) Perspectives in oncogenesis: does immunity stimulate or inhibit neoplasia? *Journal of the Reticuloendothelial Society*, **10**, 1–16.

Prehn, R. T. (1972) The immune reaction as a stimulator of tumour growth. *Science*, **176**, 170–171.

Prehn, R. T. & Main, J. M. (1957) Immunity to methylcholanthrene induced sarcomas. *Journal of the National Cancer Institute*, **18**, 769–778.

Raff, M. C. (1969) Theta-iso-antigen as a marker of thymus derived lymphocytes in mice. *Nature*, **224**, 378–379.

Raff, M. C., Nase, S. & Mitchison, N. A. (1971) Mouse specific bone marrow derived lymphocyte antigen as a marker for thymus independent lymphocytes. *Nature (London)*, **230**, 50–51.

Reiner, J. & Southam, C. M. (1967) Evidence of common antigenic properties in chemically induced sarcomas of mice. *Cancer Research*, **27**, 1243–1247.

Roitt, I. M., Greaves, M. F., Torrigiani, G., Brostoff, J. & Playfair, J. H. L. (1969) The cellular basis of immunological responses. *Lancet*, **2**, 367–371.

Römer, P. H. & Joseph, K. (1910) Experimentelle Tuberkulosestudien. *Beiträge zur Klinik der Tuberkulose*, **17**, 281–287.

Rosenau, W. & Moon, H. D. (1964) The specificity of the cytolytic effect of sensitised lymphoid cells in vitro. *Journal of Immunology*, **93**, 910–914.

Rosenthal, S. R., Crispen, R. G., Thome, M. G., Piekarski, N., Raisys, N. & Rettig, P. G. (1972) BCG vaccination and leukaemia mortality. *Journal of the American Medical Association*, **222**, 1543–1544.

Rouse, B. T., Röllinghoff, M. & Warner, N. L. (1972) Anti-O serum induced suppression of the cellular transfer of tumour specific immunity to syngeneic plasma cell tumours. *Nature (New Biology)*, **238**, 116–117.

Salvin, S. B., Sell, S. & Nishio, J. (1971) Activity in vitro of lymphocytes and macrophages in delayed hypersensitivity. *Journal of Immunology*, **107**, 655–662.

Sanderson, C. & Frost, P. (1974) The induction of tumour immunity in mice using gluteraldehyde treated tumour cells. *Nature (New Biology)*, **248**, 690–691.

Sato, H., Boyse, E. A., Aoki, T., Iritini, C. & Old, L. J. (1973) Leukaemia associated transplantation antigens related to murine leukaemia virus. The X.1 system: immune response controlled by a locus linked to H2. *Journal of Experimental Medicine*, **138**, 593–606.

Sheagren, J. N. & Monaco, A. A. P. (1969) Protective effect of antilymphocyte serum on mice, infected with *Plasmodium berghei*. *Science*, **164**, 1423–1424.

Shearer, G. M., Mozes, E. & Sela, M. (1972) Contribution of different cell types to the genetic control of immune response as a function of the chemical nature of the polymeric side chains (poly-L-prolyl and poly-DL-alanyl) of synthetic immunogens. *Journal of Experimental Medicine*, **135**, 1009–1027.

Shreffler, D. C. & David, C. S. (1975) The H_2 histocompatibility complex and the immune response region: Genetic variation, function and organization. *Advances in Immunology*, **20**, 125–195.

Simmons, R. L. & Rios, A. (1971) Immunotherapy of cancer. Immunospecific rejection of tumours in recipients of neuraminidase treated tumour cells. *Science*, **174**, 591–592.

Sjögren, H. O., Hellström, T., Bansal, S. C. & Hellström, K. E. (1971) Suggestive evidence that 'blocking antibodies' of tumour bearing individual may be antigen–antibody complexes. *Proceedings of the National Academy of Sciences, Washington*, **68**, 1372–1375.

Sm th, R. T. (1971) Immunologic interventions in cancer. In *Progress in Immunology*. ed. Amos, B. New York and London: Academic Press.

Smith, S. & Scott, M. T. (1972) Biological effects of *Corynebacterium parvum*. III. Amplification of resistance and impairment of active immunity to murine tumours. *British Journal of Cancer*, **26**, 361–367.

Snell, G. D. (1963) The immunology of tissue transplantation. In *Conceptual Advances in Immunology and Oncology*, p. 323. Hoeber.

Spector, W. G. & Heesom, N. (1969) The production of granulomata by antigen–antibody complexes. *Journal of Pathology*, **98**, 31–39.

Stockert, E., Old, L. J. & Boyse, E. A. (1971) The G–IX system—a cell surface allo-antigen associated with murine leukaemia virus; implications regarding chromosomal integration of the viral genome. *Journal of Experimental Medicine*, **133**, 1334–1355.

Stonehill, E. H. & Benditch, A. (1968) Retrogenetic expression: the reappearance of embryonal antigens in cancer cells. *Nature (New Biology)*, **228**, 370–372.

Sumner, W. L. & Foraker, A. G. (1960) Spontaneous regression of human melanoma; clinical and experimental studies. *Cancer*, **13**, 79–81.

Thompson, R. B. (1971) Lymphocyte transfer factor. A review of practical application. *European Journal of Clinical and Biological Research*, **16**, 201–204.

Thomson, D. M. P., Steele, K. & Alexander, P. (1973) The presence of tumour specific membrane antigen in the serum of rats with chemically induced sarcomata. *British Journal of Cancer*, **27**, 27–34.

Turk, J. L., Parker, D. & Poulter, L. W. (1972) Functional aspects of the selective depletion of lymphoid tissue by cyclophosphamide. *Immunology*, **23**, 493–502.

Turk, J. L. & Parker, D. (1973) Further studies on B-lymphocyte suppression in delayed hypersensitivity, indicating a possible mechanism for Jones–Mote hypersensitivity. *Immunology*, **24**, 751–758.

Turk, J. L. & Poulter, L. W. (1972) Selective depletion of lymphoid tissue by cyclophosphamide. *Clinical and Experimental Immunology*, **10**, 285–296.

Turk, J. L. & Stone, S. H. (1963) Implications of the cellular changes in lymph nodes during the development and inhibition of delayed type hypersensitivity. In *Cell-bound Antibodies*, eds. Amos, B. & Koprowski, H., pp. 51–60. Philadelphia: Wistar Institute Press.

Uhlenbruck, G. (1974) Invertebrate immunology. *Progress in Immunology*, *II*, ed. Brent, L. & Holborow, J., Vol. 2, pp. 292–296. Amsterdam: North Holland Publishing Co.

Unanue, E. R. & Cerottini, J. C. (1970) The immunogenicity of antigen bound to the plasma membrane of macrophages. *Journal of Experimental Medicine*, **131**, 711–725.

Vladiatiu, A. O. & Rose, N. R. (1974) Autoimmune thyroiditis, relation to histocompatibility (H-2). *Science*, **174**, 1137–1138.

Vogler, W. R. & Chan, Y. K. (1974) Prolonging remission in myeloblastic leukaemia by the strain Bacillus Calmette Geurin. *Lancet*, **2**, 128–131.

Warren, K. S., Domingo, E. O. & Cowan, R. B. T. (1967) Granuloma formation around schistosome eggs as a manifestation of delayed hypersensitivity. *American Journal of Pathology*, **51**, 735–756.

Wemambu, S. N. C., Turk, J. L., Waters, M. F. R. & Rees, R. J. W. (1969) Erythema nodosum leprosum: a clinical manifestation of the Arthus reaction. *Lancet*, **2**, 933–935.

Whittle, H. C., Abdullahi, M. T., Fakunle, F. A., Greenwood, B. M., Bryceson, A. D. M., Parry, E. H. O. & Turk, J. L. (1973) Allergic complications of meningococcal disease. I. Clinical aspects. *British Medical Journal*, **2**, 733–737.

Williams, G. & Castro, J. E. (1975) The diagnostic and prognostic significance of delayed hypersensitivity skin testing in patients with urological cancer. *British Journal of Urology*, **47**, 97–101.

Williams, R. M. & Moore, M. J. (1973) Linkage of susceptibility to experimental allergic encephalomyetitis to the major histocompatibility locus in the rat. *Journal of Experimental Medicine*, **138**, 775–783.

Woodruff, M. E. A. & Boak, J. L. (1966) Inhibitory effect of injection of *Corynebacterium parvum* on the growth of tumour transplants in isogeneic hosts. *British Journal of Cancer*, **20**, 345–355.

Woodruff, M. F. A., Dunbar, N. & Ghaffar, A. (1973) The growth of tumours in T-cell deprived mice and their response to treatment with *Corynebacterium parvum*. *Proceedings of the Royal Society of London B*, **184**, 97–102.

Zaleski, M. & Klein, J. (1975) A new locus (Ir-5) controlling immune responsiveness to Thy 1-1 (θ AKR) *Transplantation Proceedings*, **VII** (1) Suppl. 1, 101–108.

Zembala, M. & Asherson, G. L. (1973) Depression of the T-cell phenomenon of contact sensitivity by T-cells from unresponsive mice. *Nature*, **244**, 227–228.

Zembala, M. (1974) Inhibitory, T-cells. *Progress in Immunology*, *II*, ed. Brent, L. & Holborow, J., Vol. 3, pp. 351–354. Amsterdam: North Holland Publishing Co.

Ziegler, J. L. & Magrath, I. T. (1973) BCG immunotherapy in Burkitt's lymphoma. Preliminary results of a randomised clinical trial. *National Cancer Institute*, Monograph **39**, 199–203.

Zinsser, H. & Mueller, J. H. (1925) On the nature of bacterial allergies. *Journal of Experimental Medicine*, **41**, 159–177.

11

13
THE APUDOMAS

R. B. Welbourn   S. N. Joffe

The Apud Cell Concept

The 'apudomas' are a family of endocrine tumours which arise from apud cells and which have interesting and important relationships. Many are well known but have not in the past been recognised as being closely related.

The apud cells are distributed widely in the body and have common cytochemical characteristics clearly related to the synthesis of polypeptides and amines (Table 13.1) (Pearse and Welbourn, 1973; Welbourn et al, 1974). Their name, proposed by Pearse in 1968, is derived from the initial letters of their first three properties, namely (1) a high content of *A*mine, (2) the capacity for amine *P*recursor *U*ptake from their environment and (3) the presence of amino acid *D*ecarboxylase for the conversion of amino acids to amines. The high content of other enzymes (4) is less constant.

The ultrastructural characteristics of the apud cells (5), revealed by electron microscopy, are essentially those of all polypeptide-secreting cells and are not confined to those of the apud series. Their average diameter is 100 to 200 μm and many contain dense storage granules of their polypeptide products. The majority of gastrointestinal apud cells possess long apical processes which reach the glandular lumen, ending in tufts of microvilli, which may subserve a sensory function (Fig. 13.1).

The final characteristic (specific immunofluorescence) is assessed by the indirect or sandwich method, in which the cell containing the polypeptide antigen is brought into contact with an antibody and with an anti-antibody,

Table 13.1   Properties of apud cells

1. Fluorogenic *A*mine content
   (e.g. catecholamine, 5-hydroxytryptamine)
2. Amine *P*recursor *U*ptake
   (e.g. dopa or 5-hydroxytryptophan)
3. Aminoacid *D*ecarboxylase
4. High content of:
   (i) Side chain carboxyl groups (masked metachromasia)
   (ii) Non-specific esterases and/or cholinesterase, and
   (iii) α-Glycerophosphate dehydrogenase
5. Characteristic ultrastructure (endocrine granules)
6. Specific immunofluorescence

labelled with fluorescein. When the three substances combine in the cell a compound is formed which fluoresces under ultraviolet light (Fig. 13.2). Another technique involves labelling with the enzyme peroxidase (Fig. 13.4). The relationships between structure and function still await clarification but it is probable that the presence of many secretory granules on electron micro-

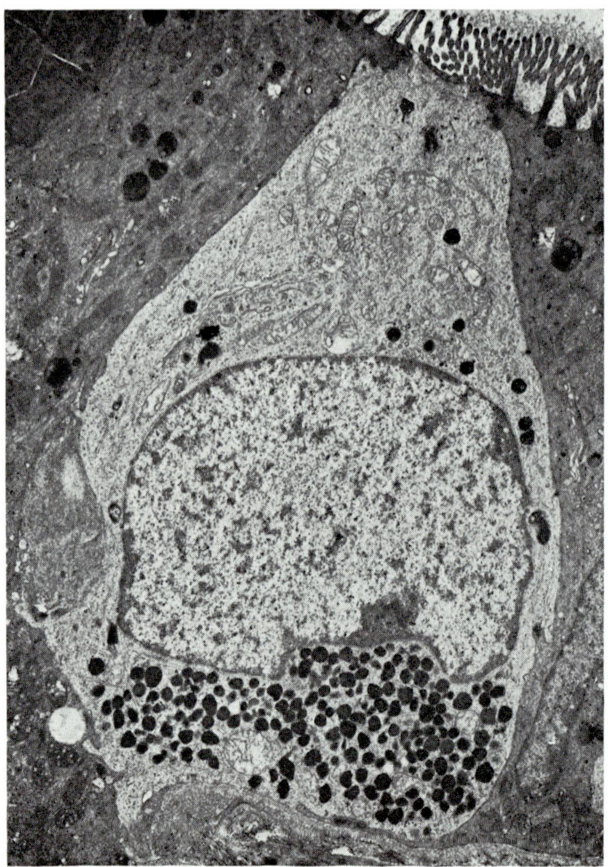

Figure 13.1 Electromicrograph of an apud cell with numerous electron dense secretory granules localised towards vascular pole and microvilli in lumen of gland. Magnification ×6300

scopy and strong specific immunofluorescence indicate storage of a polypeptide product, while absence or relative absence of these features suggests either active secretion (without storage) or a failure of synthesis.

The apud cells may be considered in two groups, namely (1) those which are known to secrete polypeptides and (2) those whose polypeptide product (if there is one) has not been identified. Some members of each group secrete amines. The first (Table 13.2) includes most of the endocrine cells of the alimentary tract, including the islets of Langerhans, and some cells of the anterior pituitary, pineal and thyroid. The second group (Table 13.3) includes cells in many parts of the body, the most important probably being in the adrenal medulla.

All these cells are being investigated intensively and knowledge about them and their products is progressing rapidly. New cells and products are being discovered and those in the second group are being moved to the first as their polypeptides are identified.

There are other polypeptide-secreting cells in the body whose relationship with the apud series is not clear. Those of the hypothalamus, which secrete the polypeptide hormones controlling the anterior pituitary, and those of the neurohypophysis (hypothalamus and posterior pituitary) which produce

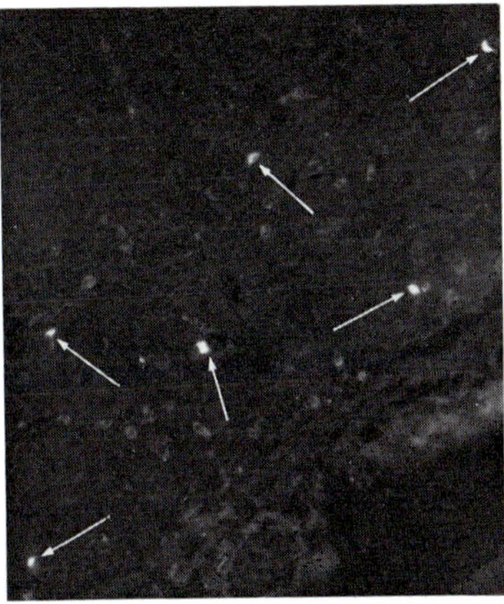

Figure 13.2   Human jejunum stained with an indirect (sandwich) immunofluorescent method using porcine anti-GIP antibody. Six GIP cells can be seen localised mainly in basal portion of gland (marked with arrows). Magnification ×83

oxytocin and antidiuretic hormone (ADH) are probably a part, but they await full investigation. The parathyroid cells are not apud in character but they are closely related to the apud series in various ways, which will be described later. The cells of the anterior pituitary which secrete glycoproteins (TSH, FSH and LH), and the endocrine cells of the kidney and placenta are probably unrelated.

At an early stage in the investigation of the apud cells it was noticed that in certain ways they were structurally and chemically similar to nerve cells. In particular, the neuroectodermal cells of the neural crest display apud characteristics from an early stage. This observation prompted Pearse in 1966 to suggest that 'the neural crest cells must be considered as possible ancestors of all the polypeptide-secreting cells of the apud series'. The cells of the adrenal medulla and sympathetic nervous system and the melanocytes of the skin have long been known to arise from the neural crest. It is now established

Table 13.2   Apud cells with known polypeptide products (together with their amine products and related orthoendocrine apudomas and syndromes)

Organs	Cells	Polypeptides	Amines	Apudomas	Syndromes
Alimentary tract					
Islets of Langerhans	B (β)	Insulin	Dopamine	Hyperplasia	Hypoglycaemia
	A (α_2)	Glucagon	or	Adenoma	Diabetes, dermatitis
	D ($\delta_1\,\alpha_1$)	Somatostatin	5-HT[a]	Carcinoma	—
		?Gastrin			Zollinger–Ellison
Stomach	G	Gastrin	—	Hyperplasia Carcinoma	Zollinger–Ellison
	AL (A-like)	Enteroglucagon	—	—	—
	D	Somatostatin	—	—	—
Duodenum and small	S	Secretin	—	—	—
intestine	D$_1$	GIP[b]	—	—	—
	EC	Motilin	5-HT	Carcinoid	Malignant carcinoid
		?Substance P			
	D	Somatostatin	—	—	—
Large intestine	D	VIP[c]	—	—	—
	EG	Enteroglucagon	—	—	—
Other sites					
Anterior pituitary	c (corticotroph)	ACTH[d]	(Tryptamine)	Hyperplasia	Cushing's Pigmentation
	m (melanotroph)	MSH[e]	(Tryptamine)	Adenoma	Acromegaly or gigantism
	s (somatotroph)	GH[f]		Carcinoma	Forbes–Albright
	l (lactotroph)	Prolactin			
Pineal	P	Melatonin	5-HT	Pinealoma	Hypogonadism
Thyroid	C	Calcitonin	5-HT	Medullary carcinoma	Medullary carcinoma

[a] 5-Hydroxytryptamine.
[b] Gastric inhibitory polypeptide.
[c] Vasoactive intestinal polypeptide.
[d] (Adreno)corticotrophin.
[e] Melanocyte stimulating hormone.
[f] Growth hormone.

Table 13.3   Apud cells without known polypeptide products (together with amine and *possible* polypeptide products, related orthoendocrine apudomas and syndromes)

Organs	Cells	Amines	Possible polypeptides	Apudomas	Syndromes
Alimentary tract					
Islets of Langerhans	D_1	—	—	—	—
Stomach	EC	?5-HT	Substance P	Carcinoid	Atypical carcinoid
Duodenum and small	I	—	VIP	—	—
intestine	K	—	GIP	—	—
	D_1	—	—	—	—
	G	—	Gastrin	—	—
Large intestine	EC	5-HT	Substance P	Carcinoid	—
	H	—	VIP	—	—
Other sites					
Carotid body	Type 1 (glomus)	Catecholamines and 5-HT	—	Carotid body tumour (chemodectoma)	—
Skin	Melanocyte	—	—	—	—
Adrenal	A (E)	Adrenaline (epinephrine)	—	} Phaeochromocytoma	Hypertension, etc.
	NA (NE)	Noradrenaline (norepinephrine)	—		
Lung	P (Feyrter)	—	VLP[a]	—	—
	EC	?5-HT	—	Carcinoid	Atypical carcinoid
Urogenital tract	U	—	Urogastrone	—	—

[a] Vasoactive lung peptide.

firmly that the apud cells of the carotid body and the thyroid and some, at least, of those of the anterior pituitary come from the same source. Evidence is accumulating that those of the alimentary tract and other sites may well do so too. The hypothalamus and posterior pituitary are of neuroectodermal but not neural crest origin, and the parathyroids, which have long been regarded as of endodermal origin, may arise from neuroectoderm also (Pearse and Takor, 1976).

If all these cells indeed arise from the neural crest (or neuroectoderm) they must have appeared between 350 and 500 million years ago in the earliest vertebrates as a distinct system of nerve cells, spreading over the neck and trunk and coming to rest largely, but not exclusively, in the endodermal tissues of the foregut and midgut and their derivatives. Although they were nerve cells originally, secreting neurotransmitter amines locally, they now respond to stimuli by secretion into the circulation either of ancestral or modified amines or of more recently developed polypeptides. They demonstrate the close relationship between the nervous and endocrine systems.

Many of the polypeptide and amine products of the apud cells are firmly established as hormones (ACTH, insulin and adrenaline, for instance). Many others, particularly those identified recently in the alimentary tract, have not yet achieved this status, and some may never do so. They are best referred to, at present, as humoral agents. A few (e.g. VIP), while not yet recognised as hormones, play major roles in disease. Those which are of clinical importance will be discussed later.

The Apudomas

The term 'apudoma' was first suggested by Szijj and her colleagues (1969) in Hungary to describe a medullary carcinoma of the thyroid which was secreting ACTH. This tumour arises from the apud C cells of the thyroid, which secrete calcitonin physiologically, while ACTH normally comes from the anterior pituitary. The significance of this apparently bizarre state of affairs will be discussed later. There is little etymological justification for the word apudoma, but it is useful because it emphasises the common characteristics of neoplastic lesions of the apud cells (Pearse and Polak, 1974; Pearse, 1975). Apudomas may be described in both biological and pathological terms. Biologically they are neoplastic lesions, derived from apud cells and thus neuroectodermal in quality, which secrete normal or modified peptide hormones or prohormones of the apud cell series and/or one or more of the apud amine hormones. Pathologically apudomas are 'endocrine' neoplastic lesions, which may take the form of hyperplasia, adenoma, adenomatous hyperplasia or carcinoma, possessing the apud cytochemical qualities, often with greater clarity than their presumptive precursor cells. They are also characterised ultrastructurally by the presence of storage granules of endocrine type, containing peptide components with or without catecholamines. These biological and pathological properties are shared by all apudomas, whether they be hyperplastic or tumorous lesions, benign or malignant.

At least half the apud cells which have been recognised are known to give rise to apudomas and new ones are being discovered frequently. Some tumours which are well known, but not recognised as such, may turn out to be apudomas. Neoplastic cells tend to be less differentiated in structure and function than their parent cells and the secretory capacity of apudomas is very versatile. Many (e.g. insulinomas and phaeochromocytomas) are *ortho*-endocrine and secrete the normal hormones of their presumptive cells of origin, but many are *para*endocrine and secrete, either instead or in addition, hormones or humoral agents which are characteristic of other apud cells. This versatility suggests that they are capable of mobilising all the primitive secretory capacity of the neural ectoderm and, in particular, of the neural crest. Some paraendocrine apudomas, like tumours of other types, secrete substances such as prostaglandins, histamine, erythropoietin and other humoral agents which are characteristic products of other non-apud cells. This property which is poorly understood is unlikely to derive specifically from their presumptive neural origin but rather to reflect a function of neoplastic tissue in general.

The apudomas constitute a large part of surgical endocrinology (Montgomery and Welbourn, 1975). The brief account which follows concentrates on recent advances in their understanding in relation to the apud concept and in other more specific details.

Identification of apudomas

Apudomas may be studied in various ways. The concentrations of poly-peptides and amines may be measured in the peripheral blood, and in the venous blood draining the tumour, by radioimmunoassay and by other methods. The tumours may be examined by conventional light microscopy, cytochemical methods, electron microscopy and immunocytochemistry, and extracts from the tumours may be analysed for their products. Specific immunocytochemistry (Fig. 13.3) will usually provide a positive result only if there is ultrastructural evidence of the presence of at least a few storage granules in each cell. The full secretory properties of an apudoma will be elucidated only if every suspected tumour is tested, not only for its presump-tive hormone, but also for as many others as possible. Hormones which are clinically 'silent' may predominate, as in calcitoninomas (medullary carci-nomas of the thyroid) and some paraendocrine tumours. Although immuno-fluorescence is the most important single technique for the diagnosis of apudomas, results are only significant when positive.

Apudomas may be named conveniently after their endocrine products. For single hormone tumours the term 'insulinoma' is well established, but others such as 'gastrinoma', 'corticotrophinoma', 'calcitoninoma', 'glucagonoma' and 'vipoma' may also be applied. To avoid unnecessary hybrids in multihormone-producing apudomas the combined pathological/histological description could well be 'apudoma secreting ACTH/MSH' and so on (Pearse, 1975).

Classification of apudomas
It is convenient to divide the apudomas into the following groups:

I. Orthoendocrine
 A. Tumours secreting normal polypeptides of their cells of origin.
 B. Tumours secreting normal amines of their cells of origin.
II. Paraendocrine
 A. Tumours of endocrine glands secreting hormones or humoral agents characteristic of other glands or cells.
 B. Tumours of organs or tissues, not usually regarded as endocrine in nature, secreting hormones or humoral agents.

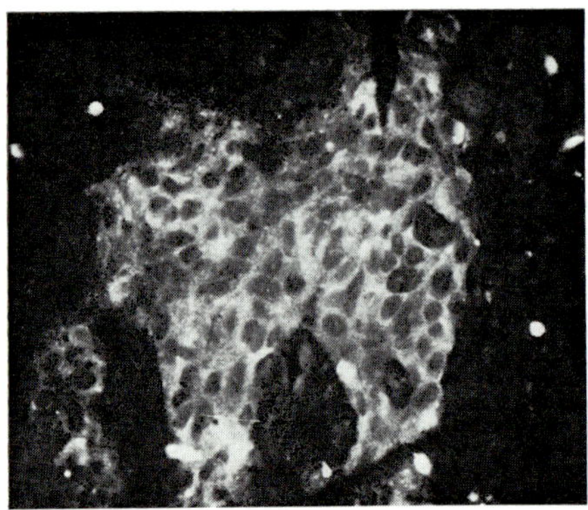

Figure 13.3   Human pancreatic insulinoma stained with an indirect immunofluorescent method using antibodies to insulin. Tumour cells appear brightly stained. Magnification × 160

III. Multiple endocrine adenopathy, in which more than one endocrine gland in the same individual is the site of neoplasia, often an apudoma, which may be orthoendocrine or paraendocrine.

IA. ORTHOENDOCRINE APUDOMAS SECRETING POLYPEPTIDES

These apudomas arise from the apud cells listed in Table 13.2 and are well known, but rare.

The Alimentary Tract

In the alimentary tract (Bonfils, 1974) the great majority of orthoendocrine apudomas develop in the pancreatic islets of Langerhans. Indeed, in the stomach and intestines no orthoendocrine polypeptide-producing tumours, other than those secreting gastrin, have yet been recognised. Those in the pancreas are often multiple. They are usually benign adenomas, less commonly malignant carcinomas, rarely adenomatous hyperplasia and, very rarely, simple hyperplasia. Carcinomas, even after metastasising, tend to run a prolonged course and provided the major symptoms can be controlled patients may survive in reasonable health for many years. The islet cells, as will be described later, are also a major site of paraendocrine apudomas.

Insulinoma (*episodic hypoglycaemia*)

Insulin-secreting islet cell tumours of the pancreas or insulinomas, causing hypoglycaemia, have been known for many years and arise from the B (β) cells. An insulinoma may be the only endocrine lesion present or may represent part of a syndrome of multiple endocrine adenopathy. Immunofluorescence may reveal the presence of insulin and/or proinsulin in the tumour and analysis of venous blood draining the tumour shows a higher concentration of insulin than that in the peripheral blood. There is no evidence that other hypoglycaemia-producing tumours, such as hepatomas and mesotheliomas, are apudomas or that they secrete insulin.

Most recent work has been directed towards earlier diagnosis and drug therapy. Delay in diagnosis may cause severe hypoglycaemic damage to the brain. The single most important step in the recognition of organic hyperinsulinism is to think of it. The clinical features are so varied and resemble those of so many diseases that the condition is often unrecognised for a long time and is at first mistaken for epilepsy, neurosis, psychosis, drunkenness, hysteria, narcolepsy or organic nervous disease. It should be considered, like phaeochromocytoma and the carcinoid syndrome, in any patient who has episodic attacks of symptoms suggesting involvement of the nervous system, especially if they occur at times of fasting.

Diagnosis has been improved greatly by the measurement of immunoreactive insulin, at the same time as glucose, in the blood. Several tests are available, which depend on the principle that normally there is a direct relationship between the blood concentrations of glucose and of insulin and that hypoglycaemia from most other causes is associated with hypoinsulinaemia. In nearly all patients with organic hyperinsulinism this relationship is lost, and high or normal (instead of low) levels of insulin accompany hypoglycaemia. The localisation of tumours in the pancreas has been improved greatly by selective angiography.

Treatment is directed towards removal of the tumour or tumours, and it must be remembered that in at least 10 per cent of patients there are two or more. If a tumour cannot be found or, usually because of malignancy, cannot be removed completely, the hypoglycaemic symptoms can usually be controlled with diazoxide. Non-resectable carcinomas can often be treated effectively for a time with streptozotocin by infusion, either intravenously or into the hepatic artery. Both drugs are toxic and may not be tolerated.

Gastrinoma (Zollinger–Ellison syndrome) (J. C. Thompson et al, 1975)

Zollinger and Ellison's original description in 1955 referred to two patients who exhibited a triad of (1) fulminant peptic ulceration, which recurred despite gastric operations, (2) gross gastric hypersecretion, and (3) non-β islet cell tumour of the pancreas. Within the next few years many more patients were reported and it was established that many of them had multiple endocrine adenopathy; that the tumours secreted gastrin (or sometimes big gastrin) and were therefore gastrinomas; that more than half of them were malignant; that they were not always in the pancreas; that gastric hypersecretion was not necessarily gross; and that the only reliable form of treatment was total gastrectomy. Since radioimmunoassay for gastrin became available the pre-operative diagnosis of the gastrinomas has been relatively easy in most cases, although in a few the level in the blood may not be high until stimulated by calcium or secretin. Patients with pernicious anaemia may have similarly high levels of gastrin in the blood, owing to the failure of acidification of the gastric antrum, but they are readily distinguished by the haematological findings and the presence of achlorhydria.

Apudomas of the pancreatic islet cells secrete gastrin (gastrinomas) and cause the Zollinger–Ellison syndrome. There has been much dispute about the cell of origin of these tumours, but the important point is that they are apudomas secreting gastrin, which could theoretically arise from any cell of the apud series. It is not certain that gastrin is a normal product of the pancreatic islets, although it may be identified in the D-cells in some pathological states. For this reason a pancreatic gastrinoma should, perhaps, be classed as a paraendocrine apudoma.

Several reported series include patients with the syndrome in whom no tumour was found, and the cause of the hypergastrinaemia and gastric acid hypersecretion was not clear. It is possible that some of these may have had hyperplasia of the G-cells of the gastric antrum, a form of G-cell apudoma, which is not excessively rare, and may cause the same syndrome as a pancreatic gastrinoma (Polak, Stagg and Pearse, 1972; Cowley et al, 1973).

It is now clear that five different types of apudoma and possibly a sixth type of lesion may produce gastrin in excess and cause variants of the Zollinger–Ellison syndrome. The five apudomas are:

Stomach   G-cell hyperplasia (Fig. 13.4),
            G-cell carcinoma
Pancreas   Islet cell tumour (adenoma or carcinoma),
            D-cell hyperplasia
Elsewhere   Carcinoma or adenoma in duodenum or hilum of spleen

The sixth lesion is parathyroid adenoma or hyperplasia, which will be discussed later.

In patients with hypergastrinaemia causing gastric hypersecretion, with duodenal or jejunal ulceration, the preoperative investigations should include

selective angiography of the pancreas for localisation of a tumour and immunofluorescent staining of antral biopsies for the diagnosis of G-cell hyperplasia.
The latter responds to antrectomy (which has usually been combined with
vagotomy), and total gastrectomy is not necessary. Gastrinomas in the
duodenum probably arise in apud cells in the mucosa and those in the splenic

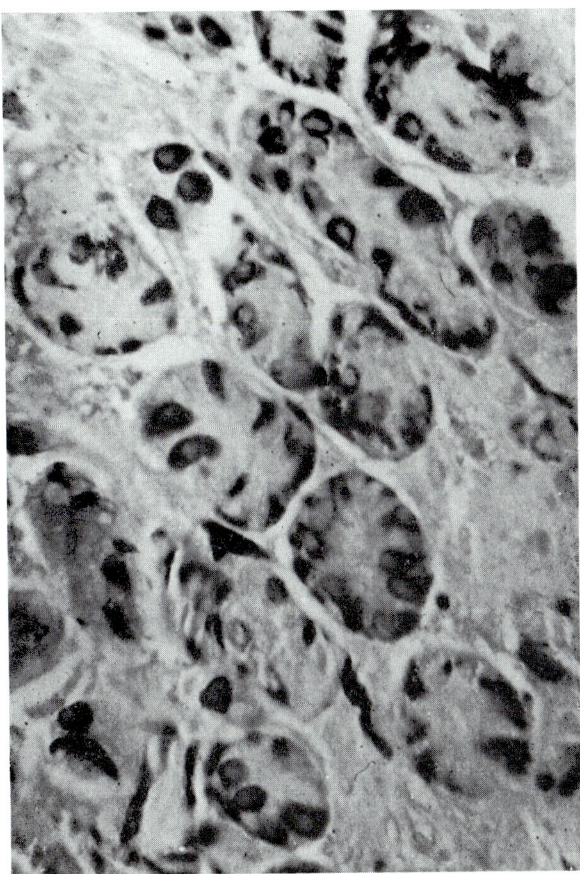

Figure 13.4   Human antrum stained with an immunoperoxidase method using antibodies
to human gastrin I. G-cells appear numerous (moderate hyperplasia) and heavily stained.
Magnification × 293

hilum in ectopic islet cell tissue. A single example of a G-cell carcinoma of
the pyloric antrum has been described (Royston et al, 1972).

Some patients, who are unsuitable or not ready for total gastrectomy, may
be treated with the H_2 receptor blocking agent metiamide, which reduces the
secretion of gastrin and of gastric acid and cures the ulceration (M. H. Thompson et al, 1975). Unfortunately it is toxic and must be used only as a last resort.

Other effective antisecretory agents (some of them hormones) are, however, likely to become available soon.

Pancreatic glucagonoma

These apudomas arise from the A (α) cells of the islets, which secrete glucagon. Although there are several reports in the literature of islet cell tumours containing hyperglycaemic material, these could not be investigated fully until the development of a radioimmunoassay for pancreatic glucagon. The first proved case, with diabetes and high concentrations of pancreatic glucagon in the plasma and in an extract of the tumour, was described by McGavran in 1966. The patient had a rash, and this clue to the diagnosis allowed nine cases to be recognised recently in the South of England (Mallison et al, 1974).

The characteristic lesion is a necrolytic migratory erythema, and any patient presenting with this lesion who is also a diabetic should be suspected of having a glucagonoma. Estimation of pancreatic glucagon in the blood and selective angiography should then confirm the diagnosis and reveal the site of the tumour(s). Several patients have been cured, at least temporarily, by removal of a tumour.

The Anterior Pituitary

Tumours or hyperplasia of the anterior pituitary cause general features, by secreting hormones in excess, and local effects, by exerting pressure on the adjacent normal tissues in the pituitary and in the hypothalamus. The lesions are nearly always benign.

Apudomas secreting corticotrophin (ACTH), which arise from the c-cells (corticotrophs), are the commonest cause of Cushing's syndrome. An almost constant companion of ACTH is the melanocyte stimulating hormone (MSH) which, when present in great excess, causes pigmentation. Although the c- and m-cells are listed separately (Table 13.2) it is uncertain whether or not they are distinct. Patients with large tumours, and especially those in whom they continue to grow after bilateral adrenalectomy, often develop severe Addisonian pigmentation.

Apudomas secreting growth hormone arise from the s-cells (somatotrophs) and cause acromegaly in adults and gigantism in adolescents.

Tumours secreting prolactin arise from the l-cells (lactotrophs) and cause the Forbes–Albright syndrome of galactorrhoea and amenorrhoea. Although they have not been studied in detail they are probably apudomas also.

It has long been believed that so-called 'chromophobe adenomas' do not secrete hormones, but cause pressure effects only. It now appears that the great majority of those in women and a few of those in men actually secrete prolactin, which may be clinically silent (Child et al, 1975), and that they are probably apudomas also.

Until recently, only two methods were used widely for the removal or destruction of pituitary tumours, namely surgical hypophysectomy by the transfrontal route and external radiotherapy, which were often used in the same patient. The disadvantages of these procedures were that the former carried an appreciable operative mortality, except in a few centres, and that the latter was not very effective. In recent years three other methods have been developed and tested thoroughly, namely external irradiation with a proton beam, transethmosphenoidal hypophysectomy and internal irradiation with radioactive isotopes. In the few centres where they are available all are yielding excellent results, but controlled trials to compare them with each other or with older methods have not been undertaken.

The Pineal

Parenchymatous pinealomas are usually associated with hypogonadism, possibly because they secrete melatonin which may inhibit gonadal function. The P-cells, from which it is derived, are apud cells and the tumour may well be an apudoma.

Calcitoninoma (Medullary Carcinoma of the Thyroid)

This apudoma, which accounts for 6 to 8 per cent of thyroid malignancies, arises from the C-cells of the thyroid and secretes large quantities of calcitonin. This hormonal excess does not in itself produce any clinical features, presumably because it stimulates a secondary hypersection of parathormone whose effects are antagonistic. The high blood levels of calcitonin, which can be further provoked by a calcium infusion or other stimuli, are diagnostic of the tumour and serial measurements of calcitonin after treatment may help to monitor the progress of the disease.

About 20 per cent of patients suffer from diarrhoea, which may be caused by a prostaglandin secreted by the tumour and which may respond to treatment with nutmeg (Barrowman et al, 1975).

Surgical removal of the affected lobe or lobes of the thyroid and of all involved lymph nodes is the only effective form of therapy, and three-quarters of the patients so treated survive five years.

These lesion may form part of a familial syndrome of multiple endocrine adenopathy and may then be diagnosed at a preclinical stage (see later).

IB. ORTHOENDOCRINE APUDOMAS SECRETING AMINES

These apudomas arise from the apud cells listed in Table 13.3 and occur in the gastrointestinal tract, the sympathetic nervous system including the adrenal medulla, and in the carotid body.

Carcinoid Tumours

These apudomas are thought to arise from the enterochromaffin (EC) cells of the gut. Most are benign and are found in the appendix after appendicectomy or incidentally in other parts of the bowel after resection. Malignant carcinoids are most common in the terminal ileum, where they are often multiple. At least one-third of patients with carcinoids of the small bowel have a second, unrelated, malignant tumour, often in another part of the alimentary tract. Occasionally the tumour forms part of a syndrome of multiple endocrine adenopathy (see later). Although malignant carcinoids metastasise to the liver and elsewhere they tend to grow extremely slowly and many patients survive in reasonable health for several (and sometimes many) years.

Most carcinoids of the midgut and its derivatives are argentaffin and secrete 5-hydroxytryptamine (5-HT) together with the enzyme kallikrein, which is responsible for the formation of bradykinin in the blood. Large malignant tumours secrete these substances in great amounts but, since they are normally inactivated in the liver (where they are carried by the portal circulation), no harm results. When large hepatic metastases develop and secrete them also, they enter the systemic circulation directly and cause the malignant carcinoid syndrome. A few carcinoids have been described in sites such as the ovary, which drain into the systemic circulation directly and cause the syndrome in the absence of metastases (Jagoe et al, 1973). Motilin (a humoral agent which stimulates gastric motility) and possibly substance P (perhaps a local hormone which stimulates smooth muscle and dilates blood vessels) have been identified as products of the small intestinal EC cells, but have not yet been found in tumours.

The syndrome is diagnosed on clinical grounds and on investigation in the laboratory. The commonest symptoms are flushing, diarrhoea and asthma and the most sinister complication is tricuspid or pulmonary stenosis. The most helpful investigation is measurement of the urinary excretion of 5-hydroxyindole acetic acid (5-HIAA), the major metabolite of 5-HT.

Treatment consists first of removal of as much of the primary tumour and the hepatic metastases as possible. Cytotoxic agents may be administered systemically or by local infusion into hepatic vessels. Cyclophosphamide, 5-fluorouracil and streptozotocin, given systemically, have caused regression of the syndrome in some patients. Infusion of 5-fluorouracil into the portal vein after ligation of the common hepatic artery, decreases the size of the liver secondaries and causes regression of the syndrome, at least temporarily, in a few. The excretion of 5-HIAA falls after resection of the tumour and often after successful treatment with cytotoxic agents. Periodic measurement gives valuable and early information about recurrence.

Drug therapy is not uniformly effective but may be helpful in the relief of symptoms. Methysergide, a 5-HT antagonist, helps to relieve diarrhoea and bronchospasm and *p*-chlorophenylalanine may relieve diarrhoea and improve appetite and wellbeing. α-Methyldopa is probably the best drug for the relief of flushing.

Carcinoid tumours of the foregut and its derivatives (stomach and bronchi) tend to secrete 5-hydroxytryptophan (5-HTP, the precursor of 5-HT) and histamine, and to cause the very severe 'atypical carcinoid syndrome'.

Carcinoid tumours at all sites, as will be described later, also form para-endocrine tumours.

Adrenal Medulla and Related Structures

The embryological relationships of the presumptive cells of origin of tumours in these sites are shown in Fig. 13.5. Sympathogonia, the most primitive cells of the neural crest, are the putative origin of the highly malig-nant neuroblastomas, while the differentiated ganglion cells, phaeochromo-

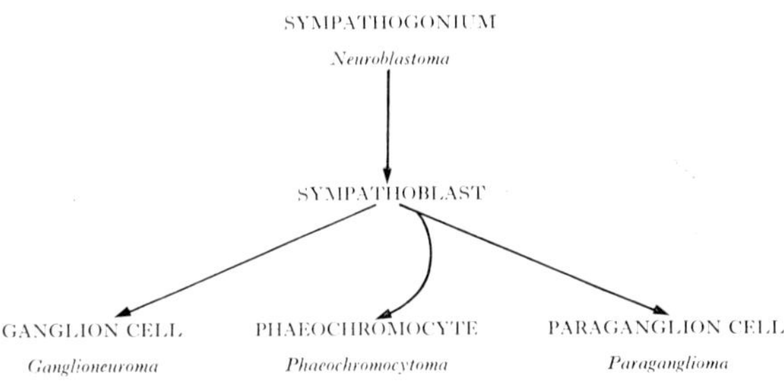

Figure 13.5   Cells of origin of adrenal medullary and related structures (cells of origin in capitals, tumours in italics)

cytes and paraganglion cells give rise to ganglioneuromas, phaeochromo-cytomas and paragangliomas respectively. Most of these tumours are benign.

All the cells of origin are apud cells and all the tumours are probably apudomas, although only the phaeochromocytomas have been studied extensively from this point of view. Nearly all phaeochromocytomas, 75 per cent of ganglioneuromas and neuroblastomas (and intermediate types of tumour), and an unknown proportion of paragangliomas are orthoendocrine and secrete excessive quantities of the catecholamines, adrenaline and/or noradrenaline. A few of these tumours are paraendocrine and secrete poly-peptides also.

Phaeochromocytoma

Phaeochromocytomas arise from phaeochromocytes in the adrenal medulla (80 per cent) or elsewhere in sympathetic nervous ganglia from the neck to the pelvis. About 99 per cent are found within the abdomen. Tumours are multiple in some 20 per cent of adult patients and in a higher proportion of children.

Most, but not all, in the adrenal medulla secrete mainly adrenaline and most elsewhere secrete mainly noradrenaline.

The symptoms are well known, the most important being arterial hypertension and sweating, which are often paroxysmal. Others, however, are many and various. Diagnosis involves measurement of the urinary excretion of vanilmandelic acid (VMA), the main metabolite of the catecholamines, which is higher than normal in 95 per cent of patients. The urinary metadrenalines and catecholamines themselves are raised in a higher proportion still. Localisation of the tumours is achieved, after α-blockade (see later) by selective arteriography and, when this fails, by selective venous sampling and measurement of catecholamines in the blood.

Phaeochromocytomas must be removed surgically. Treatment has been transformed in recent years by the use of sympathetic α-blockade before operation (and before invasive radiodiagnostic procedures) and the infusion of plasma after removal of the tumour or tumours. The rationale of these measures is that catecholamines cause constriction, not only of the arterioles (causing arterial hypertension), but also of the great veins (causing reduction of the blood volume). Failure to recognise this in the past led to severe hypotension as soon as the tumour(s) had been removed, necessitating the infusion of noradrenaline. Although therapy based on the assumption that patients are hypovolaemic is highly effective, actual measurements of blood volume in those with phaeochromocytomas frequently reveal normal blood volumes, perhaps because the methods used are too crude.

Since phaeochromocytomas are often multiple and in extra-adrenal sites, they are best approached through a long midline or paramedian incision, so that both adrenals, the whole para-aortic region and the pelvis can be explored. An exception to this rule may be made if a tumour greater than about 5 cm in diameter is seen on one side, when a lateral incision, through the bed of the eleventh rib on the left or the tenth rib on the right, gives easier and safer access. On the right side the promixity of the tumour to the inferior vena cava makes this particularly desirable. In these circumstances the peritoneal cavity should be opened and explored after removal of the tumour. If a second tumour is found it may be removed through a second appropriate incision, preferably at the same operation.

Despite preliminary α-blockade, squeezing a phaeochromocytoma causes a brisk rise in arterial blood pressure, which may be controlled with phentolamine or phenoxybenzamine intravenously. The use of β-blockers is reserved for cardiac irregularities. They are rarely needed preoperatively but are useful during the operation.

After operation urinary measurements of catecholamines and/or their metabolites should be repeated to ensure removal of all tumorous tissue. These should be delayed for about two weeks (or longer if the post-operative course is complicated) because the metabolic response to major operative stress causes increased urinary excretion for 10 days or so.

Removal of phaeochromocytomas cures all the symptoms, especially those of an episodic nature, but some degree of sustained hypertension usually persists.

Neuroblastoma and ganglioneuroma

These tumours (the former highly malignant and the latter benign) and many intermediate forms are apudomas. About three-quarters of them secrete catecholamines in sufficient quantity to increase the urinary excretion above normal, but they rarely cause general metabolic features. At operation, however, the blood pressure may rise alarmingly and they are best managed in the same way as phaeochromocytomas. Some patients have severe diarrhoea, which is cured by removal of the tumour. This may be due to the para-endocrine secretion of vasoactive intestinal polypeptide (VIP) (see later).

Paraganglionic tumours (Glenner and Grimley, 1974)

Paraganglia are found in two main regions: (1) related to the branchial arches (branchiomeric) and vagus nerves (intravagal), and (2) related to the aorta (para-aortic). All are closely associated with the sympathetic nervous system. The former include the carotid body, the glomus jugulare and the aortic body. Their main constituents are paraganglion (glomus or type 1) cells, which contain (and presumably secrete) catecholamines and 5-HT. The latter include the organ of Zuckerkandl. They contain both glomus cells and phaeochromocytes.

Branchiomeric paraganglionic tumours are probably apudomas and include carotid body, glomus jugulare and aortic body tumours. They are also called chemodectomas. They are all rare and their secretory capacity has been studied very little. It is probable that most secrete small amounts of catecholamines and 5-HT and a phaemochromocytoma-like syndrome has been observed on several occasions. Para-aortic paraganglionic tumours are either of the same type or extra-adrenal phaeochromocytomas, depending on their cell of origin.

II. PARAENDOCRINE APUDOMAS

Paraendocrine syndromes (PES) are clinical states, usually associated with hypersecretion of hormones by particular glands, but occurring in different circumstances. There are two main groups of syndromes which involve apudomas.

Paraendocrine syndromes type 1

In PES 1, tumours of endocrine glands secrete hormones or humoral agents which are foreign to their presumptive cells of origin, but characteristic of others (e.g. tumours of glands other than the anterior pituitary secrete ACTH and cause Cushing's syndrome).

The main tumours, hormones, humoral agents and syndromes are listed

Table 13.4 Paraendocrine syndromes

Tumours	Normal products of apud cells										Other
	CRH	ACTH and MSH	Prolactin	ADH	Calcitonin	Gastrin	VIP	Enteroglucagon	Catecholamines	5-HT	PTH
Of endocrine glands (PES 1)											
Apudomas											
Anterior pituitary tumours		(++)	(++)	±							
Thyroid medullary carcinoma		+			(++)						
Islet cells tumours	±	++		±		(++)	+		±	+	±
Bronchial and gut carcinoids		++			±		±			(++)	
Adrenal medullary tumours		+					±		(++)		
Other											
Parathyroid adenoma and hyperplasia		?±				?±					(++)
Of other organs (PES 2)											
Bronchial oat cell carcinoma	?±	++	±	++	±		?+			+	?±
Bronchial squamous carcinoma											+
Bronchial adenocarcinoma				?+							?±
Hepatoma and/or hepatoblastoma											±
Breast carcinoma					+						±
Cerebral tumours				+							
Renal and urinary tract tumours				±				±			
Melanoma		±					±				
Lymphatic tumours				?+							
Alimentary carcinoma											±
Syndromes	Cushing's	Cushing's and pigmentation	Galactorrhoea	Hyponatraemia	Nil	Zollinger–Ellison	WDHA	Villous hypertrophy, etc.	Hypertension, etc.	Carcinoid	Hypercalcaemia, etc.

Key: + + = Relatively common; + = Uncommon; ± = Very rare; ? = Doubtful; (+) and (+ +) = A hormone produced physiologically by the gland or cells from which the tumour is derived.

in Table 13.4. The commonest tumours are those of the islets of Langerhans, which are usually malignant when causing paraendocrine syndromes, and carcinoid tumours, especially of the bronchus. The commonest paraendocrine syndrome is Cushing's (ectopic ACTH) syndrome. These tumours may secrete their normal (orthoendocrine) hormones in addition to abnormal ones, up to a total of about six. The resulting clinical syndromes depend on the hormones or humoral agents released into the circulation, one or more of which may be 'silent'. For example, an islet cell tumour may secrete ACTH, MSH and gastrin in large quantities, producing Cushing's syndrome and pigmentation, but no gastric hypersecretion or peptic ulceration.

According to the hypothesis that apudomas arise from cells of neural crest origin, paraendocrine secretion is the result of dedifferentiation, whereby the apud cell apparatus mobilises the primitive potential of its embryological anlage and assumes the secretory properties of any members of the series. Parathyroid cells are not apud cells and parathyroid lesions are not apudomas. However, as pointed out earlier, the parathyroids may arise from neuro-ectoderm and share some fundamental properties of the derivatives of the neural crest. Other paraendocrine tumours in the thymus, ovary and adrenal cortex, secrete ACTH, parathormone (PTH), gonadotrophins and erythro-poietin. These properties cannot yet be explained.

Paraendocrine syndromes type 2

In PES 2, tumours or other lesions of organs or tissues, which are not usually regarded as endocrine in nature, secrete hormones or humoral agents characteristic of endocrine tissues (e.g. an oat cell carcinoma of the bronchus secretes ACTH or calcitonin).

The main tumours, hormones, humoral agents and syndromes are listed in Table 13.4. The commonest tumours are those of the bronchus, especially oat cell carcinoma. The commonest syndromes are Cushing's (ectopic ACTH) syndrome and the Schwartz–Bartter (ectopic antidiuretic hormone (ADH)) syndrome. Biochemical evidence of over-production of hormones is often present without a clinical syndrome of hormonal excess being recognised.

Only two of the tumours are known to be apudomas. One is the melanoma, whose cell of origin, the melanocyte, has no known secretion. The other is the bronchial oat cell carcinoma, which is regarded by some pathologists as a malignant form of bronchial carcinoid. There is no simple explanation for the secretion of polypeptide hormones by any of the other tumours. A suggestion (Warner, 1975), which could apply to any of those listed, is that the tumour cells are hybrids of two types of cell, one of them an apudoma, and that they assume the properties of both. Other paraendocrine tumours, only some of which are apudomas, may secrete hormones not of apud cell origin, such as gonadotrophins, TSH or erythropoietin. There is no ready explanation for these phenomena.

Paraendocrine Syndromes

Cushing's (ectopic ACTH) syndrome

Cushing's syndrome is the commonest form of paraendocrine syndrome of both types. The commonest causative lesions are oat cell carcinoma of the bronchus, carcinoid tumours (especially of the bronchus), epithelial carcinoma of the thymus, islet cell tumour of the pancreas, phaeochromocytoma and ovarian carcinoma. Most of these secrete ACTH and MSH, which overstimulate the adrenal cortices, rendering them hyperplastic, and cause pigmentation. Very rare tumours have been described, which secrete corticotrophin-releasing hormone (CRH), the hypothalamic hormone which stimulates the secretion and release of ACTH by the anterior pituitary.

The syndrome is usually very acute in onset, and metabolic disorders, such as hypokalaemic alkalosis and diabetes, usually precede the ordinary clinical features. The syndrome is commoner in men than in women (unlike the ordinary form), muscle wasting and weakness are usually severe, and pigmentation is common. The plasma ACTH and plasma and urinary cortisol levels are usually elevated much more than in the common form of the syndrome.

These features should lead to the suspicion of an ectopic site of ACTH secretion and to a search for the underlying tumour. Bronchial carcinoma is usually far advanced, and effective therapy is impossible. Carcinoid tumours, however, may be benign, and their removal cures the syndrome. Adrenalectomy is rarely justified, except in the case of a slow-growing tumour which cannot be eradicated.

Schwartz–Bartter (ectopic ADH) syndrome

This syndrome, caused by the secretion of the neurohypophyseal (posterior pituitary) antidiuretic hormone (ADH), is not uncommon. The most frequent cause is an advanced oat cell carcinoma of the bronchus, but several other tumours and non-tumorous conditions may be responsible.

Increased secretion of ADH, with a normal fluid intake, leads to retention of water, increased renal excretion of sodium, and hyponatraemia. When the condition is severe, the patient becomes drowsy, lethargic and confused.

If the underlying lesion can be treated, the patient excretes large amounts of dilute urine until the hyponatraemia is corrected. Symptomatic treatment involves restriction of water intake to 800 or 1000 ml daily. If this is not tolerated, fludrocortisone, 0.1 or 0.2 mg twice daily, promotes the retention of sodium and the excretion of dilute urine. It may cause depletion of potassium, which must be replaced.

The WDHA syndrome (pancreatic cholera, vipoma) (Verner and Morrison, 1974; Bloom, 1975)

In 1958 Verner and Morrison observed that two patients with non-β islet cell tumours of the pancreas, presenting with watery diarrhoea, did not develop peptic ulcers and had low gastric acid secretion. The syndrome has since been named the WDHA syndrome after the initial letters of its three principal characteristics, namely *W*atery *D*iarrhoea, *H*ypokalaemia and hypo- or *A*chlorhydria. It is rare, being about one-tenth as common as the Zollinger–Ellison syndrome, and is sometimes part of the syndrome of multiple endocrine adenopathy, type I (see later).

A non-β islet cell tumour of the pancreas is usually present and about half the tumours are malignant. Several cases have been described with bronchial (probably oat cell) carcinoma or with retroperitoneal neuroblastoma. The tumours release vasoactive intestinal polypeptide (VIP), a polypeptide humoral agent normally secreted by the small and large intestines. In large doses it causes vasodilatation, increases the blood flow to the gut, induces watery diarrhoea, reduces gastric secretion and has a strong cardiac inotropic action. These features are responsible for the clinical syndrome. In spite of the achlorhydria, the gastric mucosa appears normal, and biopsy shows no loss of parietal cells. In some patients the secretion of acid may rise during episodes of remission from diarrhoea.

Patients usually present with explosive watery diarrhoea which does not respond to simple measures. All have a low plasma potassium, ranging from 1 to 3 mEq/litre (1–3 mmol/litre) when first seen, and they often have associated hypercalcaemia, the cause of which is unexplained, but which has been cured by the removal of the tumour. Facial flushing has been observed occasionally.

The diagnosis is usually made by elimination of other possible causes of watery diarrhoea associated with hypokalaemia. Gastric secretion should be measured, preferably the 1 h basal output and the peak acid output in response to pentagastrin (6 μg/kg). Achlorhydria or hypochlorhydria would suggest the WDHA syndrome. This may be confirmed by the finding of high levels of VIP in the blood, if a radioimmunoassay is available. An attempt should then be made to identify a pancreatic or other tumour.

Treatment is directed towards finding and removing the tumour or tumours and successful results have been reported. Steroids sometimes provide temporary amelioration of symptoms. Deposits in the liver may be treated effectively by intra-arterial infusion of streptozotocin (Kahn et al, 1975).

Another group of patients (pseudo-WDHA syndrome), indistinguishable on clinical grounds from those with the WDHA syndrome, have normal blood levels of VIP and no pancreatic tumour. The cause is unknown and treatment is ineffective.

III. MULTIPLE ENDOCRINE ADENOPATHY (MEA)

The term multiple endocrine adenopathy describes a group of syndromes, often familial, in which two or more endocrine glands undergo hyperplasia or tumour formation in the same individual, either at the same time or consecutively. The glands usually exhibit hyperfunction and secrete their normal major hormones (orthoendocrine syndromes). They may, however, secrete abnormal hormones instead or as well (paraendocrine syndromes). There are two main varieties of MEA.

Multiple endocrine adenopathy type I (MEA I)

In this group the parathyroid glands are most frequently involved (90 per cent) and chief cell hyperplasia is the commonest lesion, giving rise usually to hyperparathyroidism, which is often mild. The pancreatic islet cells are also involved often (80 per cent), causing the Zollinger–Ellison syndrome, hyperinsulinism, or the WDHA syndrome, in that order of frequency. The anterior pituitary is involved next (65 per cent), causing space-occupying features of a pituitary tumour, acromegaly or, very rarely, Cushing's syndrome. Hyperplasia of the adrenal cortex, when present, is probably secondary to an ACTH-secreting tumour of the pituitary. Carcinoid tumours are not uncommon.

Many of these lesions are apudomas, and the syndrome may result from a widespread dysplasia of apud cells. However, the parathyroid lesions cannot be readily explained in this way, since the parathyroid cells are not apud in type and do not arise from the neural crest. They may, however (as mentioned already), arise from related neuroectoderm. Another possibility is that the hyperparathyroidism is secondary to hypersecretion of other hormones, for several of the intestinal hormones stimulate the secretion of calcitonin and this, in turn, promotes the secretion of PTH.

Duodenal ulceration is a common feature of the syndrome, and in patients with islet cell gastrinomas its occurrence is easily explained. However, in those without such a lesion the pathogenesis is obscure. It may be related to the hyperparathyroidism, for hypercalcaemia promotes the secretion of gastrin and this, in turn, stimulates the secretion of gastric acid. Parathyroidectomy (in patients with or without MEA I) often reduces the secretion of acid and sometimes cures duodenal ulceration. A few patients have been described in whom the parathyroids were apparently secreting gastrin (Stremple and Watson, 1974; Cassar, Cooke and Polak, 1975). If it is possible to do so, operation for duodenal ulcer should be postponed until all the endocrine lesions have been treated. It may then be unnecessary, unless the patient has a pancreatic gastrinoma, in which case total gastrectomy will probably be required.

Multiple endocrine adenopathy, type II (MEA II) (Sipple's syndrome)

In this syndrome a medullary carcinoma of the thyroid is associated with a phaeochromocytoma, hyperparathyroidism and other lesions, including subcutaneous and submucous neuromas and hyperplasia of melanocytes. The thyroid tumour produces large quantities of calcitonin which could give rise to secondary hyperparathyroidism. The whole syndrome may be regarded as an apud cell dysplasia.

The phaeochromocytoma is the lesion which requires the most urgent treatment, because investigation or treatment of other lesions may precipitate a fatal hypertensive crisis (Beaugie et al, 1975). For this reason the possibility of MEA II should be considered in all patients with medullary carcinoma of the thyroid or hyperparathyroidism, and they should be screened for the presence of a phaeochromocytoma.

Measurement of calcitonin in the blood may reveal the presence of medullary carcinoma, or a precancerous lesion, at a preclinical stage in members of affected families, even in childhood (Wolfe and Tashjian, 1974). Thyroidectomy, however, should not be undertaken lightly because the disease may run a long and relatively benign course.

CONCLUSION

The realisation that many apparently unrelated endocrine tumours can be classed together into a family, known as apudomas, provides a convenient unifying concept which increases their understanding and may in the course of time lead to more effective methods of treatment.

Many apudomas, such as carotid body tumours, await investigation of their secretory potential and others, particularly in the gut, probably await discovery. For instance, no tumours have yet been found to synthesise secretin, motilin, somatostatin or urogastrone, and it is to be hoped that awareness of these possibilities will lead to appropriate investigation of patients.

ACKNOWLEDGEMENT

We are grateful to Dr Julia M. Polak for her advice and for providing Figures 13.1 to 13.4.

REFERENCES

GENERAL

Montgomery, D. A. D. & Welbourn, R. B. (1975) *Medical and Surgical Endocrinology.* London: Arnold. (Contains full descriptions of the glands, hormones and syndromes referred to in the text, together with references.)

Pearse, A. G. E. & Welbourn, R. B. (1973) The apudomas. *British Journal of Hospital Medicine,* **10**, 617.

Welbourn, R. B., Pearse, A. G. E., Polak, J. M., Bloom, S. R. & Joffe, S. N. (1974) The apud cells in health and disease. *Medical Clinics of North America,* **58**, 1359. (These two papers are general reviews of the apud concept and apudomas and contain many references.)

Pearse, A. G. E. & Takor, T. T. (1976) Neuroendocrine embryology and the APUD concept *Clinical Endocrinology,* **5**, Suppl., 229. (A review of the embryology of apud and related cells.)

Pearse, A. G. E. (1975) Neurocristopathy, neuroendocrine pathology and the APUD concept. *Zeitschrift für Krebsforschung*, **84**, 1.

Pearse, A. G. E. & Polak, J. M. (1974) Endocrine tumours of neural crest origin: neurolophomas, apudomas and the apud concept. *Medical Biology*, **52**, 3. (These two papers provide pathological accounts of the apudomas.)

SPECIFIC

Barrowman, J. A., Bennett, A., Hillenbrand, P., Rolles, K., Pollock, D. J. & Wright, J. T. (1975) Diarrhoea in thyroid medullary carcinoma: role of prostaglandins and therapeutic effect of nutmeg. *British Medical Journal*, **3**, 11.

Beaugie, J. M., Belchetz, P. E., Brown, C. L., Frankel, R. J. & Lloyd, M. H. (1975) Report of a family with inherited medullary carcinoma of the thyroid and phaeochromocytoma. *British Journal of Surgery*, **62**, 264.

Bloom, S. R. (1975) Vasoactive intestinal peptide and the Verner–Morrison syndrome. *Gut*, **16**, 399.

Bonfils, S. (1974) Endocrine-secreting tumours of the GI tract. *Clinics in Gastroenterology*, **3**, 475. London: Saunders.

Cassar, J., Cooke, W. M. & Polak, J. M. (1975) Possible parathyroid origin of gastrin in a patient with multiple endocrine adenopathy type I. *British Journal of Surgery*, **62**, 313.

Child, D. F., Nader, S., Mashiter, K., Kjeld, M., Banks, L. & Fraser, T. R. (1975) Prolactin studies in 'functionless' pituitary tumours. *British Medical Journal*, **1**, 604.

Cowley, D. J., Dymock, I. W., Boyes, B. E., Wilson, R. Y., Stagg, B. H., Lewin, M. R. Polak, J. M. & Pearse, A. G. E. (1973) Zollinger–Ellison syndrome type 1: clinical and pathological correlations in a case. *Gut*, **14**, 25.

Glenner, G. G. & Grimley, P. M. (1974) Tumors of the extra-adrenal paraganglion system. *Atlas of Tumor Pathology*, Second Series, Fascicle G. Bethesda, Maryland: Armed Forces Institute of Pathology.

Jagoe, W. S., Gallager, N. G., Gearty, G. F. & Logan, P. J. (1973) Primary argentaffinoma of the ovary. *British Journal of Surgery*, **60**, 749.

Kahn, C. R., Levy, A. G., Gardner, J. D., Miller, J. V., Gordon, P. & Schein, P. S. (1975) Pancreatic cholera: beneficial effects streptozotocin. *New England Journal of Medicine*, **292**, 941.

Mallison, C. N., Bloom, S. R., Warin, A. P., Salmon, P. R. & Cox, B. (1974) A glucagonoma syndrome. *Lancet*, **2**, 1.

Polak, J. M., Stagg, B. & Pearse, A. G. E. (1972) Two types of Zollinger–Ellison syndrome. Immunofluorescent, cytochemical and ultrastructural studies of antral and pancreatic gastrin cells in different clinical states. *Gut*, **13**, 501.

Royston, C. M. S., Brew, D. St. J., Garnham, J. R., Stagg, D. H. & Polak, J. M. (1972) The Zollinger–Ellison syndrome due to an infiltrating tumour of the stomach. *Gut*, **13**, 638.

Szijj, T., Csapo, Z., Lasslo, F. A. & Kovacs, K. (1969) Medullary carcinoma of the thyroid associated with hypercorticism. *Cancer*, **24**, 167.

Stremple, J. F. & Watson, G. C. (1974) Serum calcium, serum gastrin, and gastric acid secretion before and after parathyroidectomy for hyperparathyroidism. *Surgery*, **75**, 841.

Thompson, M. H., Venables, C. W., Miller, I. T., Reed, J. D., Sanders, D. J., Grund, E. R. & Blair, E. L. (1975) Metiamide in Zollinger–Ellison syndrome. *Lancet*, **1**, 35.

Thompson, J. C., Reeder, D. D., Villar, H. V. & Fender, H. R. (1975) Natural history and experience with diagnosis and treatment of the Zollinger–Ellison syndrome. *Surgery, Gynecology and Obstetrics*, **140**, 721.

Verner, J. V. & Morrison, A. B. (1974) Endocrine pancreatic islet disease with diarrhoea. *Archives of Internal Medicine*, **133**, 492.

Warner, T. F. C. S. (1975) Cell hybridisation: an explanation for the phenotypic diversity of certain tumours. *Hypothesis*, **1**, 51.

Wolfe, H. J. & Tashjian, A. H. (1974) Cytological, immunological and biological studies of calcitonin in the normal human thyroid gland and in patients predisposed to medullary thyroid carcinoma. In *Endocrinology 1973*, ed. Taylor, S., p. 323. London: Heinemann.

14
THE MANAGEMENT OF LOW BACK PAIN

J. A. Mathews   D. A. Reynolds

It is estimated that seven and a half million working days are lost each year in the United Kingdom through backache (Wood and Benn, 1972). Without taking into account the cost of treating these patients, loss of earnings alone is probably in excess of £50000000 annually. In the United States every year one and a quarter million people injure their backs, and 65000 of these are left with some permanent disability (Beals and Hickman, 1972). Such is the economic measure of the problem of low back pain.

It is more than 40 years since Mixter and Barr (1934) described the detailed pathology of intervertebral disc herniation, and so brought about a new approach in the surgical management of backache. Yet, despite the optimism of earlier years, surgery has not provided a complete solution. In only a proportion of those who suffer from backache is the cause that classical combination of disc prolapse and root pressure which responds so well to decompression. The problem still remains of the patient with intractable symptoms from less clearly defined pathology.

Later advances in our knowledge have been less dramatic than this earlier contribution, but no less significant. They can be considered under several headings.

1. Diagnosis. Improved recognition of the clinical syndromes produced by progressive lumbar disc prolapse, and differentiation of other degenerative spinal disorders.
2. Differential diagnosis. Improved recognition of other spinal pathologies.
3. Treatment.
   (a) Definition of the place of non-operative management, and evaluation of non-operative techniques.
   (b) Critical evaluation of the various surgical techniques and the proper indications for their use.
4. Psychology. Definition of the importance of the emotional element in back problems.

DIAGNOSIS

It is generally accepted that the majority of patients with intermittent low back pain are experiencing symptoms resulting from self-limiting disorders of traumatic or degenerative nature. Frequently, the absence of any relevant laboratory or radiological findings forces the clinician to rely upon firstly history taking and secondly a system of examination. The usually self-limiting nature of the syndrome denies the surgeon or pathologist the opportunity to confirm his diagnostic suspicion. It is convenient to divide the features of mechanical spinal disorders into those arising from an intervertebral joint or its related structures (articular), those arising from dural tension (dural) and those arising from nerve root pressure (root) (Table 14.1). Each has its own characteristic symptoms and signs and as a lesion becomes progressively larger and more serious, so the diagnosis becomes less controversial. At one extreme there is the patient with intermittent backache and no physical signs and at the opposite the patient whose sciatica has been 'cured' by disc removal.

Table 14.1 Sites of mechanical spinal disorders (by permission of the Editor of *Rheumatology and Rehabilitation*)

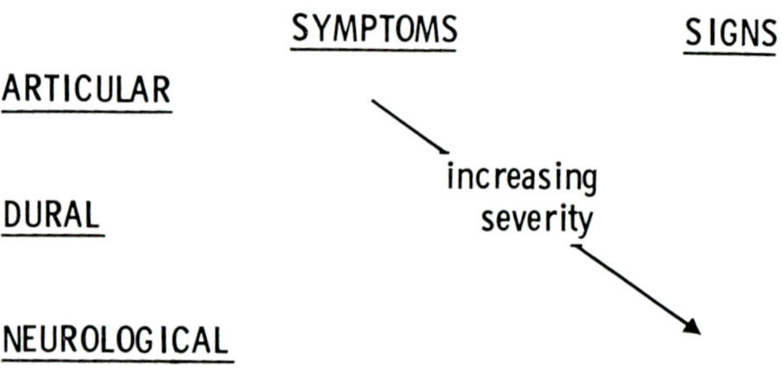

Articular: symptoms

The patient with symptoms only is in some ways in the greatest difficulty as the ability to convince the clinician that a spinal disorder exists depends entirely on the supply of an adequate history. The timing of the pain and its relationship to activities should be paid great hccd. It is reassuring to obtain a story of intermittent pain related to posture as this suggests a mechanical process; more serious (i.e. malignant, infective or inflammatory) spinal disorders are often accompanied by relentless pain or pain not related to activity. By contrast the site of pain is relatively non-specific. It can be seen (Fig. 14.1) that many of the spinal structures receive their sensory nerve supply from branches of the posterior primary ramus if they are posterior to the spine or the recurrent sinuvertebral nerve if they are intraspinal. It is unlikely that the site of referral of pain is specific to the structure involved and it is useful to adopt a system for differential diagnosis of soft tissue lesions (Cyriax, 1969). Of the posterior spinal structures several are possible causes of low back pain and can only be differentiated by eliciting appropriate physical signs.

Muscle. A muscular lesion may be suggested by finding local swelling and tenderness. Should a tender nodule be dispersed by frictions or a local anaesthetic injection, it is tempting to believe that a primary pathology has been eradicated. This is unlikely to be the case. Firstly, such a primary mechanical lesion in muscles as strong as sacrospinalis must be rare and would result only from appreciable trauma; secondly, it is possible to relieve even referred muscle spasm by local anaesthetic infiltration. The sign par excellence of a muscle lesion is pain worst on 'isometric' or 'resisted' contraction.

Ligament. Tenderness of interspinous ligaments is extremely common in patients with low backache and its significance dubious. However, when it is the only physical sign rather more notice must be taken. It may be that ligament lesions are a common accompaniment of other mechanical derangements

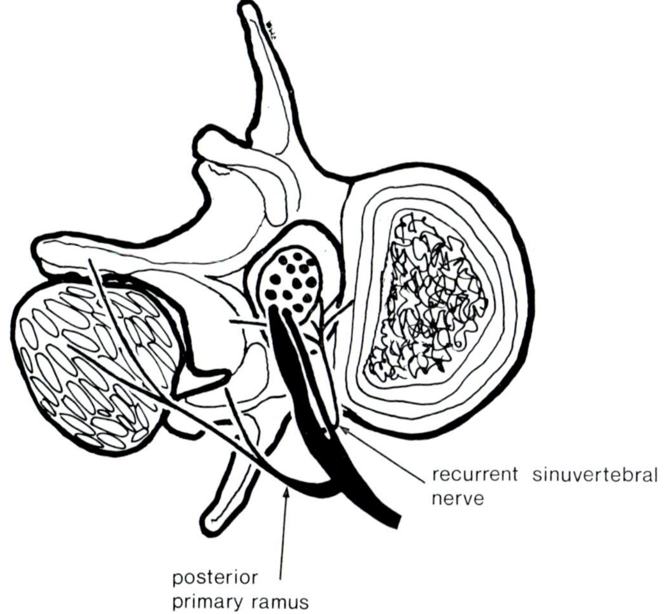

Figure 14.1   Spinal structures are supplied through branches of the posterior primary ramus or the recurrent sinuvertebral nerve

of the spine, but when they occur in isolation there will be only the local tenderness and pain when the ligament is stretched by flexion or compressed by extension.

Joint. The lumbar intervertebral joint consists of one fibrous anterior and a pair of posterior apophyseal articulations at each level. To diagnose a derangement between a pair of vertebrae with confidence requires restriction of movement but minimal lesions cause presumably pain only at extremes of range. As most derangements are asymmetrical the pattern of production of pain should be likewise.

Attempts to demonstrate sites of referral of pain were made by Kellgren (1939). Hypertonic saline was injected into a variety of soft tissues of the back of volunteers and the sites of referral of pain plotted. In general the areas of referral were of root distribution and ipsilateral, but rather more distal than expected from clinical evidence. This variance may indicate that the nature of the insult as well as its site is of importance.

Articular: symptoms with signs

When restriction of lumbar movement occurs as in osteoarthrosis or ankylosing spondylitis the restriction is classically symmetrical and involves lateral flexions particularly early. When internal derangement of an intervertebral joint takes place restriction is usually asymmetrical—the four movements (flexion, extension and two lateral flexions) examined being unequally affected. This asymmetrical restriction is again a useful and reassuring finding that the patient does not have a more serious spinal disorder. The pathological studies of Harris and Macnab (1954) indicate frequent degenerative changes in both anterior (disc) and posterior (apophyseal) joints. In the absence of serious bony defect the two are inextricably connected and both may be subject to internal derangement. It becomes impossible at this level of symptoms and signs reliably to apportion blame to one or other.

Dural: symptoms

Figure 14.1 indicates those intraspinal structures receiving sensory innervation through the sinuvertebral nerve and it can be seen that the posterior longitudinal ligament and the adjacent anterior aspect of the dural sac as well as the sheaths of the nerve roots are supplied (Wyke, 1970). It is unlikely that a patient can reliably differentiate one source of pain from another. However, Smyth and Wright (1958) have attempted to throw light on the anatomy of pain production in disc prolapse. They stimulated various structures encountered at laminectomy by leaving nylon threads in place and pulling on them when the subjects had regained consciousness. In general they found that the interspinous ligaments and ligamentum flavum were either insensitive or caused dragging sensations or vague aches, whereas pulling a nerve root produced a distinct sciatic pain. The problem of ascribing symptoms which are not accompanied by signs therefore exists with regard to the dura as it did to the articulation, but in general the evidence favours dural pain as being rather more widespread than articular pain but still ill-defined and proximal. It is believed that stimulation of the dura can provoke pain which appears to be in a different segment, the mechanism being transmission of sensory impulses through the longitudinal anastomoses demonstrated in monkeys (Stilwell, 1956) to lie along the posterior longitudinal ligament. This mechanism could explain pain felt over the lower posterior chest or abdomen in lumbar disc prolapse.

Dural: symptoms with signs

The presence of objective signs again makes interpretation of symptoms more reliable, but when signs contain a subjective factor they are a shade less helpful. The best known dural sign is the straight leg raise (Lasègue) test. In eliciting this sign it is important to raise the straight leg first on the unaffected side, and keeping the knee straight to observe the number of degrees from the horizontal at which the pelvis begins to tilt. The painful side is then raised for comparison and the level at which pain induces hamstring spasm is noted. This spasm is presumed to be induced by the approximation of the L5 or S1 nerve root to the disc protrusion. That it is produced by movement of the nerve roots is supported by the fact that foot dorsiflexion and neck flexion will often accentuate the sign. The limitation of straight leg raise by disc protrusion is not entirely mechanical—witness the effect of epidural or general anaesthesia in nullifying the sign. The usefulness and relevance of

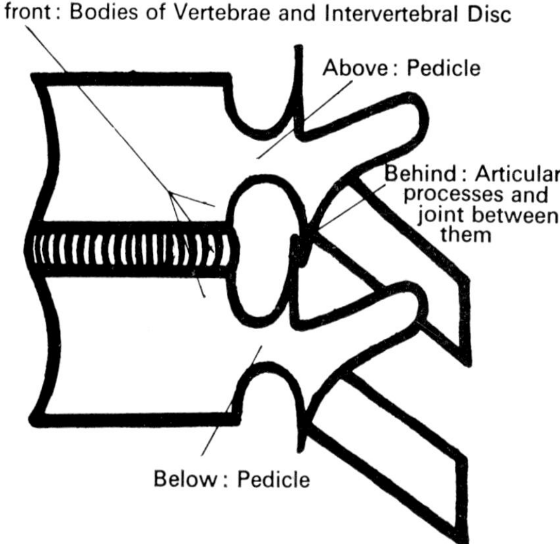

Figure 14.2   Diagram to show the relationship of the intervertebral foramen to adjacent structures (Hewitt, *Physiotherapy*, by permission of the Editor)

this sign recently has been investigated in a combined radiological and operative study (Edgar and Park, 1974). Even at the stage in progress of increasing magnitude of disc protusion that has now been reached in this description it will be clear from the description of the relationships of the intervertebral foramen by Hewitt (1970) (Fig. 14.2) that a swollen deranged apophyseal joint could theoretically be to blame as it too could cause the joint derangement and dural 'tension' signs described.

A lesser known and less commonly present dural sign is the femoral nerve stretch test (usually performed by 'prone knee flexion'). This sign depends upon the increased tension induced via the femoral nerve on the L3 and L4 nerve roots. The patient lies prone, the knee of the pain-free side is flexed and the patient asked to report any discomfort or pain. Commonly there is quadriceps discomfort but if the sign is positive the patient reports that back pain or 'the pain of which they complain' is produced.

Neurological: symptoms

Far the most common symptom in this category resulting from lumbar disc prolapse is pain, but this covers a variety of manifestations. True root pain by contrast to pain arising from intervertebral joints or even dura is more severe and distinct, usually well delineated, and conforms to the anatomical confines of the appropriate dermatome. Because the two most common roots affected are S1 and L5 the pain is usually distal and posterior in the leg, but L4 pain affecting the shin and L3 the anterior thigh and knee sometimes occur. At one extreme is the severe but self-limiting pain of nerve root interruption. This is the pain of exceptional severity and exquisitely sensitive to spinal movement or those movements causing elevation of intraspinal pressure, e.g. coughing, sneezing and straining. At the other extreme is a mild intermittent pain or similar distribution but necessitating some physical stress for its production—e.g. bending, walking, assuming unfavourable postures. Rarely the nature of the sensory insult is such that paraesthesia or numbness is an early symptom.

SPINAL STENOSIS

As in so many disorders of the musculoskeletal system, the absence of objectively abnormal physical signs forces reliance upon an accurate history, and in the context of root pain there is scope for several interesting variations. It is clearly possible for pain to be accentuated by those actions which increase the extent of the disc prolapse, e.g. repeated bending or lifting. However, pain is sometimes precipitated or aggravated by walking. Curiously, walking up-hill can be less troublesome than on the flat, suggesting that extension of the spine has a provocative action. Investigation of this phenomenon has led to recognition of a clinical entity, the syndrome referred to now as spinal stenosis (Newman, 1973).

In spinal stenosis the initial complaint is of backache precipitated by sitting, or standing, or walking. Sometimes backache is the only symptom, but classically it is followed by a combination of root pain and impairment of motor power in the legs. These neurological symptoms are relieved quickly by rest.

Early descriptions of this clinical picture referred to 'intermittent claudication of the cauda equina' as the cause. This analogy with ischaemic leg muscle claudication led some authors to postulate primary nerve ischaemia to be the underlying mechanism. Alternative suggestions included relative ischaemic anoxia on exercise, or an increase in CSF pressure distal to an intraspinal block (*British Medical Journal*, 1969). Whatever happens, neither symptoms nor signs will be present in the absence of provocation.

In many of the cases a careful radiological examination will reveal diminution in the diameters of the lumbar spinal canal. Hence the term spinal stenosis (Nelson, 1973). Congenital narrowing of the canal can be seen in achondroplasiacs (who are recognised to be prone to low back problems) and in spina bifida, but most other cases occur secondarily to degenerative changes in otherwise normal individuals. An anterior transverse osteophyte bar may be present at one or more disc levels. The stenosing effect of this may be aggravated by further narrowing from behind by extravagant osteophyte formation about the posterior joints. On clinical examination signs of these degenerative changes may be obvious, but paradoxically sometimes little or no abnormality is to be found. Myelographic findings vary from the demonstration of multiple disc prolapse in the lumbar region, to complete block. Marked attentuation of the subarachnoid space may make insertion of the needle difficult. Surgical treatment is by decompression, which must be adequate both in lateral and longitudinal directions.

Neurological: symptoms with signs

There are several points of outstanding interest in considering the neurology of the legs. The earliest and often the most persistent objective neurological deficit observed in the lumbar disc degeneration is absence of a tendon reflex. This is usually unilateral and because it is the lowest two discs which are most commonly affected it is the ankle reflex which is the more commonly impaired or absent. Its root value is S1. The only other reliably elicited tendon reflex in the leg is the knee reflex and being subserved by L3 and L4 it is much less frequently affected. The second most common root to be involved is L5 and as its tendon reflex—the great toe jerk—is only seldom detectable in normal subjects, a total L5 palsy may be unaccompanied by reflex changes. The spinal cord ends at L1 and it therefore follows that no upper motor neurone lesion or long tract signs can be caused by lumbar disc prolapse. Finally, mention should be made of the important signs of low cauda equina compression as, if unrelieved, irreversible loss of bladder control may result. These may include weakness and wasting in the conventional S1 distribution (calves and hamstrings), with S2 loss (buttocks). In addition there may be reduction of sensation in the perineum and saddle area which needs careful eliciting with the patient prone. The onset of cauda equina compression can be dramatic, requiring urgent treatment.

X-RAYS

No mention has been made so far of the value of radiographs. The disc tissue itself is radiolucent and as a gross reduction in its volume is needed to produce a detectable reduction in 'disc space' this is only rarely a helpful finding. However, indirect findings can be of help. Occasionally painful muscle spasm causes a tilt—but this can be seen more easily clinically. Most often the radiological changes are relatively late and include disc space reduction resulting from desiccation of nuclear material and the formation

12

of beak-shaped osteophytes (Fig. 14.3), whose shape is determined by the curve of the protruding disc and the periosteum elevated from the adjacent vertebral bodies. Alteration in the size or shape of the disc leads to abnormal stresses being placed on the apophyseal joints and these readily develop the changes characteristic of osteoarthrosis in synovial joints—sclerosis, osteophytosis and reduction of space.

Contrast x-rays can be of value, but each method has advantages and drawbacks (Park, 1976). Conventional oily myelography has been hallowed by experience, provides dense contrast, is confined by the dural sac (thus missing small lateral protrusions) but has a small morbidity. Radiculography uses the same route and a water-soluble medium, has inferior contrast but

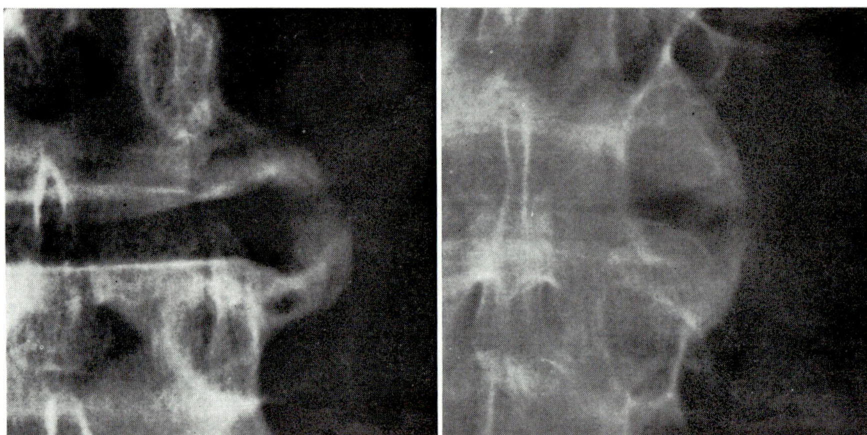

Figure 14.3   This pair of x-ray films contrasts the beak-shaped osteophyte formation around a disc prolapse (left) with the smooth annular calcification of a syndesmophyte in spondylitis (right)

better root filling and therefore better lateral discrimination. Epidurography is not confined by the dural sac and therefore can detect lateral lesions, but the inferior flow of contrast in the areolar connective tissue of the epidural space makes interpretation more difficult. Discography has the defect of poor correlation with relevant pathology as frequently evidence of multiple disc degeneration is detected. Other less proved techniques include gas contrast myelography and venography.

Perhaps the most important reason for taking plain lumbar spine x-rays in patients with backache is to try to exclude serious pathology.

DIFFERENTIAL DIAGNOSIS

The foregoing account of the mechanical form of low back pathology cannot be complete without mention of other mechanical conditions which may give rise to similar symptoms and more serious diseases affecting the spine. The list could be limitless. It is practical to consider only the conditions which occur commonly enough to be relevant to everyday clinical work with brief mention of others of particular interest at the present time.

Spondylolysis and spondylolisthesis

Classification of the various forms of spondylolysis and spondylolisthesis has contributed much to understanding and management of low back problems (Newman, 1963). Recognition of the differing natural histories of each type has made it possible to advise rational treatment.

Spondylolysis is the term used to describe a defect in a neural arch, usually of the fifth or fourth lumbar vertebra. Such defects, it is now generally agreed, are probably forms of stress fracture rather than developmental anomalies (Wiltse, Widdell and Jackson, 1975). When associated with changes of disc degeneration at the same vertebral level, the resulting instability may allow a degree of forward displacement of the affected vertebral body upon the one immediately below—spondylolisthesis. This variety of spondylolisthesis can occur at any age, even in the very young, but the patients usually are adolescents or younger adults, all active people. The degree of slip is usually minor but can become gross.

A second variety of spondylolisthesis is seen in older age groups. Vertebral slip occurs but here is always minor. It is the result of a combination of disc degeneration, and instability of the posterior articular complex arising from secondary degenerative changes. It is the earlier disc degeneration, by now well established, which is the primary lesion. Commonly the fourth lumbar vertebra moves forward upon the fifth, less frequently the fifth lumbar upon the first sacral.

Recognition of fatigue fracture as the cause of the arch defect in spondylolysis allows a logical sequence of management. In early cases where little or no slip is present healing of the fracture can occur spontaneously. The symptoms can be contained by support from a lumbosacral corset alone. Even if the defect persists symptoms may still be minimal provided there is no coincident disc problem. Occasionally it becomes necessary to overcome delay in healing of the fracture by surgical fixation and grafting of the defect thereby adding to the stability of that level. Established non-union of a defect, when associated with greater degrees of vertebral slip, can give rise to syndromes very similar to those of disc prolapse and sciatica, and spinal instability. Such late secondary changes are likely to respond only to a more radical surgical approach.

In the degenerative form of spondylolisthesis the degree of slip is usually minimal. Treatment of the symptoms is non-operative except in those very few cases where further secondary degenerative pathology such as instability or stenosis has supervened.

There remains the rare congenital form of spondylolisthesis. Here the lumbosacral vertebral pedicles are grossly defective or elongated, and give rise in early childhood or adolescence to equally gross degrees of vertebral displacement and root embarrassment. The condition is not difficult to recognise, and control usually involves major surgery.

Coccydynia

This condition of pain in the coccyx is common and troublesome. Although often regarded with exasperation by those asked to treat it, it is a cause of severe disability to those who suffer from it. The symptoms are commonly attributed to trauma, and occasionally this is clearly the cause. In such cases usually the pain resolves spontaneously, or responds to injection of steroid and a manipulation. However, most coccydynia probably is referred from the lumbosacral disc, and examination will reveal physical signs at that level. Treatment directed to the lumbosacral disc may then settle the coccydynia as well. If this is not realised, and therapy continues to be concentrated upon the coccyx alone, the symptoms are unlikely to be relieved. The patient may become obsessed with the problem to the point of hysteria. Often the situation is allowed to deteriorate so far that the coccyx is even removed, without relief. Then the emotional element may become so significant that even proper measures are unlikely to help.

Metabolic bone disease

Mention of these conditions is justified here both because of the association with backache, and because their presence is a contraindication to most of the mechanical methods of treatment used for mechanical causes of low back pain. Osteomalacia and osteoporosis share the feature that in both the amount of calcified bone is reduced and radiologically they may be indistinguishable. However, the similarity ends at this point.

Osteomalacia. This results from inadequate vitamin D to meet the body demand and consequent reduction in calcium absorbtion. Clinically this results in bone pain and tenderness and muscle weakness leading often to a waddling gait. The diagnosis is frequently missed for long periods and alternative diseases of muscles and joints are considered or the patient labelled as suffering from 'neurosis'. Sometimes the radiological features are characteristic with the appearance of Looser zones (or 'pseudo-fractures') which represent uncalcified osteoid seams. The disease may be diagnosed biochemically, the most sensitive test being elevation of the serum alkaline phosphatase; the serum calcium falls rather later. Bone biopsy may be needed to confirm the diagnosis, but Morgan (1968) in his review of the conditions regards the response to vitamin D as the ultimate confirmation.

Osteoporosis. This may result from a number of conditions which lead to a reduction of the bone matrix. It is not a disorder of calcium or vitamin D and there are no detectable biochemical abnormalities. Osteoporosis is a regular feature of ageing, particularly in the female. The common complaint is backache which is often accompanied by overt or perhaps 'micro' fractures

(Vernon-Roberts and Pirie, 1973). Clinically the patient may seem to be losing height with a developing kyphosis. Radiologically there may be wedge fractures or biconcavity ('fish-tailing') of the vertebrae—but as the latter probably depends on relatively healthy turgid intervertebral discs, it is uncommon in the elderly. Confirmation of the diagnosis in mild or moderate cases is unsatisfactory, as both x-rays and biopsies are open to subjective interpretation.

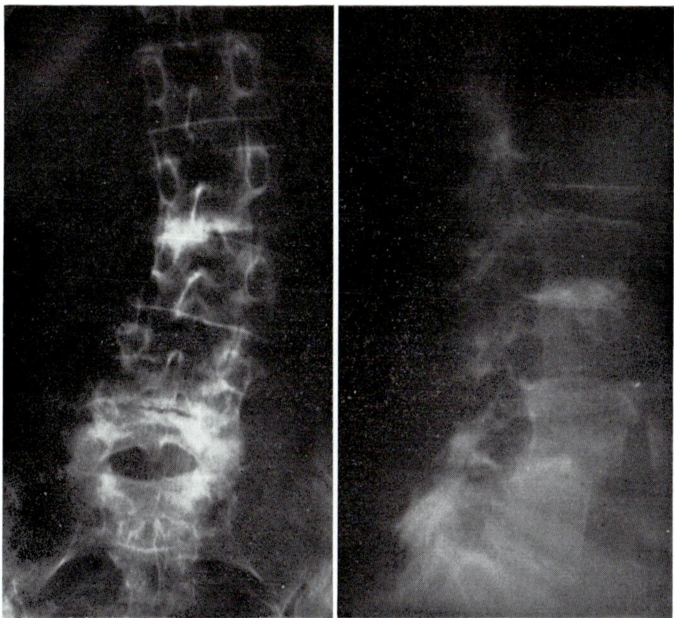

Figure 14.4   Disorganised intervertebral discs in rheumatoid arthritis

Inflammatory joint disease

Much the commonest inflammatory disease of joints is rheumatoid arthritis but clinical manifestations in the lumbar spine are uncommon and pathological descriptions even more rare. A much less common arthritic condition is ankylosing spondylitis, but it classically affects the sacro-iliac joints and lumbar spine and the pathology is well documented. Rheumatoid arthritis classically leads to inflammation of synovial joints and could therefore cause arthritis of apophyseal joints. Postmortem studies (Bywaters, 1975) have revealed also rheumatoid granulation tissue invading discs. Observation in this hospital of patients with corresponding and severe x-ray changes (Fig. 14.4) has shown the accompanying low back pain to be of rather persistent but localised nature. Ankylosing spondylitis (Cruickshank, 1960) leads to the invasion of disc material by loose vascular and fibrous tissue which later ossifies with the characteristic appearance of 'syndesmophytes' (Fig. 14.3). These patients have lengthy episodes of back pain with symmetrical restriction of movement occasionally leading to fusion. Atypical ankylosing spondylitis may occur in Reiter's disease, psoriasis and chronic intestinal disorders, and in all these forms of ankylosing spondylitis there is a strong association with the HL-A 27 antigen (Brewerton, 1975). Perhaps the critical differentiation between these ankylosing conditions and mechanical lumbar disorders is that the former tend to improve after physical activity and the restriction of movement is usually symmetrical. As in all inflammatory conditions the ESR may be raised. There is also the theoretical possibility that apophyseal joint swelling occurs, leading to dural symptoms and signs. These could be confused with lumbar disc prolapse.

Infections

The commonest organisms infecting the spine are *Mycobacterium tuberculosis* and the *Staphylococcus*.

Tuberculosis is not a rare disease (Lloyd-Griffiths, 1975) and it is not restricted to immigrant population as is commonly believed. The early symptoms can be very similar to those of a simple mechanical back problem and it is just at this stage that diagnosis is most important, since the infection can then be treated with greatest effect by chemotherapy alone. The management of later stages may involve extensive surgery (*British Medical Journal*, 1974).

Staphylococcal osteomyelitis, even when established, may mimic less ominous back problems very closely. Radiological changes are not necessarily easy to identify and characteristically appear later. The lesson to be learned is simple—to be aware of the possibility of sepsis when faced with making a diagnosis in an intractable back problem. Once such a diagnosis has been made, treatment of these conditions is straightforward and effective, often with no need to resort to surgery (Kemp et al, 1973a). Not infrequently diagnosis is made particularly difficult by the suppressive effect upon early symptoms and signs of anti-inflammatory and immunosuppressive agents being given simultaneously for other disease processes. A history of previous genito-urinary sepsis or surgery may be significant, as the venous drainage systems of both the pelvic organs and the lumbar spine are closely interconnected. In these circumstances the infecting organism may be an *E. coli*.

A new term—discitis—has been applied recently to two different clinical situations. The first is that of disc narrowing in younger children associated with back signs and symptoms, often with a limp or unwillingness to use a limb, and a raised sedimentation rate. There is argument as to whether or not this is caused by bacterial inflammation or other pathology. In general it is a self-limiting condition (Spiegel et al, 1972). 'Discitis' has also come to refer to a particularly indolent early phase of staphylococcal infection of the spine (Kemp et al, 1973a). The disease at this stage is still so isolated within the disc space that it may be difficult to establish the diagnosis by the usual serological and bacteriological means.

Brucellosis is a rare infection, but should be remembered for any patient whose work brings him into close contact with animals. Clinically, this condition in many ways mimics tuberculosis of the spine (Seal and Morris, 1974).

An epidural abscess can simulate a disc protrusion closely. Despite its rarity it is an important condition because only early recognition and operation can pre-empt permanent neurological damage. Once the diagnosis is suspected, it is capable of being established. A history of staphylococcal skin infection, or diabetes, is likely to be significant (Keon-Cohen, 1968).

Tumours

Most tumours of the spine are metastatic. Those primary tumours which do occur are not necessarily malignant. All spinal tumours can produce symptoms indistinguishable from those of a mechanical back problem, but pain from a spinal tumour can be intractable and is certainly less easy to relieve by simple rest, a treatment which nearly always settles pain of mechanical origin. Symptoms of weakness, or very early signs of paralysis combined with patchy anaesthesia are a common presentation. In children an abnormal gait or posture should raise one's suspicions, particularly in the presence of lumbar spasm and tight hamstrings (da Roza, 1964).

Posture

Lumbar backache is frequently attributed to hyperlordosis. The lordosis comes before the backache, and from this one can predict those who are likely to have back problems in later years. The most usual cause of excessive lordosis is simple bad posture, either racial, or in the droopy young, or in the older patient whose musculature has degenerated. Typically, the latter is either an ex-athlete or an over-weight multiparous woman. Hypermobility of peripheral joints has been shown to be associated with an increased incidence of non-specific backache (Howes and Isdale, 1971). Hyperlordosis is also a secondary feature of adolescent kyphosis of the thoracic spine, a common condition in both sexes. This is sometimes referred to as Scheuermann's osteochondritis, a term based upon the radiological appearances. The local symptoms in adolescents are of aching in the thoracic spine. They are self-resolving as the individual matures, but the kyphotic posture persists and it is the secondary increase in lumbar lordosis which later is associated with symptoms of low backache.

TREATMENT

To obtain a reasonably clear and rational exposition of treatments for mechanical forms of low back pain it is easiest to start by discussing lumbar disc protrusion in increasing orders of magnitude. Let it first be said that any treatment advocated must stand comparison with conventional 'rest and analgesics' hallowed by time and recognised for safety.

Rest and analgesics

Rest can be prescribed in various intensities. When the severity of symptoms is sufficient to justify absence from work or even admission to hospital, the rest should be as near absolute as is feasible. This requires the patient to remain horizontal for 24 h a day, the only exception being the use of a bedside commode if this seems less traumatic than a bedpan. It is of little importance whether the patient is supine or lies on one side, as the benefit of rest is thought to result from the lowering of intradiscal pressure; although under conditions of measurement Nachemson and Morris (1964) found variations in this pressure with altering horizontal postures, for practical purposes the most comfortable and pain-free position is almost certainly the best. It is difficult to know how long to keep the patient recumbent. A practical policy for most treatments is to try them for one or two weeks and if there is little or no improvement, to change course by adopting another regime. On the other hand it is difficult to know when it is safe to mobilise a patient after bedrest without too great a risk of recurrence, and for this reason a conservative clinician might recommend a six week spell. During bedrest it is useful to have parameters for assessing progress and as it is not advisable to sit or stand the patient upright one has to rely upon the symptom of pain or a sign such as restriction of straight leg raise. Analgesics may be given as necessary. Aspirin and paracetamol are seldom sufficient and it is usually necessary to prescribe dihydrocodeine, dextropropoxophene, or similar potency drugs. Antirheumatics may help if there is an inflammatory component to the lesion and 'muscle relaxants' also help, but probably more by their slightly sedative action.

Manipulation

Of the various accessory methods available to hasten recovery from mechanical lumbar derangements, manipulation is probably the quickest and most economical. As it is a treatment in which joints are passively moved, it is thought to be of most use in 'articular' derangement. Thus it may be safely applied to the lumbar spine when the symptoms and signs are 'articular' and possibly also when there are dural symptoms and signs. It is thought to be more likely to help in sudden or recent onset derangement rather than the gradually increasing syndrome. There are several schools of thought concerning the methods used in manipulation. There can be no doubt that the best relaxation is obtained under general anaesthesia and under these conditions relatively forceful passive movement is possible. This technique probably reduces the safety factor and removes the ability to assess progress following each manipulation. At the other extreme are the gentle passive repetitive movements favoured by some physiotherapists. This kind of technique is safe but slow and probably more useful in patients with generalised osteoarthrosis of the spine rather than a more specific disc prolapse. Between these two is a technique of rotation manipulation in which the lumbar spine is passively rotated to the end of its range, using the leg or buttock as a lever and then firmly eased through an extra range by the manipulator. The technique was investigated by Mathews and Yates (1969) and radiological evidence provided to show that this rotation technique is capable of reducing the size of a disc protrusion concurrently with relief of the patient's symptoms and signs. However, clinical trials have not so far provided evidence that manipulation is worthwhile.

Doran and Newell (1975) reported a seven-centre study of 456 patients with low back pain allocated randomly to one of four treatments. The manipulated group as a whole did no better than those given 'definitive physiotherapy', corsets or analgesics, but the overall statistics do not convey the observation that a small subgroup was dramatically relieved. It is the features which identify this group which need to be clarified. In view of the current problems of selecting patients for manipulation and the shortage of therapists, it is only reasonable to continue treatment for a week or two.

Traction

Lumbar traction is another treatment hallowed by long usage, but not yet sanctified by a good, positive, statistically validated controlled trial. Its main place seems to be in the treatment of sciatica from lumbar disc protrusion. In fact the term 'traction' covers a wide range of techniques, reviewed by Harris (1960). A cardinal fact is that the force of traction needed to exert an action upon a lumbar intervertebral disc must first overcome friction in the apparatus, friction between patient and apparatus, and then any soft tissue resistance, before affecting the disc itself. It can be calculated that with the subject on a plain, horizontal couch, approximately half the body weight being below the lumbar spine, and with a coefficient of friction between patient and couch of 0.5, that a minimum force of one-quarter the total body weight will be needed. In practice traction is applied in a variety of ways. Patients can be seen in hospital beds with traction of 10 kg applied with strapping to the lower legs. Clearly this cannot be effective on the lumbar spine but presumably has a ball and chain effect on keeping the patient in bed. In some units traction is given through a pelvic harness driven by an electrically operated machine giving intermittent forces of high value (e.g. one-third body weight). A control trial (Weber, 1973) using this 'pulsed' technique for 20 min daily for one week failed to show any benefit. A rather different technique in which traction of one-quarter body weight or more is given continuously for half an hour was investigated radiologically by Mathews (1968) and shown to be capable of both distracting lumbar vertebrae and reducing the size of disc bulges. When put to the test of a small controlled three-week clinical trial no significant advantage over placebo was found (Mathews and Hickling, 1975). However, when patients receiving placebo were changed to therapeutic levels of traction a proportion showed dramatic improvement, suggesting that criteria for selection are all important. As an overall policy it is reasonable to select a method of traction, to assess progress at weekly intervals, and if there is no clear evidence of improvement at the end of one or two weeks, to cease.

Epidural injections

Infiltration of the epidural space with weak solutions of local anaesthetic is an effective way of providing short-term relief of pain referred from local mechanical lesions. As such they can be of undoubted effect in easing a patient over the zenith of an attack of sciatica as well as occasionally providing a diagnostic test. When stronger solutions of local anaesthetic are used, a caudal block results with anaesthesiae of the lower part of the body. If a corticosteroid is added then a local anti-inflammatory effect is presumed to occur. Many enthusiastic reports of the benefit of epidural injections for sciatica have appeared often claiming relief far in excess of the known duration of action of the agents used—in fact sometimes permanent relief. Postulated mechanism of this prolonged relief include: physical dissection of adherent nerve root from the causative lesion; reduction of disc by auto-manipulation under local anaesthesia; reduction of disc bulge by hydrostatic pressure of injection (least probable). The generally accepted indication for epidural injection treatment is the presence of root pain and the more severe and constant the pain the more the temptation to inject. The appearance of a root lesion, often the time of maximum pain, is also a common indication for epidural injection.

Injections can be of large or small volume, with or without corticosteroid, and made via the lumbar or caudal route. No effective comparisons are available to evaluate the pros and cons of these variations. Beliveau (1971) compared the effect of 40 ml 0.5 per cent procaine with and without 80 mg methylprednisolone acetate injected by the caudal route for sciatica, and concluded that there was little difference save for a possible advantage of adding the corticosteroid in severe and prolonged cases. Dilke, Burry and Grahame (1973) compared injecting 80 mg methylprednisolone in 10 ml normal saline by the lumbar route with an interspinous ligamentous injection of normal saline and found the former to be superior. A beneficial effect was claimed. Occasional cases of very severe sciatica have been treated by epidural catheter injections of bupivacaine, but if prolonged for more than 48 h the risk of infection is unacceptable.

Current opinion is that epidural anaesthetic and corticosteroid injections are well worth trying for severe or intractable sciatica.

Physiotherapy

Bearing in mind that to order physiotherapy without specifying the type is like writing a prescription without naming the drug, there are those who believe that physiotherapy is essential in the management of mechanical backache. Others believe it to be irrelevant. No one would disagree that a physiotherapy department can provide a number of soothing techniques (heat, massage) which will relieve symptoms temporarily, whatever the cause. It is on the question of whether or not to prescribe exercises as well that differences occur. On the one hand it is difficult to understand how muscle strengthening can produce beneficial effects in the presence of degenerative discs, since the accompanying exertion must place increasing stress on a structure already in a precarious state. On the other hand many therapists do use carefully organised and regulated routines of exercises and claim regular success. There is no scientific basis for either view. The lesson probably is that injudicious and uncontrolled exercises are ill-advised. The number of middle-aged patients who become casualties as a result of late enthusiasm for various forms of gymnastics bears sufficient witness to the need for caution.

The corset

Surgeons usually are either strongly for or strongly against the use of the lumbosacral corset. Those who have no faith in exercises believe that where musculature cannot be improved, it must be supplemented. This applies particularly to abdominal muscles, which are responsible for keeping the sagging and stressed lumbar spine sufficiently buttressed by firm compression of the abdominal contents. A corset must be therefore inelastic.

The opposite view, held by enthusiasts of exercise therapy, is that the corset is an admission of failure, and an affliction for the patient. They point to the large numbers of patients whose corsets are discarded. However, corsets usually are rejected because of poor design or improper use, and not because they are in principle ineffective. A corset must often be worn for at least a month before it can start to have an effect upon long-standing symptoms, and in the early weeks when removed at night the backache may actually be transiently rather worse. Once such initial troubles have been overcome, a corset is likely to provide considerable relief from the most intractable backache. It seems a small price to pay for the chance of avoiding major surgery.

Chemonucleolysis

Dissolving a disc is an alternative to laminectomy and disc removal and should not, in the currect state of knowledge, be used for patients with problems of a lesser degree than would justify surgery. The substance used is chymopapain, a proteolytic enzyme extract of papaya latex which has been shown when injected to lead to hydrolysis and dissolution of degenerate disc material. Smith and Brown (1967) published the encouraging results of their first 75 treated patients and since that time the results of several larger and some comparative studies have become available (Wiltse, Widdell and Yuan, 1975; Macnab, 1973).

Ligamentous injections

A ligament is injected when it is thought to be causing painful symptoms, a situation which in theory may occur either when the ligament is primarily injured or when it has been the subject of stress secondary to a disc derangement. The diagnosis does not require restriction of movement, but should include local tenderness or pain at extremes of those movements which involve the relevant ligament. In this situation it is reasonable to inject a corticosteroid with local anaesthetic or a 'sclerosant' mixture. That most often used is a mixture of phenol, dextrose and glycerine with anaesthetic infiltrated into all the tender areas, usually on three separate occasions. Protagonists believe that strong fibrous tissue is produced and stabilises adjacent joints; others believe that the phenol renders local sensory nerve endings insensitive. Sanford (1975) has compared this type of injection with others which do not include phenol in a controlled study and has found the rate of improvement at three months to be approximately equal in all groups.

SURGERY

It is important to realise that surgical intervention plays only a small part in the overall management of low back pain. Only one in every 100 such patients attending their general practitioners eventually comes to surgery, and only one in 10000 of any population is so treated each year (Newman, 1973).

The two keystones in the surgical management of low back pain remain (1) decompression and (2) fusion. The improvements in surgical management have come from elaboration and assessment of these two basic procedures.

Decompression

The indications for decompression

Management of the emergency situation is not disputed. Signs of acute pressure upon the cauda equina require immediate decompression. However, some of the initial enthusiasm of earlier years for disc removal in less urgent circumstances has become moderated. Most surgeons today will not consider laminectomy unless there is evidence of dural tension or nerve root embarrassment. It is beginning to be understood that disc herniation and bulging is but one part of a long continuing process of mechanical back pathology. The natural outcome of back symptoms in the absence of root symptoms is probably little influenced by surgical removal of the disc material, except possibly in the youngest group afflicted, the adolescents (Bulos, 1973).

When there is root pressure, however, that particular episode in the continuing process may well be relieved by decompressive surgery. It is the progressive impairment of root conduction despite adequate conservative management that is the indication for such surgery. Intervention is called for in three clinical situations.

1. Severe sciatic pain persisting despite conservative measures, including (and this is mandatory) at least three weeks of horizontal flat bed rest.

2. A neurological defect which progresses during such bed rest.

3. Incapacitating episodes of sciatic pain (with evidence of dural tension, impairment of root conduction, or both) recurring despite intermittent successes with conservative regimes.

Techniques of decompression

The spinal column is merely another tube which can become obstructed. The standard approach to the interior of this tube is by removal of a spinous process and lamina, that is by laminectomy. In the management of low back pain it is commonly the L4/5 or the L5/S1 disc that is responsible for symptoms. Both these structures are accessible by excision of the spinous process and lamina of L5, and this, the commonest of all spinal surgical procedures, is the original approach (Armstrong, 1965).

It has been questioned whether such wide exposure is likely to give rise to problems of mechanical instability. In the belief that this was likely, the alternative limited interlaminar approach was devised, in which only adjacent parts of a lamina are removed, leaving a smallish window of entry. Those who believe that when removal of a disc is indicated its removal must be total have been slow to adopt this interlaminar approach. It is regarded as giving insufficient or, at best, too tedious, access for the necessary maximal removal of disc material. In practice it has now been demonstrated that provided the articular facets are undisturbed, the wider approach does not disturb the mechanics of the back (Jackson, 1971).

Failures of decompression

Persistence of symptoms after laminectomy usually can be attributed to a wrong indication for the operation. Poor technique, such as failure to identify correctly the disc at fault, failure to remove and identify all disc material (Macnab, 1971a,b), or damage done to a nerve root may also be responsible.

Recurrence of symptoms after a period of postoperative relief commonly is due either to reherniation of incompletely removed material, or a new herniation of a second disc at a different level. The latter is probably more common (Naylor, 1974), but even with the most meticulous and obsessive technique, total clearance of a disc at first operation may not be achieved.

A further cause of recurring or persisting root symptoms may be the formation of fibrous adhesions about the involved nerve root. Usually this is diagnosed only at second operation, in the absence of any other cause. Adhesions can be seen surrounding not only the root, but filling the whole laminectomy defect and embracing also the dura. This is the 'laminectomy membrane' (LaRocca and McNab, 1974). This membrane may or may not be a significant structure, since presumably it must exist also after successful laminectomy without causing symptoms. Formation of the membrane may be prevented by reroofing the operation defect before closure with a sheet of surgical gelatin foam. If fibrosis around a nerve root is thought to be the cause of symptoms, its clearance often is followed by only very temporary symptomatic relief. Further relapse is thought to be due to rapid reformation of the fibrous tissue, and unless this is prevented the patient is unlikely to be helped by further surgery.

Fusion

The question of when to fuse a spine for low back pain, how much to fuse, how to fuse, and whether laminectomy should always be accompanied by fusion, are still controversial even after decades of discussion. The problem is that fusion, being a last ditch procedure, is necessarily reserved for problem cases. Naturally, with such patients, there is bound to be a higher incidence of psychopathological background. In this environment, however successful a technique, the clinical result may be ambiguous. To assess such surgery objectively hitherto has been almost impossible. That it may become more possible in future is discussed later.

Fusion should be reserved for spinal instability. Determining the existence of instability, and its level, is the crux. As distinct from the grosser forms as encountered in spondylolisthesis and severe degenerative disease, minor forms of instability are almost impossible to demonstrate objectively. Radiography, even cine-radiography, usually is of little help (Macnab, 1971a). Other criteria are not clear-cut nor universally agreed. The diagnosis rests largely upon a clinical history of persistent low grade backache which, having failed to respond to any other measure, reliably is relieved while at rest (Lettin, 1967).

An extreme attempt to solve this dilemma is to adopt a policy for those undergoing laminectomy of simultaneous fusion of the lumbosacral level. However, since other experience shows that only a small percentage of laminectomy patients eventually come to be considered for spinal fusion, this particular course seems needlessly dramatic. The other extreme is never to fuse a spine on principle. This again is equally illogical, since necessarily it must deprive even that small number of patients who would respond. Opinion varies as to how this small group of patients may successfully be recognised (Campbell Connolly and Newman, 1971; Hoover, 1968a). Over the years there has been a tendency to fuse fewer spines. Experience has shown that with patience the natural history of persistent backache is to improve. It is not unusual to find that after about two years many patients find life tolerable once more (Beals and Hickman, 1972).

A well-organised prospective survey on this matter is needed. It is difficult to justify dogmatic statements about treatment when statistical knowledge of the natural history of a condition is non-existent.

If a patient fails to respond to any other treatment, has a satisfactory psychopathological background, and can be shown to be relieved of symptoms only by bed rest, then he may have 'spinal instability' and may be suitable for fusion. The problem then is to select the appropriate level for operation. While it is possible to achieve 80 to 90 per cent patient-satisfaction rates for any single level fusion, the figure probably is less than 60 per cent for two levels (Macnab and Dall, 1971) and only a very optimistic surgeon would attempt to fuse three levels. A patient with a failed fusion, especially at lumbosacral level, is likely to be worse off than if he had never been operated upon.

The techniques available for fusion of lumbar and lumbosacral vertebrae are varied. Probably the most reliable is the original cortical H-graft or bone plate wedged between or screwed to the spinous processes adjacent to the affected level and supplemented by cancellous chips (Crenshaw, 1971). The operation has to be followed by at least three months recumbency. This is uneconomic and inconvenient to both patient and hospital. For these reasons, and because suitable spinous processes are not always available after previous surgery, other techniques have been devised. In recent years the discussion has been on whether to approach this problem from the front or from the back of the spine.

Advocates of anterior fusion (Freebody, 1964) point to the mechanical advantage of a technique which leaves the graft under compression instead of under stress. An attractive approach is the transperitoneal route (Freebody, Bendall and Taylor, 1971) which calls for only a short period of postoperative recumbency, but in some hands the technique has achieved a disappointing clinical success rate (Macnab and Dall, 1971; Stauffer and Coventry, 1972a). It can also be accompanied by dangers to the presacral nerve. Both these hazards are argued to be negligible (Freebody et al, 1971) but the possible disaster, especially of producing impotence, is enough to discourage many surgeons. However, the technique is particularly useful in dealing with spondylolisthesis. Through an anterior approach only the affected level need be stabilised, whereas approached from the back it is necessary to bridge the affected vertebrae and span two levels by fusion. For infective lesions of the lumbar spine another anterior fusion, by the extraperitoneal route, is performed (Kemp et al, 1973b).

The desire to avoid lengthy postoperative recumbency has also influenced recent developments in the techniques of spinal fusion by the posterior approach. Fusions in which, in addition to posterior grafting, the posterior articular joints are ablated and stabilised by internal fixation with screws, are said to require virtually no postoperative immobilisation of the patient (Boucher, 1959; Kirwan, 1975). However, figures for clinical success rate vary widely from source to source, from some being as low as 45 per cent (Macnab and Dall, 1971). In contrast to this, advocates of the operation in its modern form claim that it compares favourably with most other methods (Kirwan, 1975).

Such screw fusions in any case are not suitable for spondylolisthesis with a great degree of displacement. Another posterior approach technique which is more versatile, and for which it is also claimed that recumbency subsequently is unnecessary, is the posterolateral fusion (Hoover, 1968b; Stauffer and Coventry, 1972a; Macnab and Dall, 1971). Adjacent surfaces of laminae, posterior joints, and also the transverse processes, are decorticated and spread with a generous dressing of cancellous bone chips obtained from the iliac crests. Such massive grafts over laminae and spinous processes are said to lead to thickening of these structures and to subsequent spinal stenosis (Macnab and Dall, 1971), and it has been suggested that the procedure is equally effective if the grafting is limited to the transverse processes alone. This is the so-called lateral mass or bilateral lateral fusion (Macnab and Dall, 1971). The plane of the transverse processes is said to be that which moves least during spinal flexion and extension (Hoover, 1968b) and it is predicted that this bony mass will become solid whether or not the patient is immobilised. However, the exposure for the procedure can be tedious and bloody (Macnab and Dall, 1971) but the technique has the advantage that it can be applied to almost any mechanical problem.

In the special case of the spondylolytic defect, where the slip of one vertebra upon another has been minimal, there has been interest in obtaining direct fusion of the defect in the pars interarticularis by graft and screw (Buck, 1970). In such a case the results are promising. The process is less tedious and disturbing than formal fusion; it is also more physiological than the rather obvious course of simple removal of the loose lamina (Amuso et al, 1970). Although this may relieve sciatic symptoms, some feel it does nothing to restore stability in a potentially unstable situation.

Fringe Operations

When there is little agreement about natural history there are bound to be strongly advocated therapies which have little scientific foundation. This is as much the case in backache as it is in any other condition. In the last decade, procedures for denervating the posterior joints, replacing disc material with a ball-bearing prosthesis, and removal of disc material by trocar, have all been advocated. So far, none has been shown to be reliably effective.

THE EMOTIONAL ELEMENT

It has long been realised that the emotional factor in a low back problem is often equal to, if not more important than, the physical factor. For this reason there has been considerable study of those failures of treatment which arise through failure to resolve a patient's psychological problems (Beals and Hickman, 1972).

Various behavioural syndromes have been blamed. Accident neurosis, the secondary gain syndrome, the accident process, traumatic neuroses, and psychoanalytical states have all been implicated. Lately, emphasis has returned to one of the original truisms of medicine, the concept of the 'whole man'.

The basis of this is hardly new. It is not diseases and injuries that need to be treated, but whole individuals suffering from the effects of these diseases and injuries. These individuals have social, economic, psychological, vocational, marital and other problems which may cause or profoundly affect their physical states. Not least among these is the duration of symptoms, unemployment and the number of previous operations already undergone. Failure to consider a single crucial variable, be it organic or otherwise, may lead to failure of a whole treatment programme.

In many cases, and particularly where reactive depression is a significant feature, the sympathetic ear and time of a good physician may be all that is needed to give the patient the necessary insight into his problem. In others, successful management requires more detailed evaluation. Particularly with problems of industrial rehabilitation, in Canada and North America it has been found that psychological techniques are of value. The use of such devices as the Minnesota Multiphasal Personality Index (MMPI), is just one example. With these methods, the ratings and predictions of the outcome of treatment made by psychologists have been shown to be superior to those made by physicians (Beals and Hickman, 1972).

In any circumstances the concept of the 'whole man' is an essential approach to the management of a back problem. It is of the greatest value when assessing those who fail to respond to therapy, in selecting patients for spinal fusion and in predicting the need for vocational back training after injury. This is not to say that when an organic cause for back symptoms exists the presence of a psychopathological problem means that surgical treatment necessarily will fail. To the patient, all backache is real. Its relief may set the scene at last for improvement in other problems.

REFERENCES

Amuso, S. J., Neff, R. S., Coulson, D. B. & Laing, P. G. (1970) The surgical treatment of spondylolisthesis by posterior element resection. A long-term follow-up study. *Journal of Bone and Joint Surgery*, **52-A,** 529.

Armstrong, J. A. (1965) *Lumbar Disc Lesions*, 3rd edn, p. 257. London: Livingstone.

Beals, R. K. & Hickman, N. W. (1972) Industrial injuries of the back and extremities. Comprehensive evaluation—an aid in prognosis and management. A study of one hundred and eighty patients. *Journal of Bone and Joint Surgery*, **54-A,** 1593.

Beliveau, P. (1971) A comparison between epidural anaesthesia with and without corticosteroid in the treatment of sciatica. *Rheumatology and Physical Medicine*, **11,** 40.

Boucher, H. H. (1959) A method of spinal fusion. *Journal of Bone and Joint Surgery*, **41-B,** 248.

Brewerton, D. A. (1975) Symposium on histocompatibility and rheumatic disease. *Annals of the Rheumatic Diseases*, **34,** Suppl. 1.

British Medical Journal (1969) Leading article. **1,** 662.

British Medical Journal (1974) Editorial. Tuberculosis of the spine. **2,** 613.

Buck, J. E. (1970) Direct repair of the defect in spondylolisthesis. *Journal of Bone and Joint Surgery*, **52-B**, 432.

Bulos, S. (1973) Herniated intervertebral lumbar disc in the teenager. *Journal of Bone and Joint Surgery*, **55-B**, 273.

Bywaters, E. G. L. (1975) Rheumatoid discitis in the thoracic region due to spread from costo-vertebral joints. *Annals of the Rheumatic Diseases*, **33**, 408.

Crenshaw, A. K. (1971) Arthrodesis of the spine. In *Campbell's Operative Orthopaedics*, 5th edn, ed. Crenshaw, A. K., Vol. 2, p. 1163. St Louis: C. V. Mosby.

Cruickshank, B. (1960) Pathology of ankylosing spondylitis. *Bulletin on Rheumatic Diseases*, **10**, 211.

Cyriax, J. H. (1969) *Textbook of Orthopaedic Medicine*, Vol. 1, p. 87. London: Biallière, Tindall and Cassell.

Da Roza, A. C. (1964) Primary intraspinal tumours: their clinical presentation and diagnosis. *Journal of Bone and Joint Surgery*, **46-B**, 815.

Dilke, T. F. W., Burry, H. C. & Grahame, R. (1973) Extradural corticosteroid injection in management of lumbar nerve root compression. *British Medical Journal*, **2**, 635.

Doran, D. M. L. & Newell, D. J. (1975) Manipulation in the treatment of low back pain: a multicentre study. *British Medical Journal*, **2**, 161.

Edgar, M. A. & Park, M. A. (1974) Induced pain patterns on passive straight leg raising in lower lumbar disc protrusion. *Journal of Bone and Joint Surgery*, **56-B**, 658.

Freebody, D. (1964) Treatment of spondylolisthesis by anterior fusion via the transperitoneal route. *Journal of Bone and Joint Surgery*, **46B**, 788.

Freebody, D., Bendall, R. & Taylor, R. D. (1971) Anterior transperitoneal lumbar fusion. *Journal of Bone and Joint Surgery*, **46-B**, 788.

Harris, R. I. & Macnab, I. (1954) Structural changes in the lumbar intervertebral disc. *Journal of Bone and Joint Surgery*, **36-B**, 304.

Harris, R. (1960) Traction. In *Massage, Manipulation and Traction*, ed. Sidney Licht. New Haven, Conn.: Elizabeth Licht.

Hewitt, W. (1970) The intervertebral foramen. *Physiotherapy*, **56**, 332.

Hoover, N. W. (1968a) Indications for fusion at time of removal of intervertebral disc. *Journal of Bone and Joint Surgery*, **50-A**, 189.

Hoover, N. W. (1968b) Methods of lumbar fusion. *Journal of Bone and Joint Surgery*, **50-A**, 193.

Howes, R. G. & Isdale, I. C. (1971) The loose back. *Rheumatology and Physical Medicine*, **11**, 72.

Jackson, R. K. (1971) The long-term effects of wide laminectomy for lumbar disc excision. *Journal of Bone and Joint Surgery*, **53-B**, 17.

Kellgren, J. H. (1939) On the distribution of pain arising from deep somatic structures, with charts of segmental pain areas. *Clinical Science*, **4**, 35.

Kemp, H. B. S., Jackson, J. W., Jeremiah, J. D. & Hall, A. J. (1973a) Pyogenic infections occurring primarily in intervertebral discs. *Journal of Bone and Joint Surgery*, **55-B**, 698.

Kemp, H. B. S., Jackson, J. W., Jeremiah, J. D. & Cook, Josephine (1973b) Anterior fusion of the spine for infective lesions in adults. *Journal of Bone and Joint Surgery*, **55-B**, 715.

Keon-Cohen, B. T. (1968) Epidural abscess simulating disc hernia. *Journal of Bone and Joint Surgery*, **50-B**, 128.

Kirwan, E. O'G. (1975) Personal communication.

Larocca, M. & Macnab, I. (1974) The laminectomy membrane. *Journal of Bone and Joint Surgery*, **56-B**, 545.

Lettin, A. W. F. (1967) Diagnosis and treatment of lumbar instability. *Journal of Bone and Joint Surgery*, **49-B**, 520.

Lloyd-Griffiths, D. (1975) Orthopaedic tuberculosis. *British Journal of Hospital Medicine*, **14**, 146.

Mathews, J. A. (1968) Dynamic discography: a study of lumbar traction. *Annals of Physical Medicine*, **9**, 275.

Mathews, J. A. & Yates, D. A. H. (1969) Reduction of lumbar disc prolapse by manipulation. *British Medical Journal*, **3**, 696.

Mathews, J. A. & Hickling, J. (1975) Lumbar traction. A double-blind control study. *Rheumatology and Rehabilitation*, **14**, 222.

Macnab, I. (1971a) The traction spur. An indicator of segmental instability. *Journal of Bone and Joint Surgery*, **53-A**, 663.

Macnab, I. (1971b) Negative disc exploration. *Journal of Bone and Joint Surgery*, **53-A**, 891.

Macnab, I. & Dall, D. (1971) The blood supply of the lumbar spine and its application to the technique of intertransverse lumbar fusion. *Journal of Bone and Joint Surgery*, **53-B**, 628.

Macnab, I. (1973) Chemonucleolysis. *Clinical Neurosurgery*, **20**, 183.

Mixter, W. J. & Barr, J. S. (1934) Rupture of the intervertebral disc with involvement of the spinal canal. *New England Journal of Medicine*, **211**, 210.

Morgan, D. B. (1968) Osteomalacia and osteoporosis. *Postgraduate Medical Journal*, **44**, 621.

Nachemson, A. & Morris, J. M. (1964) In vivo measurement of intradiscal pressure. *Journal of Bone and Joint Surgery*, **46-A**, 1077.

Naylor, A. (1974) The late results of laminectomy for lumbar disc prolapse. *Journal of Bone and Joint Surgery*, **56-B**, 17.

Nelson, M. A. (1973) Lumbar spinal stenosis. *Journal of Bone and Joint Surgery*, **55-B**, 506.

Newman, P. H. (1963) The aetiology of spondylolisthesis (with a special investigation by K. H. Stone). *Journal of Bone and Joint Surgery*, **45-B**, 39.

Newman, P. H. (1973) Surgical treatment for derangement of the lumbar spine. *Journal of Bone and Joint Surgery*, **55-B**, 7.

Park, W. M. (1976) The radiological investigation of the invertebral disc. In *The Lumbar Spine and Back Pain*, ed. Jayson, M. I. V. p. 113. London: Pitman.

Sanford, H. A. (1975) Personal communication.

Seal, P. V. & Morris, C. H. (1974) Brucellosis of the carpus. *Journal of Bone and Joint Surgery*, **56-B**, 327.

Smith, L. & Brown, J. E. (1967) Treatment of lumbar intervertebral disc lesions by direct injections of chymopapain. *Journal of Bone and Joint Surgery*, **49-B**, 502.

Smyth, M. J. & Wright, V. (1958) Sciatica and the intervertebral disc. An experimental study. *Journal of Bone and Joint Surgery*, **40-A**, 1401.

Spiegel, P. G., Kengla, K. W., Isaacson, A. S. & Wilson, J. C. J. (1972) Intervertebral disc-space inflammation in children. *Journal of Bone and Joint Surgery*, **54-A**, 284.

Stauffer, R. N. & Coventry, M. B. (1972a) Anterior interbody lumbar spine fusion. *Journal of Bone and Joint Surgery*, **54-A**, 756.

Stauffer, R. N. & Coventry, M. B. (1972b) Posterolateral lumbar-spine fusion. *Journal of Bone and Joint Surgery*, **54-A**, 1195.

Stilwell, D. L. (1956) The nerve supply of vertebral column and associated structures in the monkey. *Anatomical Records*, **125**, 139.

Vernon-Roberts, B. & Pirie, C. T. (1973) Healing frabecular microfractures in the bodies of lumbar vertebrae. *Annals of the Rheumatic Diseases*, **32**, 406.

Weber, H. (1973) Traction therapy in sciatica due to disc prolapse. *Journal of the Oslo City Hospital*, **23**, 167.

Wiltse, L. H., Widell, A. H. Jr & Jackson, D. W. (1975) Fatigue fracture: the basic lesion in isthmic spondylolisthesis. *Journal of Bone and Joint Surgery*, **57-A**, 17.

Wiltse, L. H., Widell, E. H. Jr & Yuan, H. A. (1975) Chymopapain. Chemonucleolysis in lumbar disc disease. *Journal of the American Medical Association*, **231**, 474.

Wood, P. H. N. & Benn, R. T. (1972) Statistical appendix. Digest of data on the rheumatic diseases. 3. Handicap and disability, and international comparison of morbidity and instability. *Annals of the Rheumatic Diseases*, **31**, 72.

Wyke, B. (1970) The neurological basis of thoracic spinal pain. *Rheumatology and Physical Medicine*, **10**, 356.

15
THE ANTERIOR TIBIAL COMPARTMENT SYNDROME

G. Jantet

The syndrome produced by compression of the structures in the anterior tibial compartment (ATC) of the leg is now well recognised. It is characterised by pain over the anterolateral aspect of the leg below the knee associated with failure of some or all of the structures in the ATC.

The condition was first described by Severin (1943). Mavor (1956) pointed out that the pain was superficially similar to that of intermittent claudication and could well be wrongly mistaken for it. Isolated cases of pain over the lateral aspect of the leg or of infarction of muscles were reported which were undoubtedly stages in this syndrome. More recently, the syndrome was well reviewed by Levy and Di Maria (1972) who collected 274 reports from the world literature and by Bradley (1973).

It is important to recognise this entity which exists in acute and chronic forms as the treatment is simple and very successful in the early cases but can lead to permanent foot-drop or tissue necrosis and amputation if un-recognised.

Anatomy

The leg is divided into four fascial compartments but compression is particularly liable to occur in the ATC because of the rigidity of its boundaries. The ATC lies anterolaterally between the tibia and fibula, is bounded deeply by the rigid interosseous membrane and is ensheathed by the deep fascia and the anterior intermuscular septum. It contains the extensors of the foot and toes, the anterior tibial blood vessels and the deep peroneal nerve. The anterior tibial artery which supplies all the structures in the ATC lies on the interosseous membrane and in its course in the compartment has no significant anastomoses with other arteries. Edwards (1953) has pointed out that the muscular branches of this artery must therefore be recognised as end arteries. The deep peroneal nerve is motor to the muscles in the compartment and sensory to the dorsal surface of the first interdigital space. The cutaneous branch of the superficial peroneal nerve which supplies the dorsum of the toes except the first interdigital space lies wholly outside the deep fascia ensheathing this compartment and is character-istically uninvolved in the compression syndrome.

Aetiology

The causes of this syndrome can be divided in four main groups: (1) *exercise*, (2) *traumatic*, (3) *vascular*, and (4) *various*. Reviewing 137 published reports, Bradley (1973) classified 33 per cent in the exercise group, 19 per cent in the traumatic, 38 per cent in the vascular and 10 per cent as of various causes.

The *exercise* group is associated with unaccustomed or severe exercise. In some patients in this group the clinical picture can be mild and recurrent with a *chronic* presentation but in other circumstances it is *acute* and may lead to severe complications.

The *traumatic* group may occur after fractures or soft tissue injuries not necessarily associated with arterial injuries. The syndrome has also been reported following sprains of the leg or ankle. Awareness of this possible complication should lead to its prevention by prophylactic decompression of the ATC.

The *vascular* group is associated with arterial thrombosis or emboli which may be situated in the iliac or femoral arteries and not necessarily in the anterior tibial artery. The syndrome has also been described in association with arteriovenous fistulae of the leg, in arterial by-pass procedures, in Buerger's disease and in periarteritis nodosa.

Various other conditions have been reported as the cause of this syndrome including inguinal herniorrhaphy, eclampsia, nephrosis, epilepsy, open-heart surgery, application of a brace to the leg, lumbar sympathectomy, intravenous infusions in the leg and acute generalised myopathy.

The incidence is much higher in males (95 per cent) than females and the average age of the patients, excluding those in the vascular group, is 25 years (Bradley, 1973).

Clinical Features

The most constant single feature is *pain* over the anterolateral aspect of the leg and this may or may not be followed by *weakness* of dorsiflexion of the foot or toes.

Early or mild

The *pain* over the ATC is constant but of variable intensity and if brought on by exercise persists on resting. It is characteristically made worse by attempted active or passive dorsiflexion of the toes or ankle. *Swelling* is present over the ATC with local heat and sometimes redness. *Tenderness* on palpation of the ATC at rest and on dorsiflexion of the toes or ankle is also characteristic. The presence of *weakness* of dorsiflexion of the big toe, the other toes or the foot confirms the diagnosis. The dorsalis pedis *pulse* is usually absent in the vascular group but is usually present in the other groups:

it is therefore unreliable as a confirmatory physical sign. Some *sensory loss*, selectively on the dorsum of the first web space with normal sensation of the other toes and the rest of the foot is very characteristic when present. This is an important confirmatory sign which Bradley (1973) reports as being present in 72 per cent of the patients in whom it was elicited.

Late or severe

In severe cases when the full syndrome may develop rapidly, or if the patient is seen late in the course of the syndrome, complete paralysis of dorsiflexion may be present resulting in *foot-drop* or *hallux drop*. *Anaesthesia* selectively over the first web space becomes complete and eventually *necrosis* of the skin overlying the ATC and the muscles within becomes apparent.

Exercise group

The group of patients in whom the compression syndrome is brought on by exercise presents a clinical picture quite unlike that of patients suffering from ischaemic pains of the leg on exercise (intermittent claudication) due to arterial insufficiency. In the compression syndrome the age group is commonly in the 20s, the pain is not improved by rest and in some patients may, on the contrary, be relieved by further exercise; there is usually no pulse deficit even after exercise and no clinical evidence of arterial disease; the other features described above also help to differentiate this syndrome. There is a constant history of severe or unaccustomed exercise such as route marches or athletic running in the untrained. In its mildest forms it is probably frequently misrecognised either because the victims learn spontaneously to avoid such activities or because it is misdiagnosed. The condition described as 'shin splints' or 'fresher's leg' is probably a mild form of this syndrome. The more severe acute form can occur in this group with the features described above. The patients in this group often have small muscle herniae through the deep fascia over the ATC and Mavor (1956) suggested that these were evidence of a rise in pressure in the ATC. Furthermore the condition can be brought on or aggravated by closure of the fascial 'defects' associated with these herniae.

Investigations

The diagnosis of the ATC compression syndrome is essentially clinical.
In the acute condition special investigations are unnecessary and may cause dangerous delay.
In the chronic form, arteriography may be helpful in excluding other types of pathology. Levy and Di Maria (1972) and Bradley (1973) state that plethysmography and Doppler ultrasonic testing have not been helpful. However, French and Price (1962), using the method of Wells, Youmans and Miller (1938), report that tissue pressure measurements were useful in the chronic form as this technique showed that after exercise in affected patients,

there was an abnormal and prolonged increase in tissue pressure in the muscles of the ATC. Electromyography is helpful in assessing the likelihood of recovery of muscle function and thus aids in the planning of the treatment.

Differential Diagnosis

The condition may not be suspected if mild or chronic or may be mis-diagnosed if acute. It has to be differentiated from infection, phlebitis, tenosynovitis, osteomyelitis, tibial stress fractures and anterior tibial epi-physitis (Osgood–Schlatter disease). Awareness of the syndrome and its clinical features should make recognition easier.

Pathogenesis

There is no clinical or laboratory evidence that infection or lymphatic pathology are pathogenic factors in this syndrome. Impairment of the venous return must obviously occur but this is not thought to be the main factor.

The localisation of the clinical features to the structures in the ATC, the work of French and Price (1962) showing a rise in pressure within the com-partment after exercise together with the observation that the muscles of this compartment bulge markedly on fasciotomy suggest that rise in pressure in the compartment is an important factor. The histological findings on biopsy of the affected muscles show the characteristics of ischaemia (Bradley, 1973) and not of muscle pathology or, in most cases, of pathology of the small vessels. Most authors believe that a rise in pressure is easily produced in the relatively unyielding ATC. In some patients this may lead to impairment of the microcirculation in the muscles or even the circulation in the segmental arteries supplying the muscles which, as described above, are end arteries: oedema of the ischaemic muscle follows which further increases the pressure within the ATC thus establishing a vicious circle which may lead eventually to loss of function of the structures within the ATC from ischaemia. The clinical picture thus produced can be the consequence of either paralysis of the muscles themselves or of the nerves supplying the muscles with an associated characteristic sensory loss in the first web space or a combination of both.

The other muscular compartments of the leg present a similar anatomical situation, although to a lesser degree, and similar isolated compartment compression syndromes have been described in the lateral compartment by Lunceford (1965) and in the posterior compartment by Birnstingl (1973).

In the *exercise form* of the syndrome, the rise in pressure is thought to be due to fluid retention: it is known (Wright, 1961) that in muscular activity the weight of a muscle may increase by 20 per cent from fluid retention. Thus in the affected patients, who presumably have a particularly unyielding compartment, the symptoms are brought on by severe exercise. This would also explain the presence, in some of these patients, of painful muscle herniae through the deep fascia of the ATC. The age incidence in this group, the absence of any other evidence of arterial disease (including the presence in most cases of a palpable dorsalis pedis pulse) and the good results of fasciotomy alone confirm that, in this group, the syndrome is not due to arterial disease.

In the *traumatic group* pathogenesis can easily be explained on the basis of local tissue damage leading to oedema and haematoma formation which cause a rise in tissue pressure; hypovolaemic shock may be a contributory cause resulting in muscle ischaemia.

In the *vascular forms* due to occlusion of the iliac or femoral arteries, sufficient oedema may be produced in the ischaemic muscles of the leg to result in marked rises in pressure in the muscle compartments, sufficient, particularly in the ATC, to lead to necrosis of the structures in that compartment. It is interesting that in these patients, when gangrene occurs, it is limited to the skin overlying the ATC and spares the foot, suggesting that the anterior tibial artery itself is spared but the pressure rises affect the segmental arteries and the microcirculation. The syndrome can of course be produced by occlusion of the anterior tibial artery either singly or in combination with occlusions in other arteries when the foot itself may also be affected. The pathogenesis of the syndrome in the other vascular causes in this group such as Buerger's disease, periarteritis nodosa or arteriovenous fistulae can be explained on the basis of localised muscle ischaemia and hence oedema due either to the process affecting the small arteries or to the arteriovenous shunting. Following direct arterial surgery leading to revascularisation of the muscles of the leg, reactive hyperaemia and oedema are frequent accompaniments which may well lead to a dangerous rise in pressure in a susceptible leg compartment.

An explanation of the role played by the *various* other conditions associated with this syndrome can be made in some of these conditions, such as eclampsia or epilepsy, on the basis of intense muscle exercise due to convulsions leading to an exercise form of the syndrome; oedema due to revascularisation, or ischaemia due to emboli or acute thromboses may be the explanation following open heart surgery or lumbar sympathectomy; local oedema causing a rise in tissue pressure and local ischaemia may be the explanation in those instances associated with intravenous infusions in the leg, acute generalised myopathy and the application of a brace to the leg which may have caused local trauma. No satisfactory explanation can be offered, on the evidence given, for the relationship of the other various conditions reported as associated with this syndrome.

Treatment

The complications of the ATC syndrome are probably preventable in most cases provided the condition is recognised.

The essential treatment is relief of pressure within the ATC by means of a *fasciotomy*.

Prophylactic fasciotomy

Prophylactic fasciotomy can undoubtedly save limbs in the *traumatic group*: Livingstone and Wilson (1975) advocate free use in all leg injuries of fasciotomies of the anterior and posterior tibial compartments and of the thigh.

In the *vascular group*, prophylactic fasciotomy is recommended if there is any doubt about the presence of a compression syndrome following re-vascularisation of a limb after embolectomy.

Acute ATC syndrome

In the acute form of this syndrome such as it presents in the *vascular group*, in the *traumatic group*, in the *various* associated conditions and also occasionally in the *exercise group*, the most important aspect is to recognise this clinical entity.

In the exercise group associated with unusual or very strenuous exercise, the condition is often reversible in the early stages and can be treated conservatively with cessation of all exercise and bed-rest: careful observation, however, is necessary as an emergency fasciotomy will become imperative if the condition does not respond to the conservative treatment or if it progresses. In most other patients with the acute syndrome it is probably safer to consider the condition will be progressive and to carry out an early fasciotomy as well as treating the cause when this is possible.

According to Bradley (1973) the progress of the condition from the onset of pain in the ATC to the development of muscle weakness can vary from 3 h to eight days. The onset of muscle or nerve palsy is of great prognostic importance because the results show that when fasciotomy was performed once foot drop was fully established, complete relief occurred in only 13 per cent of patients; on the other hand in the patients reported in whom the fasciotomy was performed when there was only some weakness of the anterior tibial compartment muscles, there was complete relief in all (Bradley, 1973).

Thus, decompression fasciotomy should be carried out without delay in the presence of the classical features of pain, swelling and tenderness over the anterior tibial compartment if in addition there is even a slight muscle weakness or the typical sensory loss in the first web space. Waiting for the establishment of foot drop may be disastrous. Better recognition of this syndrome will probably lead to fasciotomy at an earlier stage.

There is no clear guideline from the published reports on the length of time before irreversible changes occur in the muscles and nerves in the acute syndrome: it is not always stated whether the onset was taken as the onset of pain in the ATC or the onset of muscle weakness. This is of possible practical importance as some authors state that surgical decompression is contraindicated after irreversible changes have occurred as it will produce no improvement and may well result in secondary infection in ischaemic muscles for which the only treatment is amputation. On the other hand, other authors state that surgical decompression can be performed at any time. There is general agreement that fasciotomy is recommended until 6 h after the onset of complete foot drop. Beyond this, the management is more debatable. A fasciotomy may relieve the patient partially or completely but the risk is of infection, gangrene and inevitable amputation; on the other hand, a non-surgical approach may fail to relieve a still recoverable condition and leave the patient at the best with a permanent foot drop and at the worst with necrosis requiring amputation. In these patients serial electromyography can be of value in determining whether any potentially functioning muscle is still present.

Chronic ATC syndrome

In the chronic form of this syndrome such as is seen most commonly in the *exercise group* with pain following exercise, a warning should be given about the possible dangers of strenuous exercise and the advisability of progressive training. Such patients can undoubtedly develop the acute syndrome.

The author (Jantet) has treated two such patients with symptoms occurring in both legs which greatly limited their activities: complete relief was obtained by bilateral fasciotomies. Bradley (1973), reviewing the literature, found reports of six patients treated in similar fashion with 'excellent results'. The treatment is so simple and effective that it should probably be carried out more often than it is.

Late ATC syndrome

In patients in whom the condition is considered to be too advanced for decompression to be of any benefit or in whom decompression is performed too late, little improvement can be expected from low molecular weight dextran or from anticoagulants as the involved tissues, by this time, will be so ischaemic that none of these substances will reach them. Theoretically lumbar sympathectomy should not be of benefit either and could be harmful.

If foot drop becomes established, supports and perhaps tendon transplants or arthrodesis will be necessary. If necrosis of skin or muscle occurs, débridement may be sufficient but amputation may be necessary.

TECHNIQUE OF FASCIOTOMY

The operative technique of fasciotomy is simple and well described by De Weese and Rob (1968): it consists essentially of a 5 cm longitudinal incision two fingers' breadth lateral to the tibia beginning two fingers' breadth distal to the tibial head, through which long scissors are introduced and the deep fascia divided along its whole length.

We prefer to carry out the procedure through two such incisions (Fig. 15.1), the upper (A) as described by De Weese and Rob (1968) and a lower incision (B) in the same vertical line but placed two-thirds of the way down the leg. This ensures complete division of the fascia down to the extensor retinaculum and also ensures that the cutaneous branch of the superficial peroneal nerve which lies outside the deep fascia, is not in the path of the fascial division and inadvertently divided.

A complete skin incision along the whole length of the lateral aspect of the leg is unnecessary and short incisions minimise the danger of non-healing.

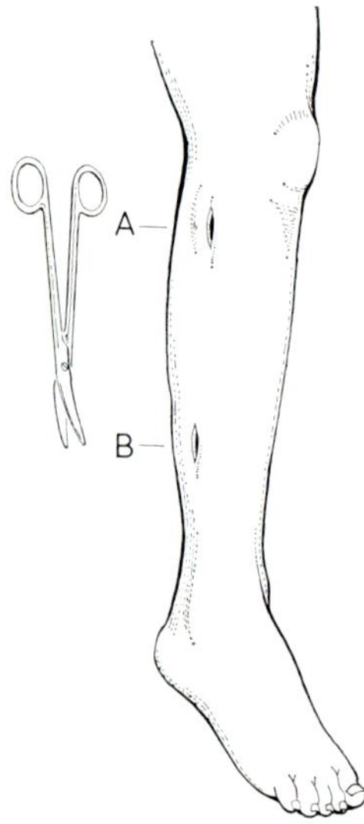

Figure 15.1   Technique of fasciotomy showing sites, A and B, of incisions and the Mayo's 21 cm (8½ in), angled scissors used

Conclusions

The anterior tibial compartment (ATC) syndrome is a definite entity which exists in chronic and acute forms. It is probably not diagnosed as often as it should be. It can lead to disability and permanent foot drop or loss of the leg. Treatment by decompression fasciotomy is simple and very effective if it is carried out before the foot drop develops. The possibility of ATC compression following trauma or leg revascularisation procedures should be borne in mind and prophylactic fasciotomy considered.

ACKNOWLEDGEMENT

My thanks are due to the Department of Medical Illustration of the Royal Postgraduate Medical School for the drawing of Figure 15.1.

REFERENCES

Birnstingl, M. (1973) Arterial injuries. In *Peripheral Vascular Surgery*, Tutorials in Post-graduate Medicine, ed. Birnstingl, M., Vol. 3. London: William Heinemann Medical Books Ltd.

Bradley, E. L. (1973) The anterior tibial compartment syndrome. *Surgery, Gynecology and Obstetrics*, **136**, 289–297.

De Weese, J. A. & Rob, C. (1968) Fasciotomy. In *Operative Surgery*, 2nd edn, ed. Rob, C. & Smith, R., Vol. 3, pp. 256–259. London: Butterworths.

Edwards, E. A. (1953) The anatomic basis for ischaemia localised to certain muscles of the lower limb. *Surgery, Gynecology and Obstetrics*, **97**, 87–94.

French, E. Z. & Price, W. H. (1962) Anterior tibial pain. *British Medical Journal*, **2**, 1290–1296.

Jantet, G. To be published.

Levy, J.-B. & Di Maria, G. (1972) Le Syndrome tibial antérieur. *Journal de Chirurgie (Paris)*, **104**, 577–590.

Livingstone, R. H. & Wilson, R. I. (1975) Gunshot wounds of the limbs. *British Medical Journal*, **1**, 667–669.

Lunceford, E. M. (1965) The peroneal compartment syndrome. *Southern Medical Journal*, **58**, 621–623.

Mavor, G. E. (1956) The anterior tibial syndrome. *Journal of Bone and Joint Surgery*, **38B**, 513–517.

Severin, E. (1943) Umwandlung des Musculus Tibialis Anterior in Narbengewebe nach Überanstrengung. *Acta chirurgica scandinavica*, **89**, 426–432.

Wells, H. S., Youmans, J. B. & Miller, D. G. (1938) Tissue pressure as related to venous pressure, capillary filtration and other factors. *Journal of Clinical Investigation*, **17**, 489–499.

Wright, S. (1961) *Samson Wright's Applied Physiology*, 10th edn, revised by Keele, C. A., Neil, E. with Jepson, J. D., p. 18. London: Oxford University Press.

16
THE SURGERY OF CORONARY ARTERY DISEASE

W. P. Cleland   Celia M. Oakley

The expectation of an infant surviving to adult life has enormously improved during this century. In the same 70 years there has been no increase in life expectancy for men after the age of 40 (Lew and Seltzer, 1970) because of a steady increase in deaths from coronary disease which despite coronary care has not yet been shown to have diminished (Blackburn, 1974). Medical measures seeming to have achieved so little, surgical approaches to the problem were tried well before the advent of open-heart techniques.

Historical Introduction

Early operations for angina were indirect and often illogical but all enjoyed a limited popularity until replaced by the next 'good idea'. These operations included sympathectomy, omentopexy or pneumopexy, internal mammary ligation and pericardial phenolisation, abrasion or poudrage. The improvements were subjective, occured in up to 70 per cent of survivors and were usually attributable to the placebo effect. Vineberg's operation of internal mammary implantation into the myocardium was introduced in 1946 but only became popular in the mid-1960s when the Cleveland Clinic group gave it some scientific credibility by using coronary angiography to localise the ischaemic area for implantation and by showing patency and connection with the coronary circulation after injection of contrast into the internal mammary arteries (Favaloro et al, 1967). The first direct attacks on obstructed coronary arteries (endarterectomy and patch grafting) (Effler et al, 1965) had limited scope and carried a high mortality, but in 1968 Favaloro followed by Johnson in 1969 reported their experience of the operation of aortocoronary bypass grafting that is used today employing reversed autogenous vein from the leg. This was the first operation to be followed by both subjective and objective evidence of successful revascularisation.

The Pathological and Natural History of Coronary Artery Disease

Only rarely is coronary artery obstruction caused by processes other than atheroma. Embolism, spasm, thrombosis, dissection, and coronary ostial

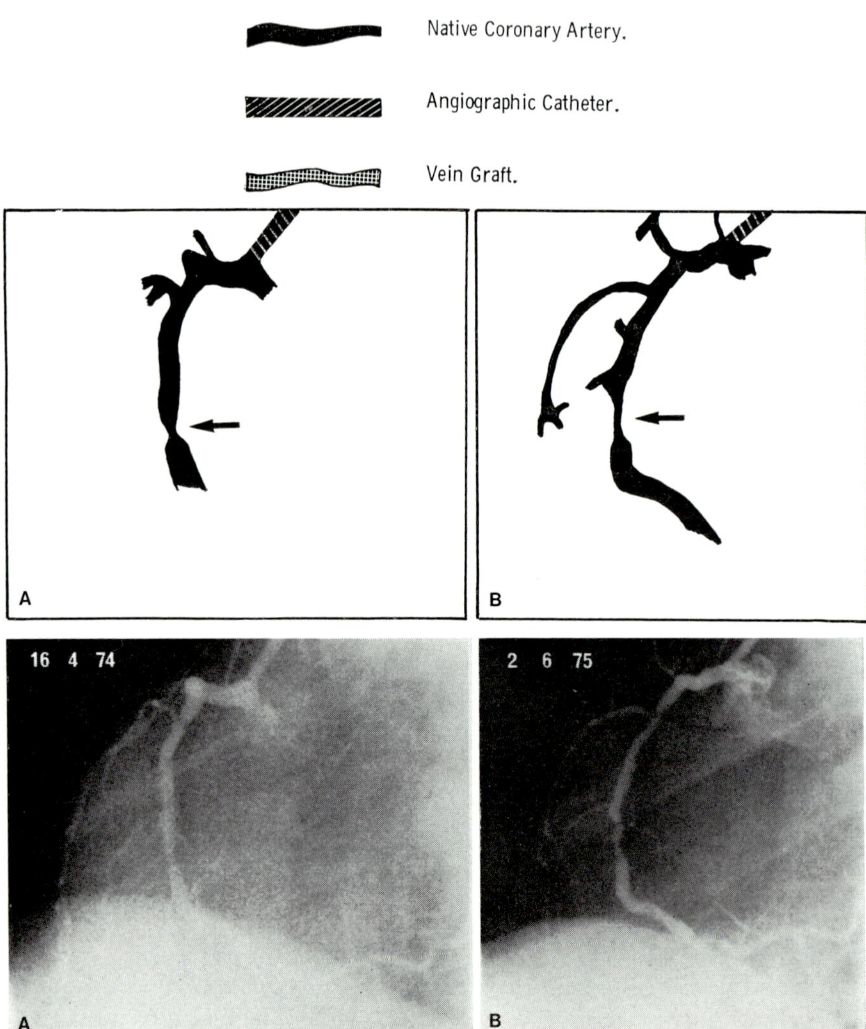

Figure 16.1 Progressive disease in the right coronary artery. Left lateral projection. The stricture in the mid-portion has progressed in 14 months from a less than 50 per cent narrowing to a greater than 70 per cent narrowing and the length of the stricture has also increased. A localised more proximal stenosis has not changed in the 14 months between the examinations. (The key to shading in the line drawing applies also to Figures 16.2, 16.3, 16.4 and 16.8)

stenosis have nevertheless to be remembered; even congenital abnormalities occasionally first cause ischaemic symptoms in adult life.

The natural history of the coronary atheromatous plaque is that of atheroma in any artery. It starts as a non-obstructive protrusion of the intima over a part of the circumference of a coronary artery, probably as a result of 'insudation' of lipid from the plasma (Walton, 1975). These plaques tend to have characteristic predilection for certain sites, for example, the mid-portion of the right main coronary artery at the origin of its main muscular branch (Fig. 16.1) and the proximal anterior descending near the origin of the first diagonal. The fatty plaque spreads both circumferentially and longitudinally, gradually acquires more fibrous tissue and obstructs the blood flow. Eventually the intima tends to ulcerate and final complete occlusion may result from secondary thrombosis. Occasionally haemorrhage into the plaque accounts for sudden decrease in luminal size and the advent of multiple subintimal haemorrhages has been described as characteristic of the patient with 'preinfarction' angina.

Usually atheroma causes coronary narrowing but sometimes the media becomes weakened in advanced disease and this can lead to a limited aneurysm or more generalised ectasia which is then usually associated with stenoses in other parts of the coronary tree.

Revascularisation surgery can at best only be an adjunct to the treatment of coronary atheroma because the latter is a progressive disorder and the *continuing* efficacy of coronary bypass grafts in an individual depends as much on the lack of development of new obstructions as on the continued patency of the grafts which themselves can become heir to the affliction. The management of the patient who has already developed symptomatic coronary artery disease (secondary prevention) should therefore be the same as that of his yet asymptomatic sons (primary prevention). This management is directed towards the provision of a more favourable internal milieu by the avoidance or removal of known 'risk factors'.

Associations and Possible Prevention
of Coronary Artery Disease

Three major 'risk factors', high blood pressure, hyperlipidaemia, and cigarette smoking, have been identified. Other predisposing attributes such as obesity, diabetes, high uric acid, high haematocrit, lack of exercise, soft water, carbon monoxide, type A personality, coffee drinking, a bad family history, and even frontal baldness have been incriminated but no direct causal relationship has been established between any of these and atheroma. Probability tables have been drawn up which enumerate the likelihood of any individual with any combination of recognised risk factors developing symptomatic coronary disease at any age and it is infrequent in clinical practice to encounter patients who have coronary atheroma in the absence of any overt risk factors. That it occurs at all underlines our continuing ignorance of basic causation. Coronary artery disease is often found to be clustered within certain families, but this may be due to a sharing of life habits and temperament as much as the inheritance of similar metabolic abnormalities and blood pressure. A taste for sporting pursuits is unlikely to be associated with obesity. Overweight is not in itself a risk factor but predisposes the individual to develop high blood pressure, high blood fats and diabetes. Similarly, diabetics are more likely than non-diabetics to suffer from hyperlipidaemia. The insurance companies have long known that the lower the blood pressure the better the life (within limits). The serum cholesterol and triglyceride concentration probably represent a similarly graded risk and the so called 'normals' within a UK or other Western population are undoubtedly 'abnormal' when the distribution curve of their blood fats is compared with that of 'normal' individuals in Japan (still relatively free from coronary disease). There is only a 10 per cent overlap, the 10 per cent with the lowest lipids in the UK overlapping the 10 per cent with the highest 'normal' lipids from Japan.

Primary prevention requires that whole populations in high risk countries start to bring up their children to eat sparingly of animal fat, avoid obesity and cigarette smoking, continue to take vigorous physical activity daily, and have their blood pressures checked from time to time.

There is yet very little information concerning the effect of the virtuous (as distinct from the 'good') life on the progression of existing coronary artery disease. While treatment may not affect the progression of an already established plaque it seems likely that the development of new plaques might be delayed. Because of the high incidence of asymptomatic coronary disease and the poor relation between angina and pathology, serial coronary angiographic studies are needed in order to study the effect of such interventions on the progression of established disease (Bemis et al, 1973; Ben-Zvi et al, 1974). Studies of secondary prevention which utilise epidemiological methods with end-points infarction and death need huge numbers and prolonged follow-up if the effect of correction of one or more risk factors is ever to be revealed.

Smoking is an independent risk factor (Rose, 1973) which may exert its adverse effect through a thrombotic rather than an atherogenic action, but nicotine does have direct effects on catecholamine and lipid metabolism and interest has also centred on higher blood carbon monoxide levels in smokers. It has been shown that cessation of smoking after myocardial infarction halved both the incidence of further infarction and of death compared with patients who continued to smoke (Wilhelmsson et al, 1975) and that the incidence of symptomatic coronary artery disease amongst those who give up smoking falls towards that in individuals who have never smoked.

Prognosis in Coronary Artery Disease

Nearly a quarter of a million people die in this country every year from cardiovascular causes. Two-thirds of these deaths are from coronary artery disease and more than half of the coronary deaths are sudden. The estimated first-year mortality from myocardial infarction is still 50 per cent: 25 per cent before reaching hospital, 15 per cent in hospital (25 per cent before coronary care), and another 10 per cent from a second infarct during the year of onset (Blackburn, 1974). Nearly half of the sudden deaths are in apparently healthy people who have never complained of recognisable ischaemic symptoms, yet nearly all of the hearts show serious obstructions of two or more major coronary arteries (Vedin et al, 1973). In other words, angina is a signal which marks the probable existence of coronary disease, but the severity of the symptom is a poor indicator of its extent or of the prognosis.

Moreover, the symptom of angina is not a specific expression of underlying coronary artery disease; it occurs when metabolic demand exceeds supply as in aortic stenosis or hypertrophic cardiomyopathy, and it can be simulated by pain due to extracardiac conditions. Up to one-quarter of patients investigated for clinically diagnosed anginal pain are found to have normal coronary arteries. Over the past few years it has become possible to link prognosis to the angiographically determined number, site and severity of coronary artery obstructions, and strikingly similar findings have emanated from many different centres (Oberman et al, 1972; Bruschke, Proudfit and Sones, 1973; Humphries et al, 1974; Webster, Moberg and Rincon, 1974). Prognosis is further influenced by the amount of left ventricular damage which has been sustained from previous infarction. It has been shown that patients with seeming angina but with normal arteries on coronary angiography have a better prognosis than 'healthy' (but unstudied) age-matched controls (Bruschke et al, 1973).

Prognosis is, then, related to the underlying disease and not to the symptom which it may or may not produce. The patient for his part is mainly or solely concerned with the symptom, and relief of it may in itself provide justification for a surgical approach.

Individuals with obstruction to the three major vessels (anterior descending, circumflex and right main) may be expected to suffer an annual mortality of 15 per cent, and nearly half of them will be dead in five years. Figures for two-vessel disease show an annual mortality of between 6 and 15 per cent, and at five years the figure is only just behind the figure for patients with three-vessel disease. The reason for this is presumably progression of obstruction in the patients with two-vessel disease and the tendency for the survival curves of observed individuals to flatten out beyond five or six years from the onset of observations. Prognosis is worst for obstruction of the left main stem coronary artery (Fig. 16.2) which carries a mortality in excess of 50 per cent in five years (Lavine et al, 1972; Bruschke et al, 1973; Lim, Proudfit and Sones, 1975). By contrast, the outlook for single-vessel disease is usually good, the annual mortality being under 2 per cent. The site of obstruction matters, proximal obstruction of the anterior descending branch of the left coronary artery carrying a higher risk (up to 7 per cent annual mortality) than single lesions of the anterior descending further down or for the right main or circumflex branches.

None of these figures have taken account of varying patterns of coronary distribution. Obstruction of the proximal anterior descending in an individual with left coronary dominance and a left ventricle which is largely supplied by it is likely to prove lethal, whereas in other individuals the anterior descending may supply only a small part of the anterior wall of the left ventricle, the apex and lateral free wall being supplied by the posterior descending

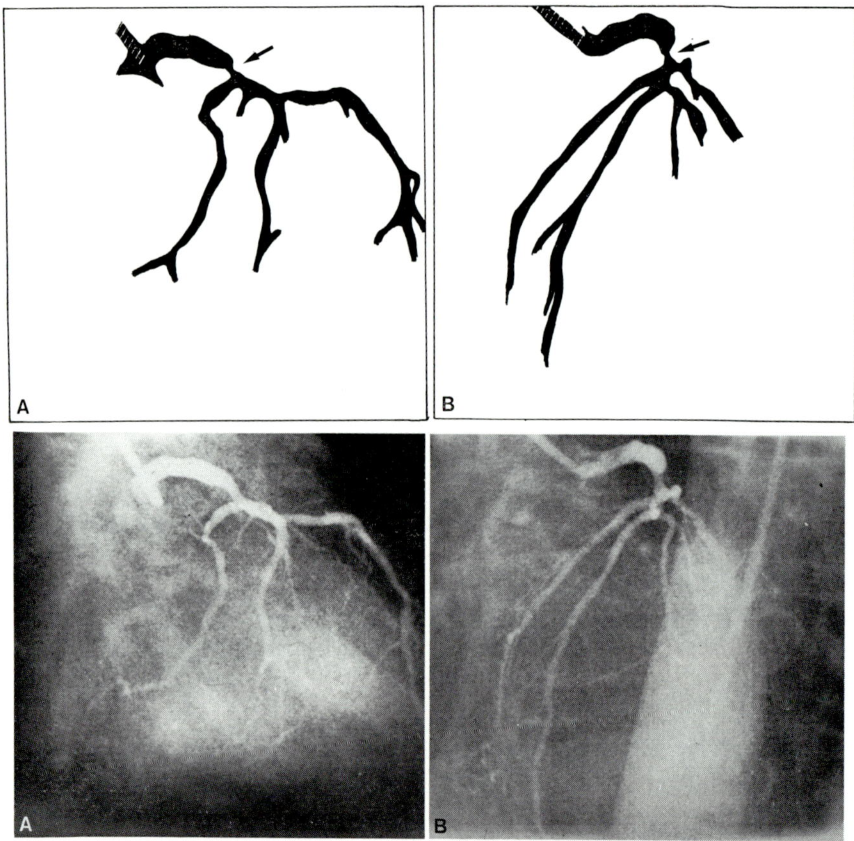

Figure 16.2   Left main stem stenosis shown (A) in the right anterior oblique view and (B) in the left anterior oblique view. There is a 70 per cent localised stricture immediately before the division of the main stem. Although there are plaques in the branches of the left coronary artery there are in this case no other significant obstructions

branch arising from the right coronary and marginal branches of the circumflex coronary arteries. Most follow-up studies on prognosis related to coronary angiographic anatomy suffer from the further disadvantage of failing to allow for the (presumably) differing rates of progression between patients in different age groups or with differing risk factors. Bruschke showed the unfavourable influence of non-obstructing plaques which may progress to flow-limiting obstruction during the years of follow-up. As with all studies based on observations of a large number of patients the conclusions have only very limited application to the individual patient. However, these are all the guidelines we have plus a common-sense approach which probably permits extreme vulnerability to be recognised. Patients with stenosis of only a single major vessel are not at much risk of dying from it unless that stenosis involves a vessel which is the main source of supply to the left ventricular myocardium usually by a dominant anterior descending. Minor plaques on other vessels should always be carefully noted because they may progress to important stenosis within a relatively short time; i.e. one-vessel disease is only benign while it remains one-vessel disease.

In considering the prognosis it has to be remembered that most of the data come from America where treatment by beta adrenergic blockade has not been widely used because of unavailability of propranolol until recently except for the treatment of dysrhythmias. In addition to being extremely effective in relieving symptoms, these drugs may themselves have a beneficial effect on prognosis. Beta blocking drugs increase cardiac efficiency so that the same physical work is achieved at less metabolic cost to the heart (1) by reduction in the heart rate response to exercise, (2) by reduction in LV systolic wall tension through reduction in blood pressure, and (3) by reduction in the velocity of contraction of the myocardium. Such treatment reduces the imbalance between supply and demand and could both reduce the chances of sudden death and the size of any infarct that occurs.

The Medical Management of Angina

The medical relief of angina depends on recognition of other diseases of the heart, particularly aortic stenosis and hypertrophic cardiomyopathy; the correction of obesity, high blood pressure, anaemia, or thyroid dysfunction; and the prescription of a beta adrenergic blocking drug. Propranolol or equivalent in a usual dose, between 80 and 160 mg t.d.s., can be expected to induce maximum benefit when used in conjunction with the nitrates. The dose chosen should keep exercise-induced tachycardia below 110 beats per minute, the resting heart rate being irrelevant. The most satisfactory nitrate drug is isosorbide dinitrate taken sublingually in 5 mg doses before any activity which normally brings on the pain. The actions of nitrates are synergistic with those of beta blocking drugs. Although nitrates cause coronary dilation this is not the method of their relief of angina because they fail to dilate the diseased portions of the vessels. The nitrate benefit stems from relaxation of smooth muscle in the capacitance veins (and to a lesser extent arterioles) so that blood is pooled peripherally, venous return is reduced, the heart gets smaller, the blood pressure falls, and the work of the heart is lessened. The fall in stroke volume and blood pressure induce a reflex tachycardia which is theoretically detrimental but which can be largely prevented if a beta blocking drug is being taken. The intelligent patient is further helped by adoption of a new life style designed to curtail deterioration in his own arterial disease and to prevent its onset in his children. We feel that it is extremely important for the ischaemic subject to become slim and as fit as possible through regular exercise up to his pain limit aided by his tablets.

Selection of Patients for
Coronary Artery Bypass Grafting (CABG)

Stable angina

Patients are usually considered for CABG because they have severe angina. Their selection for surgery then depends on the coronary anatomy.

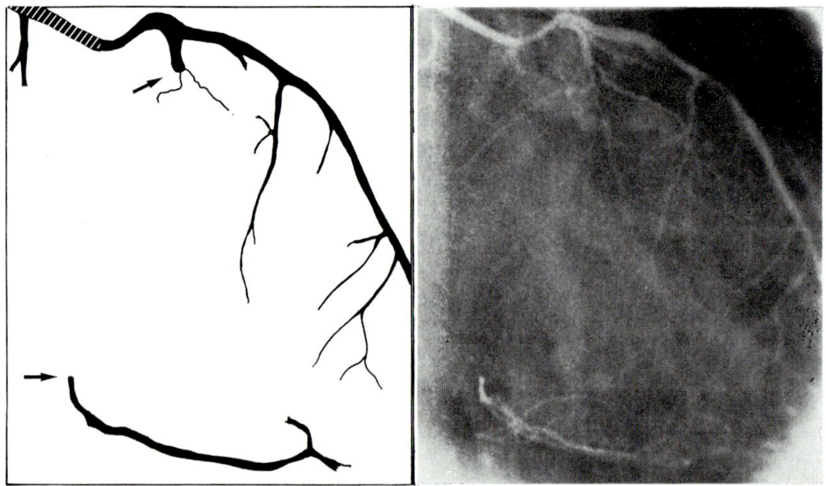

Figure 16.3   Coronary arteriogram. Right anterior oblique projection, left coronary injection showing a complete block in the circumflex 1 cm after its origin (arrowed) and retrograde filling of the right main stem as far as a complete block (arrowed)

Patients with less severe symptoms but life-threatening coronary obstructions may be advised to have surgery in the hope of improving their prognosis.

Suitability for successful CABG depends on the coronary pathology. Investigations should be directed at demonstrating all evidence of atheroma— minor irregularities and varying grades of stenosis. In addition, the condition of the vessel distal to a major obstruction is of paramount importance. The distal vessel may be filled by dye passing through the stenosis (anterograde filling) (Fig. 16.1). It may only be delineated by filling from collateral vessels which bypass the stenotic lesion (collateral filling) or it may be filled retrogradely from injection into the other coronary artery (retrograde filling) (Fig. 16.3). In all cases the condition of the distal vessel must as far as possible be determined.

Nearly half of the patients investigated with serious angina have atheroma limited to the proximal segment of a main coronary vessel. In these patients, the more distal portions of the artery may be entirely free from disease and eminently suitable for grafting. In such cases the flow of blood into the distal branches of the coronary tree (the run-off) is good and successful anastomoses are likely.

The remainder have more widespread lesions often extending along the whole length of the artery. In these cases a good anastomosis is more difficult as the vessel is abnormal and the 'run-off' is less good so that late occlusions are more likely (Bourassa et al, 1972).

The right coronary artery is often involved in a diffuse thickening of the intima which extends as a core along considerable lengths of the vessel. Fortunately, these atheromatous cores tend to tail off towards the periphery where the artery becomes relatively normal.

The state of the left ventricle has a very direct bearing on the operative mortality of bypass grafting.

While previous myocardial infarction is no contraindication to surgery, marked left ventricular dysfunction increases the operative risk and no improvement of function of fibrous areas can be anticipated. It has now become important to define the site and extent of reversible ischaemic dysfunction which may improve after revascularisation as well as to recognise areas of irreversible dysfunction caused by previous infarction. The study of left ventricular angiography after pacing stress or exercise not only high-lights the area which needs revascularisation but enables the adequacy of revascularisation to be tested postoperatively in the same manner. Conversely, areas of segmental dyskinesia seen at rest may be favourably influenced by glyceryl trinitrate (Dumesnil et al, 1975).

The ejection fraction of the LV (that fraction of the end-diastolic volume which is ejected at each beat) is usually used to judge LV efficiency. In ischaemic heart disease a reduction in the ejection fraction below the normal 60 per cent or above depends on both the amount and the site of segmental dyskinesia. When this is extensive the ejection fraction becomes impaired but may be seen to improve considerably when angiography is repeated after trinitrate (Greenberg et al, 1975).

The operative risks of patients undergoing bypass surgery with good left ventricular function vary from about 2 per cent in the best centres to 5 per cent. If a sizeable area of segmental dyskinesia is demonstrable in the left ventricular angiogram but the ejection fraction is still above 50 per cent then risks rise to between 5 and 8 per cent (Fig. 16.4). Patients with an ejection fraction below 50 per cent should still be considered provided the coronary obstructions look suitable for grafting and the severity of angina justifies an increased operative risk (which may then be as high as 12 per cent). The end-diastolic pressure in the left ventricle is a very much less useful criterion of left ventricular contractile efficiency than the ejection fraction in assessing operative risk in this context.

Patients with angina which they consider still to be troublesome and who cannot follow their normal occupations despite optimal medical therapy can be recommended for surgery. The majority of such patients have significant stenoses in more than one vessel and require more than one coronary bypass

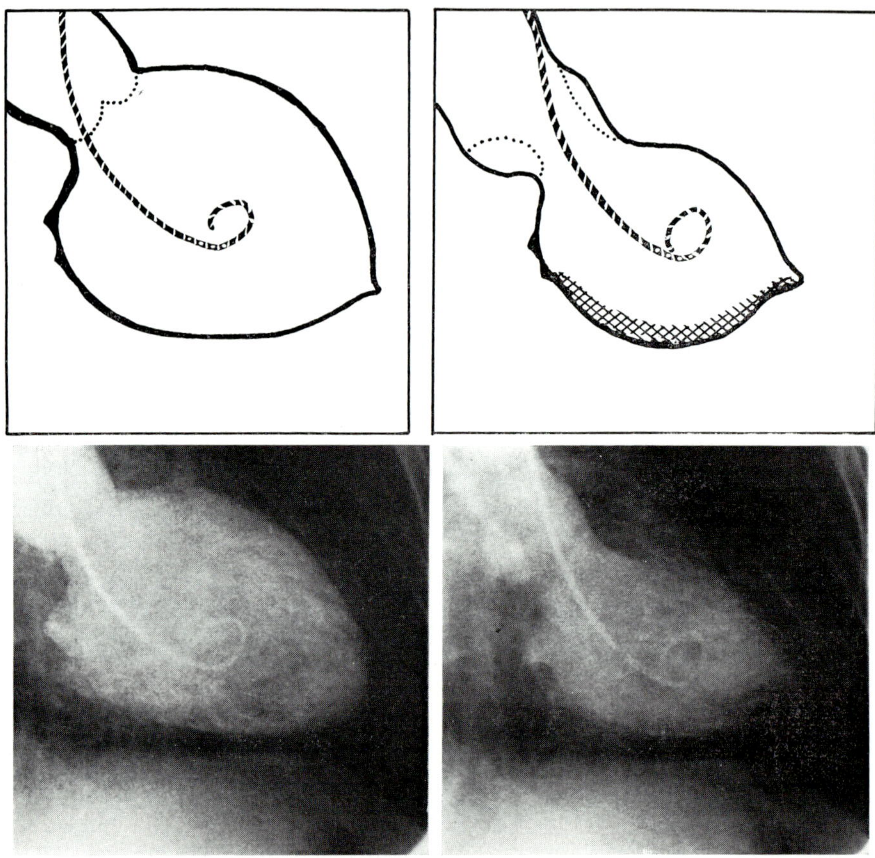

Figure 16.4   Left ventricular cine angiogram. (Same patient as Figure 16.3.) Right anterior oblique view, end-diastolic on the left and end-systolic on the right. There is a very long segment of dyskinesia involving the whole of the inferior wall as far as the apex. The immobility of the fibrous inferior wall leads to a rocking movement of the ventricle as the anterior wall contracts vigorously during systole. This is much better shown on the cine film where upward pointing of the ventricular 'toe' denotes inferior dyskinesia and downward pointing of a 'ballerina foot' denotes anterior wall dyskinesia

graft. Advice to undergo CABG for relief of severe symptoms is not contentious for suitable patients in whom the chance of worthwhile symptomatic benefit approaches 90 per cent. The relief of angina so that the patient can continue with or return to his work is a justification in itself. Operation in the hope of improving prognosis is a far more difficult problem and will be discussed in the description of surgical results. At the present time stenosis of the left main stem is considered by many to be an indication for surgical intervention.

Preinfarction angina

Preinfarction angina is here defined as angina occurring at rest, lasting often up to 20 min, but unaccompanied by diagnostic changes of infarction in either the ECG or serum enzymes. Half of these patients will develop infarction during the ensuing year, and of those patients who infarct 50 per cent will die or become permanently disabled.

The patient with preinfarction angina should be put to rest in bed and given beta blockers and glyceral trinitrate to try to undo the oxygen debt. Most patients then lose their pain. Coronary angiography should then be carried out when they are pain-free but as soon as possible, with a view to early CABG. Only a few patients fail to lose their pain and, in these patients only, coronary angiography should be undertaken without further delay. In such cases it is necessary to have the cardiac surgeon on the premises ready to go ahead with CABG immediately after the procedure. Happily, the occasions when these semi-emergency investigations are needed are uncommon.

Operative Surgery

The techniques for coronary artery bypass grafting are now well established and are fairly uniform throughout the world, although individual variation of detail occurs. Having determined that the patient's symptoms warrant surgery and demonstrated that vessels suitable for grafting distal to a serious obstruction are present and that the function of the left ventricle is not seriously impaired, the individual can be accepted for operation. The presence of a suitable saphenous vein must be confirmed. If no such vein is present, the surgeon has the choice of the rather unsatisfactory arm veins or the internal mammary artery.

Cardiopulmonary bypass is necessary. While the patient is being prepared for cannulation, the vein is isolated and its branches carefully ligated and divided. Mobilisation starts at the ankle and is extended upwards sufficiently to supply an adequate length. Occasionally veins from both sides may be required.

The coronary vessels are inspected and the sites of atheroma confirmed, as also the suitability of the distal vessel for anastomosis. Some surgeons prefer to do the aortic end of the anastomosis before instituting bypass as this will reduce the length of bypass and limit damage to blood components.

Anastomoses to the circumflex artery or its branches should be completed first as the coronary artery end of this anastomosis necessitates considerable dislocation of the heart. Anastomosis to the left anterior descending vessel and the right coronary artery can usually be completed with minimal dislocation of the heart.

Separate cannulation of cavae is preferred to a single atrial line, so that kinking and obstruction of either cava during periods of cardiac dislocation is prevented. Decompression of the left side of the heart is advisable either through a stab incision at the apex of the left ventricle or through the left atrium. The LV vent leaves a new area of scarring of variable size which is readily recognised on postoperative angiography.

On the other hand, the LV vent represents the only certain way that LV distension can be prevented, such as may occur when the heart is dislocated and the aortic valve rendered incompetent as a result. Additionally, elevation of the heart to gain access to the posterior surface is made easier if the vent can be used for elevation and stabilisation.

Cooling of the myocardium to 30°C is advised as a protection against ischaemia. Induced electrical fibrillation of the heart and periods of aortic clamping will be required to provide ideal conditions for the operation. The

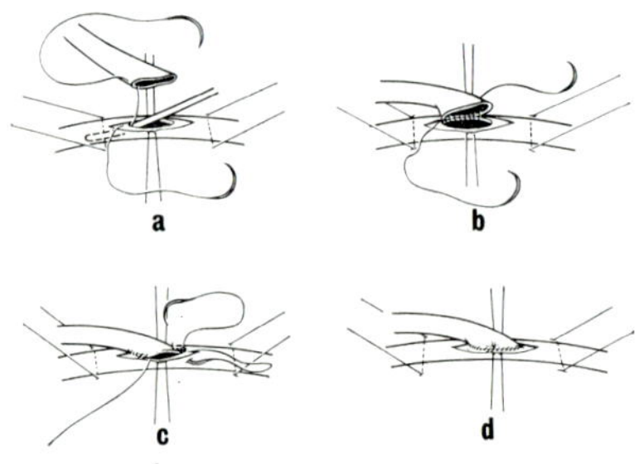

Figure 16.5 The distal veno-arterial anastomosis (a) shows exploration of coronary artery with graduated probe to determine size and levels of obstruction. The anastomosis is done with a simple over-and-over suture of 6 × 0 prolene

ideal site for anastomosis is selected, and the artery above and below is controlled by a simple stay suture.

The artery can then be incised longitudinally whilst the vessel is steadied by the stay suture and still distended with blood with the aorta not clamped. An 8 to 10 mm incision is made in the artery, forward and retrograde blood flow is determined, and the vessel explored by graduated probes to determine size and patency (Fig. 16.5).

An end-to-side veno-arterial anastomosis is then carried out using 6 × 0 prolene and a continuous simple stitch interrupted at two points in the circle.

The aortic anastomosis is effected using a side clamp and after punching out a small aperture in the aortic wall. A slightly heavier 5 × 0 prolene is usually employed in a manner similar to the distal anastomosis (Fig. 16.6).

The surgeon must ensure that the graft extends smoothly from aorta to coronary artery without tension, kinks or twists (Fig. 16.7).

Estimation of flow along the graft should be determined with an electromagnetic flow meter.

Endarterectomy and Bypass Grafting

Approximately 20 per cent of coronary arteries in need of grafting are found to be occupied by a cylindrical core of atheroma which not only reduces the calibre of the vessel but restricts the 'run-off' and makes successful grafting less likely. These lesions are much more common in the right coronary artery.

The atheromatous core starts in the proximal part of the artery usually at the site of a major plaque and extends distally for a variable distance but usually peters out towards the periphery. The core will usually extend into the branches of the main vessel for a short distance. The distal portion can often be completely enucleated using either mechanical dissection or mobilisation with small probes delivering a flow of CO_2 (gas endarterectomy).

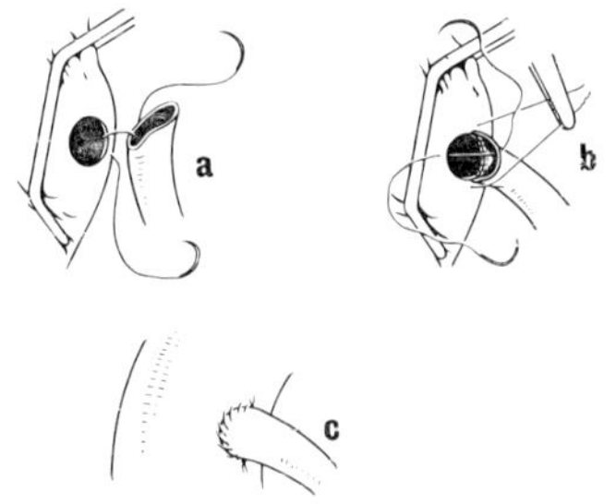

Figure 16.6 The proximal or aorto-venous anastomosis (a) shows excision of part of aortic wall and commencement of suturing. Anastomosis completed with 5×0 prolene

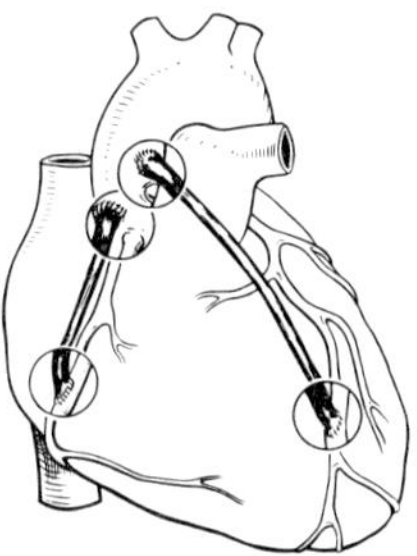

Figure 16.7 General appearances of heart after grafts of left anterior descending and right coronary arteries. The graft should lie without twists or kinks

Total endarterectomy has not been successful resulting in a high infarction rate and frequent later occlusions. Distal endarterectomy followed by grafting into the cored out vessel has given excellent results. Endarterectomy removes not only the atheroma but the intima and part of the media of the coronary vessel but the remnants still remain entirely amenable to an anastomosis.

Postoperative studies indicate that such grafts remain patent in a high proportion of cases (Yacoub et al, 1975) provided that the distal core extension into branches has been completely removed and there is good 'run-off' into the distal coronary tree.

The right coronary artery is more frequently occupied by a removable atheromatous core than are the anterior descending or circumflex vessels. Successful endarterectomy (i.e. complete removal followed by successful grafting) is much more common with right coronary lesions possibly because the branches of the main vessel are relatively few and large and more easily cleared of disease. Conversely, the anterior descending vessel is less likely to have a successful endarterectomy as it gives rise to many small but important vessels along its whole course which supply important parts of the left ventricle and are difficult to render atheroma free.

Postoperative Management

In the immediate postoperative period it is essential to maintain a good cardiac output and blood pressure so that the flow along the graft is encouraged. The blood volume should be well maintained and if the blood pressure or cardiac output tend to sag these should be boosted either with cardiac stimulant drugs (inotropic agents such as isoprenaline or adrenaline) or with a selective vasodilator such as salbutamol. These are best administered as a drip. Ventricular ectopics often occur and if frequent should be suppressed with lignocaine, either as a bolus injection of 50 to 100 mg or a drip.

Various supraventricular dysrhythmias occur occasionally and may all result in a fall of output. Atrial fibrillation can readily be dealt with by d.c shock, but if recurrent should be controlled by digitalis. Atrial flutter may respond to d.c. shock or 5 to 10 mg of intravenous verapamil. Nodal rhythms may be overcome by pacing or may respond to small doses of oxprenolol (0.5 mg i.v.).

Oral anticoagulants are started as soon as the mediastinal drains are removed and are continued for three months. There is no hard evidence that their use reduces the chances of graft occlusion but they do help the circulation of the donor leg and have reduced the incidence of postoperative pulmonary embolism.

The leg from which the vein has been removed should be encased in a pressure bandage for the first few postoperative days, and if subsequently it begins to swell an elastic stocking should be worn for some weeks until circulation has improved. Fairly rapid mobilisation of the patient is advisable with graduated exercises whilst in hospital. Once having left hospital, a course of rehabilitation designed for the cardiac or the coronary patient is advisable so that the new effort tolerance can be determined and improved. As many patients as possible should be encouraged to return to their former occupations. Any pre-existing risk factors should be rigorously controlled. Smoking should be banned and any tendency to put on weight should be discouraged. If there are cholesterol or lipid disturbances, these should be treated appropriately. Drugs designed to reduce platelet adhesiveness such as dipyridamole or aspirin are advised by some, but the evidence for their value is just not available.

Postoperative myocardial infarction

The development of new Q waves or new major conduction defects after CABG indicates muscle loss due to infarction. The incidence of these perioperative infarcts has been variously estimated between 5 and 25 per cent

(Brewer, Bilbro and Bartel, 1973; Espinoza et al, 1974; Rose et al, 1974; Assad-Morell et al, 1975). Fortunately the majority of the infarcts are small though a few are important and disabling. They may be caused by the following. (1) Distal embolism down the right coronary artery especially after endarterectomy. This usually produces inferior infarction. (2) An overlong total ischaemia time during completion of the anastomosis. (3) The creation of an island of ischaemia when a graft is placed distal to the second of two critical stenoses. The territories served by any branches coming off the main artery between the two stenoses will then not be supplied with blood either from the coronary artery at the proximal end nor retrogradely via the graft and may infarct. (4) A period of low blood pressure or low output and tachycardia postoperatively may lead to infarction in a territory served by an obstructed coronary artery which has not been successfully grafted either because no graft was attempted or because the graft has become occluded.

Factors Influencing the Outcome of Bypass Surgery

Three considerations beyond all others affect the results of surgery: the experience of the surgeon, the condition of the left ventricle which has a very direct bearing on the risks of the operation (Mundth et al, 1971; Spencer et al, 1971; Kouchoukos, Kirklin and Oberman, 1974), and the pathology of the coronary vessels which largely determines the future of the grafts themselves.

Results and Follow-up

All patients should undergo selective angiography of the grafts postoperatively. Early postoperative studies have shown a graft patency rate varying between 64 per cent in the first published series up to 96 per cent in the most recent reports (Favaloro et al, 1970; Johnson et al, 1970b; Effler et al, 1971; Spencer et al, 1971; Anderson et al, 1972; Morris et al, 1972; Walker et al, 1972; Alderman et al, 1973; Segal et al, 1973; Sheldon et al, 1973; Morch et al, 1974). Patency is related to flow rate which in turn is related to peripheral run-off. Hence the importance of a large territory of distribution in the vessel selected to be grafted (Bourassa et al, 1972) and the likelihood of failure if a graft is put into a vessel which is largely feeding a territory which has suffered infarction. Early graft occlusion is more frequent when the flow rate measured at operation is less than 20 ml/min. When postoperative studies show full bore filling of a major coronary artery territory through a graft (Fig. 16.8), then that graft will usually remain patent over the next two or three years of follow-up, which is all the time for which we have data so far. Grafts which show narrowing at the anastomotic site have a high incidence of late closure which may also involve the native vessel (McLaughlin et al, 1975). Improvement in surgical technique brings the early and late patency

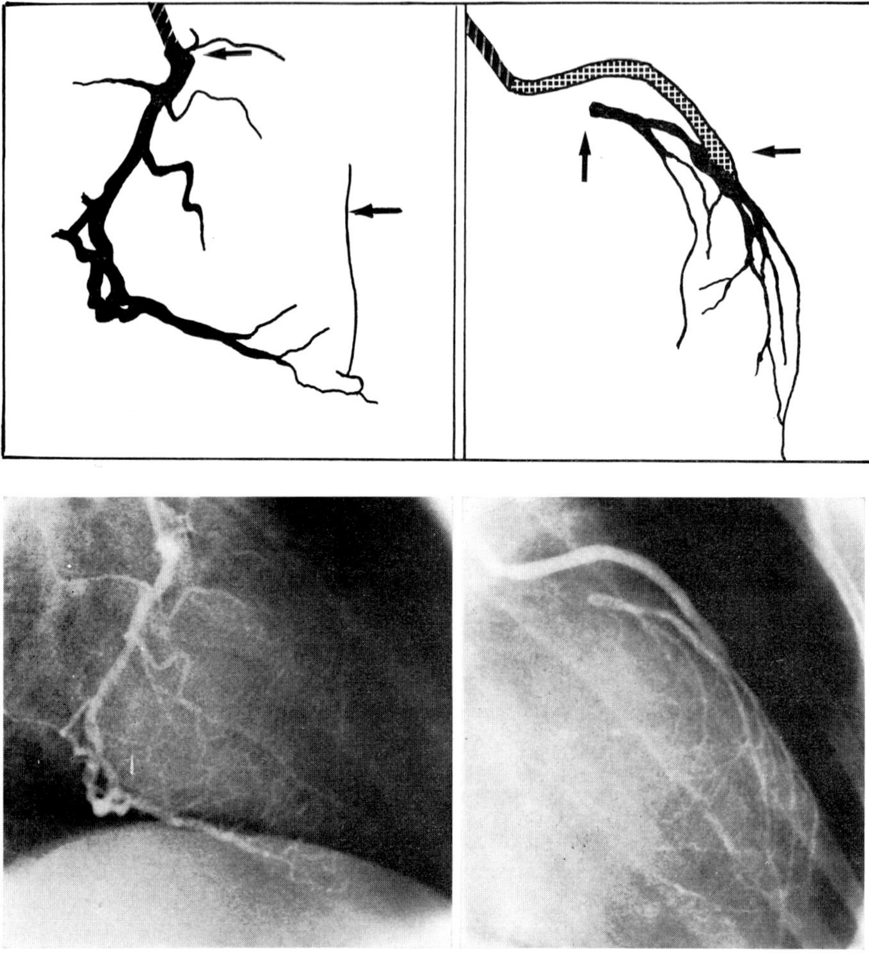

Figure 16.8   Left coronary artery injection, right anterior oblique view. On the left before operation there is only a tiny twig (arrowed) representing the first 2 cm of the anterior descending coronary artery which is otherwise not seen at all. The true circumflex in the atrioventricular groove is a large vessel and fills a diagonal branch of the anterior descending retrogradely. On the right is the postoperative contrast injection into the graft which fills the anterior descending artery seen in the same projection. The anterior descending coronary artery distal to the graft fills well with branches coursing around and down to the apex. There is also retrograde filling back up to the complete obstruction (arrowed). It can be noted that despite the unprepossessing preoperative appearance the anterior descending was in fact quite a big vessel which was capable of dilating up to a good size after grafting

rates close together. Late occlusion may be caused by a number of other factors, on whether flow is laminar or turbulent through the graft and on whether the graft itself develops atheromatous changes. Some grafts develop progressive tubular narrowing (arterialisation) and medial fibrosis (Vlodaver and Edwards, 1971) due to exposure to arterial pressures and interfering with the vein's blood supply respectively. These changes may be aggravated by rough handling of the vein, by the quality of the anastomosis and by the quantity and manner of the flow down it.

In general there is a good correlation between graft patency and relief of symptoms. Most series show that about two-thirds of patients become entirely asymptomatic following surgery while up to 90 per cent of patients show worthwhile improvement (Cannon et al, 1974). Both the surgical mortality and the success rate depend on patient selection. If only patients with well-preserved LV function are chosen then the mortality will be minimal, but many of the most deserving patients will have been turned down. It has been shown that the chances of symptomatic cure are proportional to *the number of patent grafts achieved in relation to the number needed*, this judgement being based on the pre- and postoperative coronary angiograms (Assad-Morell et al, 1975) so that it is no good leaving recognisably ischaemic territories ungrafted, and most patients require at least two grafts.

It is relevant here to mention a further determinant of graft patency which is rarely discussed in published reports. This is the attitude of surgeons towards unsuitable coronary anatomy. If only one out of three obstructed vessels appears suitable for grafting, the surgeon might attempt to graft all three, he might elect to graft only the one ideal vessel, or the patient might be offered medical treatment instead. The surgeon choosing the first option is likely to have a lower graft patency rate than the surgeon choosing the second alternative. Both surgeons will enjoy a lower rate of symptomatic 'cures' among their patients than the hypothetical third surgeon who turns the doubtful cases down. Some of the best known centres reject at least a third of cases on grounds of unpropitious coronary anatomy. Yet other surgeons, experienced in the technique, take on 'all comers', claim that very few vessels supplying surviving myocardium are ungraftable and show high graft patency rates in their patients. Selection of patients therefore depends very much on local experience but should be on the basis of planning to graft all obstructed vessels in each patient who is accepted.

Of course, the reasons for improvement need not be the relief of myocardial ischaemia through revascularisation. Relief can also come through infarction of previously viable but ischaemic muscle, through denervation of a painful area or through a placebo effect. Postoperative investigations have shown convincing evidence that most relief does come through the first mechanism but the other three mechanisms may play a variable role in some patients.

In a most relevant paper, Campeau and his colleagues (1975) compared the early and late graft patency rates between a first series of 138 patients and a second series of 100 patients. Although the patency rate at two weeks hardly differed between the two groups (86 and 92 per cent), the patency rate at one year improved from 67 to 85 per cent between the first and second series. The reduced late attrition rate was attributed to technical modifications, the second series having a much lower incidence of stenotic anastomoses. Smaller saphenous veins had been used in the second series and this would have improved flow velocity which is inversely proportional to cross-sectional area. Most interesting of all was a decreased early and late attrition rate for grafts with low measured flow rates, suggesting that technical factors are most important of all in these. Types of grafts (side to side, end to end, or y) made no difference.

The Effect of CABG on Cardiac Function

The symptomatic relief and the observation of graft patency or otherwise on postoperative graftgrams can be supplemented by objective tests of revascularisation. All of these depend on comparison of pre- and postoperative results with the patient acting as his own control. Exercise capacity may be measured pre- and postoperatively. While the onset of pain in relation to work done is subjective, the heart rate at the onset of pain or, better still, the blood pressure–heart rate product at onset of pain give a measure of maximal myocardial oxygen supply that can be compared pre- and postoperatively. Balcon et al (1974) and Chatterjee et al (1975a) have shown that following successful surgery atrial pacing could either not induce angina at all or that the heart rate at angina threshold was much higher than preoperatively. Loss of anaerobic metabolism as shown by previous lactate production reverting to lactate uptake in the coronary sinus has also been shown after successful revascularisation.

The effect on left ventricular segmental function is variable (Johnson et al, 1970a; Bourassa et al, 1972; Chatterjee et al, 1973; Moran et al, 1973; Banka, Chadda and Helfant, 1974; Hamby et al, 1974; Kennedy et al, 1974; Shepherd et al, 1974). When only resting function was tested and had been found to be normal preoperatively, then no postoperative improvement can be expected. Similarly, the scars of previous infarcts cannot be influenced. When the LV has been stressed preoperatively then segmental dysfunction can nearly always be shown, and this stress-induced segmental dysfunction which is caused by ischaemia can be removed by successful revascularisation. Loss of focal dyskinesia has been described in a series of patients with preinfarction angina (Chatterjee et al, 1972), but patients in this category are 'prestressed' and show a higher incidence of reversible segmental dysfunction on their pre-operative left ventriculograms. More recently Chatterjee (1973, 1975b) has shown similar improvement in patients with stable angina.

Although the significance of postoperative ECG changes of new infarction has been questioned, it seems likely that new Q waves mean new infarction because the development of new areas or extension of previous areas of seg-mental dyskinesia can usually be recognised on the postoperative LV angio-grams of this group of patients.

A further important influence on postoperative LV function and doubtless on future outlook after CABG is the observation that closure of vein grafts leaves a patient worse off than he was before due to the development or extension of focal ventricular dysfunction. There has also been much interest in the effect of CABG on progression of disease in the native circulation both proximal and distal to the grafts. Grafts are designed to divert blood flow round obstructions, and it is not surprising that if the surgery is successful these obstructions tend rapidly to progress to total occlusion by thrombosis. This has been shown by Aldridge and Trimble (1971), Malinow et al (1973), Griffith et al (1973), Maurer et al (1974), and McLaughlin et al (1975). If the graft subsequently becomes occluded, then it is likely that infarction will result. The rate of progression of atheroma in the distal end of the recipient artery does not seem to be accelerated if the graft is patent (McLaughlin et al, 1975). Visualisation of collateral vessels in coronary artery disease depends not only on their present size but on the pressure gradient between their ends. Thus, successful grafting brings a normal pressure into the distal territory of an artery which previously received collaterals either from its own proximal segment or from other coronary arteries. These collaterals will no longer be visualised and probably become smaller after successful re-vascularisation, but it is not known how rapidly they may expand should occlusion of the graft occur. Finally, the graft itself may develop delayed changes in it.

So for many reasons territorial revascularisation with CABG may not confer lasting benefit on account of the possibility of late occlusion of the graft and the unchecked advance of disease in the native vessels. Although many of the risk factors can be eliminated, the effects of changing habits at such a late stage of the disease on the rate of progression of the coronary atheroma remain an unknown quantity. The effect of impaired LV function on long-term results of surgery is still unknown. While greatly impaired LV function adversely affects the prognosis in patients with major coronary disease it can be argued that the same impairment of LV function would become less ominous if the threat of further infarction is lifted by successful revascularisation surgery, and this group of patients who face the highest operative risk may yet have the most to gain.

The Effect of CABG on Prognosis

The effect of CABG on prognosis remains largely unknown but it is likely to be individually highly variable and so far we cannot pick out accurately those at highest risk or those most likely to gain long lasting benefit. There are the 100 000 coronary subjects who will die each year with sudden death as their first admitted symptom. If we could only recognise them it is almost certain that CABG would improve their outlook! At the other end of the spectrum of coronary disease it is difficult to conceive that CABG could improve the survival of patients with single-vessel disease because the surgical mortality is likely to be up to 5 per cent while the annual mortality is likely to be less than 2 per cent. Exceptions would be patients with proximal stenosis of the LAD in a dominant left coronary system. It can also be argued that a single patent graft is unlikely to lift the patient into a better prognostic group, but of course this too will not be true if the graft is carrying blood into a vessel which supplies most of the left ventricular myocardium.

It is not widely agreed that CABG improves the particularly ominous prognosis of the patient with left main stem stenosis. Such patients usually also have severe obstructions in the branch vessels and may also have suffered severe left ventricular damage from infarction. Even though they represent a high risk group both for diagnostic study and for surgery, the postoperative follow-up carried out so far suggests that they live longer if treated surgically (Talano et al, 1975).

Revascularisation Surgery after Acute Infarction

The surgery of acute infarction is still in a highly developmental phase. Rarely, if ever, should infarctectomy be practised in the acute phase. Only perforation of the heart with tamponade, development of ventricular septal defect threatening life, acute papillary muscle rupture or infarction causing pulmonary oedema, indicate emergency surgery in the days following infarction.

On the face of it, coronary artery bypass grafting would seem to have no place at all after the onset of clinical infarction. The absolute warm ischaemia time of the myocardial cell is 30 min and there is no way in which a coronary bypass graft can be put in and made to function within a half-hour after the onset of infarction. This applies equally to the patient who develops an infarct as a complication of coronary angiography. However, these considerations do not apply to the ischaemic area surrounding each central zone of immediate inevitable necrosis. The fate of the borderline territory may not be determined for hours or days after the development of a cardiac infarct. Early on it may suffer from the sharp deterioration in LV function which the infarct may cause with a fall in cardiac output, blood pressure and coronary blood flow leading to extension of infarction. The consequent further decline in function and the development of oedema in the ischaemic territory may further imperil its future. This has led to strenuous efforts to prevent the spread of infarction and keep the size of any cardiac infarct to an irreducible minimum. The diversity of the measures used attest to the developmental stage we have reached. Experimentally raising the blood pressure with an alpha constrictor may limit infarction by improving coronary blood flow while it raises myocardial oxygen need. Experimentally, also beta blockers reduce the zone of necrosis by reducing myocardial oxygen demand. Unloading of the heart by a peripheral vasodilator such as nitroglycerin may reduce ischaemia from a reduction in left ventricular size and work leading to improvement in output which in turn tends to counteract the reduction in blood pressure and therefore coronary flow which might otherwise be anticipated. Multiple precordial ECG recording may be used to monitor the extent and quantitate the amount of ST segment elevation and by following this and myocardial enzyme release into the plasma the beneficial or adverse effect of such interventions may be judged.

Balloon counterpulsation still has not found an established place despite its ability to reduce left ventricular pressure work in systole but increase diastolic pressure and coronary perfusion which should make it an ideal aid. Probably its value would be proved if it were used much earlier before the establishment of cardiogenic shock indicates the loss of too much muscle to allow survival. Finally comes the question of CABG to improve the perfusion of the peripheral ischaemic territory around an infarct. Theoretically this could be lifesaving, but the risk of coronary angiography and bypass grafting in the acute phase is high and there is a danger of causing haemorrhagic infarction if reperfusion of ischaemic territory occurs too late, blood being released into dead cells across leaking capillary membranes. If such surgery is to be contemplated, then the patient should be investigated and operated with the balloon pump in situ to support the circulation.

REFERENCES

Alderman, E. L., Matloff, H. J., Wexler, L. W., Shumway, N. E. & Harrison, D. C. (1973) Results of direct coronary artery surgery for the treatment of angina pectoris. *New England Journal of Medicine*, **288**, 535.

Aldridge, H. E. & Trimble, A. S. (1971) Progression of proximal coronary artery lesions to trial occlusion after aortocoronary saphenous vein bypass grafting. *Journal of Thoracic and Cardiovascular Surgery*, **62**, 7.

Anderson, R. P., Hodam, R., Wood, J. & Starr, A. (1972) Direct revascularisation of the heart: early clinical experience with 200 patients. *Journal of Thoracic and Cardiovascular Surgery*, **63**, 353.

Assad-Morell, J. L., Frye, R. L., Connolly, D. C., Davis, G. D., Pluth, J. R., Wallace, R. B., Barnhorst, D. A., Elvebeck, L. R. & Danielson, G. R. (1975) Aortocoronary artery saphenous vein bypass surgery. *Mayo Clinic Proceedings*, **50**, 379.

Balcon, R., Honey, M., Rickards, A. F., Sturridge, M. F., Walsh, W., Wilkinson, R. K. & Wright. J. E. C. (1974) Evaluation by exercise testing and atrial pacing of results of aorto-coronary bypass surgery. *British Heart Journal*, **36**, 841.

Banka, V. S., Chadda, K. D. & Helfant, R. H. (1974) Limitations of myocardial revascularisation in restoration of regional contraction abnormalities produced by coronary occlusion. *American Journal of Cardiology*, **34**, 164.

Blackburn, H. (1974) Progress in the epidemiology and prevention of coronary heart disease. In *Progress in Cardiology*, ed. Yu, P. N. & Goodwin, J. F., Vol. III, p. 1. Philadelphia: Lea & Febiger.

Bemis, C. E., Gorlin, R., Kemp, H. G. and Herman, H. V. (1973) Progression of coronary artery disease: a clinical arteriographic study. *Circulation*, **47**, 455.

Ben-Zvi, J., Hildner, F. J., Javier, R. P., Fester, A. & Samet, P. (1974) Progression of coronary artery disease: cinearteriographic and clinical observations in medically and surgically treated patients. *American Journal of Cardiology*, **34**, 295.

Bonchek, L. I., Rahimtoola, S. H., Chaitman, B. R., Rösch, J. Anderson, R. P. & Starr, A. (1974) Vein graft occlusion. Immediate and late consequences and therapeutic implications. *Circulation*, **49–50**, Suppl. II, 84.

Bourassa, M. G., Lesperance, J., Campeau, L. & Saltiel, J. (1972) Fate of left ventricular contraction following aortocoronary venous grafts. Early and late postoperative modifications. *Circulation*, **46**, 724.

Bourassa, M. G., Lesperance, J. & Campeau, L. (1972) Factors influencing patency of aortocoronary vein grafts. *Circulation*, **45–46**, Suppl. I, 79.

Brewer, D. L., Bilbro, R. H. & Bartel, A. G. (1973) Myocardial infarction as a complication of coronary bypass surgery. *Circulation*, **47**, 58.

Bruschke, A. V. G., Proudfit, W. L. & Sones, F. (1973) Progress study of 590 consecutive non-surgical cases of coronary disease followed 5 to 9 years. Arteriographic correlations. *Circulation*, **47**, 1147.

Campeau, L., Crochet, D., Lesperance, J., Bourassa, M. G. & Grondin, C. M. (1975) Post-operative changes in aortocoronary saphenous vein grafts revisited: angiographic studies at two weeks and at one year in two series of consecutive patients. *Circulation*, **52**, 369.

Cannon, D. S., Miller, D. C., Shumway, N. E., Fogarty, T. J., Daily, P., Hu, M., Brown, B. Jr & Harrison, D. C. (1974) Long term follow-up of patients undergoing saphenous vein bypass surgery. *Circulation*, **49**, 77.

Carlson, R. G., Kline, S., Apstein, C., Scheidt, S., Blachfeld, N., Killip, T. & Lillehei, C. W. (1972) Lactate metabolism after aortocoronary artery vein bypass grafts. *Annals of Surgery*, **176**, 680.

Chatterjee, K., Swan, H. J. C., Parmley, W. W., Sustaita, H., Marcus, H. & Matloff, J. (1972) Depression of left ventricular function due to acute myocardial ischaemia and its reversal after aortocoronary saphenous vein bypass. *New England Journal of Medicine*, **286**, 117.

Chatterjee, K., Swan, H. J. C., Parmley, W. W., Sustaita, H., Marcus, H. S. & Matloff, J. (1973) Influence of direct myocardial revascularisation on left ventricular asynergy and function in patients with coronary heart disease with and without previous myocardial infraction. *Circulation*, **47**, 276.

Chatterjee, K., Matloff, J. M., Swan, H. J. C., Ganz, W., Sustaita, H., Magnusson, P., Buchbinder, N., Henis, M. & Forrester, J. S. (1975a) Improved angina threshold and coronary reserve following direct myocardial revascularisation. *Circulation*, **51–52**, Suppl. 1, 81.

Chatterjee, K., Matloff, J. M., Swan, H. J. C., Ganz, W., Kaushik, U. S., Magnusson, P., Henis, M. M. & Forrester, J. S. (1975b) Abnormal regional metabolism and mechanical function in patients with ischaemic heart disease: improvement after successful regional revascularisation by aortocoronary bypass. *Circulation*, **52**, 390.

Dumesnil, J. G., Ritman, E. L., Davis, G. D., Gau, G. T., Rutherford, B. D. & Frye, R. L. (1975) Regional left ventricular wall dynamics before and after sublingual administration of nitroglycerin. *American Journal of Cardiology*, **36**, 419.

Effler, D. B., Sones, F. M., Jr, Favaloro, R. & Groves, L. K. (1965) Coronary endarterectomy with patch graft reconstruction. Clinical experience with 34 cases. *Annals of Surgery*, **162**, 590.

Effler, D. B. (1971) Myocardial revascularisation—direct or indirect? *Journal Thoracic and Cardiovascular Surgery*, **61**, 498.

Espinoza, J., Lipski, J., Litwak, R., Dondso, E. & Dack, S. (1974) New Q waves after coronary artery bypass surgery for angina pectoris. *American Journal of Cardiology*, **33**, 221.

Favaloro, R. G., Effler, D. B., Groves, L. K., Sones, F. M. Jr & Ferguson, D. J. G. (1967) Myocardial revascularisation by internal mammary implant procedures. *Journal of Thoracic and Cardiovascular Surgery*, **54**, 359.

Favaloro, R. G. (1968) Saphenous autograft replacement of severe segmental coronary artery occlusion. *Annals of Thoracic Surgery*, **5**, 334.

Favaloro, R. G., Effler, D. B., Groves, L. K., Sheldon, W. C. & Sones, F. M. (1970) Direct myocardial revascularisation by saphenous vein graft: present operative techniques and indications. *Annals of Thoracic Surgery*, **10**, 97.

Flemma, R. J., Johnson, W. D. & Lepley, D. Jr (1971) Flow rate through coronary grafts. *Archives of Surgery*, **103**, 82.

Greenberg, H., Dwyer, E. M., Jameson, A. G. & Pinkernell, B. H. (1975) Effects of nitroglycerin on the major determinants of myocardial oxygen consumption. An angiographic and haemodynamic assessment. *American Journal of Cardiology*, **36**, 426.

Griffith, L. S. C., Achuff, S. C., Conti, C. R., Humphries, J. O., Brawley, R. K., Gott, V. L. & Ross, R. S. (1973) Changes in intrinsic coronary circulation and segmental ventricular motion after saphenous vein coronary bypass graft surgery. *New England Journal of Medicine*, **288**, 589.

Grondin, C. M., Lepage, G., Castonguay, Y. R., Meerg, C. & Grondin, P. (1971) Aortocoronary bypass graft: initial blood flow through the graft and early postoperative patency. *Circulation*, **44**, 815.

Hamby, R. I., Aintablian, A., Tabrah, I., Hartstein, M. L. & Wisoff, G. (1974) Determinants of reversibility of left ventricular function after aortocoronary bypass surgery. *American Journal of Cardiology*, **33**, 142.

Humphries, J. O., Kuller, L., Ross, R. S., Friesinger, G. C. & Page, E. E., (1974) Natural history of ischaemic heart disease in relation to arteriographic findings. *Circulation*, **49**, 489.

Johnson, W. D., Flemma, R. J., Lepley, D. Jr & Ellison, E. H. (1969) Extended treatment of severe coronary artery disease: a total surgical approach. *Annals of Surgery*, **170**, 460.

Johnson, W. D., Flemma, R. J., Manley, J. C. & Lepley, D. (1970a) The physiological parameters of ventricular function as affected by direct coronary surgery. *Journal of Thoracic and Cardiovascular Surgery*, **60**, 483.

Johnson, W. D., Flemma, R. J. & Lepley, D. Jr (1970b) Direct coronary artery surgery utilising multiple vein bypass grafts. *Annals of Thoracic Surgery*, **9**, 436.

Kennedy, J. W., Hammermeister, K. E., Hamilton, G. W. & Gould, K. L. (1974) Failure of successful myocardial revascularisation to alter left ventricular function. *American Journal of Cardiology*, **33**, 148.

Kouchoukos, N. T., Kirklin, J. W. & Oberman, A. (1974) An appraisal of coronary bypass grafting. *Circulation*, **50**, 11.

Lavine, P., Kimbiris, D., Segal, B. L. & Linhart, J. W. (1972) Left main coronary disease. *American Journal of Cardiology*, **30**, 791.

Levin, D. C. (1974) Pathways and functional significance of the coronary collateral circulation. *Circulation*, **50**, 831.

Lew, E. A. & Seltzer, F. (1970) Uses of the life table in public health. *Millbank Memorial Fund Quarterly*, **48**, 15.

Lim, J. S., Proudfit, W. L. & Sones, F. M. Jr (1975) Left main coronary arterial obstruction: long-term follow-up of 141 non-surgical cases. *American Journal of Cardiology*, **36**, 131.

Malinow, M. R., Kremkan El Kloster, F. E., Bonchek, Y. & Rösch, J. (1973) Occlusion of coronary arteries after vein bypass. *Circulation*, **47**, 1211.

Maurer, B. J., Oberman, A., Holt, J. H. Jr, Kouchoukos, N. T., Jones, W. B., Russell, R. O. Jr & Reeves, T. J. (1974) Changes in grafted and non-grafted coronary arteries following saphenous vein bypass grafting. *Circulation*, **50**, 293.

McLaughlin, P. R., Berman, N. D., Morton, B. C., McLoughlin, M. J., Aldridge, H. E., Adelman, A. G., Goldman, B. S., Trimble, A. S. & March, J. E. (1975) Saphenous vein bypass grafting. Changes in native circulation and collaterals. *Circulation*, **51–52**, Suppl. 1, 66.

Mobert, C. H., Webster, J. S. & Sones, F. M. (1972) Natural history of severe proximal coronary disease as defined by cine angiography. *American Journal of Cardiology*, **29**, 282.

Moran, S. U., Tarazi, R. C., Urzua, J. U., Favaloro, R. G. & Effler, D. B. (1973) Effects of aortocoronary bypass grafting on myocardial contractility. *Journal of Thoracic and Cardiovascular Surgery*, **65**, 335.

Morch, J. E., Morton, B. C., McLaughlin, P. R. et al (1974) Late results of aortocoronary bypass grafts in 100 patients with stable angina pectoris. *Canadian Medical Association Journal*, **111**, 529.

Morris, G. C., Reul, G. J., Howell, J. F., Crawford, E. S., Chapman, D. W., Beasley, H. L., Winters, W. L., Peterson, P. K. & Lewis, J. M. (1972) Follow-up results of distal coronary artery bypass for ischaemic heart disease. *American Journal of Cardiology*, **29**, 180.

Mundth, E. D., Harthorne, J. W., Buckley, M. J., Daggett, W. M. & Austen, G. W. (1971) Direct coronary arterial revascularisation: treatment of cardiac failure associated with coronary artery disease. *Archives of Surgery*, **103**, 529.

Oberman, A., Jones, W. B., Riley, A. P., Reeves, J. T., Sheffield, L. I. & Turner, M. E. (1972) Natural history of coronary artery disease. *Bulletin of the New York Academy of Medicine*, **48**, 1109.

Rose, G. (1973) Smoking and cardiovascular disease. *American Heart Journal*, **85**, 838.

Rose, M. R., Glassman, E., Isom, O. W. & Spencer, F. G. (1974) Electrocardiographic and serum enzyme changes of myocardial infarction after coronary artery bypass surgery. *American Journal of Cardiology*, **33**, 215.

Segal, B. L., Likoff, W., Najmi, M. & Linhart, J. W. (1973) Saphenous vein bypass surgery for coronary artery disease. *American Journal of Cardiology*, **32**, 1010.

Shepherd, R. L., Itscovitz, S. B., Glancy, D. L., Stinson, E. B., Reis, R. L., Olinger, G. N., Clark, C. E. & Epstein, S. E. (1974) Deterioration of myocardial function following aortocoronary bypass operations. *Circulation*, **49**, 467.

Sheldon, W. C., Rincon, G., Effler, D. B., Proudfit, W. L. & Sones, F. M. Jr (1973) Vein graft surgery for coronary artery disease. Survival and angiographic results in 1000 patients. *Circulation*, **47–48**, Suppl. II, 184.

Spencer, F. C., Green, G. E., Tice, D. A. & Glassman, E. (1971) Bypass grafting for occlusive disease of the coronary arteries: a report of experience with 195 patients. *Annals of Surgery*, **173**, 1029.

Talano, J. V., Scanlon, P. J., Meadows, W. R., Musgtaq, K., Pifarre, R. & Gunnar, R. M. (1975) Influence of surgery on survival in 145 patients with left main stem coronary artery disease. *Circulation*, **52**, Suppl. I, 105.

Vedin, J. A., Wilhelmsson, C., Elmfeldt, D., Tibblin, G., Wilhelmsen, L. & Werkö, L. (1973) Sudden death: identification of high risk groups. *American Heart Journal*, **86**, 124.

Vineberg, A. M. (1946) Development of an anastomosis between the coronary vessels and a transplanted internal mammary artery. *Canadian Medical Association Journal*, **55**, 117.

Vlodaver, Z. & Edwards, J. E. (1971) Pathological changes in aortocoronary arterial saphenous vein grafts. *Circulation*, **44**, 719.

Walker, J. A., Friedberg, H. D., Flemma, R. J. & Johnson, W. D. (1972) Determinants of angiographic patency of aortocoronary vein bypass grafts. *Circulation*, **45–46**, Suppl. I, 86.

Walton, K. W. (1975) Pathogenic mechanisms in atherosclerosis. *American Journal of Cardiology*, **35**, 542.

Webster, J. S., Moberg, C. & Rincon, G. (1974) Natural history of severe proximal coronary artery disease as documented by coronary cineangiography. *American Journal of Cardiology*, **33**, 195.

Wilhelmsson, C., Vedin, J. A., Elmfeldt, D., Tibblin, G. & Wilhelmsen, L. (1975) Smoking and myocardial infarction. *Lancet*, **1**, 415.

Yacoub, M. H., Fawzy, E., Anyanwu, H. & Towers, M. (1975) Combined gas endarterectomy and coronary artery bypass graft: a follow-up study. *Circulation*, **51**, Suppl. I, 182.

17
SURGERY FOR STROKE

G. W. Taylor   J. S. P. Lumley

The tragic consequences of a major stroke on the patient and his relatives demand that full consideration be given to methods of preventive or remedial treatment. Over the last two decades angiographic, surgical and autopsy studies have revealed that the majority of cerebrovascular accidents, previously labelled as intracerebral thromboses, were in fact infarctions due to embolism from areas of occlusive arterial disease. These studies have also shown that the main source of the emboli was localised atherosclerosis of the common carotid bifurcation. It is over 20 years since the first successful carotid reconstruction for stroke was reported (Eastcott, Pickering and Rob, 1954) and now the cumulative experience from many centres permits the formulation of indications for this type of surgery in reasonably precise terms.

EXTRACEREBRAL AETIOLOGY OF STROKES

Historical

The relationship between cerebral function and the extracranial vessels is reflected in the Greek derivation of the word 'carotid' which literally means 'to stupefy' or 'to plunge into deep sleep'. The pathological relationship was emphasised by Abercrombie (1828) when he likened cerebral infarction to limb gangrene, when the limb's blood supply was compromised. In 1844 Todd described a stroke in a patient with a dissecting aneurysm of the innominate artery and Virchow (1856) reported similar effects in patients with thrombosis of the carotid bifurcation. Savory (1856) was probably the first to record occlusive disease affecting the aortic arch and in 1875 the clinical features relating to obstructive aortic arch disease were detailed by Broadbent. Gowers (1875) described cerebral symptoms and the eventual death of a patient with left atrial disease and was able to demonstrate, at postmortem, that these symptoms were embolic in origin. Chiari (1905) in a classical but much neglected paper noted that 'endarteritis, chronica deformans' preferentially affected the carotid arteries. He also found that cerebral embolism originated from atheroma in the carotid bifurcation. Hunt (1914) from his clinical studies noted that transient ischaemic attacks often preceded a major stroke, but it was not until Fisher's work (1951, 1954) that the relevance of these findings to possible surgical intervention was considered.

Mechanism

Stroke syndrome can be classified into three categories, transient, developing and completed. In transient strokes the neurological defect is short lived and the patient is normal between attacks, whereas in a completed stroke some permanent neurological deficit remains. In the context of extracranial arterial disease the transient stroke is the chief indication for surgical treatment (vide infra) and the mechanism of the transient ischaemic attack (TIA) deserves further consideration.

It is now generally agreed that there are only two possible factors which could cause a TIA. These are (a) a temporary reduction of blood flow to the relevant cerebral area and (b) obstruction of the cerebral microcirculation by a small embolus which subsequently disperses.

An earlier theory that TIAs could be explained by arterial spasm (Moniz, Lima and DeLacerda, 1937) was rejected by Pickering (1948), since these symptoms are frequently retinal in origin and the retinal arteries are among the least responsive in the body.

Reduction in blood flow. This theory originally held pride of place because of the known high incidence of stroke following carotid ligation. This operation was first performed by Abernethy (1798) in a patient who had been gored by a cow (Hamby, 1952) and was subsequently frequently undertaken for the treatment of intracranial aneurysms. The stroke rate following this procedure was of the order of 30 per cent and in these instances the stroke was, of course, permanent. The relationship of blood flow reduction to the transient attack was ingeniously explained by Denny-Brown (1951) who propounded the theory of 'haemodynamic crisis'. This was based on the assumption that in a patient with an extracranial arterial stenosis sudden lowering of the blood pressure would render the stenosis 'critical' and a significant fall in blood flow through the artery would occur. When the blood pressure returned to normal levels, flow improved and the neurological signs would disappear. In support of this theory Denny-Brown and Meyer (1957) were able to produce a TIA by lowering and subsequently raising the blood pressure in an animal with a localised cerebral artery stenosis.

In clinical practice, however, Alajouanine, Lhermitte and Gautier (1960) were unable to demonstrate changes in systolic blood pressure in patients during ischaemic attacks and Kendell and Marshall (1963) failed to produce neurological symptoms by lowering the blood pressure in patients with a history of TIAs. Brice, Dowsett and Lowe (1964) demonstrated that the lumen of the internal carotid artery could be reduced by as much as 90 per cent without interference of cerebral blood flow, although this was influenced by the rate of onset of the stenosis or the presence of multiple stenoses. Russell and Cranston (1961) reported that TIAs were rare after carotid ligation. The weight of opinion thus moved to favour the microembolisation theory.

Microembolisation. The embolic theory was first suggested by Millikan,

Sieckert and Shick (1955) who postulated that small thrombi or cholesterol aggregations might be liberated from a localised patch of atheroma in the carotid area and cause temporary obstruction of the microcirculation of the retina or brain. Credence was lent to this theory by the observations of Fisher (1959) who by ophthalmoscopic examination noted the presence of retinal emboli in patients undergoing TIAs. Kollarits, Lubow and Hissong (1972) performed carotid angiography in 45 patients with transient attacks of visual disturbance and found a possible embolic source in the carotid vessels in 43 (96 per cent). It is certainly true that in many of the patients with TIAs, the carotid lesion is an ulcerated plaque of atheroma with little significant stenosis (Fig. 17.1).

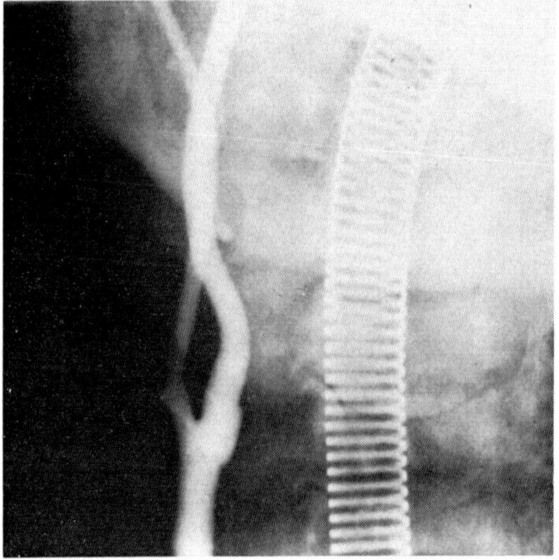

Figure 17.1   Right carotid arteriogram of a 72-year-old male patient presenting with contra-lateral TIAs. Slight irregularity of the origin of the internal carotid artery is present

It seems likely, therefore, that the majority of TIAs are due to embolisation but the haemodynamic aspect should not be totally discounted. Reivich et al (1961), in describing the subclavian steal syndrome, reported cerebral symptoms occurring during upper limb exercise, blood being diverted from the brain to the arm via the vertebral artery. Peroperative measurement of carotid blood pressure distal to a clamp site has shown that strokes are more likely to occur during clamping if the 'stump pressure' is less than 25 mmHg (Moore and Hall, 1969). Jennett, Harper and Gillespie (1966) found that in patients with intracerebral aneurysms, focal symptoms followed carotid ligation if the overall cerebral blood flow was reduced by more than 25 per cent during temporary carotid clamping. It is possible, therefore, that the flow factor may be responsible for TIAs in a small proportion of patients with carotid stenosis. The transient neurological phenomena would then presumably correspond to a period of temporary reduction in cardiac output with consequent significant reduction of flow through the narrowed carotid artery (Figs. 17.2, 17.3).

The collateral circulation becomes important in this context and accessory blood flow may occur between the external carotid and the ophthalmic artery, the meningeal and cerebral arteries, the occipital and vertebral arteries, the cervical and vertebral arteries and the occasionally encountered rete mirabile of the internal carotid artery. A persistent hypoglossal artery may occasionally

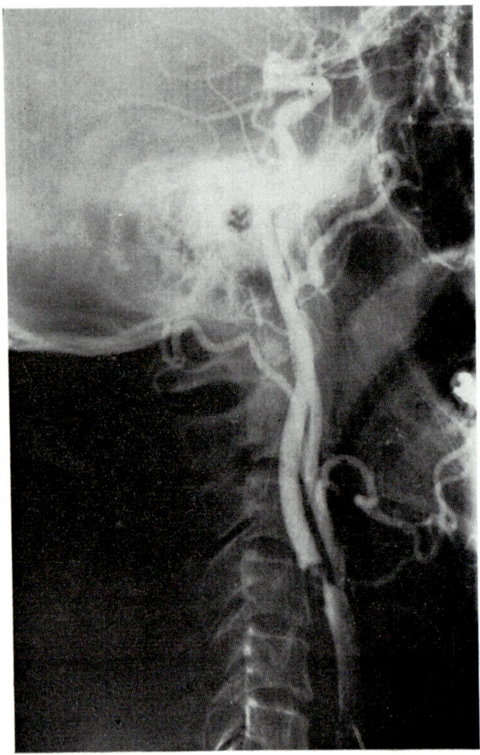

Figure 17.2   Right carotid arteriogram of a 59-year-old male patient presenting with bilateral TIAs. Marked narrowing of the origin of the internal carotid artery is present

occur and cerebral ischaemia secondary to disease of this vessel has been reported by Sutherland and Donaldson (1972). The final pathway of the collateral circulation is, however, the circle of Willis, and anatomical variation of this important anastomotic ring is not uncommon (Alpers, Berry and Paddison, 1959). Surgery may improve collateral flow and Connolly and Stemmer (1973) have reported benefit in patients with irreversibly occluded internal carotid arteries following correction of a concomitant stenosis of the external carotid origin.

Aetiology

In the large majority of patients, the aetiology of the stroke syndrome is atherosclerosis. This was confirmed in an arteriographic series from the Mayo Clinic (Houser and Baker, 1968) in which only 28 patients of 5000 were suffering from non-atheromatous disease. In over half of these patients the disease is situated at the carotid bifurcation. Other sites in decreasing order of frequency are the vertebral arteries, the left subclavian artery, the external carotid arteries, the innominate artery, the right subclavian artery, and the left common carotid artery. Other lesions occasionally responsible for neurological symptoms include: aneurysms of the brachiocephalic system,

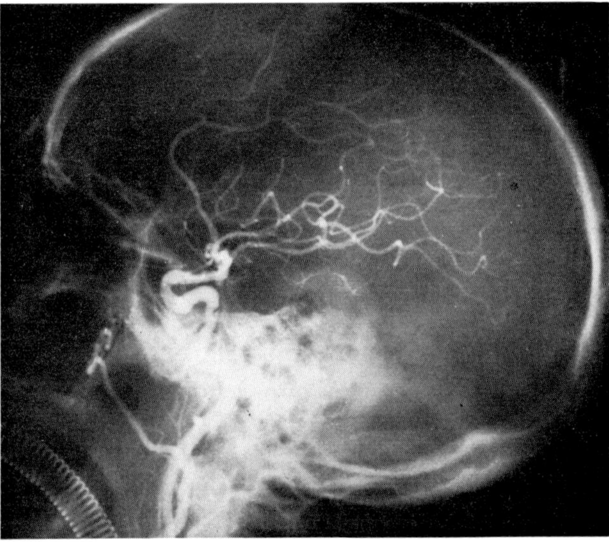

Figure 17.3 Right carotid arteriogram of a 52-year-old male patient presenting with ipsilateral TIAs and dysphasia. Irregularity and narrowing are present in the precavernous and supracavernous portions of the internal carotid artery

these being post-traumatic, mycotic, syphilitic, postradiotherapy and dissecting aneurysms, as well as atherosclerotic. Occasionally congenital or acquired arteriovenous fistulae, congenital malformations, kinks, coils and bands occur in the carotid region and these together with vascular trauma may give rise to neurological problems. A rare group of arterial conditions which have been sporadically recorded as requiring surgical treatment include fibromuscular hyperplasia, medial wall necrosis, diffuse arteritis, giant cell arteritis, scleroderma, drug-induced stenoses and adjacent inflammatory cervical nodes. Tumours in the region of the carotid bifurcation, e.g. carotid body tumours, may give rise to neurological symptoms. All cranial and extracranial vessels may be affected by extravascular factors such as hypercoagulability states and severe hypertension. Conditions giving rise to thrombosis include pregnancy, the pill, idiopathic thrombocytopenia, polycythaemia, sickle-cell anaemia, anoxia, anaemia and congestive cardiac failure. It is probable that focal neurological sequelae following severe hypotension, such as in cardiac arrest, cardiac dysrhythmia and extensive trauma only occur in patients with pre-existing asymptomatic arterial lesions.

NATURAL HISTORY OF THE ATHEROSCLEROTIC LESION

In a study of a community of 2445 people over the age of 40 years, Karp and his colleagues (1973) found 28 patients with TIAs. The incidence of this syndrome in the white population was 15.9/1000 in males and 11.5/1000 in females. A considerably higher incidence of stroke syndrome is found in patients with established arterial disease in other sites and Javid et al (1974) reported an incidence of 15 per cent in patients presenting to their vascular service with non-cerebral peripheral arterial symptoms.

Acheson and Hutchinson (1971) studied the long-term outcome in 500 patients with focal cerebral vascular disease. 349 patients had established neurological defects and 53 per cent of these worsened during the period of observation. 151 of the patients had TIAs and, of these, 62 per cent developed a complete stroke within $4\frac{1}{2}$ years. A similar study was reported by Siekert (1970) who found a 20 to 25 per cent incidence of major stroke in patients with TIAs followed over a four year period. In all reported series carotid disease has a considerably worse prognosis than vertebrobasilar. The results of these studies emphasise the considerable risk of patients with TIAs progressing to a major stroke.

Another group of patients which has received much attention with relation to possible carotid endarterectomy has been the patient with the asymptomatic carotid bruit, this being a not infrequent finding in any vascular clinic. The natural history of this group of patients was studied by Javid et al (1970) and Thompson and Patman (1970). Javid and his colleagues found that in a long-term study of 145 such patients, 11 died of a stroke, 7 died of a cardiac cause and another 7 died of unrelated causes. In 93 patients undergoing a repeat angiogram, significant changes had taken place in 51 patients and 22 of these required carotid endarterectomy. The rate of atheromatous change appeared to be directly related to hypertension, to the development of cerebral symptoms, to change in the intensity of the carotid bruit and to the degree of the original stenosis.

SELECTION OF PATIENTS FOR SURGERY

Of the three categories of stroke (vide supra) it is the TIA patient who benefits from surgical treatment of the extracranial arterial lesion. Patients with a developing stroke should not be treated surgically. Operation at this stage carries a high mortality and morbidity, from cerebral oedema secondary to revascularisation in the presence of a recent infarct. If the developing stroke concludes with a partial neurological deficit, operation can then be considered as a prophylactic measure against further extension of the stroke process. In these patients angiography and surgery should be postponed for three to four weeks to allow the initial infarct to mature. A proportion of these patients will show total occlusion of the relevant internal carotid artery and attempts to reopen the vessel are rarely successful and generally unwise. A not infrequent problem is total occlusion of the appropriate internal carotid with significant stenosis of the opposite vessel. In this group endarterectomy of the opposite 'inappropriate' artery is a useful prophylactic manoeuvre.

Thompson and Patman (1970) also advocated routine angiographic study of patients with a carotid bruit and carotid endarterectomy in asymptomatic patients with a high grade internal carotid artery stenosis. Synchronous carotid endarterectomy in patients with an asymptomatic high grade stenosis undergoing surgical treatment of abdominal aortic aneurysms or coronary artery disease was recommended by Javid et al (1974).

Patients with a dense completed hemiplegia rarely improve after carotid surgery and these patients are best managed conservatively with a programme of rehabilitation.

The value of anticoagulants in TIAs has been extensively studied by Marshall (1969). These should be used in patients with a tight stenosis awaiting surgery or when the patient is unsuitable for surgery, the lesion being inaccessible or the patient's general condition being unsatisfactory.

SYMPTOMS

Carotid disease

TIAs in the carotid distribution are usually focal in nature with para-esthesiae or weakness of one or both contralateral limbs and classically ipsilateral visual disturbance. If the dominant hemisphere is involved dysphasia will accompany the other symptoms. Visual symptoms are present in about 40 per cent of patients and are the sole disturbance in approximately 15 per cent of carotid TIAs. The degree of visual defect may range from mild blurring to significant, but temporary field loss (amaurosis fugax). Headache frequently accompanies a TIA and, after multiple episodes, patients may notice impairment of memory and concentration. TIAs are usually repetitive, but their frequency can range from multiple daily disturbances to isolated episodes many months apart. The duration of the individual attack can vary from a few minutes to several hours and rarely the neurological defect may persist for 24 h. The degree of neurological damage sustained in a completed stroke is related to the rate of onset, the duration and extent of the ischaemia and the area of brain involved. A major stroke may be accompanied by a period of unconsciousness and recovery of function, if it occurs at all, is slow and often unpredictable.

Vertebrobasilar disease

Ischaemic episodes in the vertebrobasilar territory may overlap those of the carotid distribution but they are usually less well defined. Ocular symptoms tend to be more predominant and are often bilateral; they may include optic atrophy and cataract formation. Attacks of giddiness are common and motor symptoms may be bilateral in distribution. Because ocular symptoms are frequent many reports on the condition have come from ophthalmologists. The best known of these was a report from Takayasu (1908) who described absence of upper limb pulses in a young woman with bilateral cataracts. Disease of the origins of the great vessels from the aortic arch is consequently often referred to as Takayasu's disease (Caccamise and Whitman, 1952). Other synonyms for this syndrome are Martorell's disease (Martorell and Fabré, 1944), pulseless disease (Shimizu and Sano, 1951) and perhaps the most satisfactory term—the aortic arch syndrome (Frøvig, 1946). In patients with severe stenosis of the proximal subclavian artery, arm claudication may accompany vertebrobasilar neurological symptoms due to reversal of blood flow in the vertebral artery. This constitutes the subclavian steal syndrome described by Contorni in 1960 and so named by Reivich (1961).

PHYSICAL SIGNS

In between episodes the patient with TIAs will show no neurological abnormality. In carotid disease a bruit over the carotid bifurcation is present in about 66 per cent of patients. David et al (1973) reported the angiographic findings in 417 patients with a carotid bruit. In 28 per cent of these the carotids were normal radiologically. These workers concluded that a bruit had no clear relationship to the patient's symptoms or to the angiographic findings. A possible exception to this conclusion is the presence of a characteristic high-pitched bruit which usually indicates a severe degree of arterial stenosis. Sudden loss of a previously noted high-pitch bruit (after, for instance, arteriography) implies complete occlusion of the artery and may call for urgent exploration of the lesion.

INVESTIGATION

In the preoperative evaluation of the extracranial arterial disease arteriography plays the major role. It carries with it, however, the need for experienced personnel, elaborate instrumentation and a small but definite morbidity and mortality risk to the patient. Consequently although it is an essential preoperative investigation, it must be considered an unsatisfactory screening procedure. In view of this a number of non-invasive investigations have been introduced in an attempt to detect patients with possible internal carotid artery disease and also to some extent provide additional information on cerebral blood flow and the development of collaterals. One of the early investigations was that of ocular dynanometry (Svien and Hollenhorst, 1956). The pressure device applied to the eye ball in this technique however is not without discomfort to the patient and tends to distort the globe and obliterate the curves being evaluated. The technique of oculoplethysmography (Kartchner, McRae and Morrison, 1973) provides a more sensitive measurement of arterial pressure curves. Kartchner and his colleagues suggested that bilateral ocular pulses should be recorded simultaneously, since they considered the relative timing of the two tracings was more important than absolute measurements of amplitude. These authors advised combination of this test with carotid phonangiography, the latter consisting of audiovisual analysis of cervical carotid bruit recordings, the composite diagnostic accuracy of the two tests being 91 and 86 per cent respectively in relation to arteriographic evaluation.

The doppler ophthalmic test (Brockenbrough, 1970) was introduced to assess collateral flow through the external carotid artery in the presence of internal carotid artery disease. On compression of the superficial temporal artery in the normal person an augmentation of the supraorbital flow can be detected by a doppler probe. A range from augmentation to loss of flow can be noted, this being related to the degree of occlusion in the ipsilateral internal carotid artery. The directional doppler also enables reversal of flow in this vessel to be distinguished. The doppler ophthalmic test has been studied extensively by Machleder and Barker (1972; Machleder, 1973). Care must be taken to avoid false positive results from listening over the lateral nasal artery—false positive and false negative results are unfortunately not uncommon. A negative doppler test in the presence of an internal carotid artery stenosis suggests that restoration of blood flow via the homolateral external carotid artery is minimal.

Another disadvantage of these methods is that while providing information on internal carotid artery stenosis and occlusion, they do not detect the equally important sites of ulceration and embolisation. These methods should not, therefore, be the sole form of evaluation in the symptomatic patient. A more sophisticated form of doppler scanning has been introduced by Thomas et al (1974) for mapping of the carotid bifurcation. This demonstrates by non-invasive techniques, changes such as calcification, stenosis, irregularity, kinking and flow patterns within the internal carotid artery.

Non-invasive techniques are useful in complementing angiographic studies and may be particularly valuable in assessing the postoperative patient and following up the natural history of the disease. They add a haemodynamic dimension to the angiographic assessment and they may demonstrate previously unsuspected carotid artery disease.

In the diagnosis of extracranial vascular disease it is essential to obtain biplane angiography of both carotid bifurcations. The most satisfactory pictures are usually obtained by the direct carotid stab technique, the intra-cerebral blood vessels being demonstrated simultaneously and the possibility of overlooking an intracerebral lesion diminished. This technique has the disadvantage of not demonstrating the branches of the aortic arch and the vertebral artery origins and, if symptoms suggestive of disease at these sites are present, additional arch aortography should be undertaken, preferably via the transfemoral route. It is possible that techniques will develop by which adequate carotid bifurcation views and intracerebral vascular delineation can be obtained by selective injection through the transfemoral approach, but at present schools differ in their approach to this problem.

This is generally good correlation in the interpretation of carotid bifurcation disease by the surgeon and the radiologist, particularly in advanced and roughened lesions (Gomensoro et al, 1973). The radiological diagnosis of ulceration should be suspected in the presence of penetrating niches, an irregular silhouette, the delayed wash-out of a medium in a segment of artery between areas of stenosis and well-circumscribed double density of contrast medium superimposed on the artery (Blaisdell, Glickman and Trunkey, 1974).

SURGICAL TREATMENT

Anaesthesia

Anaesthetic techniques in potential stroke patients have varied considerably and there is still no universally accepted method. Initially operations were undertaken under local anaesthesia in order to monitor the patient's neurological function during a trial period of carotid clamping. In the advent of neurological deterioration general anaesthesia was rapidly induced and the patient surface cooled to 32 to 30°C. A paper by Wells, Keats and Cooley in 1963 advocated routine general anaesthesia, hypercarbia and induced hypertension.

In the normal brain the circulation is related to the local metabolic requirements, carbon dioxide playing an important role in the regulatory mechanism (Kety and Schmidt, 1948; Patterson et al, 1955). The autoregulatory capacity of damaged brain was questioned, however, by Brawley, Strandness and Kelly in 1967; these workers considering that hypercarbia could increase the cerebral blood flow to the normal tissue but at the expense of any damaged areas, producing the so-called intracerebral steal. It could thus be postulated that induced hypocarbia would protect damaged tissue by the so-called 'Robin Hood effect' (Lassen and Pálvölgyi, 1968), blood being stolen from normal brain and increasing the blood supply to the damaged areas. Whatever technique is used adequate oxygenation is essential and every effort should be made to maintain a stable circulatory system, for autoregulation of the cerebral blood flow is lost if the systolic blood pressure falls below 60 to 80 mmHg. Controlled ventilation is advised.

Although general anaesthesia is generally used there are still some centres who advocate continued use of regional anaesthesia (Hobson et al, 1974), whereas Connolly (1973) advocated the combination of neurolept analgesia and regional anaesthesia. The latter technique enables continuous direct monitoring of the patient's cerebral state, this being more sensitive than EEG recordings or cerebral blood flow measurements. In all instances continuous blood gas analysis and intra-arterial monitoring of blood pressure are desirable.

Carotid endarterectomy

In the early 1950s, two important papers were published on carotid artery surgery. The first was by Strully, Hurwitt and Blankenberg in 1953. These workers reported an unsuccessful operation on the carotid vessels in a stroke patient. In the following year Eastcott et al reported the first successful reconstructive procedure in this group of patients and, although two successful procedures had gone unreported prior to that date (Carrea, Molins and Murphy, 1955; Thompson, 1973a), this paper has had a lasting influence on the subsequent development of surgery for this condition. The first reported endarterectomy, the present procedure of choice, was described by Cooley, Al-Naaman and Carton in 1956.

Operative procedure

The patient is placed supine with enough head up inclination to empty the cervical venous plexuses. The neck is slightly extended and the head rotated away from the operative side. A head towel is used but the appropriate ear is left exposed to be folded upward under an adhesive drape. With a high carotid bifurcation, or with disease extending well distally in the internal carotid, the incision, parallel to the anterior border of the sternomastoid, is taken superiorly to the mastoid process. A more transverse cervical incision may be used if the arteriogram demonstrates a low carotid bifurcation. Small cutaneous branches of the cervical plexus require division but the greater occipital nerve can usually be mobilised and spared. The common facial vein and occasionally the omohyoid muscle are divided to expose the common carotid artery and its bifurcation. The hypoglossal nerve is encountered superiorly in close relationship to the carotid vessel and may need to be gently mobilised by division of a branch of the occipital artery that tethers it postero-medially. The vagus nerve is frequently applied intimately to the posterior aspect of the internal carotid artery and may be inadvertently included in an arterial occlusive clamp. Temporary recurrent laryngeal nerve palsy may follow such a mishap. Mobilisation of the carotid vessels is best done by sharp dissection and with minimal disturbance in order to avoid embolisation from the area of carotid disease. If obvious thrombus is seen on the preoperative arteriogram the distal internal carotid artery should be clamped before the bifurcation is mobilised.

Diverse views exist as to the necessity of an intraluminal shunt during carotid endarterectomy. There are currently three schools of thought:

14

(a) *Shunting is unnecessary.* The 'no shunt' surgeons believe that per-operative strokes are due solely to embolisation occuring during the arterial mobilisation and that occlusion of the carotid blood flow is relatively un-important (Moore, Yee and Hall, 1973). Moreover the placement of a shunt may initiate embolism and its presence is technically restricting. Kenyon, Thomas and Goodwin (1972) advises large doses of heparin (3 mg/kg) during cross-clamping, no shunt, and neutralisation of the heparin at the completion of the endarterectomy.

(b) *Shunting should be used routinely.* Protagonists of the intraluminal shunt (Javid et al, 1974; Thompson, 1973a) believe that it is important to maintain perfusion through the carotid and that the placement of an intra-luminal shunt allows the surgeon to work in a meticulous and unhurried fashion.

Table 17.1   Operative mortality and severe stroke morbidity in patients undergoing surgery for stroke symptoms. The results of Javid et al (1974) include all forms of reconstructive surgery, the remainder relate to carotid endarterectomy

	% operative mortality	% severe stroke morbidity
Without shunt		
Bloodwell et al (1968)—347 patients, TIAs and completed strokes	5.6	4.8
Bloodwell et al (1968)—191 patients with TIAs	4.3	2.6
Young et al (1969) —137 patients with TIAs and asymptomatic patients	4.4	2.9
De Weese et al (1973)—103 patients with TIAs	1.0	5.0
With shunt		
Thompson (1973b) —537 patients with TIAs	0.7	1.5
Javid et al (1974) —1400 patients, all groups of symptoms	2.0	1.5

(c) *Shunting should be used only in selected cases.* This school advises placement of an intraluminal shunt when intraoperative measurement demonstrates poor collateral flow after carotid cross-clamping. Methods of assessment range from simple visual estimation of the back bleed from the internal carotid (Young et al, 1969) to sophisticated techniques for estimation of cerebral blood flow after carotid clamping (Boysen, 1971; Trojaborg and Boysen, 1973). The most widely used method is measurement of the blood pressure within the internal carotid distal to the point of cross-clamping. Unfortunately there is lack of agreement of the minimum level of 'stump pressure' which will permit an operation to proceed safely without the use of a shunt. Moore and Hall (1969) considered a pressure of 25 mmHg acceptable, Hayes, Levinson and Wylie (1972) 50 mmHg and Hobson et al (1974) a level of 60 mmHg. Wylie (1974) reported on 300 patients in whom shunting was only undertaken when the stump pressure was less than 50 mmHg. With this criteria shunting was required in 20 per cent of the patients and only one mild neurological deficit resulted. Further evidence on stump pressure has come from the neurosurgical field where carotid ligation is sometimes done for intracranial aneurysms. Wright and Sweet (1962) considered 50 mmHg as the minimum safe level while Leech et al (1974) reported that carotid ligation could be undertaken safely with a stump pressure of 60 mmHg or greater. Machleder and Barker (1974) studied stump pressure in a group of patients in which an external carotid to common carotid bypass had been inserted during internal carotid endarterectomy. They noted an average increase in back pressure of 20.9 per cent in this group of patients.

Other workers have measured jugular venous oxygen tension (White,

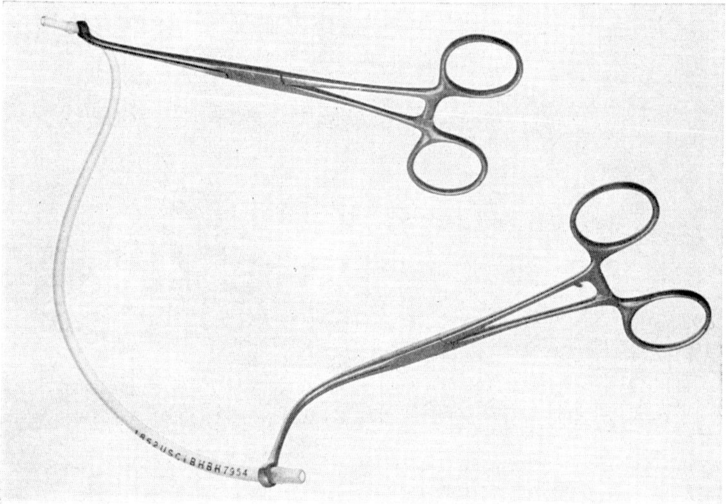

Figure 17.4   Javid shunt and associated ring clamps

Allarde and McDowell, 1967) or monitored the EEG (Perez-Borja and Meyer, 1965).

A comparison of published results from centres never using shunts and those always using them is shown in Table 17.1. It is our own practice to use an intraluminal shunt routinely. The Javid shunt (Figs. 17.4, 17.5) is an excellent device for this purpose. Constructed of flexible silastic it has a tapered bore which allows for the discrepancy in size between the common carotid and internal carotid arteries. Special ring clamps applied around the arteries hold the shunt securely in place. The proximal end is inserted into the common carotid artery first and blood allowed to flush through the shunt before the internal carotid is cannulated. This allows the escape of any fibrinous material which may have formed in the common carotid artery particularly if a carotid stab arteriogram has been recently performed. Once locked in position with the ring clamps the shunt may be safely manipulated to allow adequate access for the endarterectomy, and is removed just before completion of the arteriotomy closure. Systemic heparinisation is advised prior to carotid clamping regardless of whether a shunt is being used. An intravenous dose of 5000 to 10000 units does not usually require neutralisation at the end of the procedure.

The arteriotomy is made on the anterolateral aspect of the common carotid artery, through the bifurcation and should be extended into the internal carotid artery as far as the termination of the disease. Usually the first 1 to 2 cm of the internal carotid is opened but more extensive prolongation is sometimes required (Fig. 17.6). Blind extraction of the distal limits of the

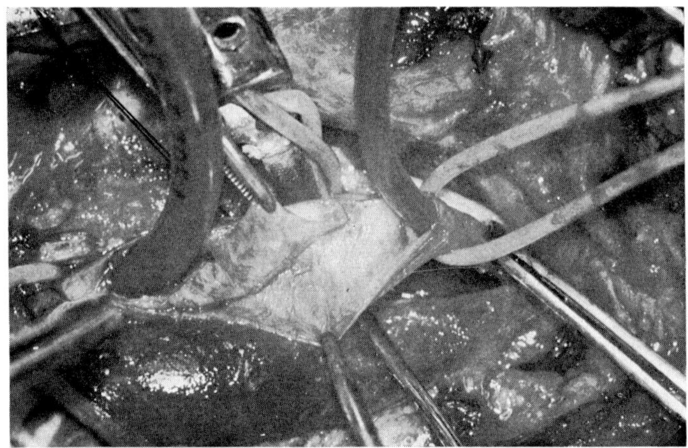

Figure 17.5 Operative photograph of a left carotid endarterectomy. The arteriotomy extends into the common and internal carotid arteries. A Javid shunt is in place, note the smooth adherent line of attachment of the distal intima

plaque should not be performed and the final junction between the endarterectomised segment and normal intima should be fashioned under direct vision. In the majority of cases the disease peters out to give a smooth transition distally and only rarely does the intima require pinning with sutures at this point.

The external carotid artery may also be associated with the stenotic process and it should be carefully endarterectomised routinely during internal carotid endarterectomy. Occasionally, in the presence of an occluded internal carotid artery, local external carotid rebore may benefit collateral circulation (Connolly and Stemmer, 1973). The arteriotomy is closed with direct continuous suture and significant narrowing rarely occurs (Angell-James and Lumley, 1974). Occasionally technical considerations contraindicate direct closure and a vein patch graft may then be used. Before the arteriotomy is finally closed all vessels are back bled and the lumen allowed to fill to exclude air bubbles. The declamping sequence is important and the external carotid and common carotid clamps are removed first. This allows the endarterectomised segment to be well flushed into the external carotid circuit and minimises the risk of minor residual débris taking the internal carotid route.

Peroperative arteriography at the completion of the procedure has been advocated by Smith (1974) and Rosental, Gaspar and Movius (1973). The technique is, however, time consuming and not always practicable. Keitzer, Lichti and DeWeese (1972) prefer monitoring with a doppler scan at the time of operation and we routinely use an electromagnetic flowmeter to confirm that the endarterectomy has achieved satisfactory haemodynamic results (Terry and Taylor, 1974).

Provided a technically satisfactory endarterectomy is done, recurrent stenosis is exceptionally rare (Blaisdell, Lim and Hall, 1967). Javid et al (1974) reported only seven cases of restenosis in their extensive experience and these

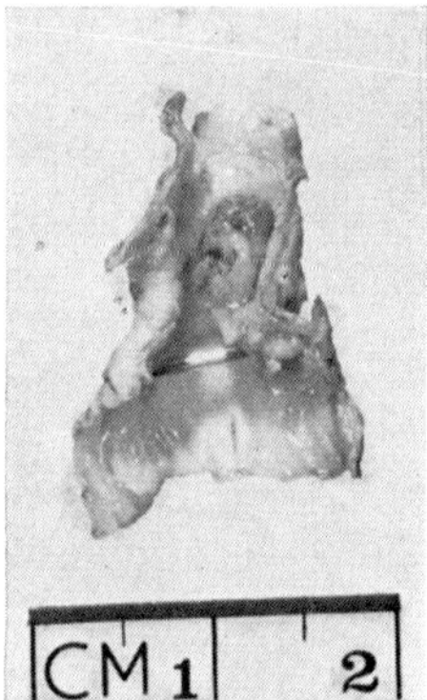

Figure 17.6 Carotid endarterectomy specimen, note the pedunculated partly adherent organised thrombus within the lumen

were thought to be due to incomplete removal of the distal segment of atheromatous plaque at the first operation. We have only encountered one case of restenosis and that was of non-atheromatous origin and occurred in a female of 31 years with a mucinoid degeneration of the artery.

The patient should be carefully monitored in the immediate postoperative period, with particular regard to the blood pressure which may be abnormally labile for the first 24 h. This is probably due to interference with sinus nerve activity either directly or by the removal of the 'stent'-like atheromatous core across the carotid bifurcation (Wade et al, 1970; Angell-James and Lumley, 1974). Reflex induced hypotension is most easily controlled by transfusion of whole blood and bradycardia by the administration of atropine. Postoperative hypertension is usually best treated conservatively or by sedation.

In patients with bilateral stenosis the symptomatic side is operated upon first. Synchronous carotid endarterectomy should not be performed and an interval of two weeks between sides is advisable.

Aneurysms of the extracranial carotid artery

Aneurysms of the extracranial carotid system are rare and Beall et al (1962) found only seven such cases in 2300 operations performed for aneurysm in their institution. Atherosclerosis and trauma are the most frequent causative factors, but occasional cases of mycotic aneurysm (Ledgerwood and Lucas, 1974), cystic medial necrosis (Barnes and Jacoby, 1962) and Marfan's syndrome (Hardin, 1962) have been reported. The common carotid artery (Fig. 17.7) is involved twice as frequently as the internal or external carotid artery (Coleman and Kittle, 1973). The usual presentation is of a symptomless

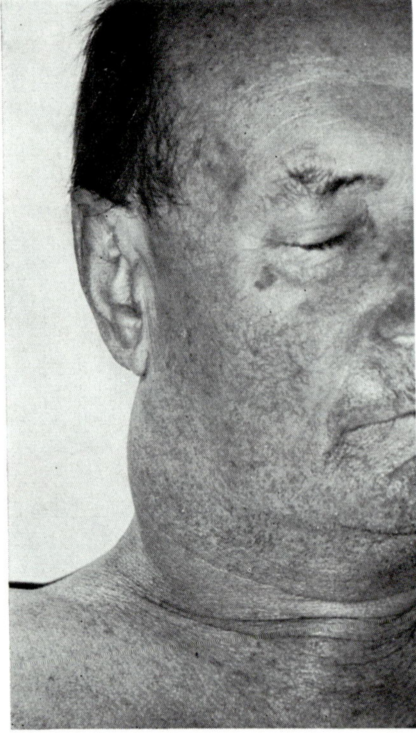

Figure 17.7 Aneurysm of the right common carotid artery. Patient presented with respiratory obstruction

pulsatile cervical mass. In this context mention should be made of the 'spurious aneurysm' which presents as a pulsating swelling above the right sterno-clavicular joint in elderly hypertensive women. This common entity is not a true aneurysm and is due to elongation and tortuosity of the innominate artery. It requires no treatment apart from control of the hypertension. True aneurysms may cause symptoms by rapid expansion or rupture. Rittenhouse, Radke and Sumner (1972) described a patient in whom a carotid aneurysm caused airway obstruction and eventual rupture into the oropharynx and we have had to undertake an emergency operation for a similar situation. Neurological symptoms may be the presenting feature secondary to cerebral embolisation by thrombus originating in the aneurysm sac (Weissman and Rankow, 1968; Boddie, 1972). Traumatic false aneurysm of the carotid system may follow either open or closed injury (Deysine, Adiga and Wilder, 1969). They enlarge slowly and the first indication of their presence may be TIAs. We have recently treated a young man who presented with a partial right-sided stroke and who had suffered a severe closed contusion of the left side of the neck in a road accident four years previously. Angiography revealed a small aneurysm of the distal left internal carotid (Fig. 17.8). Carotid aneurysm,

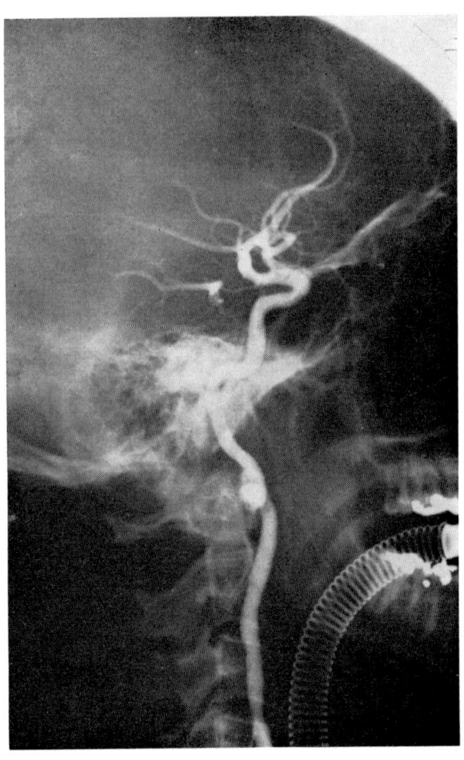

Figure 17.8 Left carotid arteriogram of a 30-year-old male patient showing an aneurysm of the internal carotid artery at the level of the atlas. The patient presented with a right sided hemiparesis and dysphasia. Four years previously he had been involved in a road traffic accident in which the left side of his neck had hit the steering wheel

untreated, carries a bad prognosis and Winslow (1926) reported that 71 per cent of 106 patients with untreated internal carotid aneurysm died of complications of the aneurysm.

Whenever possible resection of the aneurysm with restoration of continuity should be carried out (Rittenhouse et al, 1972). With common carotid aneurysms resection with end-to-end anastomosis is sometimes practicable (Kianouri, 1967; Raphael et al, 1963), but usually an interposition graft will be required. Synthetic grafts may be used but autogenous vein is probably the best material for this purpose. The commonest complication of such surgery is a cerebrovascular accident (Rittenhouse et al, 1972) and in order to minimise this risk the use of an intraluminal shunt is advised (Coleman and Kittle, 1973).

Acute carotid injuries

Involvement of the carotid arteries in trauma to the cervical region presents certain difficulties in management and the problems have been well presented in a recent report by Thal et al (1974). They discussed a series of 60 patients with carotid damage, the majority following penetrating injury, from gunshot or stab wounds: 65 per cent of these injuries occurred on the left side and 80 per cent involved the common carotid artery. Arterial laceration was the commonest injury with complete vessel transection in 18 per cent, and the presence of an enlarging haematoma was the usual indication for operation. Nineteen (32 per cent) of their 60 patients had developed a neurological deficit prior to operative treatment and this was severe in 13 (22 per cent) patients. Restoration of arterial continuity was accomplished in the majority of patients with an overall mortality of 8.3 per cent. The mortality was highest in patients with a severe preoperative neurological deficit and it is likely that revascularisation of a fresh cerebral infarct was the responsible factor. These authors suggest that in patients with carotid injury and a severe neurological deficit angiographic assessment of carotid flow should be carried out. If flow is uninterrupted it is probably safe to repair the vessel. If, however, the distal segment is not patent, repair with restoration of flow carries too great a risk of cerebral oedema and arterial ligation should be undertaken.

Other operative procedures occasionally indicated on the carotid artery are the release of bands, the resection of the diseased areas with end-to-end anastomosis, or segmental replacement, and reimplanting or refashioning of the carotid bifurcation. More extensive exposure may be obtained by detaching the sternomastoid from the base of the skull by resecting the lower portion of the parotid gland, by dividing the stylohyoid or posterior belly of the digastric muscles and by dividing the angle of the mandible. Should neurological symptoms occur in a patient with fibromuscular hyperplasia the most satisfactory form of operative treatment is carefully graded intraluminal dilation (Morris, Lechter and DeBakey, 1968).

Extra-intracerebral revascularisation

Occlusion of the internal carotid artery has until recently been considered a contraindication to surgery. Long standing occlusions are irremoval by surgical means and attempted thrombectomy of disease of recent origin carries the risk of embolising the distal carotid tree. Yet this group of patients has a 45 per cent major stroke rate within three years (Ziegler and Hassanein, 1973). In 1968 Donaghy and Yasargil gave a preliminary report of a new technique of revascularisation of the intracerebral vessels by means of the superficial temporal artery in patients with proximal occlusion of the internal carotid or middle cerebral vessels. In one of the first follow-up reports on 35 patients Austin, Laffin and Hayward (1974) found no late postoperative stroke development and such procedures may be of great value to this small but high risk group of patients.

Vertebral arteries and aortic arch

Innominate endarterectomy was first undertaken by Davis, Grove and Julian in 1956 and vertebral reconstruction by Crawford, DeBakey and Fields (1958). Initially stenoses of the great vessels at the aortic arch were treated by bypass grafting (DeBakey et al, 1958; Crawford et al, 1962). A supraclavicular approach, however, had been suggested by Lyons and Galbraith (1957) who introduced caroticosubclavian bypass procedures. In 1969 Crawford et al compared the mortality of intra- and extrathoracic corrective procedures for stenotic lesions of the aortic arch vessels and showed that the mortality of the extrathoracic procedure was only 5.2 per cent, in contrast to the mortality of 22.2 per cent in the direct approach. Harper et al (1967) advised side-to-side anastomosis of the carotid and subclavian vessels. Theories that proximal bypass procedures may steal blood from the distribution of the feeding vessel were shown to be unfounded by Lord and Ehrenfeld (1969). These authors were able to show that flow was proportionally increased in the supplying vessel to a bypass and their work has subsequently been confirmed by Barner, Kaiser and Willman (1971).

Intrathoracic procedures are now usually limited to stenosis or occlusion of more than one of the main branches of the aortic arch. In these cases the graft can usually be taken off the aortic arch with a side biting clamp for a bypass procedure, this being preferred to local endarterectomy when proximal control is usually necessary.

Moore, Blaisdell and Hall (1967) were able to disobliterate 7 of 10 common carotid artery occlusions retrogradely from arteriotomies made in the neck, while Javid et al (1974) were successful in restoring flow in all of seven similar patients. In aortic arch stenotic disease an alternative approach is to fashion uni- or bilateral axillofemoral bypass (Sproul, 1971).

Most extrathoracic corrective procedures for aortic arch stenosis involve the insertion of short dacron or longer vein bypasses. These procedures usually require exposure of one or both subclavian arteries in the root of the neck. This is obtained through a transverse incision above the medial half of the clavicle dividing platysma, the lateral head of the sternomastoid muscle and the omohyoid muscle with its adjacent pad of fat. The phrenic nerve is retracted prior to division of the scalenus anterior muscle close to its attachment on the first rib. More extensive exposure can be obtained by totally dividing the lower end of the sternomastoid and resecting the proximal portion of the clavicle. Special care must be given during the exposure of the subclavian artery, to the brachial plexus, adjacent veins and the pleura.

Heparinisation is again desirable before cross-clamping and shunting may be indicated. Occasionally the contralateral subclavian artery has to be used as the blood source for a diseased subclavian; a subclavian-to-subclavian bypass being undertaken (Finkelstein, Byer and Rush, 1972; Forestner et al, 1972). Alternatively a subcutaneous axillary–axillary bypass can be inserted (Mozersky et al, 1973). Bypass procedures may be combined with endarterectomy of one or both carotid bifurcations. Operators unfamiliar with this field should take particular care of the subclavian artery which is a very thin and an easily damaged vessel. Caroticoaxillary rather than caroticosubclavian bypass may be preferred for this reason.

Direct surgery on the vertebral artery is rarely indicated. Its contribution to total cerebral blood flow may be only one-tenth of that of the carotid system and thus an isolated stenosis is unlikely to produce cerebral symptoms by a marked reduction in cerebral blood flow. When a stenosis is accompanied by a carotid lesion, relief of the carotid lesion is usually satisfactory in alleviating the patient's symptoms (Blaisdell et al, 1969). If the symptoms are due to embolism from a vertebral stenosis then the artery may be ligated, provided alternative channels are undiseased. Endarterectomy of the vertebral artery is usually limited to the proximal 2 cm, and the origin may be endarterectomised through a subclavian arteriotomy or alternatively a venous patch may be placed across it.

RESULTS

The results of surgery for strokes have markedly improved since the introduction of these procedures in the early 1950s. Safe anaesthetic and operative techniques have been established, although as already intimated these vary in different centres. Above all, clear indications now exist as to which group of patients should be selected for surgery and the relative value of surgery over conservative treatment has been assessed in a randomised series by the joint study of extracranial arterial occlusion (Fields et al, 1970). The overall mortality in patients with TIAs in the latter series was 3.5 per cent with a 7.7 per cent postoperative stroke rate. In this combined series, however, there was marked variation between institutions and the writers concluded that the operative mortality in specialised centres should be around, or less than, 1 per cent and the morbidity less than 4 per cent in this group of patients. De Weese et al (1973) reported the five years results of 103 patients operated on for TIAs. At 30 days postoperatively 79 per cent of these patients were asymptomatic, 15 per cent had experienced an initial TIA and there were six patients with persistent neurological defects, two of them severe whereas one patient had died. Studying the same group at five years postoperatively, 34 patients had died, a quarter due to myocardial infarction. The mortality was much higher in the over 60 age group of patients and in hypertensive and diabetic patients. Six of the eight patients with combined atherosclerotic heart disease and diabetes had died in the series. Five of the patients had died of strokes, one being a patient with an infected false aneurysm at the operation site which required proximal ligation. Two of the initial six patients with persistent postoperative neurological defects had died and one of the patients had died of stroke symptoms referable to the non-operated side. Of the 68 survivors, four patients had mild strokes, two moderate and one severe, and in the five-year follow-up period, 17 patients had undergone contralateral carotid endarterectomy, 12 for TIAs and five for asymptomatic cervical bruits.

Thompson (1973b) reported on the surgical results of 537 patients with TIAs. The operative mortality was 0.7 per cent with a 1.5 per cent incidence of permanent postoperative neurological defects. There was a 5 per cent overall long-term incidence of strokes, these including fatal and non-fatal episodes. This author considered that these figures showed a seven-fold reduction of severe strokes when compared with the expected natural history of the disease. Thompson (1973b) emphasised that although the long-term mortality rates in operative and non-operative stroke patients had not been extensively studied, except by the joint study (Fields et al, 1970), the reduced postoperative rate in the operative group markedly affected the quality of life which the patients subsequently led.

De Weese et al (1973) in their series of patients with TIAs further studied improvement of their patients in relation to the initial symptomatology. Of the 88 patients who they considered presented with classical TIAs, 76 were subsequently free of these symptoms, whereas only two of the 15 patients with atypical symptoms such as dizziness, syncopy, headache, seizures and con-fusion were relieved of their symptoms by the operative procedure. Fields et al (1970) also commented on the failure of surgery to relieve non-classical symptoms. From these figures, therefore, one would conclude that surgery is the treatment of choice for patients with classical TIAs.

The work of Thompson and Patman (1970) and Javid et al (1970) on the natural history of patients with asymptomatic bruits has already been referred to. Thompson (1973a) compared conservative and surgical treatment of two groups of patients with asymptomatic bruits (the patients had not been randomly allocated). Of the 92 patients in the non-operative group over a 10 year period, 26 per cent developed TIAs and 19 per cent went on to persistent strokes. That is, 45 per cent suffered subsequent neurological symptoms. Of the operative group of 66 patients undergoing 98 elective operations for asymptomatic bruits, there was no operative mortality, there were two operative strokes, one being severe, and in the late follow-up of these patients there were two late strokes, one being severe. There was no neurological mortality in the group. From these figures Thompson advised surgical treatment of asymptomatic carotid disease where there was bilateral or progressive disease, in unilateral severe stenosis, when the disease was related to the dominant hemisphere and when the patient was young. Possible contraindications are extensive cardiac or peripheral vascular disease, multiple lesions and increasing age. Follow-up on asymptomatic patients by Javid et al (1971) showed no operative mortality, but a 3.6 per cent morbidity. Ninety per cent of these patients, however, remained asymptomatic over a six to eight year follow-up.

The necessity to perform carotid endarterectomy prior to major surgery in a patient with asymptomatic disease is less well supported, although undertaken by a number of vascular units. Treiman et al (1973) had no postoperative deaths from strokes in a group of 240 patients with asymptomatic cervical bruits undergoing surgery for abdominal aortic aneurysms. Bernhard, Johnson and Peterson (1972) reported 16 patients who underwent combined endarterectomy and coronary artery bypass procedures, with no ensuing mortality and minimal morbidity.

Surgery in the acute developing phase of a stroke is now generally not undertaken or recommended. Blaisdell et al (1969) reported a 42 per cent mortality in a group of patients operated on within two weeks of an acute episode. Possible exceptions to this rule are a sudden occlusion occurring after angiography or when a large amount of free thrombus is radiologically demonstrated at the carotid bifurcation. Immediate postoperative occlusion of an endarterectomised vessel accompanied by progression of neurological symptoms has also been advocated as an indication for further surgery by some authors (Dye and Brown, 1973). The chances of restoring patency of an occluded internal carotid vessel are increased with early operation, but so are the risks of haemorrhage into a recent infarct (Bruetman et al, 1963). Thompson, Austin and Patman (1967) were able to restore flow in an occluded vessel in 40 per cent of patients but the subsequent mortality in this situation was 6.2 per cent.

Surgery offers little in the way of recovery to the patient with an established stroke, although some degree of mental improvement has been reported by most authors and quantitated by others (Perry, Drinkwater and Taylor, 1975). When reviewing surgery in patients with completed strokes Dye and Brown (1973) reported that 35 per cent of patients improved, 20 to 30 per cent of patients were unchanged, 10 to 20 per cent were worse and the operative mortality was 15 to 30 per cent. An operative mortality rate of 45 per cent was recorded in the joint study (Blaisdell et al, 1969) in patients with an occluded carotid artery and associated residual neurological damage, when subsequent surgery was undertaken for TIAs related to the patent carotid vessel. Patterson (1974), however, found that in 23 similar patients there was no operative mortality and 17 of these patients were alive and 15 had no further symptoms 30 months later. Three patients had died and three had been lost to follow-up. Wylie and Ehrenfeld (1970) reported 70 per cent relief of symptoms in patients with unilateral occlusion and TIAs related to the contralateral carotid stenosis. The variation in these results perhaps highlights the difference between the various schools.

Experience in non-atheromatous carotid artery disease is limited and critical assessment of the results is consequently difficult. The recommendations of Rundles and Kimbell (1969) in relation to kinks, however, is that these should only be operated on if the arterial lumen is reduced by more than 40 per cent and in the absence of other possible causative lesions.

The reduced mortality of surgery for aortic arch conditions following the emphasis on an extrathoracic approach has already been mentioned. Long-term results in the subclavian steal syndrome are generally excellent. Wylie and Ehrenfeld (1970) reported that vertebral artery surgery provided 70 per cent relief of symptoms and an improvement in a further 21 per cent of these patients on five year follow-up. Javid et al (1974) reported the results obtained in 47 patients undergoing carotid subclavian bypass procedures, 12 of the patients had simultaneous carotid endarterectomies. There was no hospital mortality in the group but later thrombosis was observed in four grafts, there were two wound infections and two false aneurysms. One of the patients developed a stroke from an associated carotid endarterectomy. The result of vertebral artery surgery from the same authors showed restoration of flow in 19 of 20 patients. There was temporary aggravation of symptoms in two patients, but no mortality and no severe neurological sequelae.

CONCLUSION

Experience accumulated on surgical treatment in patients with stroke syndromes since the initiation of these procedures in the early 1950s is such that distinct guidelines can now be laid down on the advisability of surgical treatment. Surgery should be the treatment of choice in patients with TIAs and a proven extracranial stenotic lesion, and in this group of patients the operative mortality should be in the order of 1 per cent and severe neurological sequelae less than 4 per cent. Surgery should generally be avoided in the developing stroke, whereas in the patient with a completed stroke it must be realised that improvement of established neurological damage is unlikely. The treatment of TIAs contralateral to established neurological damage will depend largely on the experience and preferences of individual units. The treatment of asymptomatic stenoses remains controversial. They represent a potential stroke hazard but to justify surgical correction operative mortality should be below 1 per cent and complications no more than 2 per cent.

REFERENCES

Abercrombie, J. (1828) *Pathological and Practical Researches on Diseases of Brain and Spinal Cord.* Edinburgh: Waugh and Innes.
Acheson, J. & Hutchinson, E. C. (1971) The natural history of focal cerebral vascular disease. *Quart. J. Med.*, **40**, 15–23.
Alajouanine, T., Lhermitte, F. & Gautier, J. C. (1960) Transient cerebral ischaemia attacks in atherosclerosis. *Neurology*, **10**, 906–914.

Alpers, B. J., Berry, R. G. & Paddison, R. M. (1959) Anatomical studies of the circle of Willis in normal brain. *Arch. Neurol. Psychiat.*, **81**, 409–418.

Angell-James, J. E. & Lumley, J. S. P. (1974) The effects of carotid endarterectomy on the mechanical properties of the carotid sinus and carotid sinus nerve activity in atherosclerotic patients. *Brit. J. Surg.*, **61**, 805–810.

Austin, G., Laffin, D. & Hayward, W. (1974) Physiologic factors in the selection of patients for superficial temporal artery-to-middle cerebral artery anastomosis. *Surgery*, **75**, 861–868.

Barner, H. B., Kaiser, G. C. & Willman, V. L. (1971) Haemodynamics of carotid-subclavian bypass. *Arch. Surg.*, **103**, 248–251.

Barnes, W. T. & Jacoby, G. E. (1962) Aneurysm of the common carotid artery due to cystic medial necrosis treated by excision and graft. *Ann. Surg.*, **155**, 82–85.

Beall, A. C., Crawford, E. S., Cooley, D. A. & DeBakey, M. E. (1962) Extracranial aneurysms of the carotid artery: report of seven cases. *Postgrad. Med.*, **32**, 93–102.

Bernhard, V. M., Johnson, W. D. & Peterson, J. J. (1972) Carotid artery stenosis. Association with surgery for coronary artery disease. *Arch. Surg.*, **105**, 837–840.

Blaisdell, W. F., Clauss, R. H., Galbraith, J. G., Imparato, A. M. & Wylie, E. J. (1969) Joint study of extracranial arterial occlusion. IV. A review of surgical considerations. *J. Amer. med. Ass.*, **209**, 1889–1895.

Blaisdell, W. F., Glickman, M. & Trunkey, D. D. (1974) Ulcerated atheroma of the carotid artery. *Arch. Surg.*, **108**, 491–496.

Blaisdell, W. F., Lim, R. & Hall, A. D. (1967) Technical results of carotid endarterectomy: Arteriographic assessment. *Amer. J. Surg.*, **114**, 239–246.

Bloodwell, R. D., Hallman, G. L., Keats, A. S. & Colley, D. A. (1968) Carotid endarterectomy without a shunt. *Arch. Surg.*, **96**, 644–652.

Boddie, H. G. (1972) Transient ischaemic attacks and stroke due to extracranial aneurysm of internal carotid artery. *Brit. med. J.*, **3**, 802–803.

Boysen, G. (1971) Cerebral blood flow measurement as a safeguard during caotid endarterectomy. *Stroke*, **2**, 1–10.

Brawley, B. W., Strandness, D. E. & Kelly, W. A. (1967) The physiologic response to therapy in experimental cerebral iscaemia. *Arch. Neurol.*, **17**, 180–187.

Brice, J. G., Dowsett, D. J. & Lowe, R. D. (1964) Haemodynamic effects of carotid artery stenosis. *Brit. med. J.*, **2**, 1363–1366.

Broadbent, W. H. (1875) Absence of pulsation in both radial arteries: the vessels being full of blood. *Clin. Soc. Trans.*, **8**, 165–168.

Brockenbrough, E. C. (1970) Quoted by Keitzer et al, 1972.

Bruetman, M. E., Fields, W. S., Crawford, E. S. & DeBakey, M. E. (1963) Cerebral haemorrhage in carotid artery surgery. *Arch. Neurol.*, **9**, 458–467.

Caccamise, W. C. & Whitman, J. F. (1952) Pulseless disease: preliminary case report. *Amer. Heart J.*, **44**, 629–633.

Carrea, R., Molins, M. & Murphy, G. (1955) Surgical treatment of spontaneous thrombosis of the internal carotid artery in the neck. Carotid–carotideal anastomosis: report of a case. *Acta. Neurol. Latinoamer.*, **1**, 71–78.

Chiari, H. (1905) Ueber das Verhalten des Teilungswinkels der carotis communis bei der Endarteritis chronica deformans. *Verh. Dtsch. path. Ges.*, **9**, 326–330.

Chung, W. B. (1974) Long-term results of carotid artery surgery for cerebrovascular insufficiency. *Amer. J. Surg.*, **128**, 262–268.

Coleman, P. G. & Kittle, C. F. (1973) Aneurysms of the common carotid artery. *Surg. Clin. North. Amer.*, **53**, 231–240.

Connolly, J. E. & Stemmer, E. A. (1973) Endarterectomy of the external carotid artery. Its importance in the surgical management of extracranial cerebrovascular occlusive disease. *Arch. Surg.*, **106**, 799–802.

Connolly, J. E. (1973) Discussion in Moore et al, 1973.

Contorni, L. (1960) Il circolo collaterale vertebro-vertebrale nella obliterazione dell'arteria subclavia alla sua origine. *Minerva Chir.*, **15**, 268–271.

Cooley, D. A., Al-Naaman, Y. D. & Carton, C. A. (1956) Surgical treatment of arteriosclerotic occlusion of common carotid artery. *J. Neurosurg.*, **13**, 500–506.

Crawford, E. S., DeBakey, M. E. & Fields, W. S. (1958) Roentgenographic diagnosis and surgical treatment of basilar artery insufficiency. *J. Amer. med. Ass.*, **168**, 509–516.

Crawford, E. S., DeBakey, M. E., Morris, G. C. & Cooley, D. A. (1962) Thrombo-obliterative disease of the great vessels arising from the aortic arch. *J. thorac. cardiovasc. Surg.*, **43**, 38–53.

Crawford, E. S., DeBakey, M. E., Morris, G. C. & Howell, J. (1969) Surgical treatment of occlusion of the innominate, common carotid, and subclavian arteries; a ten year experience. *Surgery*, **65**, 17–31.

David, T. E., Humphries, A. W., Young, J. R. & Beven, E. G. (1973) A correlation of neck bruits and arteriosclerotic carotid arteries. *Arch. Surg.*, **107**, 729–731.

Davis, J. B., Grove, W. J. & Julian, O. C. (1956) Thrombic occlusion of branches of aortic arch. Martorell's syndrome: report of case treated surgically. *Ann. Surg.*, **144**, 124–126.

DeBakey, M. E., Morris, G. C., Jordan, G. L. & Cooley, D. A. (1958) Segmental thrombo-obliterative disease of branches of the aortic arch. *J. Amer. med. Ass.*, **166**, 998–1003.

Denny-Brown, D. (1951) Treatment of recurrent cerebrovascular symptoms and the question of 'vasospasm'. *Med. Clin. North Amer.*, **35**, 1457–1474.

Denny-Brown, D. & Meyer, J. S. (1957) The cerebral collateral circulation. 2. Production of cerebral infarction by ischemic anoxia and its reversibility in early stages. *Neurology*, **7**, 567–579.

De Weese, J. A., Rob, C. G., Satran, R., Marsh, D. O., Joynt, R. J., Summers, D. & Nichols, C. (1973) Results of carotid endarterectomies for transient ischaemic attack—five years later. *Ann. Surg.*, **178**, 258–264.

Deysine, M., Adiga, R. & Wilder, J. R. (1969) Traumatic false aneurysm of the cervical internal carotid artery. *Surgery*, **66**, 1004–1007.

Donaghy, P. & Yasargil, G. (1968) Extracranial blood flow diversion (abstr.) Amer. Assoc. Neurol. Surg., Chicago. Quoted Austin et al, 1974.

Dye, W. S. & Brown, C. M. (1973) Surgical correction of carotid and vertebral artery stenosis. *Surg. Clin. North Amer.*, **53**, 241–251.

Eastcott, H. H. G., Pickering, G. W. & Rob, C. G. (1954) Reconstruction of internal carotid artery in a patient with intermittent attacks of hemiplegia. *Lancet*, **2**, 994–996.

Fields, W. S., Maslenikov, V., Meyer, J. S., Hass, W. K. & Remington, R. D. (1970) Joint study of extracranial arterial occlusion. V. Progress report on prognosis following surgery or nonsurgical treatment for transient cerebral ischaemic attacks and cervical carotid artery lesions. *J. Amer. med. Ass.*, **211**, 1993–2003.

Finkelstein, N. M., Byer, A. & Rush, B. R. (1972) Subclavian–subclavian bypass for subclavian steal syndrome. *Surgery*, **71**, 142–145.

Fisher, C. M. (1951) Occlusion of the internal carotid artery. *Arch. Neurol. Psychiat. (Chicago)*, **65**, 346–377.

Fisher, C. M. (1954) Occlusion of the carotid arteries: further experience. *Amer. med. Ass. Arch. Neurol. Psychiat.*, **72**, 187–204.

Fisher, C. M. (1959) Observations of the fundus oculi in transient monocular blindness. *Neurology*, **9**, 333–347.

Forestner, J. E., Ghosh, S. K., Bergan, J. J. & Conn, J. (1972). Subclavian–subclavian bypass for correction of the subclavian steal syndrome. *Surgery*, **71**, 136–141.

Frøvig, A. G. (1946) Bilateral obliteration of the common carotid artery. *Acta Psychiat. Neurol.*, Suppl. 39.

Gomensoro, J. B., Maslenikov, V., Azambuja, N., Fields, W. S. & Lemak, N. A. (1973) Joint study of extracranial arterial occlusion. VIII. Clinical–radiographic correlation of carotid bifurcation lesions in 177 patients with transient cerebral ischemic attacks. *J. Amer. med. Ass.*, **224**, 985–991.

Gowers, W. R. (1875) On a case of simultaneous embolism of central retinal and middle cerebral arteries. *Lancet*, **2**, 794–796.

Hamby, W. B. (1952) *Intracranial Aneurysms*. Springfield, Illinois: Thomas.

Hardin, C. A. (1962) Successful resection of carotid and abdominal aneurysm in two related patients with Marfan's syndrome. *New Engl. J. Med.*, **267**, 141–142.

Harper, J. A., Golding, A. L., Mazzei, E. A. & Cannon, J. A. (1967) An experimental haemodynamic study of the subclavian steal syndrome. *Surg. Gynec. Obst.*, **124**, 1212–1218.

Hays, R. J., Levinson, S. A. & Wylie, E. G. (1972) Intraoperative measurement of carotid back pressure as a guide to operative management for carotid endarterectomy. *Surgery*, **72**, 953–960.

Hobson, R. W., Wright, C. B., Sublett, J. W., Fedde, C. W. & Rich, N. M. (1974) Carotid artery back pressure and endarterectomy under regional anaesthesia. *Arch. Surg.*, **109**, 682–687.

Houser, O. W. & Baker, H. L. (1968) Fibromuscular dysplasia and other uncommon diseases of the cervical cartoid artery: angiographic aspects. *Amer. J. Roentgenol.*, **104**, 201–212.

Hunt, J. R. (1914) The role of the carotid arteries in the causation of vascular lesions of the brain, with remarks on certain special features of the symptomatology. *Amer. J. med. Sci.*, **147**, 704–713.

Javid, H., Dye, W. S., Hunter, J. A., Najafi, H., Goldin, M. D. & Serry, C. (1974) Surgical treatment of cerebral ischaemia. *Surg. Clin. North Amer.*, **54**, 239–255.

Javid, H., Ostermiller, W. E., Hengesh, J. W., Dye, W. S., Hunter, J. A., Najafi, H. & Julian, O. C. (1970) Natural history of carotid bifurcation atheroma. *Surgery*, **67**, 80–86.

Javid, H., Ostermiller, W. E., Hengesh, J. W., Dye, W. S., Hunter, J. A., Najafi, H. & Julian, O. C. (1971) Carotid endarterectomy for asymptomatic patients. *Arch. Surg.*, **102**, 389–391.

Jennett, W. B., Harper, A. M. & Gillespie, F. C. (1966) Measurement of regional cerebral blood flow during carotid ligation. *Lancet*, **2**, 1162–1163.

Karp, H. R., Heyman, A., Heyden, S., Bartel, A. G., Tyroler, H. A. & Hames, C. G. (1973) Transient cerebral ischaemia: prevalence and prognosis in a biracial rural community. *J. Amer. med. Ass.*, **225**, 125–128.

Kartchner, M. M., McRae, L. P. & Morrison, F. D. (1973) Noninvasive detection and evaluation of carotid occlusive disease. *Arch. Surg.*, **106**, 528–535.

Keitzer, W. F., Lichti, E. L. & DeWeese, M. S. (1972) Clinical evaluation and correction of carotid artery occlusive disease. Use of the Dopler ultrasonic flowmeter. *Amer. J. Surg.*, **124**, 697–700.

Kendell, R. E. & Marshall, J. (1963) Role of hypotension in the genesis of transient focal cerebral ischaemic attacks. *Brit. med. J.*, **2**, 344–348.

Kenyon, J. R., Thomas, A. B. W. and Goodwin, D. P. (1972) Heparin protection for the brain during carotid artery surgery. *Lancet*, **2**, 153–154.

Kety, S. S. & Schmidt, C. F. (1948) The effects of altered arterial tension of carbon dioxide and oxygen on cerebral blood flow and cerebral oxygen consumption of normal young men. *J. clin. Invest.*, **27**, 484–492.

Kianouri, M. (1967) Extracranial carotid aneurysm: treatment by excision and end to end anastomosis. *Ann. Surg.*, **165**, 152–156.

Kollarits, C. R., Lubow, M. & Hissong, S. L. (1972) Retinal strokes. 1. Incidence of carotid atheromata. *J. Amer. med. Ass.*, **222**, 1273–1275.

Lassen, N. A. & Pálvölgyi, R. (1968) Cerebral steal during hypercapnia and inverse reaction during hypocapnia observed by the 133 xenon technique in man. *Scand. J. clin. Lab. Invest.*, Suppl. 102, XIIID.

Ledgerwood, A. M. & Lucas, C. E. (1974) Mycotic aneurysm of the carotid artery. *Arch. Surg.*, **109**, 496–498.

Leech, P. J., Miller, J. D., Fitch, W. & Barker, J. (1974) Cerebral blood flow, internal carotid artery pressure and the EEG as a guide to the safety of carotid ligation. *J. Neurol. Neurosurg. Psychiat.*, **37**, 854–862.

Lord, R. S. A. & Ehrenfeld, W. K. (1969) Carotid–subclavian bypass: a haemodynamic study. *Surgery*, **66**, 521–526.

Lyons, S. C. & Galbraith, G. (1957) Surgical treatment of atherosclerotic occlusion of the internal carotid artery. *Ann. Surg.*, **146**, 487–498.

Machleder, H. I. (1973) Evaluation of patients with cerebrovascular disease using the Doppler ophthalmic test. *Angiology*, **24**, 374–381.

Machleder, H. I. & Barker, W. F. (1972) Stroke on the wrong side. Use of the Doppler ophthalmic test in cerebral vascular screening. *Arch. Surg.*, **105**, 943–947.

Machleder, H. I. & Barker, W. F. (1974) External carotid artery shunting during carotid endarterectomy. *Arch. Surg.*, **108**, 785–788.

Marshall, J. M. (1969) In *Extra-cranial Cerebro-vascular Disease and its Management*, ed. Gillespie, J. A. London: Butterworth.

Martorell, F. & Fabré, J. (1944) El sindrome de obliteracion de los troncos supraaorticos. *Medicinia Clinica*, **2**, 26–30.

Millikan, C. H., Siekert, R. G. & Shick, R. M. (1955) Studies in cerebrovascular disease. V. The use of anticoagulants drugs in the treatment of intermittant insufficiency of the internal carotid arterial system. *Proc. Staff Meet. Mayo Clin.*, **30**, 578–586.

Moniz, E., Lima, A. & DeLacerda, R. (1937) Hemiplegies par thrombose de la carotide interne. *Presse Méd.*, **45**, 977–980.

Moore, W. S., Blaisdell, F. W. & Hall, A. D. (1967) Retrograde thrombectomy for chronic occlusion of the common carotid artery. *Arch. Surg.*, **95**, 664–673.

Moore, W. S. & Hall, A. D. (1969) Carotid artery back pressure: a test of cerebral tolerance to temporary carotid occlusion. *Arch. Surg.*, **99**, 702–710.

Moore, W. S., Yee, J. M. & Hall, A. D. (1973) Collateral cerebral blood pressure. An index of tolerance to temporary carotid occlusion. *Arch. Surg.*, **106**, 520–523.

Morris, G. C., Lechter, A. & DeBakey, M. E. (1968) Surgical treatment of fibromuscular disease of the carotid arteries. *Arch. Surg.*, **96**, 636–643.

Mozersky, D. J., Sumner, D. S., Barnes, R. W. & Strandness, D. E. (1973) Subclavian re-vascularisation by means of a subcutaneous axillary–axillary graft. *Arch. Surg.*, **106**, 20–23.

Patterson, J. L., Heyman, A., Battey, L. L. & Furguson, R. W. (1955) Threshold of response of the cerebral vessels of man to increase blood carbon dioxide. *J. clin. Invest.*, **34**, 1857–1864.

Patterson, R. H. (1974) Risk of carotid surgery with occlusion of the contralateral carotid artery. *Arch. Neurol.*, **30**, 188–189.

Perez-Borja, L. & Meyer, J. S. (1965) Electroencephalographic monitoring during reconstructive surgery of the neck vessels. *Electroenceph. clin. Neurophysiol.*, **18**, 162–169.

Perry, P. M., Drinkwater, J. E. & Taylor, G. W. (1975) Cerebral function before and after carotid endarterectomy. *Brit. med. J.*, **4**, 215–216.

Pickering, G. W. (1948) Transient cerebral palsy in hypertension and in cerebral embolism. *J. Amer. med. Ass.*, **137**, 423–430.

Raphael, H. A., Bernatz, P. E., Spittell, J. A. & Ellis, F. H. (1963) Cervical carotid aneurysms: treatment by excision and restoration of arterial continuity. *Amer. J. Surg.*, **105**, 771–778.

Reivich, M. (1961) A new vascular syndrome—'The subclavian steal'. Editorial. *New Engl. J. Med.*, **265**, 912–913.

Reivich, M., Holling, H. E., Roberts, B. & Toole, J. F. (1961) Reversal of blood flow through the vertebral artery and its effects on cerebral circulation. *New Engl. J. Med.*, **265**, 878–885.

Rittenhouse, E. A., Radke, H. M. & Sumner, D. E. (1972) Carotid artery aneurysm. Review of the literature and report of a case with rupture into the oropharynx. *Arch. Surg.*, **105**, 786–789.

Rosental, J. J., Gaspar, M. R. & Movius, H. J. (1973) Intraoperative arteriography in carotid thromboendarterectomy. *Arch. Surg.*, **106**, 806–808.

Rundles, W. R. & Kimbell, F. D. (1969) The kinked carotid syndrome. *Angiology*, **20**, 177–194.

Russell, R. W. R. & Cranston, W. I. (1961) Ophthalmodynonometry in carotid artery disease. *J. Neurol. Neurosurg. Psychiat.*, **24**, 281–296.

Savory, W. S. (1856) Case of a young woman in whom the main arteries of both upper extremities and of the left side of the neck were throughout completely obliterated. *Med.-chir. Trans.*, **39**, 205–219.

Shimizu, K. & Sano, K. (1951) Pulseless disease. *J. Neuropath. clin. Neurol.*, **1**, 37–47.

Siekert, R. G. (1970) Quoted Austin et al, 1974.

Smith, L. L. (1974) In discussion Chung, 1974.

Sproul, G. (1971) Femoral–axillary bypass for cerebral vascular insufficiency. *Arch. Surg.*, **103**; 746–747.

Strully, K. J., Hurwitt, E. S. & Blankenberg, H. W. (1953) Thromboendarterectomy for thrombosis of the internal carotid artery in the neck. *J. Neurosurg.*, **10**, 474–482.

Sutherland, G. R. & Donaldson, A. A. (1972) Persistant hypoglossal artery complicated by internal carotid artery stenosis. *Clin. Radiol.*, **23**, 222–224.

Svien, H. J. & Hollenhorst, R. W. (1956) Pressure in retinal arteries after ligation or occlusion of the carotid artery. *Proc. Staff Meet. Mayo Clin.*, **31**, 684–692.

Takayasu, M. (1908) A case with peculiar changes of the central retinal vessels. *Acta Soc. ophthal. Jap.*, **12**, 554.

15

Terry, H. J. & Taylor, G. W. (1974) Quantitation of flow in femoropopliteal grafts. *Surg. Clin. North Amer.*, **54**, 85–94.

Thal, E. R., Snyder, W. H., Hays, R. J. & Perry, M. O. (1974) Management of carotid artery injuries. *Surgery*, **76**, 955–962.

Thomas, G. I., Spencer, M. P., Jones, T. W., Edmark, K. W. & Stavney, L. S. (1974) Noninvasive carotid bifurcation mapping. Its relation to carotid surgery. *Amer. J. Surg.*, **128**, 168–174.

Thompson, J. E. (1973a) The development of carotid artery surgery. *Arch. Surg.*, **107**, 643–648.

Thompson, J. E. (1973b) In discussion De Weese et al, 1973.

Thompson, J. E., Austin, D. J. & Patman, R. D. (1967) Endarterectomy of the totally occluded carotid artery for stroke: results in 100 operations. *Arch. Surg.*, **95**, 791–801.

Thompson, J. E. & Patman, R. D. (1970) Endarterectomy for asymptomatic carotid bruits. *Heart Bull.*, **19**, 116–120.

Todd, R. B. (1844) Account of a case of a dissecting aneurysm of the aorta innominata and right carotid arteries giving rise to suppression of urine and white softening of the brain. *Med.-chir. Trans.* (2nd series), **27**, 301–324.

Treiman, R. L., Foran, R. F., Shore, E. H. & Levin, P. M. (1973) Carotid bruit: significance in patients undergoing an abdominal aortic operation. *Arch. Surg.*, **106**, 803–805.

Trojaborg, W. & Boysen, G. (1973) Relation between EEG, regional cerebral blood flow and internal carotid artery pressure during carotid endarterectomy. *Electroenceph. clin. Neurophysiol.*, **34**, 61–69.

Virchow, R. (1856) Cited by Hager, H. (1962) Die Diagnose der karotisthrombose durch den Augenarzt. *Klin. Mbl. Augenheilk.*, **141**, 801–840.

Wade, J. G., Larson, C. P., Hickeym, R. F., Ehrenfeld, W. K. & Severinghaus, J. W. (1970) Effect of carotid endarterectomy on carotid chemoreceptor and baroreceptor function in man. *New Engl. J. Med.*, **282**, 823–829.

Weissman, B. & Rankow, R. M. (1968) Traumatic aneurysm of the common carotid artery. *Arch. Otolaryngol.*, **88**, 543–546.

Wells, B. A., Keats, A. S. & Cooley, D. A. (1963) Increased tolerance to cerebral ischaemia produced by general anaesthesia during temporary carotid occlusion. *Surgery*, **54**, 216–223.

White, C. W., Allarde, R. R. & McDowell, H. A. (1967) Anaesthetic management for carotid artery surgery. *J. Amer. med. Ass.*, **202**, 1023–1027.

Winslow, N. (1926) Extracranial aneurysms of the internal carotid artery: historical analysis of the cases registered up until August 1st, 1925. *Arch. Surg.*, **13**, 689–729.

Wright, R. L. & Sweet, W. H. (1962) Treatment of intracranial aneurysms by carotid occlusion: correlation of late clinical follow-up with pressure recordings. *Trans. Amer. neurol. Ass.*, **87**, 158–162.

Wylie, E. J. (1974) In discussion Hobson et al, 1974. *V.S.*

Wylie, E. J. & Ehrenfeld, W. K. (1970) *Extracranial Occlusive Cerebrovascular Disease. Diagnosis and Management.* Philadelphia: Saunders and Co.

Young, J. R., Humphries, A. W., Beven, E. G. & de Wolfe, V. G. (1969) Carotid endarterectomy without shunt. Experiences using hyperbaric general anaesthesia. *Arch Surg.*, **99**, 293–297.

Ziegler, D. K. & Hassanein, R. S. (1973) Prognosis in patients with transient ischemic attacks. *Stroke*, **4**, 666–673.

18
SI UNITS

T. J. C. Cooke

A Problem in Communication

During this century there has taken place a remarkable expansion in both the pure and applied sciences, including medicine. Parallel with the rapid growth of scientific knowledge the output of books and scientific journals has mushroomed in an attempt to document and disseminate the results of research. Until recently there has been a lack of uniformity between different countries (and even within individual countries) in the presentation of published data, especially in the choice of units of measurement of physical quantities, where empiricism has often been the order of the day.

Need of Standardised Units of Measurement

By the 1950s there was a widespread feeling among scientific workers in many disciplines that the useful and indeed necessary interchange of scientific ideas would be increasingly hindered unless some uniformity were soon introduced, and they pressed for an agreed international 'standard' system of measurement. Finally in 1960, following several General Conferences on Weights and Measures under the auspices of the International Bureau of Weights and Measures, the Système International d'Unités (SI) was introduced, with widespread agreement, to replace alternative systems of measurement. This new system, which is entirely metric, is now used in most Western and industrialised countries, being taught in their schools and universities.

There has been some inertia on the part of the medical professions to transfer to the SI units of measurement, and the initial impetus has come not from clinicians but from laboratory chemists, who saw from the outset the merits of the new system. In the United Kingdom, following a period of discussions between the Department of Health and representatives of the medical profession, it has now been agreed to recommend the SI units for use in medical practice. Already most hospitals have taken steps to introduce the new system for the reporting of laboratory data, and the changeover should be completed within the next year or two. Medical editors have similarly agreed to request authors to use the SI units and nomenclature in future publications, although for a transition period the new and traditional units may both be given.

Nature of the SI Units of Measurement

The SI system is based on seven dimensionally independent basic quantities: length, mass, time, electric current, thermodynamic temperature, luminous intensity and amount of substance. Each quantity is measured in terms of a base unit, the names and symbols of which are given in Table 18.1.

Each base unit is strictly defined as a precise quantity for reference, and all other quantities may be derived from the seven base quantities in con-

Table 18.1   Names and symbols for the seven basic SI units

Physical quantity	Name of unit	Symbol for unit
Length	metre	m
Mass	kilogram	kg
Time	second	s
Electric current	ampere	A
Thermodynamic temperature	kelvin	K
Luminous intensity	candela	cd
Amount of substance	mole	mol

Table 18.2   Prefixes for SI units

Fraction	Prefix	Symbol	Multiple	Prefix	Symbol
10^{-1}	deci	d	10	deca	da
10^{-2}	centi	c	10^2	hecto	h
10^{-3}	milli	m	10^3	kilo	k
10^{-6}	micro	μ	10^6	mega	M
10^{-9}	nano	n	10^9	giga	G
10^{-12}	pico	p	10^{12}	tera	T
10^{-15}	femto	f			
10^{-18}	atto	a			

formity with physical and mathematical laws. The system is thus a logical and integral one.

Where possible quantities should be expressed in terms of base units, but appropriate multiples and submultiples of the base units exist to allow convenient presentation of data with numerical values lying in the range 1 to 999. In medical laboratory work the use of submultiples is especially appropriate, and a list of prefixes is given in Table 18.2.

Application of SI Units to Medicine

The necessary changes consequent upon the adoption of SI units in medical practice will mainly affect the reporting of quantities such as concentration, volume and pressure.

Concentration. There are two SI units of concentration, namely, mass concentration and amount of substance.

For substances whose chemical composition (and therefore also the molecular weight) is known, the new unit of 'amount of substance', i.e. the mole, will replace the older unit of mass concentration (e.g. mg/100 ml). The use of the mole, which is defined as the mass divided by the molecular weight, will have the greatest influence in laboratory reporting, for it will affect the numerical value of most substances measured, exceptions being the monovalent electrolytes where 1 mEq/l = 1 mmol/l. The use of the mole is biologically appropriate in that it permits quantitative relationships between physiologically active constituents in the body fluids to be seen clearly.

For substances of as yet undefined chemical composition, whose molecular weight is unknown, the mass concentration will remain in use. Examples of such substances include vitamin B_{12} and folate, as well as haemoglobin.

Volume. Although the cubic metre is the basic SI unit of volume, in medicine the litre will in practice be the most widely used submultiple, except in the case of haemoglobin where results will continue to be expressed in g/dl.

Pressure. For the time being blood pressure will continue to be recorded in the traditional millimetres of mercury (mmHg), but all other pressures, such as blood gases, will in future use the pascal (Pa), results being expressed in kilopascals (kPa).

Temperature. Temperature will be expressed in degrees Celsius, in which the degree interval corresponds to the centigrade scale currently in use.

Advantages of SI Units

The new units of measurement have already met with active opposition from some quarters, largely on the grounds that it involves a laborious relearning of 'normal range' values, causes confusion to ward staff attempting to decipher unfamiliar data and possibly slows up and introduces error in the treatment of patients. It is relevant, therefore, to stress the advantages of the new system.

The SI system is coherent, in that the product or quotient of any two unit quantities is the unit of resultant quantity. There is uniformity in both concept and style in the presentation of quantitative laboratory data. Furthermore, the overall number of multiples of units in use is minimised.

Implementation

Inevitably there will be a period of transition, rather than an instant changeover, to the new system. During the transition period certain problems will need to be overcome.

The change to SI units necessarily involves the recalibration of laboratory

Table 18.3   Commoner data
Key to symbols: B = Blood; P = Plasma; S = Serum

Constituent		Traditional units	SI units	Conversion factor, 'old' to new units
B	Haemoglobin	13–16 g/dl	13–16 g/dl	No change
B	Red cell count	$4.5 \times 10^6/mm^3$	$4.5 \times 10^{12}/l$	10^6
B	White cell count	4000–10000/mm^3	$4–10 \times 10^9/l$	10^6
B	Platelets	$150–400 \times 10^3/mm^3$	$150–400 \times 10^9/l$	10^6
B	PVC	41%	0.41	0.01
S	Vitamin B_{12}	200–800 pg/ml	140–590 pmol/l	0.738
P	Fibrinogen	150–400 mg/100 ml	1.5–4.0 g/l	0.01
	Acid-base parameters			
B	P_{O_2}	80–100 mmHg	10.5–13.5 kPa	0.133
B	P_{CO_2}	32–46 mmHg	4.5–6.0 kPa	0.133
B	Standard HCO_3	23–28 mEq/l	23–28 mmol/l	No change
B	Base excess	± 3 mEq/l	± 3 mmol/l	No change
P	HCO_3	24–30 mEq/l	24–30 mmol/l	No change
	Clinical chemistry			
P	Sodium	136–149 mEq/l	136–149 mmol/l	No change
P	Potassium	3.8–5.2 mEq/l	3.8–5.2 mmol/l	No change
P	Chloride	100–107 mEq/l	100–107 mmol/l	No change
P	Urea	15–40 mg/100 ml	2.6–6.5 mmol/l	0.166
P	Creatinine	0.1–1.4 mg/100 ml	9–120 μmol/l	88.4
P	Uric acid	2.7 mg/100 ml	0.1–0.4 mmol/l	0.0595
P	Calcium	8.5–10.5 mg/100 ml	2.15–2.65 mmol/l	0.25
P	Magnesium	1.4–1.8 mEq/l	0.7–0.9 mmol/l	0.5
P	Inorganic phosphorus	2.5–4.5 mg/100 ml	0.8–1.4 mmol/l	0.323
S	Total protein	6.5–8.0 g/100 ml	65–80 g/l	10
S	Albumin	3.5–5.5 g/100 ml	35–55 g/l	10
S	Globulin	2.4–3.7 g/100 ml	24–37 g/l	10
S	Bilirubin, total	0.1–0.8 mg/100 ml	1.7–13.6 μmol/l	17.1
S	Cholesterol	140–240 mg/100 ml	4.0–6.5 mmol/l	0.0259
S	Triglycerides	60–140 mg/100 ml	0.7–1.6 mmol/l	0.0113
S	Alkaline phosphatase	30–130 U/l	30–130 U/l	No change
S	Acid phosphatase, total	1–3.5 KAU	1–3.5 KAU	No change
B	Glucose, fasting	65–95 mg/100 ml	3.5–5.5 mmol/l	0.0555
S	Iron	100–130 μg/100 ml	20–23 μmol/l	0.179
S	TIBC	250–400 μg/100 ml	45–70 μmol/l	0.179
S	Transferrin	200–400 mg/100 ml	2.0–4.0 g/l	0.01
P	Cortisol	10–25 μg/100 ml	280–700 nmol/l	27.6
S	PBI	4–8 μg/100 ml	300–600 nmol/l	78.8
S	Thyroxine		55–120 ng/ml	
S	T_3		1–2 ng/ml	
P	Gastrin		0–25 fmol/ml	
	Urine constituents			
	24 h Na$^+$ output	200 mEq	200 mmol	No change
	24 h K$^+$ output	70 mEq	70 mmol	No change
	24 h urea output	25 g	410 mmol	16.6
	24 h protein	0.05 g	0.05 g	No change
	24 h calcium	0.20 g	50 mmol	250
	24 h inorganic phosphorus	1.0 g	32 mmol	32
	Creatinine clearance	70–140 ml/min	1.2–2.3 ml/s	0.0167
	5-HIAA	3–17 mg/24 h	15–88 μmol/24 h	5.23
	VMA	less than 7 mg/24 h	less than 35 μmol/24 h	5.05

Table 18.3—continued

Constituent	Traditional units	SI units	Conversion factor, 'old' to new units
Cerebrospinal fluid			
Protein	15–45 mg/100 ml	0.15–0.45 g/l	0.01
Glucose	50–90 mg/100 ml	2.7–5.0 mmol/l	0.0555
Gastric analysis			
Basal acid	3.0 ± 2.0 mEq/h	0.8 ± 0.6 μmol/s	0.2777
Maximal acid	23 ± 5 mEq/h	6.4 ± 1.4 μmol/s	0.2777
Faeces			
Fat	3.5 g/24 h	11–18 mmol/24 h	3.52

equipment, either by the makers, or by the laboratory personnel. New stationery will be required for presentation of results in the new units.

Some assistance will need to be provided during the changeover period to familiarise medical staff with the new units, allowing them to become accustomed to normal ranges in SI units. Most hospitals have already issued simple conversion tables to their staff, so that old and new units can be easily compared. For the time being, data arriving from the laboratory may actually give values in both the traditional and SI units, and some medical journals also follow this policy.

Table 18.3 lists some of the commoner haematological, biochemical and other laboratory data in both traditional and SI units, giving the appropriate conversion factors. Where possible, the values listed are those currently in use at Hammersmith Hospital; 'normal range' values will differ slightly in other laboratories.

REFERENCES

Annals of the Royal College of Surgeons (1975) Editorial. SI units: definitions, normal ranges, and conversion factors. *Annals of the Royal College of Surgeons*, **56**, 222–224.

Astrup, P. (1970) The need for a standardisation of quantities and units in clinical chemistry. *Scandinavian Journal of Clinical and Laboratory Investigation*, **25**, 1–3.

Baron, D. N. (1973) SI units in pathology: the next stage. *Journal of Clinical Pathology*, **26**, 729–730.

Baron, D. N., Broughton, P. M. G., Cohen, M., Lansley, T. S., Lewis, S. M. & Shinton, N. K. (1974) The use of SI units in reporting results obtained in hospital laboratories. *Journal of Clinical Pathology*, **27**, 590–597.

British Medical Journal (1975) Editorial: Instructions to authors. *British Medical Journal*, **4**, 6.

Ellis, G. (Ed.) (1972) *Units, Symbols and Abbreviations: A Guide for Biological and Medical Editors and Authors*. London: Royal Society of Medicine.

Royal College of Pathologists Working Party (1970) The use of SI in reporting results in pathology. *Journal of Clinical Pathology*, **23**, 818–819.

Young, D. S. (1974) Standardised reporting of laboratory data: the desirability of using SI units. *New England Journal of Medicine*, **290**, 368–373.

Young, D. S. (1975) Normal laboratory values in SI units. *New England Journal of Medicine*, **292**, 795–802.

19
THE TRAINING OF A SURGEON

Selwyn Taylor

The last 25 years have seen a revolution, albeit a bloodless revolution, in surgical training, and there has emerged a fairly well-defined and recognisable pattern in most of the English-speaking countries. The Colleges,[1] which have taken such a leading part in initiating these changes, have traditionally used the word 'training' when talking of surgery and probably advisedly, since there is a strong element of apprenticeship during this period and also the acquirement of certain manual skills. In the university the same period is referred to as the 'education' of a surgeon, but the two really refer to the same thing, it is only the nuance of interpretation that is different.

There are probably many reasons why surgical training should have gone into the melting pot in the late 1940s and have been poured into a new mould (which still retains some flexibility) during the last 25 years. First, there was a war and all that it did for anaesthesia, blood replacement and the introduction of antibiotics. Then, and perhaps most important, there was the coming of the new National Health Service in Great Britain in 1948 and this gave the opportunity for improvement in district hospitals all over the country with a consequent demand for surgeons to staff them. One has to remember that in the prewar years a great deal of surgery in the British Isles was done by general practitioners but after 1948 they had to decide which of the two disciplines they would remain in. Latterly it has been almost impossible to combine surgery with any other active part of medicine.

Town and Gown

In England the origins of training patterns in surgery are to be found in the history of those two ancient institutions which existed in the City of London more than 600 years ago, the Barbers' Guild and the Guild of Surgeons. They had a long period of rivalry and finally a rather uneasy alliance in 1540. Subsequently they broke apart once more and in 1745 an Act of Parliament established two separate companies: that of the Barbers and that of the

[1] Royal College of Surgeons of England, Lincoln's Inn Fields, London WC2; Royal College of Surgeons of Edinburgh, Nicolson Street, Edinburgh 8; Royal College of Physicians and Surgeons of Glasgow, 242 St Vincent Street, Glasgow C2; Royal College of Surgeons in Ireland, St Stephen's Green, Dublin 2.

Surgeons. In 1800 the Company of Surgeons was reconstituted by a Royal Charter into the Royal College of Surgeons in London and in 1843 this was changed to the Royal College of Surgeons of England. The present building on the south side of Lincoln's Inn Fields was started in 1800 and still remains the focal point for surgeons in England.

The object of the new College was set out in the Charter of 1800 as 'The Promotion and Encouragement of the Study and Practice of the Art and Science of Surgery'. This remains its purpose, but enormous changes have taken place and the College, which has with its associated Faculties of Dental Surgery and Anaesthetics more than 14 000 Fellows, has eight extremely active scientific departments headed by Professors conducting extensive research programmes, both in Lincoln's Inn Fields and at the College's research establishment at Downe. When one thinks about the age of departments of surgery in universities one can for the most part encompass them within the present century, and thus, at first sight, the academic heritage of surgery seems brief. But it has to be remembered that surgery and medicine are really indivisible and that medicine is one of the oldest faculties of our universities probably only antedated by Theology and of comparable antiquity with Law. Physicians, however, were not always as friendly towards their surgical colleagues as they are today, and there was a time when the physician was greeted at the front door of the manor house while the barber surgeon had to enter by the tradesmen's entrance. It is probably this distinction that encouraged surgeons to retain their old title of Mister rather than being called Doctor as they are in all other countries today outside the British Isles.

In the years before 1939 formal training for most surgeons was usually limited to studying for the primary examination of the FRCS, which was a severe hurdle in Anatomy and Physiology (the principles of Pathology being added later) and a relatively brief period of hospital experience before successful negotiation of the final Fellowship. He or she might then apply for a post on a hospital staff and the important factor was the individual with whom the trainee worked rather than the institution in which he spent his training period.

Higher Surgical Training

In the postwar years, with the enormous increase in numbers of surgeons and the growth of specialties, considerable dissatisfaction was felt with the pattern of Registrar training. Most individuals applied for whatever jobs they wished to have, or more often what they could obtain, and the pattern of training was all too often haphazard. Following a conference held at Christ Church, Oxford, in 1965 under the chairmanship of Sir George Pickering and the sponsorship of the Nuffield Provincial Hospitals Trust, there arose a genuine desire to improve the overall pattern of postgraduate training in this country. This has indeed now occurred in every branch of medicine, but it is interesting to recall that a clear pattern of higher training was pioneered by the Surgical Colleges in the first place, stimulated largely by Sir Frank Holdsworth and Professor Leslie Pyrah. This began in 1967 to be followed by most of the other major branches of medicine.

The higher training scheme which is controlled by a Joint Committee of the four Royal Surgical Colleges in Great Britain and Ireland, the Specialist Associations and the University Professors of Surgery, is based on the evolution and recognition of Higher Training Programmes which last from three to five years in each of the major surgical specialties after the pre-Fellowship requirements have been met. The intention is to provide men and women with a clear-cut (though flexible) programme in the various aspects of the specialty which they have chosen, with progressive responsibility, at the end of which they are *accredited* as fit to apply for consultant appointments. There are nine specialties; general surgery, orthopaedics, urology, neurological surgery, ophthalmology, otolaryngology, plastic surgery, paediatric surgery and thoracic surgery. There is thus an orderly pattern laid down, with possibility for wide variations in its implementation, to cover the training of a candidate who wishes to become a consultant surgeon, from the time that he qualifies as a doctor.

The Surgical Ladder

The aspirant for the post of a consultant surgeon has three main hurdles to negotiate. He has to satisfy the College that he has a sound basic knowledge in anatomy, physiology and pathology suitable for his further training in surgery. Second, he must obtain suitably approved posts in hospitals where he will get good experience in a wide spectrum of surgery and in accident work and he must then obtain the Diploma of Fellow of one of the Royal Colleges of Surgeons. Finally, he must obtain a position as a Senior Registrar (or the academic equivalent) on one of the approved higher surgical training programmes at the end of which he will be given a certificate without further examination but with annual assessment of his progress, usually through regional committee auspices. He is then able to apply for a consultant post in the knowledge that the College's assessors will regard him as having fulfilled its criteria.

To take this in more detail, the individual will, following qualification, spend a year in preregistration posts and then will spend the next two years in junior and senior resident House Officer posts where he will obtain general and specialist surgical experience. He will also be expected to have spent at least six months in an approved casualty department seeing a variety of acute emergency and accident work. If he is wise, he will, at the same time, be refreshing his knowledge in anatomy, in physiology and in pathology and to this end he may elect to attend one of the full-time courses which are provided, either at one of the Royal Colleges or elsewhere, or alternatively to attend day-release courses. With this kind of refreshment of his earlier basic science, plus the more detailed knowledge he must now have of the relevant anatomy, physiology and pathology, he can face the examiners for his Primary Fellowship examination. For those who find this particularly difficult there is an increasing number of posts now available in the country which combine a period in a casualty department or in general surgery with a spell in an anatomy department where, as a junior demonstrator, the trainee will have excellent opportunity to learn his subject. His next task is to spend two years in the grade of Surgical Registrar and if he is fortunate the post will rotate between a number of specialist departments. When he has done this he will have completed the training requirements of the four Royal Colleges of Surgeons in the British Isles for the Fellowship and he can sit his final Fellowship examination and if successful will be entitled to the letters FRCS after his name. The examination itself is a good test of clinical judgement and knowledge of surgery in general. The trainee may then spend longer in the Registrar grade gaining more experience in the kind of surgery he wants to do, while he looks round to obtain a suitable Senior Registrar appointment on one of the rotating schemes which have been approved by the Joint Committee on Higher Surgical Training.

The Specialist Advisory Committees of the Joint Committee[1] together with representatives of the university surgeons, have arranged for groups of visitors to inspect the facilities for surgical training throughout the British Isles and have recommended various rotating posts which give good experience both at university and at district hospitals. These are probably the most formative years in the young surgeon's life and he is given more and more responsibility to take decisions and to treat patients on his own initiative, while at the same time he has experienced mentors who can guide him in his further training. This is the period in his career when he should, if he wishes, become involved in research, and every encouragement is given for the individual to spend a year on a research project and, if he can afford the time, longer. This usually takes place while he is at his university hospital. It is also a very good period in which to see something of practice overseas and there are many facilities now for the individual to spend a year in the surgical department in a hospital for example in the United States or Canada, in Australasia or in certain parts of Europe and the Colleges often accept this as an integral part of the training years.

Clearly a man who has worked abroad for a year will be a more mature and probably more experienced surgeon and will be assessed as such when he comes up to obtain a consultant post. Similarly a man who hopes to obtain a position in a university hospital will be well advised to have shown his interest and ability in both the research field and in teaching before applying for such an appointment.

[1] The Joint Committee is made up of representatives from the four Royal Colleges of Surgeons in England, Edinburgh, Glasgow and Ireland and of the various Specialist Associations.

It will be seen from what has gone before that the ideal candidate, who completes all his allotted tasks on time, could theoretically have obtained his Certificate of Higher Specialist Training by the age of 32 and apply for a consultant post, but unfortunately at the present time, many candidates for vacancies at hospitals all over the country are much older than this. It is hoped, however, that as time goes by younger men will be obtaining their definitive posts by this age.

The Nine Specialties

There are nine branches of surgery which offer programmes in Higher Specialist Training. Since the requirements for each of them are different, they are sketched out here in detail as they apply to the four Royal Colleges in the British Isles.

General surgery. At least three years has to be spent as a Senior Registrar, or equivalent, in a post which has been approved and normally includes rotation between a University (Teaching) Hospital and a District (General) Hospital. A total of four years after complying with the fellowship Regulations is normally required, but there are many Registrar posts which have been inspected by the Joint Committee on Higher Surgical Training which, while being eminently suitable for part of the specialist training of four years, are not integrated in a complete programme and retrospective recognition for a year in such a post will often be given towards the total period required for accreditation.

Neurological surgery. This specialty requires the longest training period of all, five years. At least two years have to be spent as a Senior Registrar or equivalent and four years in Neurological Surgery itself after the candidate has complied with the final Fellowship requirements. The fifth year may well have been spent by the candidate in experience in the diagnosis and treatment of head injuries in an accident unit or similar post. Under certain circumstances, a period of six months may be spent in a department with special diagnostic techniques such as medical neurology or neuroradiology and this can be accepted towards the total five year period.

Ophthalmology. There is a four year training period in this specialty; at least two years must be spent as a Senior Registrar or equivalent and three years in ophthalmology after the candidate has complied with the requirements for the final Fellowship. There is a special ophthalmic FRCS examination which is usually taken in place of the FRCS in general surgery. If one of the previous years has been spent in ophthalmology, this also counts and so makes up the total of four years. Out of the four years, periods adding up to not more than one year can be spent in neurology or neurological surgery or some other approved specialty related to this discipline.

Orthopaedic surgery. There is a four year training period in orthopaedics, at least two years as Senior Registrar or in a post with equivalent responsibility and there are stipulations as to at least two years being spent dealing with the surgery of injuries of the locomotor system and two years in a post or posts devoted to elective orthopaedics in both adults and children.

Otolaryngology. As in ophthalmology, there is a special final Fellowship examination set in this discipline but this still has to be followed by a three year training period although of course it may equally follow a FRCS training period in general surgery. If the candidate has spent a year in an ENT post while working for his Fellowship, this can be counted towards his three year training and he will then only have to spend two years as Senior Registrar in the discipline.

Paediatric surgery. This is normally a three year training period and follows a FRCS which is, of course, a general surgical training. At least two of the three years have to be spent in an approved paediatric surgical department and at least one of these years must have been spent at Senior Registrar level.

Plastic surgery. The period of Higher Training for Plastic Surgery is four years, three of which are spent in the discipline itself as Senior Registrar or equivalent, but one year may count towards the total period if it has been spent in plastic surgery or a closely allied subject while the candidate was fulfilling his Fellowship regulations. It has to be remembered that nowadays plastic surgery also includes a working knowledge of the surgery of congenital anomalies, trauma including burns, faciomaxillary injuries and hand injuries.

Thoracic surgery. This also demands a four year Higher Surgical Training period and some surgeons tend to specialise in cardiac work while others devote their attention primarily to the lung and the mediastinum. At least three of the four years will be spent in the specialised discipline but one previous year may have been in thoracic work and be counted towards the higher training.

Urology. The training period is three years and this is the minimum period in the discipline which qualifies for accreditation. Most candidates spend longer than this, being at least three years in a senior registrar's post in urology and having spent at least one year previously in the specialty.

Logistics

One of the problems which faces any training programme such as that outlined above, is the fact that it is pyramidal in shape and there is a large number of house officers, a lesser number of registrars, a small group of senior registrars and finally what might be described as the élite of consultants. What happens to all the others on the ladder or on the pyramid as they approach the apex? Clearly if there were opportunities for permanent employment at grades lesser than consultant, the problem would be easier, but owing to very strong representations by the profession itself (or groups within it) in this country, such a pattern has never evolved. Thus two things may happen; there may be a relative 'wastage' of excellent trained men who cannot reach the higher echelons or there may be great delay at some of the lower levels. Thus men are seen to be doing registrar or senior registrar posts for very long periods, which was never envisaged when these schemes were evolved.

In recent years the officers of the Department of Health and Social Security have been looking long and hard at the hardships caused by such a system and they have gone some way to remedying them. There is close liaison now between the Department of Health on the one hand and the Central Manpower Committee on the other. The aim is to try to equate the number of men or women who are being trained to consultant level with the expected number of vacancies that are likely to occur. There are regular meetings between those involved in these appointments in the training programmes and there are fairly up-to-date figures now available of the likely vacancies and very accurate ones of the number of those in training for them.

Overseas Candidates

The problems outlined in the section above on logistics do not take into account the fact that there are a great many candidates who wish to come to this country from overseas and enjoy the high standard of training and teaching which they can obtain in surgery. Many of them will return to the countries from whence they came, a few will stay and some will emigrate to a third country of their choice for economic or other reasons. The presence of these candidates obviously greatly strengthens the kind of programmes that can be provided in this country, both in the quality of men who will fill the posts and by providing a group who will come for a period and then leave. There are some posts now which are reserved specifically for those who come from overseas, but because of the Race Relations Act it is not possible to advertise these as such, since it would suggest that some kind of discrimination existed. For this reason, the whole subject has become much involved of late, but a great many men and women are still visiting this country and spending a number of years in training programmes, both in teaching and district hospitals, where they obtain excellent experience and where they also give valuable help in the running of the country's health service. Unfortunately the great competition for senior registrar's posts in most of the special subjects means that many British-born and overseas-born candidates will not find the kind of programme they would like to enter. There are plans to cope with this problem at the present time, but clearly the pyramidal shape of the service will remain whatever kind of programme is introduced, and not every trainee will be able to become a consultant. It is in any case important for the maintenance of high standards that there should be competition for senior posts and most of the trainees would accept this provided that the selection of the successful is seen to be fair.

The Armed Forces

Medical officers in the armed forces have certain specific duties to perform related to the needs of their Service. Thus a naval surgeon may find himself spending a period at sea and another on an overseas station and similarly with those in the army and the air force who have specific demands made upon them which remove them from the mainstream of hospital training. Because of this it is more difficult for a service candidate to satisfy the requirements for Higher Surgical Training. The Joint Committee on Higher Surgical Training has therefore looked at this problem separately and has approved arrangements whereby candidates will be able to train partly within the Service and partly in civilian hospitals, but sometimes spending more years in the process than would normally be the case. The serviceman has advantages over the civilian in that he usually becomes a more mature citizen at an earlier stage and is trained early on to deal with emergencies of all kinds. He also has responsibilities for handling of personnel which are usually denied his civilian counterpart. It is hoped that the Services will continue to offer an attractive career for those who elect to serve in them, and that recognition of specialist training will be such as to facilitate a later return to civilian practice. The Ministry of Defence has set up a number of advisory bodies in recent years; the Armed Forces Advisory Committee on Postgraduate Medical and Dental Education in 1971 and more recently the Armed Forces Medical Advisory Board.

The European Economic Community

Now that the pattern of medical specialist training within the EEC has become clear and the Medical Directives have been signed, it is possible to see that there is a considerable gulf between the requirements for practice as a specialist in a predominantly private medical system and the requirements for appointment as a consultant in the National Health Service operating in the British Isles. Thus in Europe a surgical trainee is entitled to certain privileges as a specialist approximately two years earlier than the time at which his opposite number will have been trained to consultant level in the British Isles. It is not thought in this country that this should give any cause for anxiety nor any case for reducing our standards of what we consider is necessary for consultant status. However, there is naturally some concern among the younger surgeons training in this country that if they should wish to migrate within the EEC they might be placed at a disadvantage in comparison with their other European confrères unless some specific machinery is created for recognising a comparable specialist training. A pattern appears to be emerging, although it has not yet had final approval, in which recognition of specialist status in EEC terms would be given to those going to a country in the Community who have completed the period of training required for a Fellowship and spent at least one year in approved Higher Specialist Training. Such recognition would imply only that the trainee had received the minimum specialist training laid down in the Medical Directives and would not have relevance in this country to eligibility for appointment to a consultancy. In the British Isles the Government is likely to ask the Joint Committees of the Royal Colleges to advise the GMC on the criteria for certifying specialist qualifications in this EEC context and this also applies to other disciplines such as medicine.

What is a Surgeon?

Most of the candidates who present themselves for training in surgery are unable to give any cogent reasons why they wish to do this. This similarly applies to most of us who have spent a lifetime in the discipline. The reasons for following such a vocation are very hard to express and are probably felt very deep down in the individual.

It is important, however, that even without logical reasons for following such a discipline, individuals should not be discouraged from entering surgical training; indeed good candidates must be encouraged in every way possible if we are to maintain the standards which have for so long distinguished this country and distinguished it in such a satisfactory way from surgical practice the world over. The introduction of a regular pattern into the training of the individual is really a very great step forward from allowing candidates to apply for posts here, there and everywhere as opportunity offers and in the hope that they will obtain a suitable post at the end of it. We now have an excellent basic surgical training programme and recognised Higher Surgical Training programmes in the nine major disciplines which seem to be required for hospital care in the British Isles. We must try to make our programmes flexible and large enough to take in those candidates who want to come and join us from overseas, because they certainly give as much as they take, and make the programmes more worthwhile. Our training has to be flexible enough to include Service candidates whose careers may be very different from those of their civilian counterparts and there must be suitable provision for the man who is almost entirely interested in research or perhaps in university teaching at a high level, as well as for the surgeon who works in an isolated district hospital where his workload tends to be almost continuous and he has to show great versatility of skills. Should I have my own career over again, I would not hesitate to enter the profession of surgery once more and I only hope that I would find that the new programmes of training are as satisfying and rewarding as I found the rather haphazard ones which existed in my formative years.

In writing this account of surgical training I have in general referred to the practices of the Royal College of Surgeons of England. The statements however remain true except in minor detail for the three other British Colleges:

the Royal College of Surgeons of Edinburgh, the Royal College of Physicians and Surgeons of Glasgow and the Royal College of Surgeons in Ireland. Considerable differences in training patterns and requirements are demanded by the other English speaking Colleges: the Royal Australasian College of Surgeons, the Royal College of Physicians and Surgeons of Canada, the Colleges of Medicine of South Africa and the American College of Surgeons; but representatives of all the English speaking Colleges meet regularly. As a result of such meetings in Ottawa, Cape Town, Dublin and more recently in Edinburgh there has been virtual acceptance of criteria for the approval of Higher Surgical Training programmes being recognised in all these countries. In addition the representatives of these English-speaking Colleges agreed to recognise a year of the Higher Surgical Training programme being spent in one of the countries other than that in which the candidate was normally working. The year has to be spent in an approved post and a list of these is in active preparation in each of the countries.

Despite this very real unanimity in standards of surgical training for consultant level there remain individual differences in the titles of diploma which are awarded. In the four British Colleges the FRCS marks the point in a surgeon's career when he is ready to embark on Higher Surgical Training, and accreditation marks the completion of this. In Australasia the Fellowship is awarded towards the end of Higher Surgical Training. Perhaps one day in the future even the diplomas will be given at the same point of training, but meanwhile each country enjoys a little individuality in this matter.

ACKNOWLEDGEMENTS

I have been greatly helped in preparing this account by Mr R. S. Johnson-Gilbert, Secretary of the Royal College of Surgeons of England.

REFERENCES

Aird, I. (1961) *The Making of a Surgeon*. London: Butterworth.
Cope, Z. (1959) *The History of the Royal College of Surgeons of England*. London: Blond.
Criteria for consultants in Surgery (1974) *Annals of the Royal College of Surgeons of England*, **55**, 205–209.
Higher Surgical Training (1971) A Report published by the Joint Committee of the four Royal Colleges of Surgeons in the British Isles. A Progress Report was published in 1974.
Johnson-Gilbert, R.-S. (1974) *Royal College of Surgeons of England*. A pamphlet published by the College in Lincoln's Inn Fields, London.
Joint Committee on Higher Surgical Training (1974) *Annals of the Royal College of Surgeons of England*, **54**, 207–217.

INDEX

PRINTED BY ADLARD & SON, LTD, BARTHOLOMEW PRESS, DORKING